PATIENT CARE
in RADIOGRAPHY

WITH AN INTRODUCTION TO MEDICAL IMAGING

Ninth Edition

RUTH ANN EHRLICH, RT(R)

Radiology Faculty (Retired)
Western States Chiropractic College
Portland, Oregon;
Adjunct Faculty
Portland Community College
Portland, Oregon

DAWN M. COAKES, BS, RT(R)

Instructor and Clinical Coordinator, Radiography Program
Portland Community College
Portland, Oregon

ELSEVIER

ELSEVIER

3251 Riverport Lane
St. Louis, Missouri 63043

PATIENT CARE IN RADIOGRAPHY: WITH AN INTRODUCTION
TO MEDICAL IMAGING, NINTH EDITION

ISBN: 978-0-323-35376-2

Notices

Knowledge and best practice in this field are constantly changing. As new research and experience broaden our understanding, changes in research methods, professional practices, or medical treatment may become necessary.

Practitioners and researchers must always rely on their own experience and knowledge in evaluating and using any information, methods, compounds, or experiments described herein. In using such information or methods they should be mindful of their own safety and the safety of others, including parties for whom they have a professional responsibility.

With respect to any drug or pharmaceutical products identified, readers are advised to check the most current information provided (i) on procedures featured or (ii) by the manufacturer of each product to be administered, to verify the recommended dose or formula, the method and duration of administration, and contraindications. It is the responsibility of practitioners, relying on their own experience and knowledge of their patients, to make diagnoses, to determine dosages and the best treatment for each individual patient, and to take all appropriate safety precautions.

To the fullest extent of the law, neither the Publisher nor the authors, contributors, or editors, assume any liability for any injury and/or damage to persons or property as a matter of products liability, negligence or otherwise, or from any use or operation of any methods, products, instructions, or ideas contained in the material herein.

Previous editions copyrighted 2013 by Mosby, an imprint of Elsevier Inc., and 2009, 2004, 1999, 1993, 1989, 1985, and 1981 by Mosby, Inc., an affiliate of Elsevier Inc.

Library of Congress Cataloging-in-Publication Data
Ehrlich, Ruth Ann, 1938- , author. | Coakes, Dawn M., author.
 Patient care in radiography : with an introduction to medical imaging / Ruth Ann Ehrlich,
  Dawn M. Coakes.
 Ninth edition. | St. Louis, Missouri : Elsevier, [2017] |
  Includes bibliographical references and index.
 LCCN 2015046674 | ISBN 9780323353762 (pbk.)
 | MESH: Radiography--methods | Patient Care--methods | Technology, Radiologic |
 Professional-Patient Relations
 LCC RC78 | NLM WN 200 | DDC 616.07/572--dc23 LC
  record available at http://lccn.loc.gov/2015046674

Executive Content Strategist: Sonya Siegafuse
Content Development Manager: Jean Sims Fornango
Senior Content Development Specialist: Tina Kaemmerer
Publishing Services Manager: Jeff Patterson
Project Manager: Lisa A. P. Bushey
Senior Designer: Amy Buxton

Printed in China

Last digit is the print number: 9 8 7 6 5 4 3 2 1

REVIEWERS

Susan L. Grimm, BSRS, RT (R)
Associate Professor, Radiography
Richland Community College
Decatur, Illinois

Ly N. Hunyh, MD
Physician
PeaceHealth – Southwest Medical Center
Vancouver, Washington

Tamara E. Janak, MTD, RT(R) (M)
Instructor and Clinical Coordinator
Radiologic Technology Program
College of Southern Idaho
Twin Falls, Idaho

Carol R. Kocher, MS, RT(R) (M)
Program Director
Olney Central College
Olney, Illinois

Ingrid S. Wright
Director of Radiologic Technology
St. Johns River State College–St. Augustine Campus
St. Augustine, Florida

During the past 30 years, *Patient Care in Radiography* has expanded to meet the changing needs of students and technologists in radiography and other medical imaging modalities. It is a resource that provides an introduction to these professions and an orientation to the hospital environment. First and foremost, however, it is a fundamental text on patient care, designed and written to help radiographers meet patient needs. The reader learns to care for the patient effectively while functioning as a responsible and valuable member of the health care team from the patient introduction, through routine procedures, and the final recording of events in the medical record.

Although the primary goal is centered on patient care, concern for those who provide that care is also an essential focus in this text. Discussions of significant aspects of self-care and professional development are included in the following chapters:

- Chapter 3 incorporates important self-care concepts into the section on radiation safety.
- Chapter 4 contains discussions on career planning, malpractice prevention, and legal considerations.
- Chapter 5 describes professional attitudes and strategies for dealing with burnout and grief.
- Chapter 7 includes sections on environmental and ergonomic safety.
- Chapter 8 provides Standard Precautions and additional guidelines for infection control as recommended by the Centers for Disease Control and Prevention (CDC).

Applying these principles is critical to your well-being and your ability to provide good care to others.

NEW TO THIS EDITION

As in previous editions, the ninth edition of *Patient Care in Radiography* contains updated and new information designed to keep student and practicing radiographers current on important topics in this rapidly changing field:

- New and updated four-color images will enhance teaching and learning.

- Every effort has been made to address the content of the American Society of Radiologic Technologists (ASRT) curriculum for radiography that falls within the general scope of the text and to provide both content and learning tools that will aid in implementing the ASRT curriculum guidelines.
- Content has been updated to reflect current information and infection control guidelines from the CDC and to be consistent with Occupational Safety and Health Administration (OSHA) recommendations. This information will help to ensure the well-being of radiographers by raising practice standards in the workplace and by minimizing risks of exposure to blood-borne pathogens.
- Chapter 5 has two new tables with information on Crimes and Torts that help to clarify this content for students
- Chapter 9 has new information on Enteric Contact Precautions
- The Answer Key (now printed in the text) helps students evaluate learning

KEY FEATURES

The reading level is comfortable for the student radiographer without being overly simplistic. Again, we have done our best to retain the features that readers have appreciated in previous editions:

- Content outlines accompany each chapter.
- Smaller chapters segregate material and facilitate readability.
- Callout boxes are used to indicate key items for learning and warning boxes alert students to issues of safety.
- Step-by-step procedures are shown in photo essays, and patient care is integrated with procedural skills.
- Additional pedagogical elements, such as learning objectives, key terms, illustrations, tables, boxes, comprehensive summaries, review questions, and critical thinking exercises have been retained and improved.

These features can be incorporated into classroom objectives and activities and will also enhance the effectiveness of individual study.

The chapters of this text were designed to be used consecutively; each section builds on the preceding information. A basic glossary is included for quick reference, but please bear in mind that it is not meant to replace the more detailed definitions and discussions found in a good medical dictionary.

We hope that this book proves to be a valuable resource to you as you care for patients in the challenging field of medical imaging.

EVOLVE: ONLINE RESOURCES

The instructor resources for *Patient Care in Radiography* are available online on Evolve and consist of:

- A test bank offering more than 450 questions
- An image collection with all the images from the text
- PowerPoint slides

The student Evolve site will include an image collection, as well as check-off forms for students to use for documentation of clinical objectives related to patient care. For more information, visit http://evolve.elsevier.com/Ehrlich/radiography/ or contact an Elsevier sales representative.

ACKNOWLEDGMENTS

Suggestions by students, instructors, colleagues, and reviewers have contributed greatly to this edition and are acknowledged with our thanks. In addition to their suggestions, many students in the Portland Community College Radiologic Technology program assisted by serving as models for photography. Many thanks also to models Leslie Danford, Gregg Norman, Kay Coakes, Noah Coakes, Charlie Coakes, Sara Breithaupt, and Ron Kizziar, MD.

We are especially grateful to Dr. Ly Huynh, a radiologist with Columbia Imaging Group, for his consultation in reviewing several chapters. His expertise, insight, and suggestions have helped beyond measure. Thank you to Providence Portland Medical Center and the medical imaging staff for allowing us access to their facility when we created color illustrations. In addition, they have been an excellent and most welcome resource when questions arose about hospital policies and procedures.

We have been privileged to benefit from the photographic expertise of Jeff Watson; his technical ability is top notch, and it is applied with a sharp eye, a deep understanding of clinical practice, and a delightful sense of humor.

As always, it has been a pleasure to work with the professionals at Elsevier: Sonya Seigafuse, Executive Content Strategist; Tina Kaemmerer, Senior Content Development Specialist; Lisa A. P. Bushey, Project Manager; and the fine editorial staff at Elsevier. Our sincere gratitude to all of you!

Ruth Ann Ehrlich and Dawn M. Coakes

CONTENTS

CONTENTS

1

Introduction to Radiography

OBJECTIVES

At the conclusion of this chapter, the student will be able to:
- Name the discoverer of x-rays, state the place and date of the discovery, and describe the discovery.
- Name four other pioneers in the development of radiography and describe their contributions.
- Summarize the history and development of radiography education.
- List four essentials for the production of x-rays.
- Draw a diagram of a simple x-ray tube and label the parts.
- Briefly describe the process by which x-rays are produced in the tube.
- List five different types of electromagnetic wave radiation and identify those that are ionizing.

- List six characteristics of x-radiation.
- Define *wavelength*, *frequency*, and *velocity* with respect to a sine wave and state which of these factors is a constant.
- Describe the differences between primary radiation, scatter radiation, and remnant radiation.
- Correctly identify the essential devices found in a typical radiographic room and state the purpose of each.
- Demonstrate the vertical, horizontal, and angulation motions of an x-ray tube.

OUTLINE

KEY TERMS

amplitude	filament	latent image
anode	fluoresce	photon
attenuation	fluoroscope	photostimulable phosphor
bucky	focal spot	quantum (*pl.* quanta)
cassette	fog	remnant radiation
cathode	frequency	sine wave
collimator	grid	space charge
detent	grid cap	target
electromagnetic energy	image intensifier	Trendelenburg position
electron stream	image receptor (IR)	wavelength

The study of radiography includes many topics, and each topic is best understood when a host of others has already been mastered. Obviously, something has to come first. As you progress in your radiography education, you will discover that learning occurs somewhat like the peeling of an onion—one layer at a time will be revealed. You will visit topics again and again, each time building a broader understanding based on your previous learning and experience. The subject matter in this section is treated on an introductory level to provide a starting place for your radiography education. All these topics will be presented in depth at a later time in your program; some are the subjects of entire courses in the radiography curriculum. Eventually, this information will be woven together to provide a sound basis for clinical practice and decision making. Have patience and confidence in yourself as you take the first steps in your new profession.

Some radiography programs combine the topics of patient care with an introduction to medical imaging and instructors find that the five chapters of Part I provide a suitable beginning. The curriculum designs of other schools may include this introductory material under a different course heading. Regardless of whether the content of this chapter is a part of your current course, it may serve as a useful resource.

Entering a hospital radiology department as a student for the first time can be both exciting and bewildering. The equipment, language, and activities unique to this environment require some guidance for comprehension. A good way to introduce you to radiography might be to guide you through a medical imaging department, exploring and pointing things out. Think of this chapter as the textbook version of such a tour. But before we enter the modern world of radiology, let's take a moment to see how it all began more than a century ago.

HISTORY

Discovery of X-Rays

In the 1870s and 1880s, research involving electricity was the cutting edge of physical science, and many physicists were experimenting with a device called a *Crookes tube* (Figure 1-1), a cathode ray tube that was the forerunner of the fluorescent lamp and the neon sign. Although Crookes tubes also produced x-rays, no one detected them.

Then, on November 8, 1895, Wilhelm Conrad Roentgen, a German physicist (Figure 1-2), was working with a Crookes tube at the University of Würzburg. In his

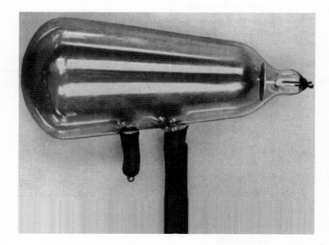

FIG 1-1 Pear-shaped Hittorf–Crookes tube used in Roentgen's initial experiments. (Courtesy of Eastman Kodak, Rochester, New York.)

darkened laboratory, he enclosed the tube with black photographic paper so that no light could escape. Across the room, a plate coated with barium platinocyanide crystals (a fluorescent material) began to glow. Roentgen noted that the plate fluoresced in relation to its distance from the tube, becoming brighter when the plate was moved closer. He placed various materials, such as wood, aluminum, and his hand, between the plate and the tube, noting variations in the effect upon the plate. He spent the next few weeks investigating this mysterious energy that he called "x ray," *x* being the symbol for the unknown. By the end of the year, Roentgen had identified nearly all the properties of x-rays known today. He was awarded the first Nobel Prize in physics in 1901 in recognition of his discovery.

> In November of 1895, Wilhelm Conrad Roentgen discovered x-rays while working with a Crookes tube in his laboratory at the University of Würzburg in Germany.

X-Ray Pioneers

Early radiography often required as long as 30 minutes to create a visible image. Over the years, many advances in this technology have reduced the time and radiation exposure involved in radiography. The early sources of

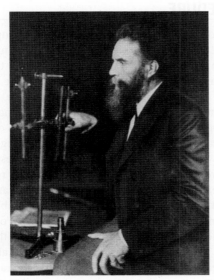

FIG 1-2 Photograph of W.C. Roentgen, the discoverer of x-rays, taken in 1906. (Courtesy Wellcome Library, London.)

electricity were not powerful enough to be efficient and could not be easily adjusted until HC Snook, working with an alternating current generator, developed the interrupterless transformer. William Coolidge designed the hot cathode x-ray tube to work with Snook's improved electrical supply. The Coolidge tube (Figure 1-3), introduced in 1910, was the prototype for the x-ray tubes of today.

Roentgen used a glass plate coated with a photographic emulsion to create the first radiograph. Soon after Roentgen's discovery was published, Michael Idvorsky Pupin demonstrated the radiographic use of fluorescent screens, now called *intensifying screens*. He used light emitted by fluorescent materials when activated by x-rays to expose photographic plates.

In 1898, Thomas Edison began experiments with more than 1800 materials to investigate their fluorescent properties. He invented the first fluoroscope and discovered many of the fluorescent chemicals used in radiography today. Edison abandoned his research when his assistant and longtime friend, Clarence Dally, became severely burned on his arms as a result of serving as a subject for many of Edison's x-ray experiments. Dally's arms had to be amputated, and in 1904 he died from his exposure. His death was the first recorded x-ray fatality in the United States.

Until World War I, glass photographic plates were used as a base for x-ray images. During the war, manufacturers of photographic plates for radiography could not get high-quality glass from suppliers in Belgium, and the U.S. government turned to George Eastman, founder of the Eastman Kodak Company, for help. Eastman had invented photographic film using cellulose nitrate, a new plastic material, as a substitute for glass. He produced the first radiographic film in 1914.

Early in the 20th century, radiation injuries such as skin burns, hair loss, and anemia began to appear in both doctors and patients. Measures were taken to

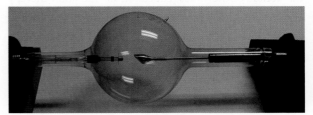

FIG 1-3 Coolidge "hot cathode" x-ray tube, prototype of modern tubes, was introduced in 1910.

monitor and limit exposures; this process is still ongoing. Lead apparel, protective barriers, and reduced exposure requirements have substantially reduced the exposure received by those involved in the use of x-rays.

> Today, because of improved technology and safety precautions, x-ray examinations are much safer for patients, and radiography is considered to be a very safe occupation.

Early Radiographers

During his early experimentation with x-rays, Roentgen produced the first anatomic radiograph—an image of his wife's hand. The first documented medical application of x-rays in the United States was an examination performed at Dartmouth College in February of 1896 of a young boy's fractured wrist.

The first radiographers were physicists familiar with the operation of the Crookes tube. As equipment for generating x-rays was installed in hospitals and physicians' offices, physicians learned to take radiographs and soon developed techniques to demonstrate many different anatomic structures. These physicians began to train their assistants to develop the photographic plates and to assist with x-ray examinations. In time, many of these assistants became skilled in radiography and were called *x-ray technicians.*

Radiography Education

On-the-job training of x-ray technicians in hospitals evolved into hospital-based educational programs. Formal classes and clinical experience were combined to provide students with the knowledge and skills needed to take radiographs and to assist with radiation therapy (x-ray treatments). As the fields of diagnostic and therapeutic radiology became more complex and specialized in the decade of the 1950s, education for radiation therapy technologists was separated from that for radiographers.

Colleges were first involved in radiography education because hospital-based radiography programs took advantage of the academic offerings at local colleges. Radiography students often attended college part-time to learn basic science subjects such as anatomy and physiology.

After World War II, with many returning soldiers wanting to attend college with the financial assistance provided by the G.I. Bill, junior colleges were developed to provide the first 2 years of academic education for university-bound students. In the 1960s, these institutions expanded and multiplied into the community college system that is currently a significant part of national public education in the United States. In the process of this expansion, more emphasis was placed on vocational education. Community colleges formed effective partnerships with companies and institutions that provided on-the-job training. Following this trend, many hospital-based radiography programs became affiliated with community colleges to provide the necessary academic courses. Some 4-year colleges and universities also began to offer educational programs in radiologic technology.

As the requirements for accreditation of educational programs in radiography have increased over the years (see Chapter 4), the organizational structure of colleges has proved to be well suited to the management of these programs. Today, colleges and hospitals still cooperate to provide education in radiography.

> Although many outstanding hospital-based programs exist, the majority of radiography programs are based in colleges.

OVERVIEW OF RADIOGRAPHIC PROCEDURE

Educational preparation provides the radiographer with the necessary knowledge and skills to confidently obtain a patient's radiographic images. To do this, the radiographer positions the patient's anatomic area of interest over the image receptor (IR) (Figure 1-4, *A*). This IR may be a traditional cassette containing film, a more sophisticated filmless system in the form of a digital radiation receptor, or a cassette containing a plate coated with photostimulable phosphors. These phosphors are crystals that store the energy of the remnant x-ray beam and release it as light when stimulated by a laser. If the IR is a cassette, it is placed on the tabletop to image small body parts, such as extremities. For larger anatomic areas, it is placed in a tray beneath the table surface. The x-ray tube position is adjusted to align the x-ray beam to the IR (see Figure 1-4, *B*). The radiographer then goes to the control booth, sets the exposure factors on the control console, and activates the exposure switch.

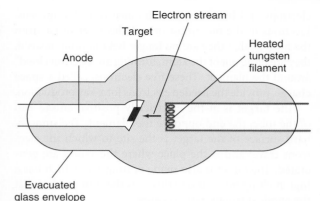

FIG 1-5 Diagram of Coolidge tube simplifies understanding of x-ray production.

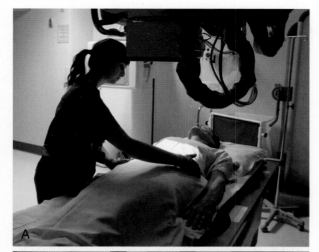

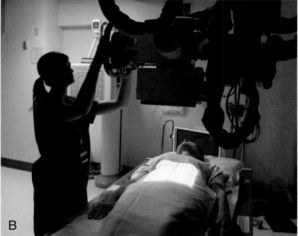

FIG 1-4 A, A radiographer aligns patient anatomy to an image receptor in a bucky tray. **B,** A radiographer aligns an x-ray tube to the patient and image receptor.

During the exposure, x-rays from the tube pass through the patient. Different types of tissue absorb different amounts of the radiation, resulting in a pattern of varying intensity in the x-ray beam that exits on the opposite side of the patient. The radiation then passes to the IR and exposes it. The IR then has a pattern of exposure that is referred to as the latent image. Depending on the type of IR, a digital image may appear immediately on a monitor, the photostimulable IR plate may be scanned by a laser in a special processor to produce a digital image, or an exposed film in a cassette may be taken to the darkroom for processing. Processing

converts the latent image into a visible one. All imaging systems include methods for identifying images with the patient's name, the date, and the name of the facility.

As you may have suspected, many details were omitted from the previous paragraphs. This is only a brief introduction to the radiographic process. Next, we consider how x-rays are produced, their physical nature, and how their various characteristics relate to the process of radiography.

X-RAY PRODUCTION

Our tour will include a close look at a number of pieces of x-ray equipment. To better appreciate their purposes, it will be helpful to understand how x-rays are produced. There are four basic requirements for the production of x-rays:
1. A vacuum
2. A source of electrons
3. A target for the electrons
4. A high potential difference (voltage) between the electron source and the target

The container for the vacuum is the x-ray tube itself (Figure 1-5), sometimes referred to as a *glass envelope*. It is made of borosilicate glass (Pyrex) to withstand heat and is fitted on both ends with connections for the electrical supply. All the air is removed from the tube so that gas molecules will not interfere with the process of x-ray production.

The source of electrons is a wire filament at the electrically negative cathode end of the tube. It is made of the element tungsten, a large atom with 74 electrons orbiting around its nucleus. An electric current flows through the filament to heat it; this accelerates the movement of the electrons and increases their distance from the nucleus. Electrons in the outermost orbital shells get so far from the nucleus that they are no longer held in orbit; instead, they are flung out of the atom, forming an "electron cloud" around the filament. These free electrons, called a space charge, provide the needed electrons for x-ray production.

The target is at the electrically positive anode end of the tube, the end opposite the filament. The smooth, hard surface of the target is the site to which the electrons travel and is the place where the x-rays are generated. The target is also made of tungsten, which has a high melting point and withstands the heat produced at the anode during x-ray exposure.

The voltage required for x-ray production is provided by a high-voltage transformer. The two ends of the x-ray tube are connected in the transformer circuit so that, during an exposure, the filament or cathode end is negative and the target or anode end is positive. The high positive electrical potential at the target attracts the negatively charged electrons of the space charge, which move rapidly across the tube, forming an electron stream. When these fast-moving electrons collide with the target, the kinetic energy of their motion must be converted into a different form of energy. The great majority of this kinetic energy is converted into heat (>99%), but a small amount is converted into the energy form known as *x-rays*.

> When fast-moving electrons collide with the target of an x-ray tube, the kinetic energy of their motion is converted into other forms of energy: heat and x-rays.

ELECTROMAGNETIC ENERGY

X-rays are among several types of energy described as electromagnetic energy, or electromagnetic wave radiation. They have both electrical and magnetic properties, changing the field through which they pass both electrically and magnetically. These changes in the field occur in the form of a repeating wave, a pattern that scientists call a *sinusoidal form* or sine wave.

Several characteristics of this waveform are significant. The distance between the crest and valley of the wave (its height) is called the amplitude (Figure 1-6). More important to radiographers is the distance from one crest to the next, or wavelength (Figure 1-7). The frequency of the wave is the number of times per second that a crest passes a given point.

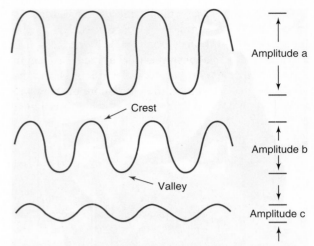

FIG 1-6 These three sine waves are identical except for their amplitudes. (From Bushong SC: *Radiologic science for technologists,* ed 10, St Louis, 2013, Mosby.)

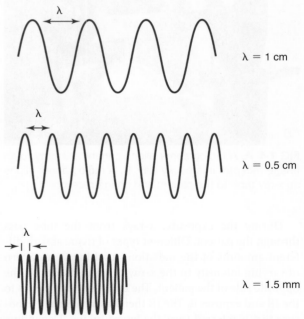

FIG 1-7 These three sine waves have different wavelengths. The shorter the wavelength, the higher the frequency. (Note that the symbol for wavelength is the Greek letter lambda—λ.) (From Bushong SC: *Radiologic science for technologists,* ed 10, St Louis, 2013, Mosby.)

Because all electromagnetic energy moves through space at the same velocity—approximately 186,000 miles/sec, which is 30 billion (3×10^{10}) cm/sec—it is apparent that a relationship exists between wavelength and frequency. When the wavelength is short, the crests are closer together; therefore more of them will pass a given point each second, resulting in a higher frequency. Longer wavelengths will have a lower frequency; this can be expressed mathematically as follows:

Velocity (v) = Wavelength (λ) × Frequency (f)

The more energy the wave has, the greater will be its frequency and the shorter its wavelength. We can therefore use either wavelength or frequency to describe the energy of the wave. In radiologic science, wavelength is more often used to describe the energy of the x-ray beam. The average wavelength of a diagnostic x-ray beam is approximately 0.1 nanometer (nm), which is 10^{-10} (0.00000000001) m, or approximately one billionth of 1 inch.

The wavelength of electromagnetic radiation varies from exceedingly short (shorter than that of diagnostic x-rays) to very long (more than 5 miles). This range of energies is known as the *electromagnetic spectrum;* it includes x-rays, gamma rays, visible light, microwaves, and radio waves (Figure 1-8). Radiation with a wavelength shorter than 1 nm (10^{-9} m) is said to be *ionizing radiation* because it has sufficient energy to remove an electron from an atomic orbit. X-rays are one type of ionizing radiation.

The smallest possible unit of electromagnetic energy (analogous to the atom with respect to matter) is the **photon,** which can be thought of as a minute "bullet" of energy. Photons occur in groups or bundles called **quanta** (singular, **quantum**).

> The smallest possible unit of electromagnetic energy is the photon, which can be thought of as a minute "bullet" of energy.

CHARACTERISTICS OF RADIATION

Because x-rays and visible light are both forms of electromagnetic energy, they share some similar characteristics. Both travel in straight lines, and both have an effect on photographic emulsions. When film is used,

Applications:	Wavelength:	
Therapeutic x-ray	1/100,000 nm	Ionizing
	1/10,000 nm	
Gamma rays	1/1000 nm	
	1/100 nm	
Diagnostic x-ray	1/10 nm	
	1 nm	
Ultraviolet rays	10 nm	Nonionizing
	100 nm	
Visible light	1000 nm	
Infrared rays	10,000 nm	
	100,000 nm	
	1/1000 m	
Radar	1/100 m	
	1/10 m	
	1 m	
Television	10 m	
Radio	100 m	
	1 nanometer = 10^{-9} meters	

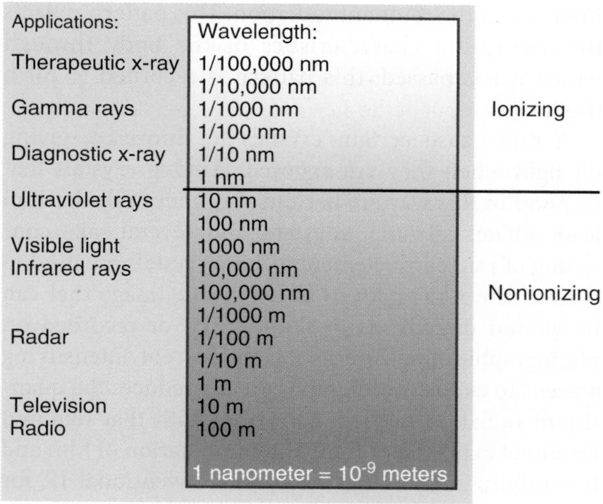

FIG 1-8 Electromagnetic spectrum.

the photographic effect of x-rays is important in the production of radiographic images. It is also important to remember because accidental exposure can occur when film is placed near x-ray sources.

Both x-rays and light have a biologic effect; that is, they can cause changes in living organisms. Because of their greater energy, x-rays are capable of producing more harmful effects than light. Unlike light, x-rays cannot be refracted by a lens. The x-ray beam diverges into space from its source until it is absorbed by matter.

Unlike light, x-rays cannot be detected by the human senses. This fact may seem obvious, but it is important to consider. If x-rays could be seen, felt, or heard, we would have an increased awareness of their presence and radiation safety might be much simpler. Because they are undetectable, however, safety requires that you learn to know when and where x-rays are present without being able to perceive them.

X-rays can penetrate matter that is opaque to light. This penetration is differential, depending on the density and thickness of the matter. For example, x-rays penetrate air readily. There is less penetration of fat or oil, even less of water, which is approximately the same density as muscle tissue, and still less of bone. The effect on the x-ray beam caused by passing through matter is called **attenuation**. X-rays that have passed through the body are referred to as **remnant radiation** or exit radiation. Attenuation results in the absorption of a portion of the radiation and produces a pattern of intensity in the remnant radiation. This pattern reflects the absorption characteristics of the body through which it has passed; this pattern is recorded to form the image.

X-rays cause certain crystals to **fluoresce,** giving off light when they are exposed. Among crystals that respond in this way are barium platinocyanide, barium lead sulfate, calcium tungstate, and several salts consisting of rare earth elements. These crystals are used to convert the x-ray pattern into a visible image that can be viewed directly, as in fluoroscopy, or recorded on photographic film. The use of fluorescent intensifying screens to expose radiographs greatly reduces the quantity of radiation needed, compared with that required for direct exposure of film. The combination of film and intensifying screens has been the conventional IR for decades, but is now largely replaced by filmless technology that produces digital images. This topic is explored further in Chapter 2.

THE PRIMARY X-RAY BEAM

X-rays are formed within a very small area on the target (anode) called a **focal spot.** The actual size of the largest focal spot is no more than a few millimeters in diameter. From the focal spot, the x-rays diverge into space, forming the cone-shaped *primary x-ray beam* (Figure 1-9). The cross section of the x-ray beam at the point where it is used is called the *radiation field*. A photon in the center of the primary beam and perpendicular to the long axis of the x-ray tube is called the *central ray*.

The x-ray beam size is restricted by the size of the port, the opening in the tube housing. Attached to the housing is the **collimator,** a device that enables the radiographer to further control the size of the radiation field.

SCATTER RADIATION

When the primary x-ray beam is attenuated by any solid matter, such as the patient or the x-ray table, a portion of its energy is absorbed. This results in the production of scatter radiation (Figure 1-10). Scatter

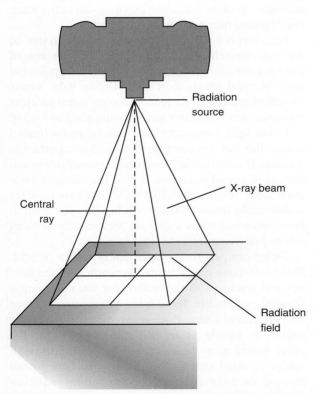

FIG 1-9 A cross section of the x-ray beam is called the *radiation field;* an imaginary perpendicular ray at its center is called the *central ray*.

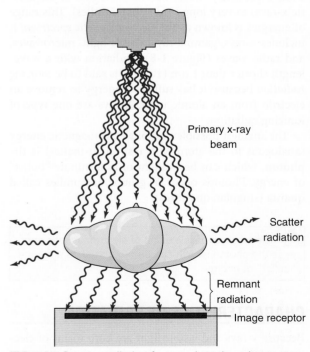

FIG 1-10 Scatter radiation forms when the primary x-ray beam interacts with matter. (From Bushong SC: *Radiologic science for technologists*, ed 10, St Louis, 2013, Mosby.)

radiation generally has less energy than the primary x-ray beam, but it is not easily controlled. It emanates from the source in all directions, causing unwanted exposure to the IR and posing a radiation hazard to anyone in the room.

> 📌 Scatter radiation is the principal source of occupational exposure to radiographers.

The characteristics of primary radiation, scatter radiation, and remnant radiation are summarized for comparison in Table 1-1.

RADIOGRAPHIC EQUIPMENT

X-ray rooms vary in design, depending on their purpose. For example, a room dedicated to upright chest radiography might not have an x-ray table because the patients in this room would be standing for their examinations, not lying down. A room designed for doing gastrointestinal examinations would be equipped for both radiography and fluoroscopy. This dual-purpose equipment is described later in this chapter. A typical room designed for general radiography (Figure 1-11) is suitable for many different types of x-ray examinations. In a hospital setting, the room will be fairly large, perhaps 18 × 20 feet in size, with wide doors to accommodate hospital beds and stretchers. Physical features will include the radiographic table, the x-ray tube and its support system, an upright IR cabinet against one wall, and a shielded control booth that contains the control console.

The X-Ray Tube

The x-ray tube is the source of the radiation. Modern multipurpose x-ray tubes (Figure 1-12) are dual focus tubes. Their cathode assemblies contain two filaments, one large and one small (Figure 1-13). Each is situated in a focusing cup that directs its electrons toward the same general area on the target portion of the anode. When the small filament is activated, its electrons are directed to a tiny focal spot on the target. The small filament and focal spot provide finer image detail when a relatively small exposure is appropriate—for example, when imaging a small body part such as a toe or wrist. The large filament provides more electrons and is aimed at a somewhat larger target area. The combination of large filament and large focal spot is used when a large exposure is required, such as for radiographs of the lumbar

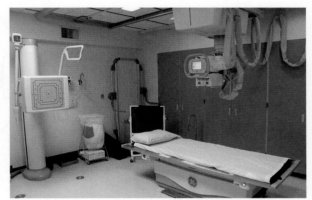

FIG 1-11 A typical room designed for general radiography.

TABLE 1-1	X-Ray Beam Attenuation		
	Definition	**Travel Pattern**	**Energy Level**
Primary Radiation	The x-ray beam that leaves the tube and is not attenuated, except by air.	Its direction and location are predictable and controllable.	Its energy is controlled by the kilovoltage setting.
Scatter Radiation	Radiation is scattered or created as a result of the attenuation of the primary x-ray beam by matter.	It travels in all directions from the scattering medium and is difficult to control.	Generally, it has less energy than the primary beam.
Remnant (Exit) Radiation	What remains of the primary beam after it has been attenuated by matter.	Because the pattern of densities in the matter results in differential absorption, this pattern is inherent in remnant radiation.	The pattern of intensity of remnant radiation creates the radiographic image.

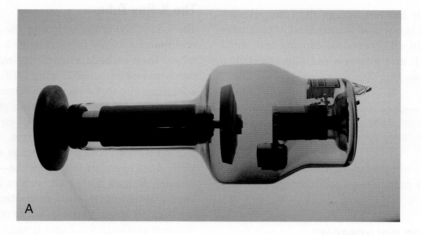

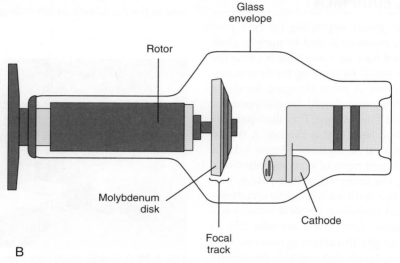

FIG 1-12 Modern rotating-anode x-ray tube.

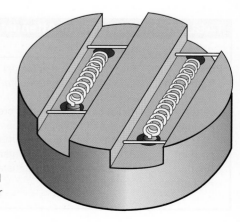

FIG 1-13 Dual focus x-ray tube has focusing cups with large and small filaments. (From Long B, Frank E, Ehrlich RA: *Radiography essentials for limited practice,* ed 4, St Louis, 2013, Saunders.)

spine or the abdomen, because the large filament provides more electrons and the large focal spot can better handle the resulting heat at the anode. The anode is disk-shaped and rotates during the exposure (Figure 1-14), distributing the anode heat over a larger area than the focal spot itself and increasing the heat capacity of the tube. It is the rotation of the anode that causes the whirring sound heard just before and after the exposure.

X-Ray Tube Housing

The x-ray tube is located inside a protective barrel-shaped housing (Figure 1-15). The housing incorporates shielding that absorbs radiation that is not a part of the useful x-ray beam. The housing protects and insulates the x-ray tube while providing a base for the attachments that allow the radiographer to manipulate the x-ray tube and to control the size and shape of the x-ray beam.

X-Ray Tube Support

The tube housing can be either attached to a ceiling-mounted tube hanger or mounted on a tube stand. Both types of mountings provide support and mobility for the tube. A tube hanger (Figure 1-16) is suspended from the ceiling on a system of tracks to allow positioning of the tube at locations throughout the room. This ceiling mount is useful when positioning the tube over a stretcher or when moving the tube for use in different locations. A tube stand is a vertical support with a horizontal arm that supports the tube over the radiographic table. The tube stand rolls along a track that is secured to the floor (and sometimes also the ceiling or wall), permitting horizontal motion.

A system of electric locks holds the tube support in position. The control system for all, or most, of these locks is an attachment on the front of the tube housing. To move the tube in any direction, the locking device must be released. Moving the tube without first releasing the lock can damage the lock, making it impossible to secure the tube in position.

> 📌 Do not attempt to move the x-ray tube without first releasing the appropriate lock.

Typical tube motions (Figure 1-17) include the following:
- Longitudinal—along the long axis of the table
- Transverse—across the table, at right angles to longitudinal
- Vertical—up and down, increasing or decreasing the distance between the tube and the table
- Rotation—allows the entire tube support to turn on its axis, changing the direction in which the tube arm is extended
- Roll (tilt, angle)—permits angulation of the tube along the longitudinal axis and allows the tube to be aimed at the wall rather than the table

A **detent** is a special mechanism that tends to stop a moving part in a specific location. Detents are built into tube supports to facilitate placement at standard locations. For example, a vertical detent will indicate when the distance from tube to IR is 40 or 48 inches, common standard distances. Other detents provide "stops" when the transverse tube position is centered to the table and when the tilt motion is such that the central ray is perpendicular to the table or to the upright IR cabinet.

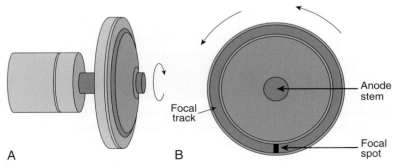

FIG 1-14 Rotating anode. Electrons strike the anode in the tiny focal spot area, but the heat is spread around the entire focal track of the spinning anode face. **A,** Side view. **B,** View from cathode. (From Long B, Frank E, Ehrlich RA: *Radiography essentials for limited practice,* ed 4, St Louis, 2013, Saunders.)

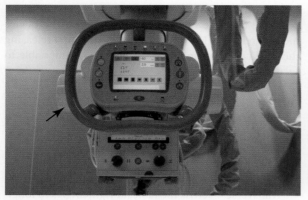

FIG 1-15 The tube housing *(arrow)* shields the tube and provides mounting for tube motion controls and collimator.

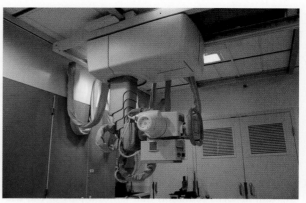

FIG 1-16 Ceiling-mounted tube support.

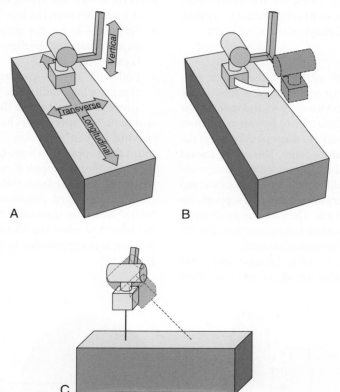

FIG 1-17 Tube motions. **A,** Longitudinal, transverse, and vertical. **B,** Rotation. **C,** Angulation. (From Long B, Frank E, Ehrlich RA: *Radiography essentials for limited practice,* ed 4, St Louis, 2013, Saunders.)

Collimator

Another attachment to the tube housing is the collimator, a boxlike device mounted beneath the port, the opening of the housing. Collimators allow the radiographer to vary the size of the radiation field and to indicate with a light beam the size, location, and center of the field. There is usually a centering light that also helps to align the IR (Figure 1-18). Controls on the front of the collimator allow the radiographer to adjust the size of each dimension of the radiation field. The collimator

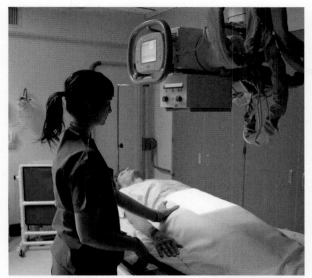

FIG 1-18 Collimator light defines the radiation field and aids in the alignment of the bucky tray.

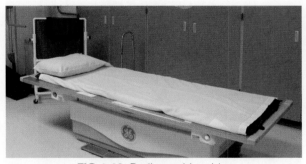

FIG 1-19 Radiographic table.

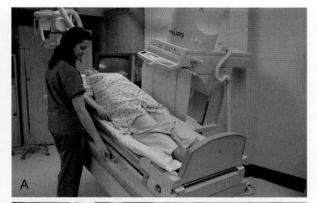

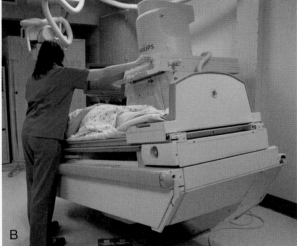

FIG 1-20 The hydraulic fluoroscopic table tilts to change the patient's position. **A**, Semiupright position. **B**, Trendelenburg position.

has a scale that indicates each dimension of the field at specific source-image distances. A timer controls the collimator light, turning it off after a certain length of time—usually 15 to 30 seconds. This helps to avoid accidental overheating of the unit by prolonged use of its high-intensity light.

Radiographic Table

The radiographic table (Figure 1-19) is a specialized unit that is more than just a support for the patient. Although the table is usually secured to the floor, it may be capable of several types of motion: vertical, tilt, and "floating" tabletop.

For vertical table motion, a hydraulic motor, activated by a hand, foot, or knee switch, raises or lowers the height of the table. This motion allows the lowering of the table so that the patient can sit on it easily and permits the table to rise to a comfortable working height for the radiographer. Adjustments to exact stretcher height can be made to facilitate patient transfers. There will be a detent at the standard height for routine radiography. This standard table position corresponds to indicated distances from the x-ray tube. Because it is important that standard tube–IR distances be used, it is necessary to return the table to the detent position after lowering it for patient access. Not all tables are capable of vertical motion.

A tilting table (Figure 1-20) also uses a hydraulic motor to change position. In this case, the table turns on a central axis to attain a vertical position; this allows the patient to be placed in a horizontal or vertical position or at any angle in between. The table can also tilt in the opposite direction, allowing the patient's head to be lowered at least 15 degrees into the **Trendelenburg position.** A detent stops the table in the horizontal position. Tilting is an essential feature of fluoroscopic tables and may also be a feature of a radiographic unit.

Special attachments for the tilting table include a footboard and a shoulder guard system to provide safety for the patient when tilting the table (Figure 1-21). Pay particular attention to the attachment mechanisms so that you will be able to apply these devices correctly when needed.

> **!** Before tilting a patient on the table, always test the footboard and shoulder guards to be certain that they are securely attached.

The motor that tilts the table is powerful and can overcome the resistance of obstacles placed in the way. Many step stools and other pieces of movable equipment have been damaged because they were under the end of the table and out of view when the table motor was activated. Such a collision can also damage the table motor.

> **!** Be certain that the spaces under the head and foot of the table are clear before activating the tilt motor.

A floating tabletop allows the top of the table to move independently of the remainder of the table for ease in aligning the patient to the x-ray tube and the IR. This motion may involve a mechanical release, allowing the radiographer to shift the position of the tabletop, or it may be power-assisted, activated by a small control pad with directional switches. Power-assisted movement is usual for fluoroscopic tables.

Grids and Buckys

You will recall from an earlier part of this chapter that when primary radiation encounters matter, such as the patient or the x-ray table, the resulting interaction produces scatter radiation. Most of the scatter produced during an exposure originates within

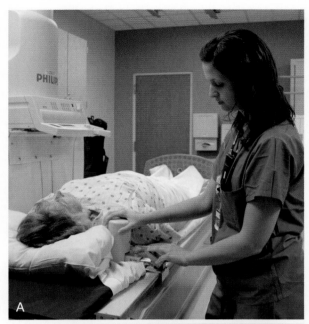
A

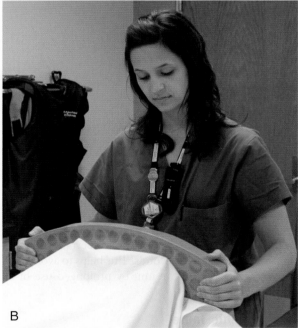
B

FIG 1-21 Table attachments must be secured carefully for patient safety before tilting the table. **A,** Shoulder guard. **B,** Footboard.

the patient. This scatter radiation causes **fog** on the radiographic image, a generalized exposure that compromises the visibility of the anatomic structures. **Grids** and **buckys** are devices to prevent scatter radiation from reaching the IR.

> 📌 Grids and buckys prevent scatter radiation from reaching the IR and producing fog that degrades the image.

A bucky is usually located beneath the table surface; it is a moving grid device that incorporates a tray to hold the IR (Figure 1-22). The entire unit can be moved along the length of the table and locked into position where desired. The grid that is incorporated into the bucky device is situated between the tabletop and the IR (Figure 1-23). It is a plate made of tissue-thin lead

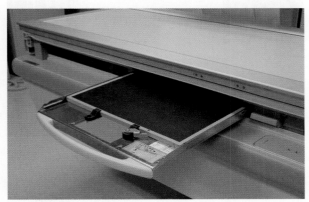

FIG 1-22 The bucky tray holds the image receptor within the x-ray table.

strips, mounted on edge, with radiolucent interspacing material (Figure 1-24). The strips must be carefully aligned to the path of the primary x-ray beam, so precise alignment of the x-ray tube is essential. In most radiographic units, the grid moves during the exposure. The purpose of moving the grid is to blur the image of the thin lead strips so that they are not visible on the radiograph. When the table has a floating tabletop, the bucky mechanism and IR tray do not move with the tabletop.

Stationary grids that do not move during the exposure serve the same purpose as a bucky. A grid can also be incorporated into a device called a **grid cap,** which is a grid mounted in a frame that can be attached to the front of an IR for mobile radiography and other special applications.

Grids or buckys are generally used only for body parts that measure more than 10 to 12 cm in thickness. (The average adult's neck or knee measures 12 cm.) When a grid is not needed, the IR is placed on the tabletop.

> 📌 Grids or buckys are generally used only for body parts that measure more than 10 to 12 cm in thickness.

Upright Image Receptor Units

The upright bucky or grid cabinet is a device that holds the IR in the upright position for radiography (Figure 1-25). It is adjustable in height and can incorporate either a bucky or a stationary grid. When a stationary grid is included, this device can be referred to as a *grid cabinet;* when the grid moves during the exposure, the device is called an *upright bucky.* Even if the table tilts to the upright position, it is common to have a separate upright unit for some examinations, such as those

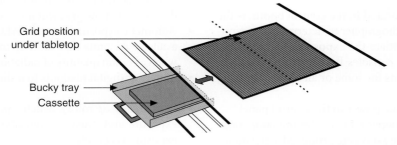

Grid position under tabletop

Bucky tray

Cassette

FIG 1-23 The bucky device for scatter radiation control incorporates a tray for the image receptor and is mounted under the tabletop. Note that the lead strips are parallel to the long axis of the table. (From Long B, Frank E, Ehrlich RA: *Radiography essentials for limited practice,* ed 4, St Louis, 2013, Saunders.)

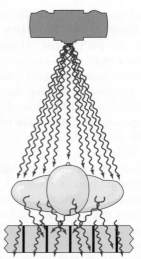

FIG 1-24 Lead strips in the grid absorb scatter radiation emitted from the patient; remnant radiation passes through the grid and exposes the image receptor.

of the cervical spine and the chest. When the patient is sitting or standing at the upright bucky, the tube is angled to direct the x-ray beam toward the IR. The distance may be adjusted to 40, 48, or 72 inches, depending on the requirements of the procedure.

Transformer

Cables from the tube housing connect the x-ray tube to the transformer, which provides the high voltage necessary for x-ray production. Some transformers look like a large box or cabinet, which may be located within the x-ray room. Newer transformer designs are much smaller and can be incorporated into the control console.

Control Console

The control console, located in the control booth, is the access point for the radiographer to determine the exposure factors and to initiate the exposure (Figure 1-26). Radiographic control consoles have buttons, switches, dials, or digital readouts for some or all of the following functions:

- Off/On—controls the power to the control panel
- mA—allows the operator to set the milliamperage, the rate at which the x-rays are produced; determines the focal spot size
- kVp—controls the kilovoltage, and thereby the wavelength and penetrating power, of the x-ray beam
- Timer—controls the duration of the exposure

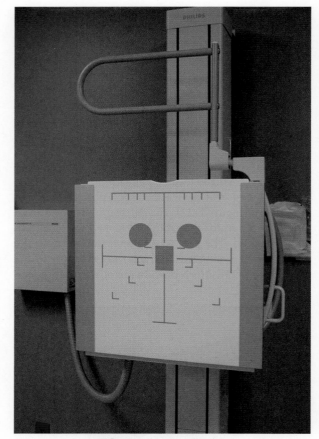

FIG 1-25 Upright bucky.

- mAs—some units have an mAs control instead of mA and time settings; the mAs (the product of mA and time) determines the total quantity of radiation produced during an exposure
- Bucky—activates the motor control of the bucky device so that the grid will move during the exposure
- Automatic exposure controls (AECs)—special settings available on units that allow termination of exposure when a certain quantity of radiation has reached the IR
- Meters or digital readouts to indicate the status of the settings
- Prep (ready or rotor) switch—prepares the tube for exposure and must be continuously activated until exposure is complete
- Exposure switch—initiates the exposure and must be continuously activated until the exposure is complete
- Accessories—other controls may also be present, depending on the equipment and its specific features

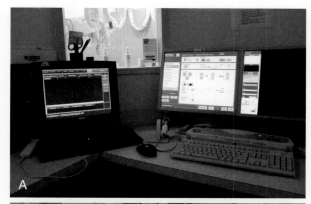

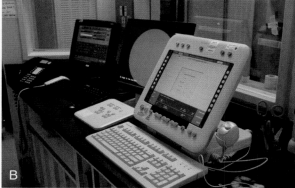

FIG 1-26 Examples of x-ray control consoles. A, Simple computerized radiographic controls. B, Controls for filmless radiography with digital fluoroscopy.

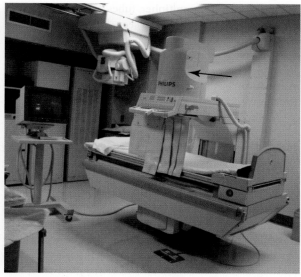

FIG 1-27 Typical radiographic/fluoroscopic unit. The tower *(arrow)* contains the image intensifier.

view various anatomic areas. Because the fluoroscopic image was dim, dark adaptation was required and the procedure was performed in a darkroom.

> A fluoroscope is an x-ray machine designed for direct viewing of the x-ray image. This equipment permits the radiologist to view and record x-ray images in motion in real time.

FLUOROSCOPY

Whereas routine radiography produces still or *static* images, fluoroscopy permits the viewing of *dynamic* images or x-ray images in motion. Fluoroscopy is usually performed by radiologists with the assistance of radiographers. Fluoroscopic procedures are a routine aspect of every radiographer's clinical education.

Fluoroscopic Equipment

A **fluoroscope** is an x-ray machine designed for direct viewing of the x-ray image. This equipment permits the radiologist to view and record radiographic images in motion in real time. Early fluoroscopes consisted simply of an x-ray tube mounted under the x-ray table and a fluorescent screen mounted over the patient. The physician watched the radiographic image on the screen while turning the patient into the desired positions to

Modern equipment is far more sophisticated. Most fluoroscopic units are properly called *radiographic/fluoroscopic* (R/F) units because they can be used for both radiography and fluoroscopy. This is convenient because most fluoroscopic examinations also have a radiographic component. "Spot films" are taken during fluoroscopy to record the image as seen on the fluoroscope. Depending on the age of equipment, cassettes, roll film, or digital systems can be used to record fluoroscopic images. The fluoroscopic tube is used to expose spot films and image areas of interest. After the fluoroscopic portion of the study is completed, additional images can be taken using an overhead tube for comprehensive visualization of the entire anatomic region.

The radiation required for a fluoroscopic study has been greatly reduced by the use of the **image intensifier.** This electronic device is in the form of a tower that fits over the fluoroscopic screen (Figure 1-27). Inside is a series of photomultiplier tubes that brighten and enhance the image formerly seen by looking directly at the fluoroscopic screen. The enhanced image is digitized or photographed by a video camera to provide direct viewing on a video monitor. A computer or video recorder can be used to make a record of the entire study. The fluoroscope and spot film device can be moved out of the way when the table is used for radiography.

The control console of an R/F unit is more complex than that of a basic radiography unit. There must be separate mA and kVp settings for the control of the radiographic (overhead) and fluoroscopic (under table) tubes, and special settings for spot film radiography. The radiologist activates the fluoroscope intermittently during an examination. When the fluoroscope is activated so that x-rays are being produced, a timer on the control advances and an alarm sounds after a preset period, usually 5 minutes. This warning is a reminder to reduce fluoroscopy time, and thus minimizes the radiation exposure received by all involved.

> **!** When the fluoroscope is activated so that x-rays are being produced, a timer on the control advances and an alarm sounds after a preset period, usually 5 minutes. This warning is a reminder to reduce fluoroscopy time, and thus minimizes the radiation exposure received by all involved.

Radiographer's Duties in Fluoroscopic Examinations

For a fluoroscopic examination, the duties of the radiographer can include the following:

- Taking the patient's history, including information on the success of dietary or bowel cleansing preparation (see Chapter 17)
- Filling out necessary preprocedural paperwork such as Contrast Media Consent, Time-Out, and Patient Education forms
- Assisting the patient to undress and don a gown
- Explaining the procedure to the patient
- Taking and processing any required preliminary images
- Setting the control panel correctly for fluoroscopy and spot film radiography
- Positioning the patient for the start of the procedure
- Preparing the equipment for fluoroscopy, including attaching the footboard and shoulder guard.
- Entering patient data into the computer for digital imaging, if applicable
- Loading the spot film device, if applicable
- Preparing contrast agents as needed
- Assisting the radiologist as needed, which can involve helping the patient assume various positions; assisting the patient and/or the radiologist with the contrast medium; changing spot film cassettes as needed; loading, unloading, and identifying roll film; or electronically managing digital images
- Taking follow-up radiographs
- Providing postprocedural care and instructions to the patient

Your orientation to the fluoroscopy suite may be to observe or assist with fluoroscopic studies of the gastrointestinal tract. These x-ray examinations of the stomach or the bowel are described in detail in Chapter 17. Other examinations involving fluoroscopy are discussed in Chapters 17, 19, 20, and 21.

SUMMARY

- W.C. Roentgen discovered x-rays in Würzburg, Germany, in 1895, while experimenting with a Crookes tube.
- Other x-ray pioneers included Edison (experimented with many phosphors), Snook (invented the interrupterless transformer), Eastman (made the first x-ray film), and Coolidge (invented the hot cathode x-ray tube).
- Radiography education began in hospitals as physicians trained their assistants to help with x-ray examinations. Hospital-based programs still exist, but most radiography education today takes place in college programs affiliated with medical centers.
- A simple x-ray tube contains a vacuum, a filament to provide a source of free electrons, and a target at which the electrons are directed. When a high voltage is applied to the tube, the free electrons collide with the target, decelerate suddenly, and produce both heat and x-rays.

- X-rays are a form of electromagnetic energy that occurs in units called *photons*. Photons occur in bundles called *quanta*. X-ray energy occurs in a sine wave form, changing the field through which it passes both magnetically and electrically.
- Electromagnetic sine wave characteristics include amplitude, wavelength, frequency, and velocity. The wavelength multiplied by the frequency equals the velocity (the speed of light).
- The characteristics of x-rays are similar to those of light except that x-rays cannot be refracted by a lens, are not detectable by the human senses, and are capable of ionizing matter.
- The primary x-ray beam is that which exits the x-ray tube and is unattenuated except by air; its location and direction are predictable and controllable.
- Scatter radiation is that created by the interaction between radiation and matter; it travels in all directions from the scattering medium and is difficult to control.
- Remnant radiation is what remains of the primary beam after it has been attenuated by the patient; its pattern of intensity represents the pattern of absorption and is the pattern that creates the radiographic image.

- Ceiling mounts or tube stands support x-ray tubes and provide a means to secure them in position. Tube motions include horizontal, vertical, angulation, and rotational movements.
- A collimator is a device attached to the x-ray tube housing for the purpose of controlling the field size; it has a light that indicates the location of the field, the location of the central ray, and the alignment of the x-ray beam to the IR.
- Grids and buckys are devices placed between the patient and the IR to prevent scatter radiation from fogging the image; they are located beneath the top of the radiographic table, in upright cabinets, and in grid caps for mobile radiography.
- The control console is the access point for the radiographer to control the exposure settings and initiate the x-ray exposure. Certain settings and readings are typical of all control consoles and should be recognized and understood by radiographers.
- Fluoroscopes are special x-ray machines that permit viewing of the x-ray image in motion in real time. Radiographic units are often combined with fluoroscopes, and fluoroscopic examinations often have a radiographic component.

REVIEW QUESTIONS

1. X-rays were discovered in 1895 in:
   A. the United States
   B. England
   C. Germany
   D. China
2. The inventor of the hot cathode x-ray tube was:
   A. Crookes
   B. Roentgen
   C. Coolidge
   D. Edison
3. The majority of radiography education programs are based in:
   A. colleges
   B. clinics
   C. hospitals
   D. the Internet
4. A cassette containing a photostimulable phosphor plate is one form of:
   A. fluoroscope
   B. image receptor

   C. grid device
   D. transformer
5. Which of the following is not a basic requirement for the production of x-rays?
   A. A vacuum
   B. A source of electrons
   C. A photostimulable phosphor
   D. A target
6. When fast-moving electrons collide with the target of an x-ray tube, the kinetic energy of their motion is converted into x-rays and:
   A. a space charge
   B. heat
   C. potential difference (voltage)
   D. scatter radiation
7. Of the following types of electromagnetic energy, which has the shortest wavelength?
   A. Radio waves
   B. Gamma rays

C. Microwaves
D. Ultraviolet light

8. Which of the following is not an accurate statement regarding the characteristics of x-rays?
    A. They can penetrate matter that is impenetrable to light.
    B. They can be refracted by a lens.
    C. They have an exposure effect on photographic emulsions.
    D. They cannot be detected by the human senses.

9. The characteristic most often used to describe the energy of an x-ray beam is its:
    A. velocity
    B. space charge
    C. wavelength
    D. amplitude

10. An x-ray beam that has been attenuated by matter is called:
    A. remnant radiation
    B. primary radiation

C. secondary radiation
D. scatter radiation

11. A device used to indicate the location of the radiation field and to control its size is called a:
    A. grid
    B. collimator
    C. transformer
    D. control console

12. An x-ray machine that permits viewing of the x-ray image in motion in real time is called:
    A. a control console
    B. a fluoroscope
    C. a collimator
    D. a bucky

Answers can be found in the Answer Key on pages 429-431.

■ CRITICAL THINKING EXERCISES

1. Crookes and others worked with Crookes tubes before Roentgen did. Why didn't one of them discover x-rays? What important characteristics did Roentgen display during and after the discovery?

2. When did your radiography program begin? How does its history correspond with the history of radiography education in this chapter?

3. List characteristics of x-rays that are similar to those of light and those that are different. Which characteristics of x-rays are useful in radiography?

4. Compare and contrast radiography and fluoroscopy.

2

Image Quality Factors

OBJECTIVES

At the conclusion of this chapter, the student will be able to:

- Define *milliamperage* and state its significance with respect to radiographic exposure.
- Explain the significance of exposure time with respect to optical density.
- Explain the significance of mAs with respect to image quality.
- Describe the effects of an increase in kVp with respect to both the x-ray beam and the radiographic image.
- State the content and purpose of an x-ray technique chart.
- Define *OID* and state its significance with respect to radiographic quality.

- Explain the effect of an increase in source-image distance on both optical density and image detail.
- List three types of image receptor system and describe each.
- List the two types of image distortion and state the cause of each.
- Differentiate between images that exhibit high contrast and those with low contrast.
- List factors that influence image contrast.
- List possible causes of poor image detail.

OUTLINE

Factors of Radiographic Exposure
Exposure Time
Milliamperage
Kilovoltage
Distance
Technique Charts
Image Receptor Systems
Cassettes and Intensifying Screens

Film
Film Processing
Filmless Radiography
Image Quality
Optical Density
Image Contrast
Image Detail
Distortion

KEY TERMS

automatic exposure control
  (AEC)
computed radiography (CR)
digital radiography (DR)
distortion
exposure index number (EI)

exposure time (T)
image contrast
image detail
kilovoltage (kVp)
milliamperage (mA)
milliampere-seconds (mAs)

object-image distance (OID)
optical density (OD)
picture archiving and
  communication system
  (PACS)
source-image distance (SID)

As radiographers are responsible for controlling the quality of the images they produce, it is important to understand the terms used to discuss image quality and the factors that can be changed to influence the appearance of the image. This chapter provides an introduction to image quality factors and the language you will need to learn more about this important aspect of radiography.

FACTORS OF RADIOGRAPHIC EXPOSURE

The four prime factors of radiographic exposure are exposure time (T), milliamperage (mA), kilovoltage (kVp), and source-image distance (SID). Each factor contributes to the amount of exposure impacting the image receptor (IR), and each has an effect on radiographic quality. When you have learned the basics of these four factors, we will consider how they affect radiographic quality and examine additional factors affecting the appearance of the image.

Exposure Time

Exposure time is a measure of how long the exposure will continue and is measured in units of seconds, fractions of seconds, or milliseconds (thousandths of seconds). Electronic timers provide a wide range of possible settings, allowing the radiographer to precisely control the length of exposure. Together with milliamperage (see following section), exposure time determines the total quantity of radiation that will be produced. When a variation in the quantity of exposure is desired, the exposure time is varied. Because a longer exposure time results in the production of more x-rays, when all other factors are equal, a longer exposure time will produce a darker radiographic image. A decrease in exposure time will result in less radiation exposure and a lighter image. Patient dose is directly proportional to exposure time.

> Exposure time is a measure of how long the exposure will continue and is measured in units of seconds, fractions of seconds, or milliseconds. When all other factors are equal, a longer exposure time will produce more exposure and a darker radiographic image; a shorter exposure time will result in less radiation exposure and a lighter image.

Exposure time settings can vary from as short as 1 millisecond (msec) (0.001 second) to as long as several seconds. Some units have automatic timers called automatic exposure control (AEC). These devices terminate the exposure when a specific quantity of radiation has reached the IR. Units with AEC have special controls related to this process.

Milliamperage

Milliamperage (mA) is a measure of the current flow rate in the x-ray tube circuit. It determines the number of electrons available to cross the tube and thus the rate at which x-rays are produced. Think of mA as an indication of the number of x-ray photons that will be produced per second. Thus, the mA setting will determine how much time is required to produce a given amount of x-ray exposure. High mA settings are used to shorten the needed exposure time when motion during a longer exposure would likely cause blurring of the radiographic image.

The number of possible mA settings is limited and is usually in whole numbers that are divisible by 50 or 100. For example, a typical radiographic unit may have the following mA settings: 50, 100, 200, 300, 400, and 500. Some x-ray machines are capable of producing as much as 1000 or 1500 mA.

> Milliamperage (mA) is a measure of the current flow rate in the x-ray tube circuit. It determines the number of electrons available to cross the tube and thus the rate at which x-rays are produced.

The relationship between mA and exposure time is simple. When the mA is multiplied by the exposure time, the product is given in units of milliampere-seconds (mAs). The mAs indicates the amount of radiation in the exposure. Exposures made with the same mAs quantity will be similar in appearance, regardless of the quantities of mA and time used. For example, an exposure made at 100 mA and 0.1 sec. would produce the same amount of radiation as an exposure using 200 mA and 0.05 sec. Both exposures equal 10 mAs, but the second exposure is a shorter and its image is less likely to be blurred if the patient moves.

> The product of mA and time is milliampere-seconds (mAs), which is an indicator of the total quantity of radiation produced in the exposure. This relationship is represented by the following formula:
>
> $$mA \times Time (seconds) = mAs$$

Most control consoles today provide the option of setting the mAs directly, while older models usually require the operator to set mA and exposure time separately. The mAs settings for various applications commonly range between 1 and 500.

Changing the mA has other effects as well. In dual focus tubes, specific mA stations control each filament. In general, mA settings of 150 or lower use the small filament and the small focal spot, while mA settings of 200 or higher are associated with the large filament and large focal spot. On controls that permit the operator to select the mA setting, each setting will have an indication of which focal spot is associated with it. Controls that provide mAs selection without specific mA settings will have a separate means of selecting focal spot size.

In addition to varying the focal spot size, changes in mA will affect the amount of heat that accumulates in the anode during the exposure and will be a cause for concern when very large exposures are required. As a rule, an x-ray tube can handle larger exposures when the desired mAs is obtained with a lower mA setting and a longer exposure time, assuming the same focal spot is used in both cases.

Kilovoltage

The **kilovoltage,** or **kilovoltage peak (kVp),** is a measure of the potential difference across the x-ray tube. One kilovolt is equal to 1000 volts. Kilovoltage determines the speed of the electrons in the electron stream; this determines the amount of kinetic energy each electron has when it collides with the target and therefore determines the amount of energy in the resulting x-ray beam. This energy is expressed by the wavelength of the photons. X-ray photons with shorter wavelengths have more energy and are more penetrating than those with longer wavelengths. For this reason, an increase in kVp results in a more penetrating x-ray beam; this will cause more exposure to the IR, because a higher percentage of the x-rays produced will pass through the patient and reach the receptor. For this reason, an increase in kVp will produce a darker image, whereas a decrease in kVp will produce a lighter image.

> ✒ Kilovoltage (kVp) is a measure of the potential difference across the x-ray tube. An increase in kVp results in a more penetrating x-ray beam and a greater degree of exposure to the IR, producing a darker image.

Changes in kilovoltage will also cause other changes to the image. Because the differential penetration of the x-ray beam will be affected by wavelength, the contrast of the image will also change. As a result, the degree of difference between the darker and lighter areas of the image will be affected. Somewhere between no penetration and total penetration of the subject is the optimal amount of differential penetration that will show a contrast in exposure between the various features of the subject. The amount of kVp that produces optimal penetration varies with the examination. This concept is discussed in the section on Image Quality later in this chapter.

Kilovoltage settings for typical radiographic units range between 40 kVp and 150 kVp in increments of 1 or 2 kilovolts. Low kVp settings are used for small body parts. For example, 50 to 60 kVp is commonly used for radiographic examinations of the hand, wrist, or foot. Spine radiography typically uses settings between 75 and 100 kVp, and settings greater than 100 kVp can be used for chest radiography and for studies of the digestive tract that use barium sulfate as a contrast agent.

Distance

The distance between the source of the x-ray beam (the tube target) and the IR is referred to as the **source-image distance (SID).** This distance is a prime factor of exposure because it affects the intensity of the x-ray beam. Radiation intensity can be considered as the number of photons per square inch striking the surface of the IR. Because the x-ray beam diverges from its source, the size of the beam expands as the distance from the source increases. As the total quantity of x-ray photons in the beam spreads out, there are fewer photons in any given area (Figure 2-1).

The change in x-ray beam intensity that results from changes in the SID is expressed by the *inverse squares law,* which states that the intensity of the radiation is inversely proportional to the square of the distance. The inverse squares law is expressed mathematically in this equation:

$$\frac{I_{orig}}{I_{new}} = \frac{SID^2_{new}}{SID^2_{orig}}$$

Note in Figure 2-1 that, as the distance is doubled, each dimension of the radiation field is doubled; therefore the radiation field is four times greater in area. As a result, the number of photons per unit area within the field is

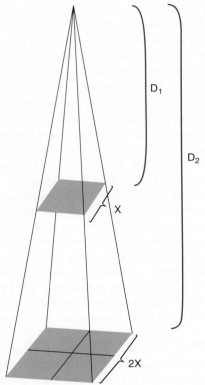

FIG 2-1 Source-image distance affects radiation field size and radiation intensity.

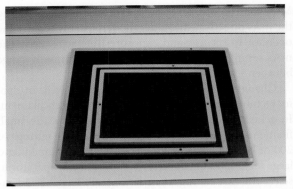

FIG 2-2 Radiographic cassettes come in a variety of sizes. They are lined with intensifying screens that are held in contact with both sides of the film.

one fourth the original amount. Likewise, if the distance were tripled, the field area would be increased in size ninefold (i.e., 3^2), and the radiation intensity would be one ninth the original amount.

> The distance between the tube target and the IR is referred to as the source-image distance (SID). The inverse squares law states the relationship between radiation intensity and the SID: radiation intensity is inversely proportional to the square of the SID.

Of course, as the radiation intensity changes, exposure to the IR will also change. To maintain the same degree of image darkness when the SID changes, the mAs must be adjusted correspondingly. The formula for this adjustment is:

$$\frac{mAs_{orig}}{mAs_{new}} = \frac{SID^2_{orig}}{SID^2_{new}}$$

As you will learn later when you study x-ray technique calculations in more detail, this formula will enable you to maintain a given radiation intensity, and therefore a given image appearance, when changing the SID. For example, this formula will result in a fourfold increase in mAs when the SID is doubled. This increase in mAs compensates for the reduction in radiation intensity that occurs with the SID increase, with the result that the radiation intensity is unchanged.

Technique Charts

A technique chart located near the control console usually provides the radiographer with a listing of recommended mAs and kVp settings, as well as the SID, for each of the various body parts for different sizes of patients. Some control consoles have anatomic programming. These computerized units are preprogrammed with the required exposure settings for the selected body part and size.

IMAGE RECEPTOR SYSTEMS

Cassettes and Intensifying Screens

The cassette (Figure 2-2) serves as the film holder during the radiographic procedure. It provides a light-tight, rigid structure to protect the film and also houses the intensifying screens. Most cassettes contain two intensifying screens, one front and one back, and the film is placed between them. Intensifying screens are plates coated with phosphors (fluorescent crystals) that emit light when exposed to x-rays. Their purpose is to reduce the amount of exposure required to produce a satisfactory image on film. Without intensifying screens, as much as 50 to 100 times more exposure would be needed to adequately expose film. Intensifying screens greatly reduce patient dose and also reduce the output capacity requirements of x-ray generators and x-ray tubes

> Intensifying screens are fluorescent plates that line cassettes. Their purpose is to reduce the amount of exposure required to produce an image on film.

Most phosphors in current use are salts from rare earth elements. When exposed to x-rays, they emit green, blue, blue-violet, or ultraviolet light, depending on the specific phosphor. The type of crystal, the size of the crystals, and the thickness of the phosphor layer determine the amount of exposure required. Larger crystals and thicker layers require less exposure. Screens with finer crystals and thinner layers produce sharper image detail. Most radiography departments that use screens have at least two types: "fast" screens with larger crystals for routine use, and "detail" or "extremity" screens that have smaller crystals and require more exposure. The detail screens are used only for relatively small parts, such as hands and feet, where fine detail is most important. They are used only on the tabletop, not with grids or buckys. A third type is used in some departments for chest radiography, where the screen–film combination produces low-contrast images (images with more shades of gray) to improve the visualization of the lungs, airway, and vascular structures.

Each cassette has a small area where there is no intensifying screen and where exposure is blocked from the film by lead foil. This area is reserved for the photographic imprint of the patient identification; it is indicated on the front of the cassette by the position of the identifying label.

If your department uses film/screen cassettes, it is important that you become familiar with the types of screens used so that you can select cassettes correctly and use them with the appropriate exposure factors. Cassettes are marked according to the type of screens

they contain, and the technique chart will state which screens are appropriate with a given set of exposures.

Intensifying screens are expensive and easily damaged. Damaged areas, dirt, or stains on the screens prevent light from exposing the film and result in artifacts on the image. For these reasons, it is important to avoid touching the screens and to keep the film processing area free of dust and dirt.

Film

Radiographic film is manufactured with a particular sensitivity to the light emitted by intensifying screens. Green-sensitive film is used with screens that emit green light, blue-sensitive film is matched with blue light–emitting screens, and ultraviolet light–emitting screens are paired with film that is sensitive to ultraviolet light. Film for routine radiography has emulsion coating on both sides of the base so that the film responds to the light from both intensifying screens. This system decreases the required exposure by half. Both sides of the film are therefore identical; there is no right or wrong side to a sheet of double-emulsion film.

IRs, including film and cassettes, come in standard sizes. You will work more effectively in the clinical area when you have learned to recognize them at a glance. The most common sizes are the following:
- 8 × 10 inches (20 × 25 cm)
- 10 × 12 inches (25 × 30 cm)
- 11 × 14 inches (28 × 35 cm)
- 7 × 17 inches (18 × 43 cm)
- 14 × 14 inches (35 × 35 cm)
- 14 × 17 inches (35 × 43 cm)

Film Processing

Film must be stored correctly to avoid fog, a generalized exposure that reduces image contrast. A good storage area is clean, cool, and dry and is protected from radiation and processing chemical fumes. Film boxes should stand on edge with the expiration date visible. This date is checked to ensure that older film is used before its expiration date.

To avoid artifacts resulting from improper film handling, be sure that your hands are clean and dry, and touch only the corners of the film when removing it from the cassette. Avoid bending and crimping the film by allowing it to hang vertically when holding it with only one hand. To place it horizontally, use both hands and hold the film on opposite corners.

> ✎ To avoid artifacts resulting from improper film handling, be sure that your hands are clean and dry, and touch only the corners of the film.

In a conventional processing system, the exposed cassette is taken to the darkroom, where the film is removed and fed into the automatic processor in near darkness. Patient identification can be stamped on the film using a daylight system that identifies the film either outside the darkroom while it is still in the cassette, or inside the darkroom after the film is removed from the cassette. After the film has entered the processor, the cassette is reloaded with fresh film from the film bin, which is a storage unit located under the counter. A safelight provides just enough illumination to see where things are located. A tone or a red light on the processor will indicate when it is safe to feed another film or to turn on the lights.

Cassettes are often passed to and from the darkroom without opening the door by using a pass box. This compartment is installed in the darkroom wall and has two sets of doors: one set inside the darkroom and one set in the outside wall. Because the inner and outer doors cannot be opened at the same time, cassettes can be transferred while the darkroom remains dark. The pass box has two compartments: one for exposed cassettes awaiting processing, and one for the unexposed cassettes that have been reloaded and are ready for use. It is essential to designate specific locations for cassettes based on their exposure status, because it is not possible to determine whether the film is exposed by looking at the cassette. Only by following the established routines can radiographers be confident that a cassette is unexposed and ready for use, or that previously exposed images will not be damaged by exposing them a second time.

Filmless Radiography

Most major imaging centers have converted to filmless systems for much of their radiographic imaging. Compared with conventional systems, filmless systems save space, time, and processing chemicals, and have the added advantages of producing digital electronic images. There are two basic types of filmless radiography: **computed radiography (CR)** and **digital radiography (DR)**.

The IR for CR is an imaging plate that consists of photostimulable phosphors. It is exposed in a special

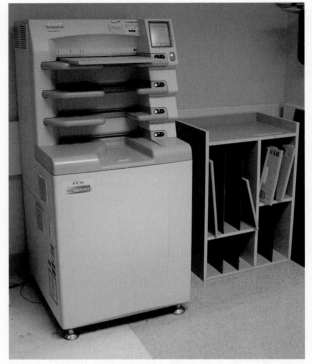

FIG 2-3 Image processor for filmless computed radiography system.

cassette using conventional radiographic equipment. The radiographer inserts the exposed cassette into a special processor (Figure 2-3) and selects the type of examination from a menu so that the image will be processed correctly. A small beam from a high-intensity laser in the processor converts the latent image to a visible one that is captured by a photomultiplier tube similar to those used in fluoroscopic image intensifiers. The photomultiplier tube emits an electronic signal that is digitized and stored in a computer. The image can then be displayed on a high-resolution monitor. Hard copies can be produced using a laser film printer.

DR does not use conventional equipment. Special radiographic tables and upright cabinets contain radiation receptors that react to the pattern of the remnant radiation and transmit a digital signal directly to the computer system, producing an image instantaneously on a monitor. No cassettes and no processing are involved.

📌 There are two basic types of filmless radiography: computed radiography (CR) and digital radiography (DR). CR systems use conventional x-ray equipment with a cassette containing a photostimulable phosphor that must be processed in a laser device to create a digital image. DR systems have radiation receptors within the radiographic table or upright cabinet that transmit digital signals directly to the computer system.

Because both CR and DR imaging systems automatically adjust the visual quality of the image, there is no telltale darkness or lightness of the image to indicate overexposure or underexposure as in film/screen imaging systems. For this reason, digital processing systems usually display an exposure indicator number on the monitor, also referred to as an **exposure index (EI) number,** *S number,* or other number, depending on the equipment. This number must be monitored by radiographers to ensure that exposures are of diagnostic quality and are not excessive.

❗ Radiographers using digital imaging systems must monitor exposure index numbers in order to use adequate exposures for image quality and avoid excessive exposure to patients.

Once stored in the computer system, digital images from either CR or DR systems are organized and cataloged and can be accessed on monitors from multiple locations connected to the system network. These digital images can be manipulated electronically to enhance visibility. Analog images (conventional radiographs) can be added to the system by scanning them with a laser device called a *film digitizer.*

The computer hardware and software technology used to manage digital images in hospitals and health care facilities is called a **picture archiving and communication system (PACS).** These systems provide archives for the storage of images from all digital imaging modalities, connect images with patient database information, facilitate printing of images or transfer them to CD-ROM media, and display both images and information at work stations throughout the network as needed. A PACS may include transmission equipment for teleradiology, allowing images to be viewed in remote locations, such as a physician's home, and receiving images from remote locations such as outlying clinics. PACS technology can transmit images over telephone lines and via the Internet.

📌 The computer hardware and software technology used to manage digital images is called a picture archiving and communication system (PACS). These systems provide archives for the storage of images from all imaging modalities, connect images with patient database information, facilitate laser printing or transfer to CD-ROM media, and display both images and information at work stations throughout the network as needed.

IMAGE QUALITY

The more exposure received by a specific portion of the IR, the darker that portion of the image will be. The visibility of the radiographic image depends on two factors: the overall blackness of the image and the differences in blackness between the various portions of the image. The clarity and sharpness of the image are also important, as is the degree to which the image is a true representation of the subject. These features make up the four elements of radiographic quality: density, contrast, detail, and distortion.

Optical Density

The overall blackness of the image is referred to as the **optical density (OD),** often referred to as *radiographic density.* When the OD is optimal, the image is both dark enough and light enough to see the anatomic details clearly on the view box or monitor. Figure 2-4 shows radiographs of varying optical density. In conventional film/screen systems, OD is controlled by the exposure factors, primarily the mAs. Because exposure darkens the image, an increase in mAs will result in a darker radiograph, whereas a decrease will cause it to be lighter. In filmless radiographic systems, the radiographic density of the image is controlled by the computer; a change in exposure factors will not darken or lighten the image. An increase or decrease in exposure can only be detected by looking at the exposure indicator number.

📌 The overall blackness of the image is referred to as the *optical density* (OD). In conventional film-screen systems, OD is controlled by the exposure factors, primarily the mAs.

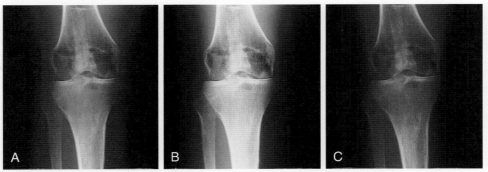

FIG 2-4 Radiographs of a phantom knee demonstrate differences in radiographic density. **A,** Optimum density. **B,** Underexposed. **C,** Overexposed.

Take care not to confuse radiographic density with tissue density, which refers to the mass density of anatomic parts. Whereas increased optical or radiographic density indicates that the image is darker, an increase in tissue density will result in an image that is lighter. To avoid errors, try not to use the word *density* without an appropriate descriptor.

Image Contrast

The difference in the OD of adjacent structures within the image is referred to as the **image contrast.** Even when an image has the proper OD, it is possible for structures to be too similar in density to be easily distinguished from one another. Figure 2-5 shows radiographs with high, low, and optimal contrast. Note that the high-contrast image has a black-and-white appearance. Structures in the gray areas are easily distinguished, but no details can be seen in the very dark or very light portions of the image. The low-contrast image has an overall gray appearance, and the structures tend to blend into one another. The optimal-contrast image shows details within all areas of the image, although the contrast in some areas is less pronounced.

Kilovoltage is the primary contrast control factor, but radiographic contrast is influenced by a number of other factors as well. These factors include the nature of the subject, the characteristics of the film or the IR, and the amount of scatter radiation impacting the IR. High kilovoltage produces an x-ray beam that penetrates more completely, leaving no white areas in the image. The dark, easily penetrated portions of the subject are not quite as dark when the kVp is high because less mAs is needed to obtain the desired radiographic

density. When more (higher) contrast is desired, the kVp is decreased. Because this will result in less penetration by the x-ray beam, a beam of greater intensity is needed, and the mAs must be increased. Contrast is best evaluated when the overall radiographic density is optimal.

> The difference in the optical density of adjacent structures within the image is referred to as the *image contrast.* Kilovoltage is the primary contrast control factor, but radiographic contrast is influenced by a number of other factors as well.

Image Detail

The third element of image quality is **image detail.** This term refers to the sharpness of the image. When detail is high, the edges and lines that make up the image are crisp and precise; with low detail, these lines and edges are less distinct and appear somewhat blurred or out of focus. Among the factors that affect image detail are the distance between the source of x-rays and the IR (the SID) and the distance between the object and the IR, referred to as the **object-image distance (OID).** Increasing SID sharpens the image, whereas increasing the OID reduces sharpness. Other factors include the size of the screen crystals and the thickness of the phosphor layer when intensifying screens are used, the size of the pixels in digital systems, the x-ray tube focal spot size (the smaller the focal spot the greater the detail), and whether the patient is able to hold still during the exposure.

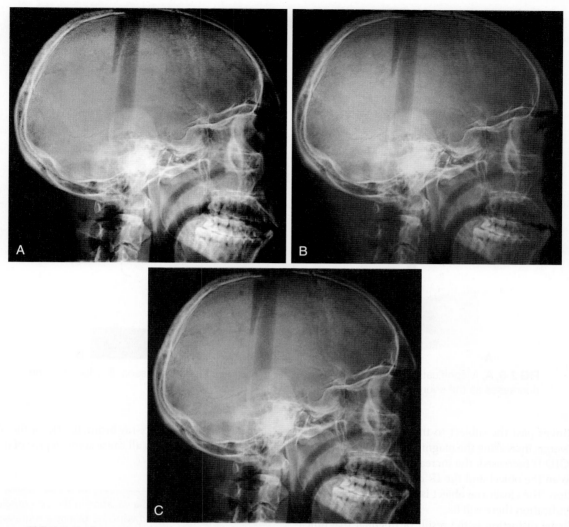

FIG 2-5 Radiographs of a phantom skull demonstrate differences in radiographic contrast. **A,** High contrast. **B,** Low contrast. **C,** Optimal contrast.

> 📌 *Image detail* refers to the sharpness of the image. Among the factors that affect image detail are the SID, the OID, the intensifying screens or the size of the pixels in digital systems, the focal spot size, and patient motion.

Distortion

The fourth element of image quality is **distortion.** This term refers to a variation in the size or shape of the image compared with the object it represents. Size distortion is always in the form of magnification and all radiographic images are magnified to some degree. The factors that affect magnification are the OID and the SID. The angulation of the diverging x-rays that define the edges of a subject affects the degree of magnification (Figure 2-6). When the x-ray tube is farther from the IR, the central, more parallel rays will define the subject, resulting in less magnification. When the SID is shorter, the rays that define the subject are those that diverge at a greater angle, increasing the magnification. As the x-ray beam

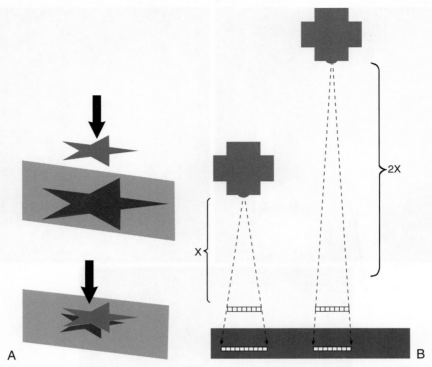

FIG 2-6 **A,** Magnification is decreased as the object-image distance decreases. **B,** Magnification decreases as the source-image distance increases.

continues past the subject to the IR, the rays continue to diverge, increasing the magnification. Likewise, when the OID is increased, the increased angle of divergence between the object and the IR causes increased magnification. The closer the object is to the receptor, the less magnification there will be.

Shape distortion is the result of unequal magnification of various parts of the subject. The least shape distortion occurs when the plane of the object is parallel to the plane of the IR and the central ray is perpendicular to it. Angulation of the x-ray beam, the IR, or the object in relation to the IR will all cause some degree of distortion (Figure 2-7).

> Distortion refers to a variation in the size or shape of the image compared with the object it represents. SID and OID control magnification distortion. Shape distortion is caused by misalignment of the tube, part, and IR.

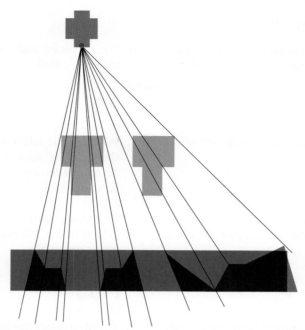

FIG 2-7 Radiographic Distortion. Distortion is minimized when the subject is parallel to the image receptor and the central ray is perpendicular to the film. Shape distortion results when there is angulation of the x-ray beam in relation to the subject or image receptor.

SUMMARY

- The prime factors of radiographic exposure are time, mA, kVp, and SID.
- Exposure time is the length of the exposure measured in seconds or portions of seconds.
- Milliamperage (mA) is a measure of the electron flow rate across the x-ray tube; it determines the rate of exposure.
- The milliampere-seconds (mAs) indicate the total quantity of exposure; mAs is the product of the mA and the exposure time.
- Technique charts indicate the prime factors for various examinations and for various patient sizes.
- IR systems may consist of film and intensifying screens, or may be of the filmless type.
- Two types of filmless systems are computed radiography (CR) and digital radiography (DR). Filmless systems create digital images that can be viewed, stored, modified, and transmitted via computer.
- The four elements of image quality are optical density (OD), image contrast, image detail, and distortion.

- OD is the darkness of the image; it is influenced by all the exposure factors, but is controlled primarily by varying the mAs.
- Image contrast is the difference in OD between adjacent portions of the image. This contrast is essential for the eye to differentiate one structure from another. Contrast is primarily controlled by kVp, but is also influenced by the subject and the amount of scatter radiation impacting the IR.
- Image detail, also called *definition,* is the sharpness of the lines that define the image. Without sufficient definition, the image appears blurred and small details are not clearly visualized.
- Distortion is variation in the size or shape of the image compared with the object it represents. Magnification distortion is affected by both SID and OID. Shape distortion occurs as a result of misalignment of the body part, IR, and x-ray tube.

REVIEW QUESTIONS

1. The four prime factors of radiographic exposure are exposure time, milliamperage, kilovoltage, and:
   A. optical density
   B. source-image distance
   C. object-image distance
   D. image detail

2. The prime factor that controls the wavelength of the x-ray beam is:
   A. milliamperage
   B. exposure time
   C. kilovoltage
   D. object-image distance

3. The prime factor that controls the rate at which x-rays are produced is:
   A. exposure time
   B. kilovoltage
   C. milliampere-seconds
   D. milliamperage

4. The mAs value of an exposure is varied to provide control of:
   A. optical density
   B. image contrast
   C. image detail
   D. radiographic distortion

5. The imaging system that provides an instantaneous digital image on a monitor is called:
   A. digital radiography
   B. computed radiography
   C. film-screen radiography
   D. anatomical programming

6. The hardware and software for managing digital images is called:
   A. PACS
   B. CR
   C. DR
   D. AEC

7. Which of the following factors is not affected by a change in the mA setting?
   A. optical density
   B. anode heat
   C. OID
   D. radiation intensity

8. Which of the following factors is used to control image contrast?
   A. mA
   B. SID
   C. OID
   D. kVp

9. The inverse squares law states that radiation intensity is inversely proportional to the square of the:
   A. mA
   B. SID
   C. T
   D. kVp

10. A variation in the size or shape of the image in comparison to the object it represents is called:
    A. distortion
    B. image contrast
    C. definition
    D. density

Answers can be found in the Answer Key on pages 429-431.

CRITICAL THINKING EXERCISES

1. Explain the significance of the x-ray wavelength in the production of radiographic images.
2. Compare the relative advantages and disadvantages of CR and DR imaging systems.
3. Explain the difference in purpose between AEC and anatomic programming in the determination of x-ray exposures.
4. Explain the difference between optical density and tissue density.

Radiation Effects and Safety

OBJECTIVES

At the conclusion of this chapter, the student will be able to:

- Use appropriate units when discussing the measurement of x-radiation.
- Describe events that can occur on a cellular level as a result of radiation exposure.
- List four characteristics of a cell that affect its radiation sensitivity according to the Laws of Bergonié and Tribondeau.
- State the characteristics that are significant in categorizing radiation effects.
- Contrast stochastic radiation effects with deterministic effects.
- List and describe the three types of deterministic short-term radiation effects.
- Explain why stochastic radiation effects are difficult to identify and measure.

- List documented latent effects of low doses of ionizing radiation.
- Explain the significance of gene dominance with respect to genetic radiation effects.
- Describe how changes in time, distance, and shielding affect radiation exposure.
- Demonstrate practices that minimize occupational x-ray exposure.
- Explain the ALARA principle.
- List the methods used to reduce patient exposure to radiation.
- Describe the risks of radiation exposure during pregnancy with respect to both patients and health care workers.

OUTLINE

Radiation Units and Measurement
Biologic Effects of Radiation Exposure
    Short-Term Somatic Effects
    Long-Term Somatic Effects
    Genetic Effects
Radiation Safety

Personnel Safety
Personal Monitoring
Effective Dose Limits
Patient Protection
Gonad Shielding
Radiation and Pregnancy

KEY TERMS

ALARA principle
centigray (cGy)
coulombs per kilogram (C/kg)
deterministic
dominant
dose equivalent
dosimeter
erythema
free radicals

genetic effects
Gray (Gy)
hematologic
long-term effects
mutation
optically stimulated
    luminescence (OSL)
radiation absorbed
    dose (rad)

radiation equivalent in
    man (rem)
recessive
Roentgen (R)
short-term effects
Sievert (Sv)
somatic effects
stochastic
weighting factor (WF)

This chapter builds on your understanding of the nature of radiation by introducing radiation measurement, radiation effects, and radiation safety. These topics will be essential to your work as a radiographer and are covered in greater detail later in your curriculum.

RADIATION UNITS AND MEASUREMENT

Radiation measurements can be made in two different, but related, systems: the traditional (British) system, still sometimes used in the United States, and the Système Internationale (SI) units established by the International Commission on Radiation Units in 1981. These units and their relationships are summarized in Table 3-1.

The traditional unit of radiation exposure is the **Roentgen (R or r)**, a measurement of radiation intensity in air. The Roentgen is equal to the quantity of radiation that will produce 2.08×10^9 (more than 2 billion) ion pairs in 1 cm^3 of dry air. The SI unit for measuring radiation intensity is **coulombs per kilogram (C/kg)**, specifying the quantity of electrical charge in coulombs produced by the exposure of 1 kg of dry air. One Roentgen equals 2.58×10^{-4} (0.000258) C/kg.

The C/kg and R units are useful for measuring the quantity of radiation present, but are not useful dose measurements. The dose varies with the depth of measurement and the quantity of radiation energy absorbed in the exposed tissue. To measure therapeutic radiation doses, as well as specific tissue doses received in diagnostic applications, the traditional unit is **radiation absorbed dose (rad)** and is equal to 100 ergs (an energy unit) per gram of tissue. One Roentgen of exposure will result in approximately 1 rad of absorbed dose in muscle tissue. The SI unit for dose measurement is the **Gray (Gy)**. One Gray equals 100 rad, and conversely, 1 rad equals 1 **centigray (cGy)**.

The biologic effect of radiation exposure varies according to the type of radiation involved and its energy. Equal doses of various types of radiation, as measured in Gray or rad, will not necessarily result in equal biologic effects. Some radiation workers, such as engineers in nuclear power plants, nuclear submarine construction workers, or technologists in nuclear medicine laboratories, may be exposed to several types of radiation with unequal levels of biologic effect. Neither the radiation measurement units (coulombs per kilogram and Roentgen) nor the dose units (Gray and rad) are useful units for measuring the occupational dose of combined radiations with different levels of effects.

To simplify the process of measuring occupational dose, a **weighting factor (WF)** is assigned to each type of radiation based on its absorbed energy in a mass of tissue and its relative biologic effect compared with x-rays. Formerly, weighting factors were called *quality factors*. The weighting factors for different types of ionizing radiation are listed in Table 3-2. For example, note that alpha particles have a WF of 20, because 1 Gy of alpha particles causes biologic effects that are approximately equal to those produced by 20 Gy of x-ray energy. The absorbed dose is multiplied by the WF to obtain the **dose equivalent**. The resulting SI unit is the **Sievert (Sv)**. Thus, the worker exposed to 1 Gy of alpha particles would receive 20 Sv of occupational exposure.

$$Gy \times WF = Sv$$

TABLE 3-1	Radiation Units	
	SI Units	**Traditional (British) Units**
Exposure units	Coulombs per kilogram (C/kg) $1\ R = 2.58 \times 10^{-4}$ C/kg	Roentgen (R) Quantity of radiation that will produce 2.08×10^9 ion pairs in 1 cm^3 of air
Dose units	Gray (Gy) 1 Gy = 100 rad	Radiation absorbed dose (rad) 100 erg per gram of tissue
Dose equivalent units	Sievert (Sv) Sv = Gy × WF 1 Sv = 100 rem	Radiation equivalent in man (rem) rem = rad × WF

TABLE 3-2	Radiation Weighting Factors
Radiation Type	**Radiation Weighting Factors**
Photons	1
Electrons and muons	1
Protons and charged pions	2
Alpha particle, fission fragments, heavy ions	20
Neutrons (energy dependent)	A continuous function of neutron energy

Summarized from the International Commission on Radiological Protection (2007).

The British unit used to measure dose equivalents is the **radiation equivalent in man (rem)**; it is determined by multiplying the dose in rad times the WF:

$$rad \times WF = rem$$

and

$$1\ Sv = 100\ rem$$

 The dose equivalent is equal to the dose times the WF.

Because the radiation quantities involved in diagnostic radiology are so small, radiographers commonly use units that are 1/1000 of the common unit (for example, millisieverts [mSv]). A chest radiograph can result in a skin entrance dose of 0.15 mSv, or 15 mrad. The most common unit for the calculation of radiation doses in the United States has become the centigray (0.01 Gy). As the United States converted to the SI system, the centigray was the first and easiest unit to convert because it is equal to the rad, the dose unit in the British system.

> The most commonly used dose unit in the United States is the centigray (cGy); 1 cGy = 1 rad.

Students often find it confusing to determine which radiation units should be used in a given situation. This choice is made more difficult by the tendency of many radiographers to use the traditional Roentgen, rad, and rem units interchangeably. This does not cause serious inaccuracy when speaking only of diagnostic x-rays, because exposure to 1 R of x-ray energy will result in approximately 1 rad in muscle. Because the WF of diagnostic x-rays equals one, 1 rad is also equal to 1 rem.

In general, the reason for the measurement determines which unit is the most appropriate. The coulombs per kilogram and Roentgen units are used to measure the presence of x-radiation without any reference to its absorption or attenuation—that is, the quantity of radiation present in air. For example, these units can be used to measure the output of an x-ray machine or determine the radiation level in the hallway during an x-ray exposure in the adjacent room.

The Gray and the rad are used to measure radiation dose. These units are used to prescribe radiation therapy. The amount absorbed by a specific tissue is what is being measured; therefore a statement indicating the part of the body involved usually modifies the dosage unit. For example, a radiation oncologist may prescribe a therapeutic dose of 5040 cGy to the breast. This dose can be delivered in a series of 28 treatments involving 180 cGy each. A research report might state that a patient who undergoes a routine chest radiograph receives an average thyroid dose of 4 mrad. The laboratory that processes personal radiation monitor badges will report occupational dose in dose equivalent units, usually in millisieverts.

BIOLOGIC EFFECTS OF RADIATION EXPOSURE

As mentioned in the previous chapter, x-rays can ionize substances by removing electrons from their orbits. This process results in a free, negatively charged electron and leaves the remainder of the atom with a positive charge. When human beings are irradiated, ionization can occur to any part of a living cell, such as the material that makes up its membrane, the water within the membrane, or the DNA that makes up the cell's chromosomes and directs its activity. The initial ionization can produce a domino effect, causing ionization in the surrounding area. Exposure also creates **free radicals** (temporary molecules and parts of molecules with electrical charges). Free radicals can interact directly with the DNA or produce toxic substances that are injurious to DNA.

Most effects of exposure are extremely short-lived because electrons find new homes in the orbits of other atoms and the balance of charges returns to normal. Free radicals combine to form more stable compounds. Occasionally, however, the damage is not instantly resolved. A cell may be damaged to such an extent that it cannot sustain itself and subsequently dies. Cell death is an insignificant injury unless a large number of cells is involved. Cells may sustain damage that requires several days for the body to repair. The body produces special enzymes that function to repair the DNA protein molecules. A cell can be damaged in such a way that its DNA programming is changed and it no longer behaves normally. This type of injury can eventually result in the runaway production of new, abnormal cells, causing a cancerous tumor or malignant blood disease.

The relative sensitivity of different types of cells is summarized in the Laws of Bergonié and Tribondeau, which state that cell sensitivity to radiation exposure depends on four characteristics of the cell:

1. *Age.* Younger cells are more sensitive than older ones.
2. *Differentiation.* Nonspecialized cells are more sensitive than highly complex ones.
3. *Metabolic rate.* Cells that use energy rapidly are more sensitive than those with a slower metabolism.
4. *Mitotic rate.* Cells that divide and multiply rapidly are more sensitive than those that replicate slowly.

According to these laws, we see that blood cells and blood-producing cells are highly sensitive. Cells in contact with the environment are simple, have relatively short lives, and are highly sensitive. These cells include those of the skin and the mucosal linings of the mouth, nose, and gastrointestinal tract. Some glandular tissue is also particularly sensitive, especially that of the thyroid gland and the female breast. The tissues of embryos, fetuses, infants, children, and adolescents tend to be more sensitive than adult tissues because of their younger age and their higher metabolic and mitotic rates. Nerve cells, which have a long life and are highly complex, are much less vulnerable to radiation injury. Cortical bone cells are also relatively insensitive.

Radiation effects are classified in various ways. **Short-term effects** are those observed within 3 months of exposure and are associated with relatively high radiation doses (greater than 50 cGy). Short-term effects can be further categorized according to the body system affected: central nervous system, gastrointestinal, and **hematologic** (blood-related) effects. **Long-term effects,** sometimes referred to as *latent effects,* may not be apparent for as many as 30 years. **Somatic effects** are those that affect the body of the irradiated individual directly, whereas **genetic effects** occur as a result of damage to the reproductive cells of the irradiated person and may be observed as defects in the children or grandchildren of the irradiated individual.

Short-Term Somatic Effects

Short-term radiation effects are predictable, and the quantity of exposure required to produce them is well documented. These effects are classified as **deterministic.** Deterministic effects (formerly called nonstochastic somatic effects) occur only after a certain amount of exposure and the severity of the effect depends on the dose.

> Deterministic radiation effects are short-term somatic effects associated with high-dose exposures. They are predictable and their severity is dose dependent.

One observable short-term effect is a reddening of the skin called **erythema.** This phenomenon is sometimes called a *radiation burn.* In the early days of radiation use, the amount of radiation necessary to produce reddening of the skin was called the *erythema dose.* It was the first unit used to measure radiation exposure.

Other short-term effects from doses in excess of 50 cGy have been observed and studied in radiation therapy patients and in the victims of radiation accidents and atomic bomb blasts. This is vastly more exposure than is delivered by diagnostic x-ray machines. Extremely high doses produce central nervous system effects such as seizures and coma that can result in death in a short period of time. Lesser doses will result in radiation sickness, a gastrointestinal effect in which the mucosal lining of the digestive tract is damaged, breaks down, and becomes infected by the bacteria that normally inhabit the bowel. These victims also have a compromised immune system because of the death of white blood cells and are unable to fight the infection. Radiation sickness is usually fatal, and suffering may be prolonged. A lesser dose, affecting primarily the blood and blood-forming organs, results in hematologic effects, including anemia and a compromised immune system. The victims are prone to infectious diseases that can be fatal, depending on the radiation dose and the severity of the disease process. One way that scientists describe the risk of high-level radiation exposure is to calculate the whole-body radiation dose that is lethal to 50% of the irradiated population within 30 days—a calculation that is abbreviated as LD 50/30. The LD 50/30 for humans is approximately 3 Gy.

Long-Term Somatic Effects

In this discussion, *long-term* refers to the length of time between the exposure and the observation of the effect. The time required for long-term effects to manifest is generally considered to be 5 to 30 years, with the greatest percentage occurring between 10 and 15 years. In contrast to the predictable nature of short-term effects, long-term effects are apparently random, and there is no threshold amount of exposure that must be received for them to occur. Effects of this type are termed **stochastic.**

The likelihood of stochastic effects is greater when the dose is increased, but there is no correlation between the dose and the severity of the effects. They can occur as the result of repeated small doses, such as those used in radiography.

> Stochastic radiation effects are random, long-term effects associated with low-dose exposure. Their likelihood is dose dependent and the severity of the effect is random.

The percentage of observable effects from the radiation involved in typical x-ray examinations is extremely low, and the risk to any single patient is minimal. Most of us take greater risks every day when we drive our cars or walk across busy streets. Nevertheless, there is a risk of long-term effects that has been demonstrated by studying large populations over long periods. The incidence of certain conditions is greater when results for irradiated groups are compared with those of nonirradiated control groups.

Long-term radiation effects are not easily identified as such because they occur years after the initial exposure and because the same effects also occur in the absence of radiation exposure. Only extensive research with large populations (epidemiologic studies) and computer analysis can demonstrate the role of radiation in causing these effects. In other words, radiation causes increased risk of these effects, but the effects cannot be predicted for any one individual. Although the individual risk may be extremely small, increasing the exposure to the entire population poses public health risks that require the attention and concern of everyone involved in applying ionizing radiation to human beings.

The documented latent effects of low doses of ionizing radiation include the following:

- *Cataractogenesis.* The formation of cataracts, or clouding of the lens of the eye, is an effect that concerns radiologists and radiographers who work extensively in fluoroscopy and those who perform other work that involves repeated exposure to the eyes.
- *Carcinogenesis.* There is an increased risk of malignant disease—particularly cancer of the skin, thyroid, and breast—and leukemia (a group of malignant blood diseases associated with radiation exposure).
- *Life span shortening.* A study of the life span of radiologists who died during a 3-year period before 1945

showed that they had shorter life spans than did physicians who did not use radiation in their practices. This group included radiologists who had used radiation since the early days of x-ray science. Additional research has confirmed the link between life span shortening and radiation exposure, but recent studies show that occupational exposure no longer has a measurable effect on the life spans of radiologists.

Genetic Effects

Genetic effects in the form of changes or **mutations** to the genes can be caused when the ovaries or testes are exposed to ionizing radiation. In females, all the ova cells that an individual will ever produce are present in an immature state at birth. Because no new egg cells are produced as the individual ages, the effect of radiation exposure to the ovaries is cumulative. The genetic effects of radiation to the testes are manifest for a longer term than may at first be presumed, because damage to the stem cells that produce the sperm can result in the continued production of sperm with the genetic mutation. The majority of genetic mutations are considered negative, or less well suited to the survival of the individual than nonmutated cells.

Because reproductive cells have only half the number of chromosomes found in all other cells, each parent contributes one chromosome to each pair in the new individual, and nature makes the choice as to which gene of each pair will affect the characteristics of the offspring. Genes that are expressed are said to be **dominant,** and those that are not expressed are called **recessive.** Mutated genes are usually recessive and therefore do not manifest their characteristics in the offspring. Both dominant and recessive genes, however, occur in the reproductive cells of the offspring and may be transmitted to future generations.

> Genes that are expressed are said to be *dominant,* and those that are not expressed are called *recessive.* Mutated genes are usually recessive.

As an increasing percentage of the population is exposed to radiation from natural, environmental, occupational, and health care sources, there is an increased likelihood that individuals will be conceived with a mutation of both genes in a strategic pair, resulting in some type of deformity or maladaptation. Public health officials and governments are highly concerned about preserving the integrity of the population's gene pool by minimizing harmful, defect-causing radiation. This concern should motivate those who apply ionizing radiation to humans to minimize gonad doses in every way possible. Gonad shielding for this purpose is addressed later in this chapter.

Genetic effects from mutations caused by x-ray exposure have long been demonstrated in animal research. Interestingly, few genetic effects have been confirmed by the continuing research into the Japanese populations affected by the atomic bombs dropped on Hiroshima and Nagasaki during World War II, and in other studies of human populations.

RADIATION SAFETY

Clearly, exposure to x-rays creates some risk for patients and radiographers. It is an essential part of your education and your ethical responsibility to be knowledgeable about radiation safety and to use this knowledge to avoid all unnecessary radiation exposure to your patients, your coworkers, and yourself. A comprehensive course on the subject of radiation biology and radiation safety will be a part of the curriculum in your radiography program.

Personnel Safety

Radiographers can be exposed to radiation either from the primary x-ray beam or from the scatter radiation that results from the interaction of the primary beam with the patient or other material in its path. Because radiographers are considered to be "occupationally exposed individuals," they may be prohibited from activities that would result in direct exposure to the primary x-ray beam. This could mean that they are not allowed to hold patients or image receptors during x-ray exposures and must stand clear of the path of the primary x-ray beam during fluoroscopic and mobile radiographic examinations. These activities are controlled by state regulations.

As explained in Chapter 1, scatter radiation is ambient radiation in the x-ray room during an exposure. Radiographers are not exposed to any significant amount of this radiation in a typical radiographic room when they stand well behind the protective lead barrier of the control booth. The exposure increases when the radiographer assists with fluoroscopic procedures or uses mobile x-ray equipment. The three principal methods used to protect x-ray equipment operators from unnecessary radiation exposure are *time, distance,* and *shielding.*

Time

The amount of exposure received is directly proportional to the time spent in a scatter radiation field; therefore the occupational dose is decreased when this time is minimized. For example, a radiographer may shorten the time of exposure by stepping into the control booth during fluoroscopic procedures when not required to be near the patient.

Distance

The second method involves using distance. Increasing the distance between yourself and a radiation source decreases your exposure in proportion to the square of the distance; therefore small increases in distance have a relatively large effect. Mobile x-ray units have long cords on the exposure switches, enabling the radiographer to get as far from the radiation source as possible while making an exposure.

Shielding

The third method is shielding, which is by far the most common method of dose reduction used by radiographers. The lead wall of the control booth provides the primary barrier and is the radiographer's principal defense. Other types of shielding include lead aprons, gloves, goggles, and thyroid shields (Figure 3-1). These types of shielding can be worn during fluoroscopic procedures and mobile radiographic examinations.

An essential part of your clinical education will be learning to protect yourself and your coworkers from

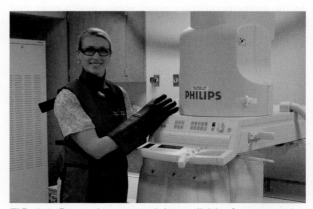

FIG 3-1 Protective apparel is available for protection during fluoroscopic and mobile radiographic examinations.

unnecessary radiation exposure. This includes doing a safety check before each exposure—making certain that all personnel are properly protected and that the door is closed before initiating exposures.

Personal Monitoring

Devices for monitoring radiation exposure to personnel are called **dosimeters.** Radiation workers who are issued single badges for monitoring whole-body dose should wear them in the region of the collar with the label facing out. When a lead apron is worn, the dosimeter should be outside the lead apron. Technologists who work with fluoroscopy may wear two badges, one on the collar outside the lead apron and one at the waist that is under the apron. The two dosimeters should be distinguished by color or icons indicating their intended locations. Personnel who are issued dosimeters should wear them at all times when working in radiation areas and should keep them in a safe place, away from radiation, when off duty. In addition to whole-body badges, ring dosimeters can be worn by nuclear medicine technologists and others whose work results in more exposure to the hands than to the body.

Monitoring dosimeters using **optically stimulated luminescence (OSL)** technology are the most common type of monitoring dosimeter currently used in health care situations (Figure 3-2). Aluminum oxide is the radiation detector in this device, which is processed using a laser. OSL dosimeters can measure small doses precisely and can be reanalyzed to confirm results. They are accurate over a wide dose range and have excellent long-term stability.

Radiation monitor badge service laboratories provide dosimeters, processing services, and reports, and keep permanent records of the radiation exposure of each person monitored. Service can be arranged on a weekly, monthly, bimonthly, or quarterly basis. Personnel who receive relatively high doses of occupational exposure change their badges most frequently. Dosimeters cannot accurately measure total exposures that are extremely small. For this reason, personnel who receive very small amounts of exposure will obtain more accurate measurements with less frequent badge changes. Personnel involved in diagnostic radiography who are always or nearly always in a control booth during exposures are usually best monitored with a quarterly service. A monthly service is a better choice for those who work in fluoroscopy and those who perform bedside radiography.

Service companies provide an extra dosimeter in every batch that is marked *Control*. The purpose of this dosimeter is to measure any radiation exposure to the entire batch while in transit. Any amount of exposure measured from the control badge will be subtracted from the amounts measured from the other badges in the batch. The control badge should be kept in a safe place, away from any possibility of x-ray exposure. It should never be used to measure occupational dose or for any other purpose.

Radiation badge service companies need to know the name and date of birth of all persons to be monitored so that all the records can be accurately identified. If there has been a history of previous occupational radiation exposure and the dose is known, this information should also be provided so that the record will be complete and accurate. Exposure reports are sent to the subscriber for each batch, and an annual summary of personal exposure is also provided. Radiation workers should be advised of the radiation exposure reported from their badges and should be provided with copies of the annual reports for their own records. Employees exposed to ionizing radiation should not leave their employment without a complete record of their radiation exposure history. Employers are required to provide this information.

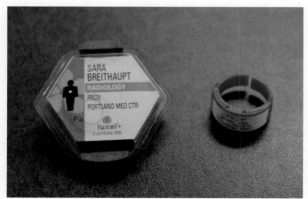

FIG 3-2 The current generation of personal dosimeters is the optically stimulated luminescence type.

Radiographers should monitor their exposure reports on a regular basis and maintain a record of their exposure history.

Effective Dose Limits

The ALARA principle is the guiding philosophy associated with all radiation use that involves exposure to humans—both patients and workers. It states that all radiation exposure to humans should be limited to levels that are *as low as reasonably achievable.*

The effective dose limit system is used to calculate the upper limit of occupational exposure that is permitted in specific circumstances. For occupationally exposed personnel, the upper effective dose (ED) limit is 50 mSv (5 rem) per year. This limit applies to workers older than 18 years who are not pregnant, and it is assumed to be a whole-body dose. These limits apply to occupational exposure only, and not to exposure that workers may receive as a result of imaging or tests related to their own health care.

> For occupationally exposed personnel, the upper ED limit is 50 mSv (5 rem) per year.

The ED system also states a retrospective or cumulative dose limit that is equal to 10 mSv (1 rem) times the worker's age. For example, a 30-year-old worker with no previous occupational exposure would have a cumulative ED limit of 300 mSv (30 rem); this is referred to as the *rem bank.* The worker is permitted to exceed the annual limits by small amounts as long as the rem bank is not depleted.

The ED system also specifies dose limits for specific body organs and tissues. For example, workers who receive exposure to their hands while their bodies are protected may wear ring or wrist dosimeters. A higher dose limit is established for this limited exposure.

The established ED limits ensure that the safety of radiation workers is comparable with that of workers in other safe occupations. The risk from the allowable exposure is considered to be insignificant. The occupational dose received by radiographers is usually well below the established limit.

The upper boundaries of the occupational dose were formerly referred to as the *maximum permissible dose.* This term is now out of favor because it implies that exposure in excess of the lowest achievable dose is permissible. The ALARA principle must be applied in conjunction with the use of ED limits. It is important for radiographers not to be complacent simply because their dose is below the limit. Radiation control agencies require the occupational dose to be kept to the lowest levels that are reasonably achievable.

Patient Protection

The topic of patient protection will be addressed repeatedly in various contexts throughout your education in radiography. You will be able to understand this more completely at a later date. For now, you should be aware that radiographers are responsible for minimizing the radiation exposure to patients. The following methods are used to minimize patient dose:

- *Avoid errors.* Double-check requisitions and patient identification so that the right patient gets the right examination.
- *Avoid repeated exposures.* Establish good routine procedures and follow them strictly so that careless errors do not necessitate repeat exposures. Note, however, that unsatisfactory images must be repeated. Radiation safety cannot be used as a reason for failing to produce a satisfactory examination.
- *Collimate.* Use the smallest radiation field that will encompass the area of clinical interest. In no case should the size of the radiation field be greater than the size of the IR.
- *Use the highest kVp that is consistent with acceptable image quality.* Patient dose is directly proportional to the mAs. High kVp permits using the lowest possible mAs to obtain an acceptable exposure. The combination of high kVp and low mAs is referred to as a "low-dose" exposure.
- *Ensure at least 40 inches of source-image distance.* This practice limits patient exposure from tube housing leakage and collimator scatter.
- *Use fast IRs. When using film and screens,* use the fastest receptor that is consistent with the required image quality.
- *Provide shielding for the gonads, eyes, breasts, and thyroid as appropriate.*

Gonad Shielding

The purpose of gonad shielding is not so much to protect the patient as to limit the genetic effects of radiation on the gene pool of the population. Lead shields that prevent unnecessary radiation to the reproductive organs are required when the patient is of reproductive age or younger, whenever the gonads are within the primary radiation field, and when a shield will not interfere with the examination. Generally, this rule applies to most patients younger than 55 years. A shield device consisting of at least a 0.5-mm lead equivalent is placed between the x-ray tube and the patient. Shields attached to the collimator (shadow shields) can be positioned by viewing their shadows within the collimator light field. Shields placed on or near the patient's body are referred to as *contact shields* and are somewhat more effective than shadow shields. Both types meet the legal requirements for gonad shielding.

Figure 3-3 demonstrates the placement of shields for both males and females. The top of the male shield is placed 0 to 1 inches inferior to the symphysis pubis. The lower edge of the female shield is placed 0 to 1 inches superior to the symphysis pubis. When positioning gonad shielding, it is helpful to remember that the pubic symphysis is at the same level as the greater trochanter of the femur, which avoids the necessity of palpating the pubic symphysis for proper shield placement.

> **!** Lead shields that prevent unnecessary radiation to the reproductive organs are required when the patient is of reproductive age or younger, whenever the gonads are within the primary radiation field, and when a shield will not interfere with the examination.

RADIATION AND PREGNANCY

It has long been recognized that radiation exposure poses specific risks to the developing embryo or fetus. In general, we know that radiation during pregnancy can result in spontaneous abortion, congenital defects in the child, an increased risk of malignant disease in childhood, and an increase in significant genetic abnormalities in the children of parents who were exposed *in utero*.

Animal studies first alerted scientists that radiation could cause spontaneous abortion of the developing embryo and increase the rate of congenital abnormalities seen in those that survived to birth. These findings have been confirmed in humans by studying the pregnancies of women who survived the atomic bomb blasts of Hiroshima and Nagasaki during World War II and the nuclear accident at Chernobyl in the Ukraine in 1986. Studies of smaller groups of women exposed to

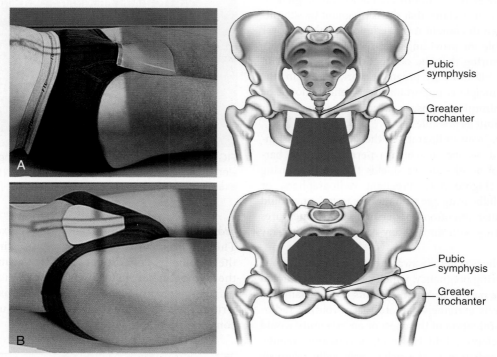

FIG 3-3 A, The male shield is placed in the midline with its top margin 1 inch inferior to the pubic symphysis. **B,** The lower edge of the female shield is placed at or near the superior margin of the pubic symphysis. It is centered in the midline, halfway between the level of the anterior superior iliac spine and the symphysis pubis. Note that in both males and females, the pubic symphysis is at the level of the greater trochanters. (Photographs from Long BW, Rollins JH, Smith BJ: *Merrill's atlas of radiographic positioning & procedures*, ed 13, St Louis, 2016, Mosby. Line drawings from Long B, Frank E, Ehrlich RA: *Radiography essentials for limited practice*, ed 3, St Louis, 2010, Saunders.)

radiation as a result of diagnostic and therapeutic procedures confirm that radiation in excess of 5 cGy to the uterus is cause for some level of concern. In the 1950s, Alice Stewart, an English researcher, demonstrated a 14-fold increase in the incidence of childhood leukemia among children who had been exposed to radiation *in utero* as a result of x-ray pelvimetry examinations in the third trimester of pregnancy.

The greatest risks for spontaneous abortion, fetal death, and significant birth defects exist when significant levels of exposure occur during the first trimester of pregnancy (that is, the first 3 months of gestation). The embryo is most vulnerable to radiation injury while the tissues are in the process of differentiation. Unfortunately, this creates the greatest hazard at a time when a woman may not yet be aware she is pregnant.

Radiation control agencies address the issue of radiation exposure to pregnant radiation workers. The ED limit of whole-body radiation for the pregnant worker is 50 mSv over the 9-month course of the pregnancy. When a worker declares that she is pregnant by submitting a written document to her employer, the employer is responsible for providing fetal radiation monitoring and for ensuring that the occupational dose does not exceed the ED limit for pregnant workers. Again, the ALARA principle is important. Every effort should be made to minimize exposure, keeping the dose as far below the limit as possible.

For a pregnant radiographer, the safest work assignment would be one in which a permanent lead barrier (control booth) always shields the worker during exposures (Figure 3-4). Pregnant radiographers, or those of childbearing age who may be pregnant, should pay particular attention to personal safety measures when assisting with fluoroscopy or using mobile x-ray equipment.

The public is generally aware that x-radiation is to be avoided during pregnancy, which can lead to irrational fears on the part of pregnant patients or their families. The chance is extremely remote that a routine radiographic examination of the chest or an extremity would harm a developing child. However, examinations requiring direct radiation to the pelvis, especially relatively high-dose fluoroscopic studies or computed tomography (CT) scans of the abdomen or lumbar spine, should be cause for concern.

Radiation control regulations require that female patients of childbearing age be advised of potential

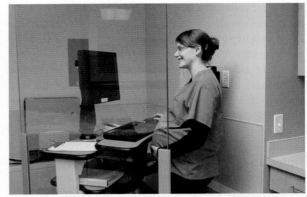

FIG 3-4 The lead barrier of the control booth protects a pregnant radiographer.

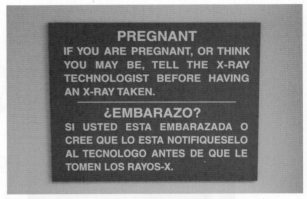

PREGNANT
IF YOU ARE PREGNANT, OR THINK YOU MAY BE, TELL THE X-RAY TECHNOLOGIST BEFORE HAVING AN X-RAY TAKEN.

¿EMBARAZO?
SI USTED ESTA EMBARAZADA O CREE QUE LO ESTA NOTIFIQUESELO AL TECNOLOGO ANTES DE QUE LE TOMEN LOS RAYOS-X.

FIG 3-5 Signs in dressing rooms and imaging suites can alert patients to the potential hazards of radiographic examination when pregnant.

radiation hazards before radiographic examination. This requirement is usually met by posting signs in the radiology department advising women to tell the radiographer before the examination if they may be pregnant (Figure 3-5). These signs should be written in all the languages commonly used in the community.

> ⚠ Examinations of pregnant women are a cause for concern when they require direct radiation to the pelvis, especially relatively high-dose fluoroscopic studies or computed tomography (CT) scans of the abdomen or lumbar spine.

The patient's physician is in the best position to be aware of an early pregnancy. The patient's history may indicate the possibility of pregnancy, and specific questions to rule out pregnancy should be a part of any medical history that precedes the ordering of pelvic x-ray examinations. In practice, however, the possibility of pregnancy may not even be considered. This is especially true in cases of accident or injury for which the emergency department or office visit is brief and the history is limited to the injury complaint. For this reason, *it is essential for the radiographer to consider the possibility of pregnancy in any female of childbearing age.* Ask specific questions to determine that the patient's physician has addressed the issue of pregnancy before ordering the examination. Female patients of childbearing age may also be asked the date of their last menstrual period to determine whether there is a possibility that they may be pregnant. A date more than 1 month back could indicate a possible pregnancy. A woman is least likely to be pregnant during the first 10 days of the menstrual cycle, with the onset of menstruation considered to be day 1.

If pregnancy is a possibility, an early pregnancy test, easily and quickly performed in the physician's office, may clarify the situation. If the patient is pregnant and the proposed x-ray examination involves direct pelvic radiation, the physician must weigh up the potential risks and benefits of the examination and discuss them with the patient before proceeding with the study. In the case of minor or chronic complaints, it is common to delay the examination until after the child is born.

If x-ray examinations of a pregnant patient must be done, modifications in the procedure can help to minimize the dose to the embryo or fetus. If the part to be examined is not the abdomen or pelvis, the area can be shielded with a lead apron. If the abdomen or pelvis is to be evaluated, the number of exposures, the size of the radiation field, or both, may be minimized, resulting in less radiation exposure than that required for a routine procedure. The decision to do a limited study and the determination of the exact limitations to be imposed are the prerogatives of the radiologist.

▌ SUMMARY

- The traditional or British system of units and the Système Internationale (SI) are used to measure radiation. In the British system, exposure is measured in Roentgens (R), dose is measured in rad, and dose equivalents are measured in rem.
- The SI units for these measurements, respectively, are coulombs per kilogram (C/kg), Gray (Gy), and Sievert (Sv); 1 Gy equals 100 rad, and 1 Sv equals 100 rem.
- Cellular responses to radiation exposure range from no effect to cell death. While the great majority of cellular injuries is repaired by enzymatic action, cell damage from the direct or indirect action of the x-ray beam can have a negative effect on cell function and reproduction.
- The laws of Bergonié and Tribondeau define the characteristics of cells that affect their sensitivity to radiation injury: age, differentiation, mitotic rate, and metabolic rate.
- Radiation effects can be categorized as somatic or genetic, short-term or long-term, and deterministic (predictable) or stochastic (random).
- Effects from high doses tend to be somatic, short-term, and predictable, whereas low-dose effects are long-term and randomly unpredictable, and the risk of their occurrence is extremely small.
- Safety from radiation exposure requires radiographers to avoid contact with the primary x-ray beam; use time, distance, and shielding to minimize exposure; and monitor exposure using dosimeters.
- Protecting the patient from unnecessary radiation exposure involves taking care to avoid errors, using low-dose techniques, and shielding sensitive tissues.
- The effective dose (ED) limiting system sets limits for occupational exposure. Special rules and limits apply to pregnant radiation workers.
- The ED system is used in conjunction with the ALARA principle, which states that all radiation exposure to human beings should be as low as reasonably achievable.
- When exposing women of childbearing age to x-rays, precautions must be taken to avoid any inadvertent exposure to an embryo; they include posting signs, asking patients about the possibility of pregnancy, and sometimes using early pregnancy tests.
- Special care must be taken to minimize exposure when x-rays are necessary during pregnancy.

REVIEW QUESTIONS

1. The product of dose in Grays times the WF is equal to the dose equivalent, which in the SI system is measured in units called:
   A. rem
   B. Roentgens
   C. rad
   D. Sieverts

2. One centigray (cGy) is equal to:
   A. 100 rad
   B. 100 Sv
   C. 1 rad
   D. 1 R

3. The laws of Bergonié and Tribondeau state that the sensitivity of cells to radiation injury depends upon four principal factors. These factors are cell age, cell complexity, the rate of replication, and:
   A. the rate of energy use by the cell
   B. the cell's location within the body
   C. the rate at which the dose is delivered
   D. the weight of the individual

4. Short-term, predictable radiation effects typically occur as a result of:
   A. high doses of radiation exposure, such as those received in radiation therapy
   B. low doses of radiation, such as those received in diagnostic imaging
   C. occupational radiation exposure
   D. low-dose exposure during pregnancy

5. The term *radiation sickness* refers to:
   A. occupational radiation effects
   B. congenital illness owing to genetic effects
   C. short-term gastrointestinal effects
   D. any stochastic effect

6. The effective dose-equivalent limit for whole-body occupational radiation exposure to nonpregnant radiation workers older than 18 years is:
   A. 1.25 Gy per year
   B. 5.0 Gy per year
   C. 5.0 mSv per year
   D. 50 mSv per year

7. Long-term radiation effects that are apparently random, and have no threshold amount of exposure that must be received for them to occur, are termed:
   A. somatic
   B. genetic
   C. occupational
   D. stochastic

8. Genes that are expressed in the individual are said to be:
   A. mutated
   B. dominant
   C. random
   D. recessive

9. Which of the following is a type of personal radiation dosimeter?
   A. SID
   B. kVp
   C. OSL
   D. OID

10. When a pregnant patient requires abdominal or pelvic radiography, the decision to do a limited study and the determination of the exact limitations to be imposed are the prerogatives of the:
    A. patient's physician
    B. radiologist
    C. patient
    D. radiographer

Answers can be found in the Answer Key on pages 429-431.

CRITICAL THINKING EXERCISES

1. Using the laws of Bergonié and Tribondeau, explain why certain cells are more sensitive to radiation and why some are less so. Give examples of each type.
2. List the three principal methods used to protect radiographers from unnecessary radiation exposure, and explain how each method is applied in practice.
3. What should a radiographer do to prevent inadvertent exposure to an embryo or fetus?
4. Explain the purpose of gonad shielding, list the requirements for gonad shielding, and describe the correct placement of shields for males and females.

4

The Health Care Delivery System

OBJECTIVES

At the conclusion of this chapter, the student will be able to:

- Compare and contrast the different types of health insurance with regard to benefits, route to care, and cost coverage.
- Explain the general organizational structure within a health care facility.
- Diagram the typical organizational structure of the medical imaging department.
- Describe the radiographer's role in relation to the radiologist, the referring physician, the hospital administration, nursing personnel, and other hospital staff.
- List three different types of professional organizations and explain their purposes and their benefits for the medical imaging community and its employees.

- Explain the purpose of the RadCARE bill and its current status in the legislative process.
- List three ways in which a radiographer can contribute to the advancement of radiologic technology.
- Describe the current job outlook for radiographers in relation to geographic location, salary, and advancement opportunities.
- Define *profession* and describe how the Practice Standards for Medical Imaging and Radiation Therapy apply to professionalism.

OUTLINE

Today's Health care Delivery System
  Health care Insurance and Benefit Systems
  Health care Facilities
The Health care Team
  Physicians
  Hospital Organization and Management
Services and Roles in the Imaging Department
Radiography as a Profession
  Professionalism

Professional Organizations
Practice Standards
Education
Credentials
Continuing Education
Employment Outlook
Career Ladder
Accreditation

KEY TERMS

Accreditation

Affordable Care Act (ACA)

American Registry of Radiologic Technologists (ARRT)

American Society of Radiological Technologists (ASRT)

credentials

diagnostic

fee-for-service

fellow

health maintenance organization (HMO)

hospitalist

intern

managed care system

Medicaid

Medicare

mission statement

practice standards

preferred provider organization (PPO)

radiologist

resident

therapeutic

TODAY'S HEALTH CARE DELIVERY SYSTEM

In earlier generations, patients with serious illnesses were often cared for at home. The doctor was summoned by telephone and brought his black bag to the bedside. The patient usually got better, and only in the most critical instances did a patient go to a hospital. A substantial part of the treatment was the application of common sense and supportive care. With the discovery of antibiotics and more sophisticated medical and surgical treatments, simple measures gave way to intensive treatment protocols. Today, after years of professional treatment for even the slightest discomfort, there is less incentive to take personal responsibility for prevention and self-care, and there is often a reluctance to rely on simple remedies. The inappropriate and excessive use of medications such as antibiotics has reduced their effectiveness. The steadily increasing costs of this approach have forced us to adopt new ways of coping with disease and health maintenance. For these reasons, health care is returning to many of the preventive measures and natural treatments that were once part of the medical knowledge in most households. Prevention is an important part of the solution, because it is more affordable than the costs of treating disease.

The delivery of health care can be viewed in many ways. Crisis intervention is one approach, in which the patient or client seeks help only when unable to manage alone. As soon as the emergency has passed, the former lifestyle is usually resumed. In comparison, the health maintenance or preventive health care system attempts to promote well-being and avoid the need for medical intervention. It encourages good nutrition, exercise, vaccinations, and health screening tests, such as mammograms. A preventive system promotes self-care that avoids such habits as smoking and the use of recreational drugs. Potential health problems are identified before they manifest as illnesses. Illnesses are treated promptly, before they become chronic or life threatening.

These two approaches are not mutually exclusive, because each deals with different points on a line drawn between optimal health and fatal illness called the *health–illness continuum*. On one end of this line, you may find a healthy patient required to obtain a chest radiograph for employment purposes. On the other end of the spectrum, you could encounter a critically ill patient whose examination might provide lifesaving information. Because patients in the imaging department may fall anywhere along this health–illness continuum, you must be both empathetic and flexible in your approach to widely varying needs. Any measures you can take to promote health will help to reduce hospital stays and prevent the duplication of services; this increases both cost-effectiveness and patient satisfaction.

Health care Insurance and Benefit Systems

Until 40 years ago, most health care was provided on a fee-for-service basis. Under this system, insurance companies reimburse patients for the costs of their health care within the limits of the policy, and the patient is responsible for any costs not covered. Patients can seek care from their choice of physicians and hospitals. Because private physicians may provide a more personal service and greater continuity of care under this system, many individuals find this kind of care reassuring and are willing to pay a high premium for this type of insurance coverage.

As health care and hospital services became more technical and more expensive, health insurance premiums and uninsured charges began to cost more than many individuals could afford. In an effort to deliver more affordable care, health maintenance organizations (HMOs) were formed. These organizations provide complete and comprehensive health care for the cost of the premium and a small fee called a *copayment* for each visit. HMOs control costs by promoting good health and by providing care in specified facilities only. The physicians and other professionals who provide this care may be salaried employees of the organization. Physician assistants and nursing practitioners may provide many aspects of care formerly provided by physicians only.

If you belong to an HMO and have a health concern, the first person you see is your primary health care provider, who may be a physician or perhaps a nurse practitioner (a nurse with advanced education and credentials for providing primary care). If your condition necessitates additional diagnostic attention or care, you will be referred to a secondary provider. This provider may be a specialist such as an ophthalmologist, a gynecologist, or a radiologist. At times, your condition may be serious enough to warrant care within a hospital setting, which is called *tertiary (third-level) care*. Your primary care provider will coordinate your treatment and provide follow-up care after you are discharged from the hospital.

By promoting good health, the HMO tries to reduce the average cost of health care for all its members. Regular physical examinations, immunizations, weight control, treatment for hypertension, and other forms of preventive care, such as fitness programs, and classes on health-related topics, are typically included among the benefits of these organizations. This preventive care system is in direct contrast to crisis intervention or episodic care, in which you see your physician only when you are ill. An inherent part of an HMO system is that patients are expected to become more involved in meeting their own health care needs. They seldom have the ongoing, one-to-one relationship with a primary care provider that was once common with a family doctor.

As HMOs succeeded and became more popular, many private physicians and hospitals cooperated to form managed care systems. These systems allow private hospitals and physicians to provide private services while also providing care through insurance plans that operate as HMOs or PPOs. PPO stands for preferred provider organization, a system that offers care at reduced rates within an established network of providers. Managed care systems save money by limiting access to expensive services when they are not needed. Their benefits vary from modified fee-for-service programs to comprehensive HMOs.

To relieve unnecessary crowding in emergency departments and provide more cost-effective care, a system evolved to treat patients who need urgent care or minor surgery for conditions that are not immediately life-threatening. These facilities are called *immediate* or *urgent care clinics* and *surgicenters*. At urgent care clinics, patients are seen without waiting several days for an appointment. These centers treat acute but minor illnesses and accidents. Conditions such as broken fingers, middle ear infections, and upper respiratory infections can be seen quickly and treated effectively in such centers. Surgicenters are outpatient surgical facilities. Patients are admitted in the early morning for minor procedures such as a simple hernia repair and are released to home care the same evening. The charges involved are less than those for the use of a major surgical suite and a subsequent overnight hospital stay.

Despite these changes, the health care delivery system has had difficulties in coping with the escalating costs of diagnostic procedures and hospital care. Health insurance rates have soared, and the number of families unable to afford health care has increased dramatically. One outcome is that many low-income families have turned to emergency departments to provide care for all kinds of illnesses. This crisis intervention model of care is expensive on a per-patient basis, and because many of these patients are unable to pay, the cost is spread over the entire span of hospital care.

In an effort to relieve the pressure on hospital emergency departments and provide more cost-effective care, the Affordable Care Act* (ACA, often called "Obamacare") became law in 2010. Its stated purpose was to ensure that all Americans were covered by health insurance. Under this law, employers are required to provide health insurance for their fulltime employees when they employ more than 50 workers. Federal and state insurance exchanges facilitate the purchase

---

*For further information, please see http://www.hhs.gov/healthcare/rights/

of health insurance through private companies and administer a federal program that provides subsidies for this insurance according to the ability to pay. Penalties in the form of fines are assessed for the failure to carry adequate health insurance and are administered by the Internal Revenue Service.

Medicare, a federal health insurance program in the United States, covers a portion of the medical care costs for those 65 years and older. Medicare offers four plans: Part A, Hospital Coverage; Part B, Medicare Insurance; Part C, Medicare Advantage Plans; and Part D, Prescription Drug Plans. Part A insurance covers a portion of a subscriber's inpatient care costs in hospitals or services from other facilities that provide skilled nursing care, home health care and hospice. Part B helps to cover other medically necessary services and preventive health care measures, such as doctor visits, radiographs, and laboratory tests, on an outpatient basis. The Medicare Advantage Plans are offered by private companies to provide subscribers with both Part A and B insurance, and frequently also prescription drug coverage. The patient's Medicare benefit is applied to pay for these policies, and when there is an additional premium cost it is deducted from their Social Security payments. These policies may take the form of HMOs, PPOs, or fee-for-service plans, to provide subscribers with the maximum amount of choice and flexibility.

The federal government also provides funds to assist the indigent through a program called Medicaid. Persons must fall within a designated group, recognized by the federal and state governments, in order to be eligible for partial or full Medicaid funding. Each state sets its own guidelines for services and eligibility; examples of the designated eligibility groups include age, income and resources, disability, and US citizenship. A considerable percentage of the financial reimbursement to health care facilities for services comes from Medicare and Medicaid.*

Consumers need to know how to use the coverage available, because insurance programs vary greatly and are often subject to change. Should you be referred to an emergency department for a sudden illness, or is there an urgent care center? Does your policy cover radiographs and medication? It pays to be an informed and assertive consumer.

*For further information, please see http://www.medicare.gov and http://www.cms.gov/home/medicaid.asp.

If benefits are not used correctly, or if care is not implemented with the proper coding and documentation, the insurance company may deny coverage for the care received and patients may be faced with large, unexpected bills.

Health care Facilities

Hospitals can be owned and operated as either public or private agencies. Public hospitals and health care facilities are operated by federal or local governments. Military hospitals and facilities for veterans operated by the Department of Veterans Affairs are examples of federal agencies. Counties, cities, and communities may provide public health care services, including hospital care. Many hospitals are privately owned. These may be not-for-profit institutions, such as those owned by religious or charitable groups, or proprietary hospitals, which are health care businesses run for a profit. Although there are still independent hospital institutions, many hospitals are members of a hospital system that cooperates to cut costs by sharing the use of highly technical equipment and by purchasing supplies in volume.

The role of the hospital in relation to the community it serves is reflected in its mission statement, a one- or two-paragraph declaration of the institution's basic philosophy and primary goals. This statement provides guidance for the decisions that govern the activities of the facility. An example of a mission statement for a hospital system belonging to a religious order is in Box 4-1.

Many patients currently receive care in outpatient clinics, whereas only a few years ago they would have been admitted to a "short stay" ward for minor surgical procedures or invasive diagnostic procedures, such as colonoscopies. Hospitals often include outpatient clinics for certain services such as well-baby checkups and follow-up care for oncology patients. Many public health departments also provide clinics, especially for prenatal and pediatric care.

BOX 4-1   Mission Statement for a Hospital System Belonging to a Religious Order

Providence Health System continues the healing ministry of Jesus in the world of today, with special concern for those who are poor and vulnerable. Working with others in a spirit of loving service, we strive to meet the health needs of people as they journey through life.

Our mission is carried out by employees, volunteers, physicians, and others who work together in a spirit of service that reflects our core values.

Patients with chronic diseases may receive home health care provided by the health department or by an HMO or managed care system. Others may be cared for in extended care facilities, often called *nursing homes,* or in a foster care facility. Foster care is sometimes provided in private homes. Skilled nursing facilities provide care for patients during their convalescence when professional help is necessary for rehabilitation, but the services of a hospital are no longer required. Medicare, Medicaid, and state health programs help to defer the expenses of care in skilled nursing facilities, foster care, or long-term residential facilities for the elderly and infirm.

THE HEALTH CARE TEAM

Patients are the most important people in the health care community. They come to us for help in preserving health and solving health-related problems, and all the efforts of the health care team should be directed toward meeting these needs. You will be an important member of this team; therefore it will be helpful

to become acquainted with other team members and their functions in the hospital. Although you may see patients in physicians' offices, outpatient clinics, or other health care settings, most of your clinical experience will occur in a hospital, the setting on which this book is focused.

Physicians

Patients may be brought directly to the hospital for emergency care. Many patients are sent to the hospital by a doctor known as the *referring physician.* On admission, the referring physician may also serve as the *attending physician* who provides direction for hospital care, or another physician may be assigned to the case. The attending physician is responsible for assessing the patient's needs and prescribing therapeutic procedures to promote health.

The attending physician may determine that the expertise of one or more specialists would be helpful in the patient's diagnosis or treatment, and may refer the patient to a specialist for consultation. Common specialty areas are listed in Table 4-1.

TABLE 4-1	Abbreviated List of Medical Specialties
Specialty	**Functions**
Emergency department physician	Specializes in trauma and emergency situations; a triage expert in disaster situations
Family practice physician	Treats individuals and families in the context of daily life
Gastroenterologist	Diagnoses and treats diseases of the gastrointestinal tract
Geriatrician	Specializes in problems and diseases of elderly persons
Gynecologist	Treats problems and diseases of the female reproductive system
Hospitalist	Specialist, often an internist, who treats patients in a hospital setting
Internist	Specializes in the medical care and treatment of adults
Intensivist	Specialist, often a pulmonologist, who treats patients in the intensive care unit
Obstetrician	Specializes in pregnancy, labor, delivery, and immediate postpartum care
Oncologist	Specializes in tumor identification and treatment
Ophthalmologist	Diagnoses and treats problems and diseases of the eye
Otorhinolaryngologist	Specializes in conditions of the ear, nose, and throat
Pathologist	Specializes in the scientific study of the alterations in the body caused by disease and death
Pediatrician	Specializes in the care, diagnosis, and treatment of diseases affecting children
Pulmonologist	Specializes in diagnosis and treatment of diseases of the lungs
Psychiatrist	Specializes in diagnosis, treatment, and prevention of mental illness
Radiologist	Specializes in diagnosis by means of medical imaging
Surgeon	
Abdominal	Specializes in surgery of the abdominal cavity
Plastic	Restores or improves the appearance and function of exposed body parts
Neurologic	Specializes in surgery of the brain, spinal cord, and peripheral nervous system
Orthopedic	Diagnoses and treats problems of the musculoskeletal system
Thoracic	Specializes in surgery involving the chest

The physicians who practice in the hospital form the medical staff. Depending on the institution's size and organization, this group may also include **interns** (recent medical school graduates gaining practical experience), **fellows** (licensed physicians receiving advanced training), and **residents** (licensed physicians in an educational program to become certified in a specialty area).

In recent years, the **hospitalist** specialty has become an option for physicians who choose to treat hospitalized patients only. They serve as the attending physicians for inpatients, freeing primary care physicians from hospital duties so that they can better manage their outpatient practices. Hospitalists practice in groups, providing 24-hour availability within the hospital. They are experts at dealing with conditions that require hospitalization and are familiar with the staff, services, and procedures of the institution. On discharge, the patient returns to the care of the primary care physician.

Hospital Organization and Management

The hospital is governed by an executive board that establishes the goals, policies, and financial plans for the hospital and hires the director or administrator. One of the responsibilities of the board is to extend the privilege of staff membership to qualified physician applicants and to organize the staff to cooperate in making the rules that govern professional activities. Many of these rules relate to standards of care and medical records.

The administration must see that suitable facilities and equipment are provided, and that a staff of well-trained professional, technical, and support personnel is present. Figure 4-1 shows a typical organizational structure for a hospital and the lines of authority and responsibility that form the chain of command for the health care team.

The hospital may have one or more assistant administrators who have clearly defined areas of responsibility for several departments. They do not need any specific training or experience in the areas under their direction because their expertise is in health care management. These administrators rely on departmental supervisors for decisions and communication at the level where specialization is required.

Each department has a chief or supervisor whose education and expertise relate directly to the area of responsibility. For example, the supervisor of a hospital pharmacy is a registered pharmacist, whereas the supervisor of the radiology department is usually a radiographer. Each supervisor leads a group of skilled employees who carry out the department's goals.

Some departments meet patient needs directly. Nursing service, for example, provides patient care by implementing nursing care decisions, implementing the physician's orders within the framework of hospital policies, and communicating plans for patient care and physician orders to other departments. Some typical hospital departments are listed in Table 4-2. Note that some are categorized according to whether their functions are **diagnostic** (related to identification of patient problems) or **therapeutic** (devoted to treatment). Still other departments serve patients indirectly by providing support services, such as

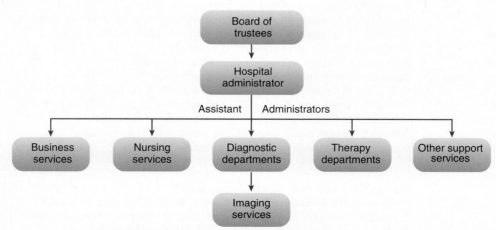

FIG 4-1 Simplified example of hospital organizational chart.

purchasing, central supply, and laundry. Social service departments may support patients and their families by providing a hospital chaplain, a trained counselor, or a translator. These departments also coordinate with other agencies and services as needed when a patient is discharged or transferred. Many hospitals also have auxiliary groups consisting of volunteers who tend to the special needs of patients and their families. Large institutions often include research and education departments as well as separate departments or clinics for providing outpatient services.

The names of departments and where they fit into the chain of command vary with the institution's size and its management philosophy. It is useful to study the organizational chart of the clinical facilities affiliated with your radiography program.

Few patients use the services of all departments, but the well-being of most patients requires the cooperative efforts of many team members. You can gain a better understanding of how the team functions by focusing your attention on a fictional scenario that describes the hospital stay of one patient (Box 4-1).

TABLE 4-2   Some Typical Hospital Departments

DIRECT PATIENT SERVICES			
General	**Diagnostic**	**Therapeutic**	**Support Services**
Admissions	Computed tomography	Dietary	Accounting
Emergency	Electrocardiography	Occupational therapy	Central/sterile supply
Nursing service	Electroencephalography	Oncology	Human resources
Social services	Magnetic resonance imaging	Physical therapy	Housekeeping
Chaplain/counseling services	Nuclear medicine	Respiratory therapy	Laundry
	Pathology (medical laboratories)	Surgery	Medical records
	Radiography		Purchasing
	Sonography		Security

CASE STUDY 4-1   Health Care: A Team Effort

Judy Colton was brought to the emergency department with acute back pain and was admitted to the hospital. Dr. Evans, a hospitalist, became her attending physician, consulting on behalf of her family physician. Dr. Evans requested a lumbar myelogram to assist in the diagnosis and planning of an effective course of treatment. The examination request was actually a referral to a specialist, the radiologist, for a diagnostic consultation. Dr. Evans wrote the order in Ms. Colton's chart, and a nurse made arrangements for the procedure.

A patient transporter brought Ms. Colton and her chart to the radiology department, where the radiographer greeted her and checked the chart to confirm the order. The radiologist explained the procedure and the radiographer assisted the radiologist to perform the examination. Clean linen used during the examination was provided by the hospital laundry. The radiographer processed the images, checked them on the monitor for quality, and cleared them with the radiologist before releasing the patient. The radiographer completed the examination by entering the patient and examination data into the radiolo-

gy information system. The requisition was scanned and sent with the images to the picture archiving and communication system so that the images could be interpreted by the radiologist and a report dictated. Another radiographer assisted by helping to move the patient. The transporter then took Ms. Colton to the computed tomography (CT) department for a postmyelogram follow-up scan and then returned her to the care of the nursing service. Dr. Evans was then able to confirm the diagnosis of a herniated intervertebral lumbar disk.

Dr. Evans contacted Dr. Ortiz, a neurosurgeon, who recommended a type of spinal surgery called a *laminectomy* and ordered an MRI examination to assist with the preoperative evaluation.

The radiologist dictated reports of the imaging studies which were electronically converted to text. Then the reports were reviewed and electronically signed off. Once approved, they were posted on PACS and on Ms. Colton's electronic chart.

After the surgery, Ms. Colton received medication for pain from the hospital pharmacy. As soon as her condition

Continued

permitted, physical therapy was implemented with the help of other team members.

Members of the business office staff used information from the various departments to prepare the billing, and copies were sent to Ms. Colton and to her insurance company. The payment received helped to support the many services rendered by the hospital, including the purchase of imaging supplies and the radiographer's salary.

During a random sampling taken to ensure that hospital regulations had been followed and to gather statistics about hospital services, Ms. Colton's chart was reviewed by a medical staff committee. Her chart was then stored for future reference, because it could be needed to assist with her future care. The images and reports are part of Ms. Colton's medical record and were archived with her other medical records. A summary of her hospital stay was sent to her family physician, who provided follow-up care after she was discharged from the hospital.

This case is a simplified representation of a hospital stay.

How many departments shared responsibility for Ms. Colton's care?

What types of communication were required to coordinate the team's efforts?

Were any of the team members unnecessary or unimportant?

SERVICES AND ROLES IN THE IMAGING DEPARTMENT

The department where you receive your clinical experience in radiography may be called the *radiology department*. Since the early use of x-rays in medicine, *radiology* has been the term applied to the science of medical imaging. As technology has added new imaging methods to the medical repertoire, radiologists have incorporated them into their practices and within existing radiology departments. Because some of the new imaging modalities do not involve the use of x-rays, some radiology departments have been renamed *diagnostic imaging departments*. This text uses the two terms interchangeably.

Whether it is called *radiology* or *diagnostic imaging,* this department provides various diagnostic services that relate directly to the patient, and its typical administrative structure is set out in a diagram in Figure 4-2. Radiologists are physicians who specialize in diagnostic imaging. They are members of the medical staff and serve as consultants in one or more of the imaging modalities in radiology. The line of responsibility for radiologists goes through the medical staff organization. Radiologists play a major role in establishing the standards of care and technical quality within the department, in addition to performing many examinations with the assistance of radiographers (Figure 4-3). A radiologist must interpret each examination and provide a report to the referring physician (Figure 4-4).

The radiology services in a modern hospital can be divided among several departments under the supervision of a radiology manager who works with the radiologists, radiation safety officers, physicists, and the hospital administration to establish policies and budgets for the various imaging departments.

The radiology manager may also supervise several groups of employees, such as those in radiography, nuclear medicine, ultrasound, cardiovascular angiography, computed tomography (CT), and magnetic resonance imaging (MRI). Under the manager's direction, groups of employees may be referred to as *teams*. The team approach to management is popular because it rewards cooperative effort and encourages team members to work together for the benefit of the patient. This book focuses primarily on the radiography department team. , Chapter 22 provides an introduction to other imaging modalities and the corresponding aspects of patient care.

The lead radiographer, sometimes called the *department coordinator* or *chief technologist,* manages the day-to-day activities in the radiography department. He or she also schedules the staff of radiographers and support personnel in this area and orders the necessary supplies. The division of responsibility between the lead radiographer and the radiology manager varies with the institution. The lead radiographer is often promoted from the ranks of staff radiographers because of technical expertise and supervisory capability. The exact titles for these positions vary greatly among institutions.

Staff radiographers may report directly to the chief radiographer or to a lead radiographer or team leader responsible for a given area. In practice, they also work and communicate directly with radiologists rather than along the established chain of command.

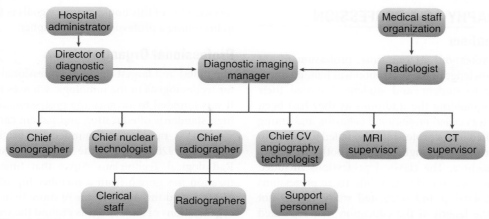

FIG 4-2 Typical organizational structure of the medical imaging department. Actual titles may vary. *MRI*, Magnetic resonance imaging; *CT*, computed tomography.

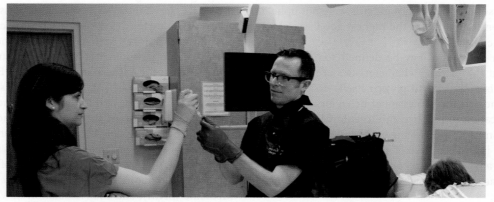

FIG 4-3 Radiologists perform many examinations with a radiographer's assistance.

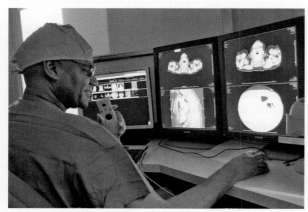

FIG 4-4 A radiologist interprets each imaging study and provides a report to the referring physician.

Imaging departments also require support staff. Depending on the size of the department and the organization of the hospital, the support personnel may include administrative assistants, receptionists, biomedical technologists, equipment maintenance engineers, medical secretaries, and transportation service personnel. There may also be an information systems manager with a staff to maintain patient and image files, with the computerized images organized in a picture archiving and communication system.

Good communication systems depend on the ability of all team members to relay information systematically, preventing essential details from being overlooked. As you begin to understand each team member's responsibilities, you will appreciate the cooperation and communication lines that help the team function smoothly.

RADIOGRAPHY AS A PROFESSION

Professionalism

What is a profession? At one time, profession meant "calling." Knowledge of the profession was handed down from master to student, and students honored their teachers by upholding the traditions as they had been taught. This was called *professional behavior,* and young people accepted into a profession who failed to live up to its highest principles brought shame to both themselves and their teachers. The classical professions included medicine, law, and the clergy. While these professions required scholarship and dedicated study, it was not necessarily the length of the education that separated the professions from other occupations. The nature of the work required professionals to place a high value on their service to others—both the client and the community would suffer if the high standards were not upheld. Commitment to truth and the highest good were hallmarks of the professional.

Today, a profession may be defined somewhat differently, but the primary characteristics are similar. A profession is organized to govern itself—to effectively set the standards for professional behavior, education, and qualification to practice and to enforce those standards within its ranks. Having a peer review journal or publication is also expected of a profession, because this allows it to advance and to continually review and challenge the basis of the knowledge on which it functions.

> ⚡ A profession is not only a field of study, but also the application of specialized knowledge to benefit others.

Radiographers and other radiologic technologists, working primarily through their principal professional organization, the **American Society of Radiologic Technologists (ASRT)**[†], have brought medical imaging technology to a professional level. As a professional radiographer, your work must focus on your patients and your efforts must be devoted to providing quality service. One of this book's primary goals is to assist you in becoming a professional radiographer.

Professional Organizations

The oldest and largest national professional association for technologists in the radiologic sciences is the ASRT. It was founded to advance the profession and promote high standards of education and patient care. Fourteen visionary x-ray pioneers founded the original organization in 1920, calling it the American Association of Radiological Technicians. Since that time, the organization has grown from a membership of 46 to over 152,000, and the ASRT is one of more than 70 national organizations of technologists around the world that are members of the International Society of Radiographers and Radiologic Technologists. Other organizations of imaging technologists, some of which are affiliated with the ASRT, serve those with specific professional interests. For example, the American Health care Radiology Administrators (AHRA) provides a network and resources for technologists with administrative positions, whereas the Association of Collegiate Educators in Radiologic Technology (ACERT) and the Association of Educators in Imaging and Radiologic Sciences (AEIRS) provide forums to meet the needs of technologists and others who teach in this field. Organizations also exist for those involved in imaging modalities other than general radiography, such as the Society of Diagnostic Medical Sonography (SDMS), the Society of Nuclear Medicine (SNM), and the Association of Vascular and Interventional Radiographers (AVIR). Some of these imaging specialty organizations, such as the SNM, are international organizations with membership categories for physicians, technologists, and others.

The ASRT is the only nationally recognized professional society representing all the radiologic technologists in the United States. It reaches radiographers on the local level through the affiliated state societies. These affiliates must conduct their business according to ASRT standards, and each state society elects a board of directors to conduct the society's business. State societies also sponsor continuing education programs and have roles similar to those of the national organization.

The ASRT governance structure includes a House of Delegates, a Board of Directors, and a Commission. The House of Delegates is the legislative body of the organization, with 166 eligible delegate positions, including affiliate delegates elected or appointed by the state

---

[†]Information about the ASRT, membership applications, and copies of the ASRT documents mentioned in this chapter are available directly from the ASRT. Write to the ASRT at 15000 Central Ave SE, Albuquerque, NM 87123-3917. Telephone: 800-444-2778 or 505-298-4500. Fax: 505-298-5063. Or visit the ASRT website at http://www.asrt.org.

societies, national chapter delegates elected by the membership at large, and military chapter delegates. Chapter delegates represent the different areas of practice in the radiologic sciences, including management and education, and imaging and therapeutic professionals in the military. The role of the House of Delegates is to debate and vote on issues that have a major impact on professional practice.

The Board of Directors is the governing body and consists of the chairman, president, vice president, president-elect, and secretary-treasurer, plus the speaker and vice speaker of the House of Delegates. The first five members of the board are elected by the membership at large, and the remaining members by the House of Delegates. The role of the board is to consider and act on issues that relate to the business functions of the ASRT.

The commission comprises a seven-member panel with backgrounds in administration, education, and extensive professional practice. The commission is appointed by the Board of Directors. The role of the commission is to review issues relative to professional practice, business, and governance, and to refer these to either the house or the board for consideration and action.

ASRT serves its membership in many ways, including making significant contributions to education, professional advancement, legislation, and public relations. The ASRT also appoints technologist representatives to other organizations and committees whose work is significant to the profession.

As far as education is concerned, the ASRT provides guidelines for the organization, correct operation, and curriculum design for programs in the various imaging modalities. In addition, the ASRT sponsors educational conferences and self-study materials for technologists. The ASRT publishes two peer-reviewed scientific journals, *Radiologic Technology* and *Radiation Therapist,* and a magazine, the *ASRT Scanner,* which covers timely topics and key issues in the radiologic sciences. The organization also reviews and approves educational programs for continuing education and maintains continuing education records for members, providing copies of these to members annually.

The ASRT actively supports legislation to protect the public from excess radiation exposure by inadequately trained workers. This includes efforts to mandate state licensure and to set minimum standards for both the accreditation of educational programs and granting credentials to individuals who administer radiation.

The voluntary federal minimum educational standards for the practice of radiological technology form part of the Consumer-Patient Radiation Health and Safety Act of 1981. The ASRT has been instrumental in attempting to amend this act through the introduction of the Consumer Assurance of Radiologic Excellence (CARE) Bill into the U.S. Congress in 2001. It was passed in the U.S. Senate in 2006 and reintroduced into the House of Representatives in early 2007, passed in 2009, and was then referred back to the Senate for approval. In August 2010, the Senate committee referred it to the Committee on Health, Education, Labor and Pensions where it languished. In 2013 it was reintroduced to both Houses of Congress. If enacted, this legislation will impose mandatory education and credentialing standards for everyone who uses ionizing radiation or magnetic resonance as well as for those who plan and deliver radiation therapy. States that fail to meet these standards will lose Medicare and Medicaid reimbursement for radiologic procedures.

Through its public relations program, the ASRT promotes awareness of the profession and the duties of radiographers. To commemorate the anniversary of the discovery of x-rays, the ASRT sponsors the annual National Radiologic Technology Week during the first full week of November. This observance honors the contributions of radiologic technologists to the health care field.

Practice Standards

The ASRT has worked for many years to attain professional status for radiological technologists. To meet this goal, the ASRT has developed a written statement that describes the radiographer's duties and responsibilities. This document, titled *The Practice Standards for Medical Imaging and Radiation Therapy*, defines the clinical practice, technical activities, and professional responsibilities of imaging and therapeutic professionals. *The Practice Standards for Radiography* are set out in Appendix A. These standards include desirable and achievable levels of performance against which actual performance can be assessed. Because of its general format, the standards can be adapted to any area of practice and region of the country. The practice standards can be used by radiology managers to develop job descriptions and performance appraisals, and in the case of medical malpractice or negligence claims, a lawyer can use this document to determine an acceptable level of care and to show whether this professional standard has been met.

Education

Hospitals, community colleges, and universities offer approved education programs in radiography, with a minimum program length of 2 years; some last as long as 5 years. All these programs must meet the same rigorous standards for academic excellence and clinical experience.

Hospital-based programs provide a comprehensive academic and clinical curriculum under the sponsorship of one or more health care institutions. They usually require a time schedule of at least 40 hours per week, with a portion of this time reserved for formal classes and the remainder devoted to clinical practice. Graduates receive a diploma or certificate of completion.

Community college programs usually provide a more comprehensive academic curriculum and are affiliated with hospitals that provide the requisite clinical experience. Although more time may be spent in academic activities than in hospital-based programs, clinical experience continues to occupy more than half a student's time. Graduates are awarded an associate's degree.

University programs may require at least a 4-year commitment with a greater portion of the student's work devoted to academic courses. These programs lead to a bachelor's degree and may also qualify the graduate for advanced postgraduate programs.

Credentials

In the field of radiologic technology, credentials such as registration, permits, certificates, and licenses all refer to documents that attest to the qualifications of an individual.

The **American Registry of Radiologic Technologists (ARRT)** is a national organization of appointees from both the ASRT and the American College of Radiology (ACR). The ACR is an organization of physician specialists in radiology affiliated with the American Medical Association. The ARRT establishes the minimum standards for certification in the various imaging specialties and radiation therapy. Applicants must have high school diplomas or the equivalent and must have completed an approved education program in radiologic technology, to be eligible to take the certifying exam. Applicants must also meet *ethical requirements*. The ARRT conducts qualifying examinations that entitle the applicants who pass to use the designation *Registered Technologist* (RT) in association with their names. The ARRT conducts primary specialty examinations in radiography

(R), nuclear medicine (N), radiation therapy (T) and MRI, and permits the use of these abbreviations with the RT designation. Postprimary specialty examinations are offered in CT, MRI, mammography (M), cardiac-interventional technology (CI), vascular-interventional radiography (VI), quality management (QM), sonography (S), vascular sonography (VS), breast sonography (BS), bone densitometry (BD), registered radiologist assistant (RRA), and radiology practitioner assistant (RPA). At the present time, post-primary certification is not required to practice MRI, CT, or other special modalities with the exception of mammography.

Certification by the ARRT is recognized nationally, and to some degree internationally, as a standard qualification to practice radiologic technology and is a prerequisite for employment in this field by most accredited institutions in the United States. Once certified, you must renew your registration annually with the ARRT by paying a nominal fee. Each year before your birth month, you will be sent a renewal form and a questionnaire to complete, documenting your current employment status and eligibility for renewal. Proof of 24 credits of continuing education is required every 2 years.

> Certification by the ARRT is an important goal for student radiographers.

Licensure refers to the granting of "official permission" and is a prerogative of state governments. All states have laws requiring a driver's license and licenses to practice medicine and nursing. State licensure of radiologic technologists began in the early 1970s when laws were enacted in New York, New Jersey, and California. Now many states and territories have a license requirement for practicing radiologic technology, and several others have licensure bills pending. These laws vary greatly. If the pending federal legislation is enacted, all states will require licensure and this will be granted to any person certified by ARRT who applies and pays a fee.

Radiographers may also be required to have certification in other specific areas. For example, the State of Washington requires the completion of an approved 7-hour course on human immunodeficiency virus (HIV) infection. Additional examples include the periodic CPR certification required of all patient care personnel in most hospital settings and venipuncture certification that may be required for personnel who draw blood or administer intravenous fluids and medications. These certification requirements provide incentive to maintain competencies and document qualifications.

Some states issue permits to practice radiologic technology under limited circumstances or in limited scope. These permits do not require the same high standards that are necessary for ARRT certification or licensure. Limited permits may allow a public health nurse, certified medical assistant, or orthopedic assistant to take chest and extremity radiographs. To obtain a permit, an applicant must demonstrate knowledge of radiation safety and technical expertise in a limited area of radiography.

Continuing Education

In radiologic technology, as in any rapidly changing technological field, continuing education is essential to stay abreast of current trends and maintain competencies. This also is an important professional responsibility.

Many options for continuing education are available to the radiographer. Hospitals, colleges, and professional organizations all provide educational opportunities for radiographers to keep up with current developments and expand their skills. Education can take the form of courses, classes, workshops, seminars, and other group experiences, but there is also a variety of materials available for individual learning and self-study (Figure 4-5). The ASRT provides self-study materials for continuing education, which helps individuals who cannot attend

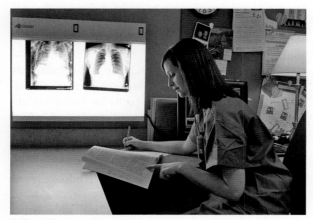

FIG 4-5 A radiographer earns continuing education credits through independent study.

classes or those who wish to study subjects that are not otherwise immediately available.

In addition to the continuing education requirements for the renewal of ARRT certification, states may also require continuing education as a condition for license renewal. In some states, such as Texas, the renewal of ARRT certification is accepted as proof of the required continuing education for renewing a state license.

When you are required to provide evidence of continuing education, be sure to determine in advance whether the education you plan to receive is approved and accredited for this purpose. Keep an accurate record of your continuing education activities, including any documentation of participation that you receive. Documentation is valuable even if it is not immediately required, because it may help you later in qualifying for a promotion or a new position.

Failing to maintain competency, licensure, registration, or any required additional certification places the employer and the employee at risk and may result in the loss of employment and professional reputation. Knowing the credentials required in a given situation and maintaining current credentials are important professional responsibilities. A violation of state licensure laws can result in fines and imprisonment.

Employment Outlook

Historically, the demand for radiographers has been cyclical and has changed with fluctuations in the economy and in the health care industry. The Bureau of Labor Statistics has predicted that by the year 2022, 275,000 radiographers will be needed—48,600 more than in 2010—an increase of 21%, which is a more rapid growth than average. This prediction is largely based on the increased needs that will occur as a result of the ACA requirement for every person to have health insurance, but there are several other important reasons to anticipate a demand for radiographers. Aging baby boomers, a large segment of our society, will be making more hospital visits and using more diagnostic services, including medical imaging. In addition, aging radiographers will be retiring at a faster rate than new radiographers can enter the profession. Currently, most radiographers are over 30 years of age. In addition, continued improvements in equipment and technology will create more opportunities for radiographers to specialize in advanced imaging areas, and this will create openings in general radiography. Expanding health care facilities will also contribute to the continued need for radiographers. The passage of the CARE Bill will have an effect on the demand for qualified and registered technologists because employers will no longer be able to hire individuals who have no formal education or certification to perform medical imaging examinations.

Radiographers entering the profession will have geographic mobility and salaries that are competitive with other health care professionals. Radiographers will have the freedom to work anywhere in the country and hold either a permanent or temporary position; they will be able to work in a variety of settings from physicians' offices to major medical centers.

Career Ladder

Many possibilities exist for radiographers to achieve promotion and advancement, depending on their interests, skills, experience, and education. At this point, it may be fun to speculate about how your career will develop into the professional life that is right for you. Giving some thought to the possibilities now may help you to begin setting professional goals and to recognize opportunities that may present themselves later.

As a staff radiographer gains experience and demonstrates ability, the first promotional step is likely to be the position of lead technologist, team lead, or coordinator. A lead technologist supervises the work in a specific area or on a given shift. Excellence in clinical performance and a demonstrated ability to relate well to other team members may qualify a radiographer for this position.

The position of department manager varies significantly with the size of the institution and department. In small hospitals, the position of lead technologist may be similar to that of the manager in a large medical center. Department managers need supervisory skills and an understanding of the operations of the entire institution so that they can align the needs and contributions of the department to the mission of the organization. In most cases, education and experience beyond those needed to practice radiography are required.

The title of radiology director designates the supervisor of a large diagnostic imaging department. This executive must have management ability and experience. The position usually requires a bachelor's or master's degree in health care administration or the equivalent experience.

The position of educator in radiologic technology usually requires advanced education (a degree in a related field) plus at least 3 years of clinical experience. This position can involve classroom, laboratory, and clinical work. Experience and further study can lead to advanced positions in education, such as program director or dean of health sciences.

Commercial positions in radiology also exist. A strong technical background and good interpersonal skills may qualify a radiographer as a representative of a company that sells radiographic equipment, supplies, or both. Commercially employed radiographers may perform technical services such as the repair and maintenance of equipment. They may provide education and problem-solving consultation to customers of companies that manufacture imaging systems. Alternatively, they may be involved in the direct marketing of imaging equipment to the radiologists and administrators who make major purchasing decisions. Employers may provide specialized training for these positions to qualified radiographers.

Opportunities also exist for qualified radiographers to work in research and development positions as employees of either corporations or educational institutions.

Technologists who provide services in special imaging departments may be recruited from the ranks of radiographers. Skills in CT, MRI, mammography, and angiography can be learned on the job and through independent study. It is up to each state's regulating body to determine whether technologists need to be certified to practice within a specialized modality. Specialty certification in these areas is granted by examination through the ARRT.

The specialty areas of radiation therapy, nuclear medicine, and sonography can be entered directly through educational programs for these technologies or through formalized programs open to technologists with any of the primary certifications.

Current trends indicate changes in baccalaureate degree programs in radiologic technology that will provide advanced clinical career paths for technologists. Four-year degree programs in radiologic technology have traditionally offered a broad general education, often with curriculum options in health care management or education, but the clinical credentials conferred by these programs have been equal only to those received by community college graduates. More recently, however, several colleges and universities have developed degree programs leading to advanced clinical competencies and credentials. Graduates of these programs are given various titles such as advanced practice technologist, RT clinical specialist, radiologist assistant (RA), and radiology practitioner assistant (RPA). They may qualify to supervise the work of other technologists, make decisions about the quality of images, and perform procedures such as fluoroscopy, venography, and arthrography under the direct supervision of a radiologist. Recognizing the value and popularity of these programs, the ASRT has developed a curriculum guide for a baccalaureate program leading to qualification as a radiologist assistant.

ACCREDITATION

Accreditation is a process that applies to institutions and results in documentation attesting to the attainment of certain minimum standards. Hospitals seek accreditation by The Joint Commission, formerly the Joint Commission on Accreditation of Health care Organizations (JCAHO), which indicates that the institution meets the criteria for equipment, staff, safety, funding, management, and patient care. This credential is required for the hospital to receive Medicare payments and insurance payments from many private carriers.

> The Joint Commission certifies that a health care institution meets certain minimum standards. This credential is required for the hospital to receive reimbursement from Medicare and other health insurance programs.

The Centers for Medicare and Medicaid Services is the federal agency that administers Medicare and Medicaid. Hospitals and other health care providers that wish to receive reimbursement for services under these federal programs must submit applications and provide documentation of the appropriate credentials and accreditation.

The independent agency responsible for program accreditation in radiologic technology and radiation therapy technology is the Joint Review Committee on Education in Radiologic Technology (JRCERT). It is made up of members appointed by the ASRT, ACR, and AERS. The JRCERT establishes minimum educational standards, conducts inspections, and grants accreditation to programs that comply with the standards.

The accreditation of colleges and universities is the province of state and regional agencies and attests to certain standards of education in the accredited institutions. It is the basis for determining the value of the diplomas granted as well as the value of credits transferred from one institution to another.

The accreditation processes for hospitals and schools involve a periodic self-assessment in which the institution evaluates its objectives, outcomes, resources, strengths, and weaknesses and documents how it meets the established criteria for quality in its field. This activity is followed by an on-site visit by accrediting agency representatives during which interviews, physical surveys, and document reviews are used to assess the institution. The accreditation process provides insight that allows the institution to strive for improvement while assuring quality service for the consumer.

SUMMARY

- The health care delivery system is a vast network of government agencies, profit-centered corporations, charitable organizations, and practicing professionals who deliver care under several different types of systems—some that provide crisis intervention and others that emphasize individual responsibility and preventive health care. The continually rising cost of health care has caused major changes in the health care delivery system over the past 60 years.
- The health care team is a dedicated group of physicians and hospital personnel that meet patient needs and provide services in a hospital setting.

- Radiographers and other imaging technologists are valuable and respected members of this team.
- The hospital administration is organized to keep the team functioning smoothly and meet patient needs. Its guiding philosophy is defined in its mission statement.
- In imaging departments, one or more radiologists interpret images and perform imaging procedures. They are members of the hospital medical staff.
- The imaging department is supervised by a radiology director, manager, or lead technologist. Staff radiographers may report directly to the manager or to a team leader. They also receive direction from radiologists outside the established chain of command.

■ SUMMARY—cont'd

- A profession is a field of study that applies specialized knowledge to benefit others. Professions are organized to govern themselves, set standards of behavior, education and qualification to practice, and to enforce those standards. Professional organizations usually hold meetings, publish journals, and adopt a code of ethics. Radiologic technology is considered a profession, and the American Society of Radiologic Technologists (ASRT) is the oldest and largest and professional organization for the radiologic sciences.

- The CARE bill has been introduced in the U.S. House of Representatives and has passed into the U.S. Senate with the support of the ASRT. If and when it becomes law, federal voluntary standards for qualifications to practice radiography will be replaced by mandatory requirements. States that do not comply will not receive funds for Medicare and Medicaid payments.

- Education for radiographers involves study and clinical experience in a program accredited by the Joint Review Committee on Education in Radiologic Technology that may range in length from 2 to 5 years and qualify the graduate for a diploma, an associate's degree, or a bachelor's degree.

- The American Registry of Radiologic Technologists (ARRT) is a certifying body composed of representatives appointed by the ASRT and the American College of Radiology (ACR). This organization provides examinations, certification, and registration renewal for qualified applicants. Certification by the ARRT is the principal qualification to practice radiography in the United States and is recognized by all state agencies that license radiographers. The ARRT provides several primary certifications for various imaging modalities and postcertification specialty qualifications for a number of others.

- Continuing education is a requirement for renewal of the ARRT registry and for license renewal in many states. Professional organizations provide opportunities to obtain continuing education credits, and participation in continuing education programs is an important professional responsibility.

- Radiographers who secure a job in the profession will have relative job security, geographic mobility, and salaries competitive with other health care professionals as a result of the high demand for imaging specialists in health care for the foreseeable future.

- The career ladder affords opportunities for professional growth and the pursuit of a variety of individual interests.

- Accreditation of an institution is a review and inspection process that documents the attainment of minimum standards. The Joint Commission is the accrediting organization for hospitals and medical centers in the United States. The accreditation of medical imaging education programs is provided by the Joint Review Committee on Education in Radiologic Technology.

■ REVIEW QUESTIONS

1. The only recognized professional society open to all radiologic technologists in the United States today is the:
   A. AVIR
   B. AHRA
   C. ASRT
   D. AARP

2. Fee-for-service–type health insurance is often appealing to patients because:
   A. the insurance company will reimburse the patient for covered costs
   B. the patient does not have to pay the cost above what is covered by insurance
   C. patients can seek care from their choice of physicians and hospitals
   D. all of the above

3. The nationwide increase in patient visits to the emergency department is principally due to:
   A. convenient hours
   B. a lack of doctors who make house calls
   C. lower costs per visit than doctors' offices
   D. the inability of patients to obtain low-cost health insurance

4. Medicare Advantage Plans help to cover health care costs for which type of patients?
   A. low-income families
   B. seniors older than 65 years
   C. homeless persons
   D. immigrants to the United States

REVIEW QUESTIONS—cont'd

5. The day-to-day scheduling of staff in the radiography department is the responsibility of the:
   A. radiologist
   B. lead radiographer or manager
   C. department secretary
   D. admitting clerk
6. A pulmonologist who practices exclusively in a hospital intensive care unit may be referred to as:
   A. a lung specialist
   B. an internist
   C. an intensivist
   D. a thoracic surgeon
7. The designated eligibility groups for Medicaid are recognized by the _____, although the _____regulates who falls within these eligibility groups.
   A. federal government; state government
   B. state government; federal government
   C. state and federal governments; state government
   D. state and federal governments; federal government
8. The *Practice Standards for Medical Imaging and Radiation Therapy* may be used:

   A. to develop job descriptions and performance appraisals
   B. by a lawyer to determine negligence or malpractice
   C. both A and B
   D. neither A nor B
9. The ASRT has approximately how many members?
   A. 120,000 to 130,000
   B. 130,000 to 140,000
   C. 140,000 to 150,000
   D. 150,000 to 160,000
10. Which criterion does The Joint Commission (the accrediting agency for hospitals) *not* use to certify that a hospital meets certain minimum standards?
    A. Education
    B. Equipment
    C. Safety
    D. Funding

Answers can be found in the Answer Key on pages 429-431.

CRITICAL THINKING EXERCISES

1. Is access to health care a right, regardless of the ability to pay? Describe how hospitals respond to this question, and explain how their response affects the cost of health care.
2. Draw a diagram of the organizational structure of your imaging department, and insert the names and position titles of the personnel.
3. Contrast the purposes of the ARRT with those of the ASRT. Why are both organizations important to the profession of radiologic technology?

5

Professional Roles and Behaviors

OBJECTIVES

At the conclusion of this chapter, the student will be able to:

- State three reasons why a study of professional behavior is important to the radiographer.
- List three aspects of self-care that demonstrate responsible behavior by the radiographer.
- Describe *empathetic care* and provide a strategy for providing such care when the situation is difficult for you.
- Define ethics and list the ethical principles that apply to radiographers.
- Discuss professional communications, including sensitivity, appropriateness, and the rationale for confidentiality.
- List and explain three theories that provide guidance for right action. List the steps in ethical analysis and use these steps to analyze an ethical dilemma.
- List four patient rights that the radiographer is responsible for protecting.
- Discuss the ethical handling of genetic information and why this can be a sensitive ethical issue.

- Define *Informed Consent* and list the legal requirements for a valid informed consent document.
- Define the terms *negligence* and *malpractice*.
- List three specific acts of intentional misconduct and three acts of unintentional misconduct that may occur in radiology departments.
- Discriminate between misconduct that is criminal and that which would be considered a tort.
- Define the legal terms plaintiff, defendant, *res ipsa loquitur,* battery, assault, libel, slander, borrowed servant, and *respondeat superior.*
- Locate the portions of a paper chart containing information relevant to diagnosis, history, current status, laboratory reports, radiology reports, allergies, and medications.
- List five reasons for keeping accurate medical records.
- Describe the radiographer's responsibility for malpractice prevention and for reporting both unusual occurrences and misconduct.

OUTLINE

Job Satisfaction
Self-Care
Empathetic Care
Burnout
Care of Supplies and Equipment
Participation in Professional Activities
Professional Behavior
Morals and Ethics
Standards of Ethics for Radiographers
Ethical Judgments and Conflicts
Patient Rights
Considerate and Respectful Care

Information
Privacy and Confidentiality
Informed Consent
Right to Refuse Treatment or Examination
Death with Dignity
Legal Considerations
Crimes: Felonies and Misdemeanors
Torts
Medical Information and Records
Effective Documentation
Medical Recording on Computers
Responsibilities for Record Keeping

KEY TERMS

advance directive   ethical analysis   misdemeanor
assault   ethics   moral agent
battery   false imprisonment   negligence
chart   felony   plaintiff
charting   Health Insurance Portability and   radiology information
chronic   Accountability Act (HIPAA)   management system (RIMS)
defendant   libel   slander
empathy   malpractice   tort

JOB SATISFACTION

Most students choose to study radiography because it is a caring, helping profession, but it takes more than good intentions to be a good radiographer. The stressful demands of clinical practice often tend to overshadow humanitarian considerations. The patient's needs may be overlooked while you are coping with highly technical material unless you make an effort to learn from the beginning to handle both at once.

Your work will be the most satisfying when your contributions and the personal contacts they involve are genuine and sincere. Performing tasks because you enjoy them will make your work more productive and much less stressful.

Self-Care

Health is a state of physical, mental, and social well-being, and being healthy implies that you are capable of promoting health. Health professionals are responsible for their own well-being and are also expected to serve as health role models for their patients and members of the community. Take care not to project an attitude that announces, "Do as I say, not as I do." This attitude undermines our credibility in the eyes of the people we most want to help.

An unhealthy radiographer is not a good health role model and cannot function effectively for both physical and psychological reasons. To help others, we must first meet our own physical and mental needs. Certain needs are universal and can be listed and ranked in importance (Figure 5-1). Any unmet need causes stress and prevents an optimal state of well-being.

Our most basic needs are foremost until they are adequately satisfied. As we achieve satisfaction on one level, the needs of the next level occupy our attention. Self-actualization is the state in which a person welcomes tension and effort as a stimulus to creativity and self-expression. Your need for esteem and self-actualization may be the reason why you are a student in this program. Constructively meeting our needs for well-being, knowledge, and self-esteem enables us to function more fully and remain free from self-preoccupation at those times when the patient requires our full attention.

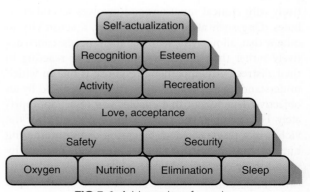

FIG 5-1 A hierarchy of needs.

Because many patients have a lowered resistance that makes them especially vulnerable to infection, a radiographer who is ill should stay at home. However, because the team is counting on full attendance, every effort should be made to prevent illness. Everyone occasionally experiences powerful emotional states, such as grief or acute anxiety, and such stresses can make you more susceptible to illness. Whenever possible, you should stay at home to deal with such problems until some resolution is reached, because anxiety and stress can prevent you from properly fulfilling your responsibilities.

Recommendations for the practice of good nutrition and exercise habits may sound trite, but these practices are rewarded with less time lost from work and an increased sense of well-being. In addition, the knowledge and practice of the principles of body mechanics (see Chapter 7) will help you avoid the types of injuries that can result from lifting and moving patients or equipment. Preventive health measures are equally important. The precautions discussed in Chapter 9 have been developed to help prevent disease transmission from patient to patient and from the patient to you. Such precautions are only effective when you understand and practice the principles and use the necessary personal protective equipment.

Radiation exposure over the course of a career can have serious health consequences for you if the proper precautions are not observed. Chapter 3 provides an introduction to safe practice, and your curriculum will include an extensive study of radiation protection. Adherence to radiation safety practices is another important aspect of self-care.

Empathetic Care

Job satisfaction depends on your ability to deal effectively with clinical situations and involves several attributes. One such attribute is empathy, a sensitivity to others that allows you to meet their needs constructively rather than merely sympathizing or reacting to their distress. An empathetic response is one in which understanding and compassion are accompanied by an objective detachment that enables you to act appropriately. For example, you could express sympathy for the victim of a tragic accident by crying or by smothering him with pity. A more productive expression of empathy would show concern and care while quickly and accurately providing the images that could assist in a rapid diagnosis and treatment.

Beginning students often express concerns such as, "What will I do if the patient vomits? I just know I'll get sick too!" or "I faint at the sight of blood." As you gain confidence and experience, you will learn to deal with an emergency first and let your knees shake later. Focusing on the patient while projecting a calm, reassuring attitude will be your best reinforcement.

By focusing on patient needs you will be able to respond calmly and assertively if patients act inappropriately. It may seem strange or frightening when an individual responds to stress and anxiety by becoming hostile or even threatening. These actions are often coping mechanisms patients use to feel in control of a situation. Maintaining a composed, objective attitude is most effective in dealing with such patients. Overt sexual expressions by patients are encountered infrequently, and usually indicate anxiety by patients who no longer feel sexually functional because of their current physical state. With this in mind, you can be less judgmental while setting limits on patient behaviors. In other words, you can refuse to accept the behavior while continuing to reassure and care for the patient.

Burnout

Health care workers are particularly susceptible to a condition known as *burnout*. Burnout is a response to the chronic strain of dealing with the constant demands and problems of people under our care. This emotional overload can be exacerbated by personal problems and by unreasonable workplace demands. Burnout typically causes exhaustion, dissatisfaction, anxiety, and eventually apathy. Burned-out workers often experience depersonalization and may tend to withdraw. When required to relate to others, their attitude may be hostile. The decline in job performance may be severe enough to jeopardize employment. Victims of burnout are also subject to health problems and are likely to abuse substances such as tobacco, caffeine, and alcohol.

If you are working long hours and work seems to be the entire focus of your life, it is wise to examine your motivation. Positive motivation characterizes the individual who works for positive results. Even when this person works very hard, enthusiasm is maintained. Hard workers with positive attitudes could be called *work enthusiasts*. Those with a negative motivation, however, work to avoid negative consequences such as losing their jobs or dealing with the unpleasant aspects of their personal lives. These workers are often referred to as *workaholics*.

The likelihood of burnout is decreased by paying attention to the aspects of self-care discussed earlier in this chapter. Stress relief is also important. Humor is a stress reliever that helps us connect with others, and difficult situations have less power to defeat us when we can laugh at them. Humor also increases creativity and has health benefits. Other forms of stress-relief, such as exercise, hobbies, and meditation, are also good habits to practice regularly. Stress is diminished when we remember that occasional mistakes are bound to happen and that no one is perfect.

Care of Supplies and Equipment

Hospitals must stock tremendous quantities of supplies to function effectively. In such an environment, it is easy to assume that free access implies free use, but in truth someone must pay the bill. Added to the purchase price of each item is an overhead factor that may be two- or threefold the item's basic value. For example, when a portable grid is damaged, the cost of replacement includes not only the price of the grid plus the overhead costs for shipping, but also the proportional cost in work hours of the stock clerk, receiving clerk, purchasing agent, and accountant, as well as the administrators who supervise these employees.

Medical equipment is expensive, and proper care is required to ensure that its value is preserved and that it is available when needed. The misuse of equipment or supplies, or their diversion for personal use, wastes money and increases health care costs. The radiographer who avoids such waste is demonstrating a high standard of ethical behavior.

Participation in Professional Activities

Health care professionals value the acquisition of additional skills and regularly expand their knowledge. Those who are content with the status quo quickly find that the profession marches on without them. Standard practice changes rapidly, and today's knowledge will soon be out of date. Textbooks often contain information that is valid when the manuscript is completed but is outdated by the time the book is published. Formal and informal continuing education also helps us to maintain interest in our work and to avoid the boredom and routine that are detrimental to our emotional health.

In the area of professional growth, cooperation is often more productive than individual effort. The American Society of Radiologic Technologists (ASRT) has 54 affiliate societies—one in each state and one each in the District of Columbia, the city of Philadelphia, and the territories of Guam and Puerto Rico. There are also many district groups within the state societies. These groups provide occasions for radiographers to become acquainted, share problems and ideas, hear speakers, present papers, and exhibit their work. Professional associations advance the profession while providing opportunities for members to help each other. Members can further a profession's goals while developing leadership skills through chairing committees, holding office, and participating in business and educational sessions.

The importance of scientific contribution should be emphasized. Professionals often respond to problems or new situations by developing new methods of performing their work, and many of these ideas can be helpful to others. We owe a large debt to those who have advanced the art and science of our profession. We can acknowledge these gifts and receive recognition and a sense of belonging through our own contributions.

PROFESSIONAL BEHAVIOR

Litigation has become so common in our society that it is especially important for health care workers to become familiar with the moral, ethical, and legal implications of their actions. For many of us, the terms *moral, ethical,* and *legal* seem almost interchangeable. In practice, however, they have somewhat different applications.

Morals and Ethics

Personal morality is based on the lessons of right and wrong that were taught to us at an early age. As we grow older, we expand our understanding of these principles and apply them in a general way to other circumstances. The customs, beliefs, and rules of our formative years play an important part in our decision making. Morals provide an internal motive that governs our relationships with others and permits us to live together in harmony.

Lawrence Kohlberg studied and wrote on the subject of moral development in the 1970s, and his description of the stages of moral development is called *Kohlberg's theory.* Kohlberg's work describes how individuals learn morality first through experience with obedience and punishment. In time, they learn to behave morally to gain acceptance and approval. An advanced state of moral development is characterized by a principled conscience that recognizes the value of morality to society and to the human condition. More recently, the researcher Carol Gilligan has applied Kohlberg's moral developmental research principles to the differing preferences between the sexes. Female subjects indicated that there was more emphasis on the significance of caring in the moral development of women, as compared with a greater emphasis on justice in the moral development of men.

The beliefs that we share with our community about values and duties constitute the *societal morality* that influences the laws, customs, and moral components of our culture. As stated in the *Declaration of Independence,* our founding fathers believed that "all men are created equal" and that they are entitled to "life, liberty, and the pursuit of happiness." These concepts form the central core of our societal morality as a nation.

Group morality refers to the moral principles that apply specifically to certain groups of people. For example, professionals have certain duties to clients and the public that do not apply to the population in general. The moral duties of physicians were defined in ancient Greece in the Hippocratic Oath. Examples of group morality for today's health professionals include the duties of providing due care, maintaining professional competence, and maintaining the confidentiality of patient information.

Ethics is a branch of philosophy that can be defined as a systematic reflection on morality. The application of ethical principles to specific human activities may be thought of as "applied morality." Ethical actions are behaviors that fall within the accepted principles of right and wrong. There are a number of different analytical approaches to answering ethical questions. If you are fortunate to have a course in ethics as part of your education program, you will have the opportunity to explore the thought processes used by ethicists to arrive at conclusions. Basically, these approaches consider the proper response to any situation, measured against the standard of a deep respect for the dignity of all life and for the environment.

Group ethical behavior includes the duties and obligations placed on us by our profession. Ethical questions that arise in the practice of professions have been considered and addressed by most professions and their organizations. The essential principles of ethical behavior for the group are stated in a document called a *code of ethics*. Because professionals have important moral duties, they are responsible for knowing and honoring the principles of ethics that govern their professional activities.

Although the application of moral, ethical, and legal standards may be confusing, there are a few clear differences. Our moral principles instill a sense of right and wrong and a desire to do the right thing. Professional ethics define correct moral behavior in the context of performing professional duties. Laws are the means used by a government to enforce commonly accepted moral standards in the interests of society. When injured individuals believe that we have caused them harm by failing to fulfill our moral or professional responsibilities, laws exist to provide remedies. These laws ensure that the rights of carelessly or unjustly injured parties are protected by the courts.

 Professional ethics define correct moral behavior in the context of performing professional duties.

Standards of Ethics for Radiographers

A code of ethics is the hallmark of a profession because it signifies high principles of professional behavior and a willingness by the profession to control its own conduct. As stated earlier in this chapter, most professions have their own codes of ethics that govern their behavior. The *Standards of Ethics for Radiologic Technologists* is a two-part document that includes the *Code of Ethics,* an aspirational document, and the *Rules of Ethics,* a more specific list of standards.

ASRT Code of Ethics

The ASRT Code of Ethics, set out in Box 5-1 appears on the ASRT website, www.ASRT.org. Developed and jointly adopted by the ASRT and American Registry of Radiologic Technologists (ARRT), it establishes broad principles of professional conduct. Specific behaviors to achieve these ends are detailed in the Practice Standards in Appendix A. Some principles of the ASRT Code of Ethics are self-explanatory, and some are expanded in other sections of this chapter. Four of them (the third, fifth, seventh, and ninth principles) are not discussed elsewhere in this chapter and deserve additional attention.

The third principle requires radiographers to put aside all personal prejudice and emotional bias when rendering professional services. This is more difficult than it may first appear. Most of us can easily identify prejudice in others, but our own biases or judgments are beyond our awareness and are justified as "only common sense." We all have natural preferences that can result

---

BOX 5-1   American Society of Radiologic Technologists Code of Ethics

1. The radiologic technologist conducts herself or himself in a professional manner, responds to patient needs and supports colleagues and associates in providing quality patient care.

2. The radiologic technologist acts to advance the principal objective of the profession to provide services to humanity with full respect for the dignity of mankind.

3. The radiologic technologist delivers patient care and service unrestricted by concerns of personal attributes or the nature of the disease or illness, and without discrimination on the basis of sex, race, creed, religion or socioeconomic status.

4. The radiologic technologist practices technology founded on theoretical knowledge and concepts, uses equipment and accessories consistent with the purpose for which they were designed, and employs procedures and techniques appropriately.

5. The radiologic technologist assesses situations; exercises care, discretion and judgment; assumes responsibility for professional decisions; and acts in the best interest of the patient.

6. The radiologic technologist acts as an agent through observation and communication to obtain pertinent information for the physician to aid in the diagnosis

and treatment of the patient and recognizes that interpretation and diagnosis are outside the scope of practice for the profession.

7. The radiologic technologist uses equipment and accessories, employs techniques and procedures, performs services in accordance with an accepted standard of practice, and demonstrates expertise in minimizing radiation exposure to the patient, herself or himself, and other members of the health care team.

8. The radiologic technologist practices ethical conduct appropriate to the profession and protects the patient's right to quality radiologic technology care.

9. The radiologic technologist respects confidences entrusted in the course of professional practice, respects the patient's right to privacy, and reveals confidential information only as required by law or to protect the welfare of the individual or the community.

10. The radiologic technologist continually strives to improve knowledge and skills by participating in continuing education and professional activities, sharing knowledge with colleagues, and investigating new aspects of professional practice.

Revised and adopted by The American Society of Radiologic Technologists and the American Registry of Radiologic Technologists, February 2003.

---

in discriminatory treatment if we are not fully aware of them. With which patients do you feel most comfortable? Men? Women? Those of your own race? Those older than the age of 16? Younger than 65? Middle class? Do you feel greater compassion for a patient with a heart problem than one with a sexually transmitted disease?

Once we identify the areas in human relationships in which we feel most at ease, it becomes apparent that we are less at ease in other situations and would prefer to avoid them altogether. It is instructive to pay attention to how we deal with patients who fall outside our "comfort zone." Sometimes we tend to act in a more friendly or solicitous way to cover up our feelings, while at other times we may remain aloof, appearing to be preoccupied. A lack of interest or concern is unacceptable; feigned concern is never the same as the real thing. Faithfulness to the spirit of the third principle requires a high degree of self-awareness and presents a serious professional challenge to the radiographer.

The fifth principle addresses the issue of professional responsibility, implying that radiographers are truly

professional because they are sufficiently educated and experienced to be capable of independent discretion and judgment. Within the scope of our professional activity, we are expected to make decisions and to be accountable for our decisions. An important aspect of this responsibility is an awareness and acceptance of our limitations. Although our responsibilities can vary with the working environment, regular duties should be specified in written job descriptions and be consistent with the scope of practice authorized by one's credentials as permitted by law and institutional policy. The Standards of Practice provide guidance with respect to these duties and responsibilities. It is in no one's best interest to perform tasks without sufficient knowledge or to undertake a responsibility without being adequately qualified. This principle also holds the radiographer accountable for errors committed under the orders of another person if the radiographer knew, or should have known, that the order was in error.

The seventh principle requires radiographers to adhere to accepted practices and make every effort to protect themselves and all patients and staff from exposure to unnecessary radiation. The ethical implications of this issue are important. When a radiographer violates this principle, there is no telltale evidence. The negative consequences of other breaches of ethics may be immediate, but the latent and genetic effects of unnecessary radiation may not be apparent for 10 to 30 years, or even for several generations. Making every effort to minimize exposure to radiation—despite difficult patients or added time constraints—requires good habits and a strong ethical commitment to radiation protection.

The ninth principle relates to confidentiality in a health care setting, one of the cardinal concepts in all codes of ethics relating to health care. The confidentiality of conversations between patients and their physicians is considered so important that, along with communications to lawyers and the clergy, it is protected by "legal privilege." As a result, the professional cannot be required to divulge such information, even when it is of material value in a court of law. Although the information provided to a radiographer is not legally privileged, radiographers often hear conversations between patients and their physicians and have access to confidential information contained in patient charts. You may witness circumstances in which patients are unable to preserve their dignity and behave in ways that would embarrass or shame them if known to friends or family members. Many patients do not want it known that they are ill or have been hospitalized, and others may wish to keep their diagnosis confidential. Information that may seem of no consequence to you may constitute a highly sensitive issue for the patient.

Any breach of confidence, even if no names are mentioned, could be interpreted by others as an indication that you do not respect professional confidence. Betrayals of confidence cause mistrust of the health care team and may prevent patients from revealing facts essential to their care. In addition, the violation of protected health information is grounds for termination from the institution.

The patient's right to confidentiality is not violated by appropriate communications among health care workers when the information is pertinent to the patient's care. It is justifiably assumed in such a case that the transfer of information is for the patient's benefit, and that all personnel involved are bound by the ethics of confidentiality. Appropriate communications are those directed privately to those who need the information. Conversations about patients must never be held in public areas such as waiting rooms, elevators, or cafeterias.

The ethics of patient-staff communication also require sound judgment and restraint to avoid exposing patients to the radiographer's personal concerns or the problems of the hospital staff. Using the patient as a sounding board for complaints or gossip is inexcusable.

Rules of Ethics

As mentioned previously, the Standards of Ethics for the profession as published by ARRT also include Rules of Ethics. These rules are mandatory, specific standards of minimally acceptable professional conduct for all registered technologists and applicants for certification by the ARRT, and they are enforceable by the ARRT. The Ethics Committee and the Board of Trustees of the ARRT handle challenges to the Rules of Ethics through established administrative procedures. These rules are published in their entirety by the ARRT and are found on the ARRT website (www.ARRT.org). They prohibit the following practices:

1. Use of fraud or deceit to obtain employment or credentials.
2. Dishonest conduct with respect to the ARRT examination.
3. Conviction or no-contest plea to a felony, gross misdemeanor, or misdemeanor (with the exception of speeding or parking infractions).
4. A failure to report to the ARRT that legal or ethical charges are pending against the person in any jurisdiction.
5. The failure or inability to practice the profession with reasonable skill and safety. Practicing outside the scope of practice authorized by one's credentials.
6. Any professional practice that is illegal, contrary to prevailing standards, or that creates an unnecessary danger to the patient.
7. The delegation, or acceptance of any delegation, of professional functions that might create an unnecessary danger to a patient.
8. Any actual or potential inability to practice radiologic technology safely by reason of:
   • Illness, use of alcohol or drugs, or any physical or mental condition, or
   • Adjudication of mental incompetence, mental illness, chemical dependency, or posing a danger to the public
9. Revealing privileged communication except as permitted by law.

10. Engaging in any unethical conduct such as deceiving, defrauding or harming the public, or the willful or careless disregard for the health, welfare, or safety of a patient. Actual injury need not be established.

11. Engaging in conduct with a patient that is sexual or could be interpreted as sexual, or in any verbal behavior that is seductive or sexually demeaning or exploiting to a patient or former patient. This includes unwanted sexual behavior, verbal or otherwise.

12. Knowingly engaging in or participating in abusive or fraudulent billing practices.

13. The improper management of patient records, such as failure to maintain records, or any actions that may result in a false or misleading record.

14. Assisting a person to engage in the practice of radiologic technology without current and appropriate credentials.

15. Violating a state or federal narcotics or controlled-substance law.

16. Providing false or misleading information directly related to the care of a patient.

17. Making a false statement to the ARRT or failing to cooperate with an investigation conducted by the ARRT or the Ethics Committee.

18. Engaging in dishonest or misleading communication with respect to one's education, experience, or credentials.

19. Failing to report to the ARRT any violation or probable violation of any rule of ethics by any registered technologist or applicant for certification by the ARRT.

20. Failing to immediately report information concerning an error made in connection with imaging, treating, or caring for a patient.

Ethical Judgments and Conflicts

The process of ethical analysis is a method of evaluating situations in which the correct action is in question. Although some situations may be obviously unethical and unacceptable to almost anyone, circumstances often present conflicts between values, and the best solution is not immediately apparent. In the face of an ethical dilemma, you must be prepared to assess the problem objectively and come to a conclusion that you can implement and defend. Ethical analysis is a process involving four basic steps:
1. Identify the problem.
2. Develop alternate solutions.

3. Select the best solution.
4. Defend your selection.

You may realize that there is a problem before you have fully identified it. Identifying the problem means that you can state the conflict clearly. It may be helpful to write it down. It is important to consider every aspect of the problem, to be certain that you have all the pertinent information, and to be confident that your information is accurate. Do not rush this process. A competent identification of the dilemma is essential to its successful resolution.

Once the problem is well defined, the next step is to proceed with the development of alternative solutions. In this part of the process, we think of as many potential solutions as possible. This is a brainstorming exercise in which no judgments are made. View the problem from the perspective of everyone involved. Include not only the interests of individuals, but those of your institution, your profession, and society as a whole.

Only after you have an exhaustive list of possible resolutions does the next step in the process begin—the selection of the best alternative. This is the most challenging part of the analysis, in which you weigh the alternatives and render a judgment as to which is best. In this process, you will need to eliminate choices that have positive attributes and possibly one or two that you particularly like.

When the best alternative has been selected, you should be prepared to explain your choice based on the standards that influenced your decision. By what standard, then, should the alternatives be judged and defended?

Both moral principles and ethical theories provide guidelines for determining whether actions are right or wrong. No one system serves adequately for all occasions. Although religious literature and educational systems may have instilled moral rules, there is no comprehensive list of moral principles that is universally accepted and available as a resource. Ethical theorists have tried to codify moral rules into sets of generally accepted principles, but they are not all in agreement.

Ethical theories differ depending on whether any judgment of right and wrong is based on the essential nature of an action (nonconsequentialism) or its consequences (consequentialism).

These two types of ethical theory provide an example of the classic debate over whether the end justifies the means. The consequentialist believes that an action is right if the outcome is good. For example, speeding is good if the outcome is that I arrive at work on time; it is bad if there is a negative outcome, such as an accident. The nonconsequentialist might argue that speeding is always bad because it is against the law and because it places you and others at risk.

Modifications to the traditional ethical theories are increasingly being used to analyze and defend actions related to quality patient care. Social contract theory holds that certain persons or groups have relationships that contain inherent expectations, duties, and obligations. For example, patients expect radiographers to minimize exposure to radiation, and radiographers expect patients to cooperate by holding still during the procedure. An intentional or careless failure to meet these expectations could be seen as a violation of the social contract. Of course, the contract is not written and there are no clear sanctions when it is broken.

The ethics of care reflect a viewpoint that could be considered *situational ethics*. This theory recognizes that right actions for a patient in any given situation may be wrong for other patients or other circumstances. A caring ethic demands moral judgments that reflect community values such as respect, patience, tact, and kindness. Related to the care theory is the theory of virtue-based ethics. This theory places a value on virtues—admirable character traits such as caring, faithfulness, trustworthiness, compassion, and courage.

Rights-based ethics emphasize the rights of individuals in a democratic society to be shielded from undue restriction or harm. The rights of some individuals place duties on others. For example, a patient's right to competent and compassionate care places a duty on the radiographer to provide such care. Rights-based ethics are appealing because they seem to clarify our duties and define accountability. Unfortunately, there is a potential for conflict between what professionals see as their duty and what patients may claim as their rights.

Principle-based ethics, also called *principlism,* is a widely accepted standard for selecting and defending solutions to ethical dilemmas in health care communities. Six moral principles, sometimes called *ethical principles,* are accepted as guides to right action that should be respected unless there is a compelling moral reason not to do so. The six principles are:

1. Beneficence—goodness; actions that bring about good are considered right.
2. Nonmaleficence—no evil; an obligation not to inflict harm.
3. Veracity—truth; an obligation to tell the truth.
4. Fidelity—faithfulness; an obligation to be loyal or faithful.
5. Justice—fairness; an obligation to act with equity.
6. Autonomy—self-determination; respecting the independence of others, and acting with self-reliance.

Now, consider the dilemma of Melanie Baines and evaluate her problem using ethical analysis.

CASE STUDY 5-1   Ethical Analysis

As Melanie Baines waited for the surgeon to call for an x-ray in the operating room, she stood quietly behind Dr. O'Brien, the anesthesiologist. A large vertical drape across the patient's shoulder region separated Dr. O'Brien from the view of the surgeon and others in the room with the exception of Melanie. Twice Ms. Baines noticed that Dr. O'Brien disconnected the tubing between the anesthesia machine and the patient and inhaled deeply over the tube. When she moved the C-arm fluoroscopy unit into position over the patient, she noticed that Dr. O'Brien seemed startled to see her. He apparently had not been aware that she was behind him. While this seemed strange, she thought little about it until the following week when Jon, a staff technologist and coworker, mentioned that Dr. O'Brien had fainted during an open hip reduction procedure and

been replaced by a nurse anesthetist. "I hope he's all right," said Jon. "He sure is a nice guy."

Identifying the Problem

Ms. Baines suspects that Dr. O'Brien has become addicted to anesthetic gas. She also considers that he may have been inhaling oxygen from the anesthesia machine. Although Ms. Baines sometimes works in the operating room, she is not a member of the surgical department staff and does not have a place in its chain of command. She hardly knows Dr. O'Brien. She does not know whether others who work with Dr. O'Brien may have identified a problem and reported it. However, Dr. O'Brien's actions that Ms. Baines observed and the subsequent fainting spell raise concerns about the safety of patients under his care and about his own well-being.

Developing Alternate Solutions

Ms. Baines considers the dilemma and lists the following possible actions:

- Do nothing at all.
- Ask around the hospital grapevine and try to ascertain whether anyone knows the cause of Dr. O'Brien's fainting spell.
- Discuss this issue with her supervisor, George Bell.
- Make an appointment to discuss her concerns with the surgical supervisor.
- Talk to Dr. O'Brien and urge him to submit to treatment.
- Send an anonymous note to the chairperson of the medical staff.
- Send a signed note to the chairperson of the medical staff.
- Write a letter to the Board of Medical Examiners.

Select the Best Solution

Is there a solution that will protect Dr. O'Brien's reputation, especially if Ms. Baines's suspicion is unfounded?

How could the rights of Dr. O'Brien's patients be affected by her actions? Does she have a duty to judge Dr. O'Brien's actions? Is there any way to confirm or refute her suspicions without spreading rumors or slandering him?

Defend Your Selection

The basic principle of nonmaleficence is often expressed as, "First, do no harm." Because the potential for harm to Dr. O'Brien's patients may be great, Ms. Baines must act. Principle five of the ARRT Code of Ethics states, "The radiologic technologist assesses situations; exercises care, discretion and judgment; assumes responsibility for professional decisions; and acts in the best interest of the patient." This is clearly a case that calls for Ms. Baines's discretion, judgment, and sense of responsibility. Which course of action best fits this description? Defend your answer.

Ethical analysis is being used increasingly to solve institutional problems. When several individuals have analyzed the situation, the next step may be to seek resolution through discussion, which leads to consensus. Once the question is resolved, action can be taken. The person responsible for implementing the ethical decision is called the **moral agent.**

Ethical conflicts may be troubling when the ethics of the group are not compatible with our personal beliefs. For example, there are health professionals who find that caring for some patients with acquired immune deficiency syndrome offends their personal sense of morality because they disapprove of the lifestyle in which the disease may have been acquired. For others, the conflict between their religious beliefs and the legal right of a patient to receive an abortion may be a problem. Professionals must not permit issues of personal morality to supersede the group moral duty to provide quality patient care. Although ethical standards may pose personal moral challenges, these standards assure us that professional ethical judgments can be made that will hold true for everyone in similar circumstances. These standards test whether a specific behavior will support the values and duties of the profession. If you experience frequent ethical conflicts that cannot be resolved, you may need to find a new position or career that conforms more closely to your own moral standards.

PATIENT RIGHTS

A major ethical concern for radiographers is to protect patient rights at all times. Considerable emphasis is placed on consumer advocacy in our society, and this value is especially significant in health care. There are many different statements of patient rights, and patient rights legislation is currently pending in the U.S. Congress. The patient rights statement of the American Hospital Association, now called *The Patient Care Partnership,* is set out in Box 5-2. This statement replaces the AHA's Bill of Rights as a plain-language brochure that informs patients about what they should expect during a hospital stay with regard to rights and responsibilities. It is available in multiple languages at www.aha.org.

Considerate and Respectful Care

Foremost is the right to considerate and respectful care. This statement is self-explanatory and is essentially the same professional behavior prescribed by the second and third principles of the Code of Ethics for Radiologic Technologists. It applies to all patients, regardless of their status.

BOX 5-2   American Hospital Association Patients' Rights Statement

The Patient Care Partnership: Understanding Expectations, Rights, and Responsibilities

When you need hospital care, your doctor and the nurses and other professionals at our hospital are committed to working with you and your family to meet your healthcare needs. Our dedicated doctors and staff serve the community in all its ethnic, religious, and economic diversity. Our goal is for you and your family to have the same care and attention we would want for our families and ourselves.

The sections explain some of the basics about how you can expect to be treated during your hospital stay. They also cover what we will need from you to care for you better. If you have questions at any time, please ask them. Unasked or unanswered questions can add to the stress of being in the hospital. Your comfort and confidence in your care are very important to us.

What to Expect During Your Hospital Stay
High-Quality Hospital Care
Our first priority is to provide you the care you need, when you need it, with skill, compassion, and respect. Tell your caregivers if you have concerns about your care or if you have pain. You have the right to know the identity of doctors, nurses, and others involved in your care, and you have the right to know when they are students, residents, or other trainees.

Clean and Safe Environment
Our hospital works hard to keep you safe. We use special policies and procedures to avoid mistakes in your care and keep you free from abuse or neglect. If anything unexpected and significant happens during your hospital stay, you will be told what happened, and any resulting changes in your care will be discussed with you.

Involvement in Your Care
You and your doctor often make decisions about your care before you go to the hospital. Other times, especially in emergencies, those decisions are made during your hospital stay. When decision-making takes place, it should include:

Discussing Your Medical Condition and Information about Medically Appropriate Treatment Choices
To make informed decisions with your doctor, you need to understand:
- The benefits and risks of each treatment.
- Whether your treatment is experimental or part of a research study.
- What you can reasonably expect from your treatment and any long-term effects it might have on your quality of life.
- What you and your family will need to do after you leave the hospital.

- The financial consequences of using uncovered services or out-of-network providers.
- Please tell your caregivers if you need more information about treatment choices.

Discussing Your Treatment Plan
When you enter the hospital, you sign a general consent to treatment. In some cases, such as surgery or experimental treatment, you may be asked to confirm in writing that you understand what is planned and agree to it. This process protects your right to consent to or refuse a treatment. Your doctor will explain the medical consequences of refusing recommended treatment. It also protects your right to decide if you want to participate in a research study.

Getting Information from You
Your caregivers need complete and correct information about your health and coverage so that they can make good decisions about your care. That includes:
- Past illnesses, surgeries or hospital stays.
- Past allergic reactions.
- Any medicines or dietary supplements (such as vitamins and herbs) that you are taking.
- Any network or admission requirements under your health plan.

Understanding Your Healthcare Goals and Values
You may have healthcare goals and values or spiritual beliefs that are important to your well-being. They will be taken into account as much as possible throughout your hospital stay. Make sure your doctor, your family, and your care team know your wishes.

Understanding Who Should Make Decisions When You Cannot
If you have a signed healthcare power of attorney stating who should speak for you if you become unable to make healthcare decisions for yourself, or a "living will" or "advance directive" that states your wishes about end-of-life care; give copies to your doctor, your family and your care team. If you or your family need help making difficult decisions, counselors, chaplains, and others are available to help.

Protection of Your Privacy
We respect the confidentiality of your relationship with your doctor and other caregivers, and the sensitive information about your health and healthcare that are part of that relationship. State and federal laws and hospital operating policies protect the privacy of your medical information. You will receive a Notice of Privacy Practices that

---

BOX 5-2 American Hospital Association Patients' Rights Statement—cont'd

The Patient Care Partnership: Understanding Expectations, Rights, and Responsibilities

describes the ways that we use, disclose, and safeguard patient information and that explains how you can obtain a copy of information from our records about your care.

Preparing You and Your Family For When You Leave the Hospital

Your doctor works with hospital staff and professionals in your community. You and your family also play an important role in your care. The success of your treatment often depends on your efforts to follow medication, diet, and therapy plans. Your family may need to help care for you at home.

You can expect us to help you identify sources of follow-up care and to let you know if our hospital has a financial interest in any referrals. As long as you agree that we can share information about your care with them, we will coordinate our activities with your caregivers outside the hospital. You can also expect to receive information and, where possible, training about the self-care you will need when you go home.

Help with Your Bill and Filing Insurance Claims

Our staff will file claims for you with healthcare insurers or other programs such as Medicare and Medicaid. They also will help your doctor with needed documentation. Hospital bills and insurance coverage are often confusing. If you have questions about your bill, contact our business office. If you need help understanding your insurance coverage or health plan, start with your insurance company or health benefits manager. If you do not have health coverage, we will try to help you and your family find financial help or make other arrangements. We need your help with collecting needed information and other requirements to obtain coverage or assistance.

While you are here, you will receive more detailed notices about some of the rights you have as a hospital patient and how to exercise them. We are always interested in improving. If you have questions, comments, or concerns, please contact _____.

Information

The patient also has a right to information, but this does not obligate the radiographer to provide any and all the information that may be requested. Radiographers must be prepared to explain radiographic procedures and to identify themselves and the radiologists. Patients have the right to copies of their billing records, medical records, and radiographic images. When these records are requested, they should be provided according to the established policies of the institution.

> Questions regarding diagnosis, treatment, and other aspects of care must be referred to the patient's physician.

Privacy and Confidentiality

Privacy

The right to privacy implies that the patient's modesty will be respected and that every effort will be made to maintain the patient's sense of personal dignity. The radiographer must remember that many common procedures, such as enemas, threaten the patient's modesty and dignity. Patients are likely to be much more sensitive in these situations than the health care workers who perform these procedures daily.

Physicians or health care workers should not be left alone with patients of the opposite sex in a physical examination setting that requires undraping the patient or examining the genitalia or female breasts. A chaperone, preferably the same sex as the patient, should be present. The main reason for this practice is to ease the patient's mind if he or she fears such an encounter and to provide a witness in case the patient later claims to have been assaulted or touched in an unprofessional manner. Many institutions have policies for these situations, and physicians usually prefer to be chaperoned even when no such policy exists. The radiographer should be aware of the institution's policies and sensitive to the needs of others in this regard.

Students and others not required for any procedure must have the patient's permission to be present. Taking photographs for any other purpose than the patient's care also requires written consent. Photographs taken outside this exception could violate the institution's photography policy, as well as the patient's privacy.

Confidentiality

The right of privacy also includes the expectation of confidentiality introduced earlier in this chapter.

The Health Insurance Portability and Accountability Act (HIPAA) was enacted under the U.S. Department of Health and Human Services (HHS) to protect the privacy rights of patients. In April 2003, hospitals were required to provide protection for patients concerning the release of individual financial and medical information without their written consent. No information may be released to employers, financial institutions, or other medical facilities without the specific permission of the patient. In brief, this law requires the following:

1. The patient must receive a clear, written explanation of how the health provider may use the disclosed information.
2. The patient will be able to see, and copy records, and request amendments.
3. A history of routine disclosures must be available to the patient.
4. Health care providers must obtain consent before sharing routine information on treatment, payment, and health care operations. Separate authorization is needed for non-routine disclosures and non-health purposes.
5. Patients have the right to request restrictions on the use and disclosure of their information.
6. Patients may file complaints with a provider or with the HHS about any violations of these rules.

Your hospital and radiology department will have specific written procedures to ensure compliance with HIPAA standards. It is your duty to familiarize yourself with these procedures and to apply them conscientiously. The following practices are examples of specific applications of HIPAA standards as they are used in some institutions:

- No schedules or other documents that include patient names may be posted in public areas.
- Only the first names of patients may be used when summoning them from public areas. Avoiding the use of last names is preferred to preserve a degree of anonymity.
- All health record information used for statistical or research purposes must be depersonalized by eliminating any names, numbers, codes, or biometric identifiers associated with a specific person.
- When the release of medical information is authorized, only the specific information designated in the authorization may be included in the release. A copy of the authorization must be kept on file.

- Only specific individuals trained in HIPAA compliance are allowed access to protected health care information.
- All computer files that contain or may contain patient information must be encrypted. Secure access is required for this data.

Genetic Information

The question of who has access to the information contained in an individual's genetic code poses questions relating to confidentiality and patient rights. In June 2000, the Human Genome Project reported that, for the first time, human beings are able to read their own genetic make-up. The human genome is essentially the instruction on how to build and operate a human being. This incredible achievement brings us closer to identifying and potentially altering the genes responsible for the transmission of genetically-based diseases. For example, research into cancer-suppressing genes offers a new approach to the treatment of many kinds of tumors.

These discoveries open up an entire new world of research and potential treatment, but they also open the door to new ethical dilemmas. Many genetically based diseases are relatively rare, but present long-term care problems with extremely high medical costs. Should everyone be screened for these diseases? Should families with a history of these diseases be compelled to undergo screening? What actions should be considered if a fetus is tested and found to have inherited a serious familial disease? Should prenatal genetic screening be as much a part of prenatal care as blood pressure screening?

These questions will continue to pose ethical problems as genetic counseling becomes a more frequent component of health care. Physicians, social workers, and others with training in this sensitive field will be used with increasing frequency to help patients make informed decisions about genetic questions.

Some institutions give patients the opportunity to opt out or give permission for their biologic material to be used in conjunction with their health information for anonymous genetic research purposes. Forms for patients to indicate their preferences in this regard are accompanied by a notice describing the institution's policy with respect to genetic privacy.

Informed Consent

Although patient consent for routine procedures is given on admission and is implied by the continued acceptance of hospital care, informed consent is necessary for any procedure that involves substantial risk or is considered experimental. Certain imaging procedures, such as myelograms and arteriograms, require that the patient receive a full explanation of the procedure and its potential risks and benefits. The patient and a witness then sign a consent form. The patient's signature is usually witnessed by the person providing the explanation. For some procedures, providing information and obtaining consent is the physician's duty, but for patients undergoing most routine procedures, a staff member provides the necessary form and an explanation on the physician's behalf.

When it is your duty to obtain informed consent, be sure that you fully understand the procedure and its risks and benefits so that you can adequately explain them to the patient and answer any questions. If the patient asks a question you cannot answer, seek the correct answer before continuing, because an improper response may invalidate the consent. Medically trained interpreters should be used when the patient does not speak, read, or write English. The legal implications of informed consent cannot be overemphasized. Successful litigation has been based on a lack of compliance with the following guidelines:

- Patients must receive a full explanation of the procedure and its risks and benefits and sign the consent form before being sedated or anesthetized.
- A patient must be competent to sign an informed consent.
- Only parents or legal guardians may sign for a minor.
- Only a legal guardian may sign for a mentally incompetent patient.
- Consent forms must be completed before being signed. Patients should never be asked to sign a blank form or a form with blank spaces "to be filled in later."
- Only the physician named on the consent form may perform the procedure. Consent is not transferable from one physician to another, not even to an associate.
- Any condition stated on the form must be met. For example, if the form states that a family member will be present during the procedure, the consent is not valid if the family member is not there.
- Informed consent can be revoked by the patient at any time after signing. This is an invocation of the patient's right to refuse examination.

A typical consent form is reproduced in Appendix B. The radiographer is responsible for knowing which procedures require written consent and for checking the chart to be certain that these forms are completed properly before beginning any examination for which informed consent is required.

Right to Refuse Treatment or Examination

Patients have the right to refuse treatment, which also implies the right to refuse an examination. When a patient chooses to exercise this right, you must not proceed with the study.

> Note that signing an informed consent form does not invalidate the patient's right to refuse treatment once the procedure has begun.

Consent can be revoked at any time during the procedure. If this occurs, take time to find out why the patient is unwilling to continue, because this may be a response to a temporary discomfort and not an objection to the procedure itself. If the patient still refuses to complete the procedure, comply gracefully and allow the patient to leave or return to the nursing service. Notify the attending physician.

Death with Dignity

Although the right to die is not specifically mentioned in the *Patient Bill of Rights*, it has received considerable public attention in recent years. A patient's right to die presents a potential ethical conflict between the health care worker's commitment to do everything possible to preserve and prolong life and the responsibility to relieve suffering, respect patient choice, and honor the patient's right to die with dignity. The news media have focused their attention on the debate over whether physicians may assist the death of qualified terminally ill patients, and several states have passed, or will be passing, laws permitting this practice. Only three states presently allow patients control over their final days: Oregon, Washington, and Vermont. There is a wide array of definitions and beliefs, along with some passionate opinions, within this debate.

As a separate issue, the resuscitation of patients for whom there is a reasonable expectation of recovery is considered to be medically and ethically correct, but sometimes heroic measures may only serve to prolong a patient's suffering, causing emotional distress to the family and great financial cost to the family or the public. This issue has become important because modern technology has made it possible to sustain life indefinitely by providing artificial life support to individuals who would not otherwise survive.

When the patient's condition is terminal, or when chronic illness or suffering has resulted in a substantial decrease in quality of life, the physician and the patient (or the patient's family, if the patient is incompetent) may agree to a "no-code" or do not resuscitate (DNR) order. This means that if death is imminent, no effort at resuscitation is to be attempted. When a DNR order is instituted, a notation is made in the patient's chart so that everyone involved in the patient's care is aware of the order. Intubation (placing a breathing tube in the trachea) to provide assisted respiration by means of a mechanical ventilator is another aspect of artificial life support. While this treatment is often instituted in combination with other resuscitation procedures, it is sometimes indicated to prevent the need for resuscitation. An order that reads *DNR/DNI* stands for "do not resuscitate/do not intubate," and indicates that neither resuscitation nor intubation is to be undertaken.

Many patients have an **advance directive,** which is an outline of specific wishes about the medical care to be given in the event that the individual loses the ability to make or communicate decisions. Copies of these directives are usually given to the family physician and an attorney or family member and should be part of the medical record.

Another way for individuals to influence decision making about their health care is to appoint a personal representative (durable power of attorney for health care). This action enables a trusted person to act on the patient's behalf if and when the patient is unable to communicate his or her wishes. The designated person is empowered to sign a valid informed consent form and should be aware of the patient's wishes, values, and beliefs about life-sustaining treatments in a wide range of situations.

To avoid any confusion or contention at critical times, all members of the immediate family should be informed when an advance directive is executed or when a health care representative is appointed.

LEGAL CONSIDERATIONS

Laws are legal requirements for behavior. Laws govern the practice of health care delivery, the practice of radiography, and certain interpersonal interactions. In general, laws can be divided into two categories: criminal and civil.

Criminal law deals with offenses against the state or society at large. Crimes may be further differentiated according to gravity or importance. A serious crime is called a **felony** and may be punished by imprisonment. A less significant crime is called a **misdemeanor** and is usually punishable by a fine or by imprisonment for less than 1 year.

Civil law deals with the rights and duties of individuals with respect to one another. A civil wrong committed by one individual against the person or property of another is called a **tort.** Lawsuits pursued under tort law claim that the **plaintiff,** the suing party, has been injured in some way by the **defendant,** the party being sued. Civil lawsuits seek damages rather than punishment; they are satisfied by court-ordered payment to the injured party by the defendant. In other words, civil law allows compensation to be paid to individuals who have been injured by a noncriminal act.

Crimes: Felonies and Misdemeanors

Criminal acts committed by radiographers could include either felonies or misdemeanors. Thefts and some drug-related crimes, for example, are felonies. Violations of laws that regulate practice, such as licensing requirements or scope of practice limitations, are usually classified as misdemeanors. Fraud or misrepresentation with respect to one's credentials or qualifications may be classed as a felony or misdemeanor, depending on the circumstances. Violations of criminal law could make it impossible for you to obtain professional standing or employment as a radiographer in the future. Table 5-1 summarizes these criminal acts.

Torts
Intentional Misconduct

Civil lawsuits alleging personal injury are becoming increasingly common in the health care field. The torts involved can fall into one of two categories: intentional misconduct or negligence. The intentional torts that occur in a hospital setting include assault, battery, false imprisonment, invasion of privacy, libel, and slander (defamation of character). Torts are summarized in Table 5-2.

False imprisonment is the unjustifiable detention of a person against his and/or her will. This becomes an issue when the patient wishes to leave and is not allowed to do so. It is acceptable to use physical immobilization when appropriately applied for safety reasons with the patient's permission. For example, hospitals have policies requiring the use of side rails on stretchers and hospital beds at night. The least restrictive immobilizer that

TABLE 5-1 Crimes and Their Potential Punishments

Crime	Definition	Example(s)	Punishment
Felony	A serious crime, violent or non-violent	Murder, arson, fraud, manslaughter, aggravated assault, grand theft, kidnapping	Death, or imprisonment longer than 1 year
Misdemeanor	Less significant crime	Trespassing, petty theft, vandalism, disorderly conduct, simple assault, reckless driving, public intoxication	Fine and/or imprisonment for less than 1 year, jail time, probation, community service
Torts	A civil wrong committed by one individual against the person or property of another	See Table 5-2	

TABLE 5-2 Torts: Intentional and Unintentional Misconduct

Type	Definition	Example(s)	Penalty
Intentional Misconduct: **Malicious Intent:**			
Assault	The threat of touching in an injurious way	Threatening an adult or pediatric patient to remain still for an exam	Lawsuit, court order to pay monetary damages, loss of license, potential unemployment
Battery	Unlawful touching of a person without his/her consent	A radiograph taken against the patient's will or on the wrong patient	
False Imprisonment	Unjustifiable detention of a person against his and/or her will	A patient wants to leave and is prevented from doing so	
Invasion of Privacy	Intrusion into a patient's private affairs, disclosure of private information, use of the patient's name falsely or for personal gain	Confidentiality has not been maintained or when the patient's body has been improperly and unnecessarily exposed or touched	
Libel & Slander	Malicious spreading of information that causes defamation of character or loss of reputation. Libel (written), slander (verbal)	Breach of confidentiality, speaking negatively about a patient, or documenting a negative comment about the patient in the chart	
Unintentional Misconduct: **Not intentional or deliberate:**			
Malpractice	Professional negligence; an act of negligence in the context of a relationship between a professional person and a patient/client	Error in diagnosis, complications resulting from a procedure, insufficient communication with the patient	Lawsuit, individual and/or hospital ordered to pay monetary damages, loss of license, potential unemployment
Negligence	Neglect or omission of reasonable care or caution. The radiographer is held to the standard of care and skill of the "reasonable radiographer" in similar circumstances (includes gross negligence, contributory negligence and corporate negligence)	Two patient identifiers were not checked prior to beginning a procedure and the wrong patient was x-rayed.	Lawsuit, individual and/or hospital ordered to pay monetary damages, loss of license, potential unemployment

Continued

TABLE 5-2   Torts: Intentional and Unintentional Misconduct—cont'd

Type	Definition	Example(s)	Penalty
Gross Negligence (Higher degree of negligence than ordinary negligence)	A negligent act that involves "reckless disregard for life or limb"	Performing professional services while intoxicated	Greater penalty than ordinary negligence. Punitive (punishment) damages may be assessed.
Contributory Negligence	An act of negligence in which the behavior of the injured party contributed to the injury	A patient is injured in a fall after being instructed not to get up from a chair.	Less severe penalty than in the absence of the injured party's negligent act.
Corporate Negligence	When the hospital as an entity is negligent	Health care worker suffers from hepatitis B following a needle stick because there is no established protocol in the organization to ensure reporting and treatment in this situation.	Monetary damages awarded to injured party.

provides adequate safety should be used. The inappropriate use of either immobilizers or physical restraints, however, may constitute false imprisonment. Reasonable judgment must be used to decide whether restraints are necessary. Hand or leg restraints are used only when the patient's physician orders them (see Chapter 10).

Invasion of privacy charges can result when confidentiality has not been maintained or when the patient's body has been improperly and unnecessarily exposed or touched. The significance of confidentiality is reemphasized here. Hospitals and their employees may be liable if they disclose confidential information obtained from a patient or contained in his/her medical record. If the information disclosed reflects negatively on the patient's reputation, one may also be liable for defamation of character. The protection of the patient's modesty is vitally important and is noted throughout this text as it pertains to specific procedures. Liability can also result if photographs are published without a patient's permission.

Libel and **slander** refer to the malicious spreading of information that causes defamation of character or loss of reputation. Libel usually refers to written information, and slander is more often applied to verbal communication. It should be clear that a breach of confidentiality is not only unethical, but may also provide sufficient grounds for a slander suit against the radiographer.

Assault is defined as the threat of touching in an injurious way. Note that the person need not be touched in

any way for assault to occur. If the patient feels threatened and is made to believe that he or she will be touched in a harmful manner, an assault charge may be justified. To avoid this possibility, the radiographer must explain what is to occur and reassure the patient in any situation where the threat of harm may be an issue. Never use threats to force the cooperation of either adult or pediatric patients.

Battery is defined as unlawful touching of a person without consent. If the patient refuses to be touched, that wish must be respected. Even the most well-intentioned touch may fall into this category if the patient has expressly forbidden it. This should not prevent the radiographer from placing a reassuring hand on the patient's shoulder as long as the patient has not forbidden it and when there is no intent to harm or to invade the patient's privacy. However, a radiograph taken against the patient's will or on the wrong patient could be construed as battery. This emphasizes the need for consistently double-checking the patient's identity and being certain that proper informed consent has been obtained for procedures that require it.

Intentional misconduct as discussed in this section often causes emotional distress in addition to any harm caused directly by the misconduct. For this reason, charges of intentionally inflicting emotional distress may be added to any of these other charges. Occasionally, such a charge may be made on its own merit without being accompanied by other charges of misconduct.

Unintentional Misconduct

Unintentional torts include negligence and malpractice. Negligence refers to the neglect or omission of reasonable care or caution. In the relationship between a professional person and a patient or client, the professional has a duty to provide reasonable care. An act of negligence in the context of such a relationship is defined as professional negligence or malpractice. The radiographer is held to the standard of care and skill of the "reasonable radiographer" in similar circumstances.

> The standard of reasonable care is based on the doctrine of the reasonably prudent person. This standard requires a person to perform as any reasonable person would perform under similar circumstances.

You may also hear the terms *gross negligence, contributory negligence,* and *corporate negligence.* Gross negligence is a negligent act that involves "reckless disregard for life or limb." It denotes a higher degree of negligence than ordinary negligence and results in more serious penalties. Contributory negligence is an act of negligence in which the behavior of the injured party contributed to the injury. Corporate negligence applies when the hospital as an entity is negligent.

To legally establish a claim of malpractice, a claimant must prove to the court's satisfaction that four conditions are true:

1. The defendant (person or institution being sued) had a duty to provide reasonable care to the patient.
2. The patient sustained some loss or injury.
3. The defendant is the party responsible for the loss.
4. The loss is attributable to negligence or improper practice.

The doctrine of *res ipsa loquitur* literally means "the thing speaks for itself." This doctrine is sometimes applied when negligence and loss are so apparent that they would be obvious to anyone. For example, if a patient who has had surgery is demonstrated to have a surgical instrument inside his body at the surgical site, the fact of the instrument's presence establishes the negligence of the surgeon.

Although a patient may sustain some loss, the court must be convinced that the loss is a result of negligent care or treatment before the patient is entitled to damages. Usually a determination of negligence is based on whether the usual standards and procedures were followed. However, a patient may prove that someone was negligent, but not be entitled to damages unless it can be demonstrated that a loss occurred as a result. Nonetheless, it is inexcusable to be complacent about negligence simply because there was "no harm done," or to be callous about loss just because the accepted and established procedures were followed.

Because malpractice lawsuits against physicians and hospitals are becoming increasingly common, the rates for malpractice insurance coverage have soared. This topic is of serious concern to all health professionals. There has been much discussion concerning whether radiographers should carry malpractice insurance. Hospitals carry liability insurance that covers the negligence of employees acting in the course of their employment. Radiographers must familiarize themselves about the extent of malpractice coverage in their institutions.

Traditionally, there has been a tendency to place legal responsibility on the highest authority possible. For instance, according to the legal doctrine of *respondeat superior* ("let the master respond"), the employer is liable for employees' negligent acts that occur in the course of their work. The liability by one person or agency for the actions of another is called *vicarious liability.* According to the doctrine of the "borrowed servant," a physician may be liable for wrongful acts committed by hospital employees under the physician's orders. Under these doctrines, the actions of radiographers may result in lawsuits against their employers or against the physicians with whom they work.

In recent years, however, the "rule of personal responsibility" has been increasingly applied. This means that each person is liable for his or her own negligent conduct. Under this rule, the law does not allow the wrongdoer to escape responsibility, even though someone else may be legally liable as well. Although radiographers themselves are seldom named specifically in malpractice lawsuits, the rule of personal responsibility has resulted in some unfavorable judgments against radiographers as individuals.

Some believe that the increasing application of the rule of personal responsibility places the radiographer in legal jeopardy, and for this reason they should be protected by their own liability insurance policies. The ASRT sponsors the provision of professional liability coverage on a group basis, which indicates that this organization believes such coverage is important. The possibility of losing personal assets such as one's home may provide motivation for joining such a plan.

MEDICAL INFORMATION AND RECORDS

Effective Documentation

Effective documentation of information about patients and their care marks the professional who acknowledges efficient record keeping as a means to meet ongoing patient needs. Attention to clerical details may seem to be a nonprofessional function, but dates, account numbers, chart numbers, Social Security numbers, and similar data are necessary for your institution and the patients it serves. While different forms and types of data are used to meet the needs of various departments, certain terms are commonly used. Charting refers to any records you are expected to add to a document for the patients chart.

In most imaging departments, the majority of record keeping is done with requisition forms or within a computerized radiology-specific ordering system, both of which usually have a limited area for documentation. A chart usually refers to a more extensive compilation of information, such as an emergency department record, the chart brought with a patient who is hospitalized, or an online record.

The forms may vary according to your institution or department, but any written records you initiate must be accurate, pertinent, and legible. These medical records include not only written information on the condition of the patient, medications, and treatments, but also laboratory results, radiographs, and any other information that pertains to the health and welfare of the patient.

Medical Recording on Computers

Health care providers today use computers extensively for clerical functions (Figure 5-2). Unlike in the business world, where every individual in an office has a personal computer, it is more common in hospitals and radiology suites for computers to be strategically located and for the staff to use any computer that is convenient. Under these circumstances, using the computer system for personal communications is inappropriate. Your ability to log on to a hospital computer may be protected by a password or barcode identification that must be scanned. These systems are used to maintain the security of all information stored on the computer network. The files and types of information that you are authorized to access may be limited.

> Be sure to log off your computer workstation when you are finished using the computer to prevent unauthorized access to confidential medical records. Never give out your password or lend your barcode to anyone.

Access to a patient's *e-chart*, or electronic medical record, supplies basic information about the patient, such as the room number, birth date, medical record number, and next of kin, as well as the diagnosis, test results, treatment, and other observations pertinent to patient care. Computers are also used for scheduling, generating requisitions, billing, or entering charges when procedures have been completed. However, computers are only capable of using the information provided to them. If data are incorrect or incomplete, the computer may not be able to right the error and may reject the entire entry. Most hospitals provide in-service instructions applicable to their computer systems.

Responsibilities for Record Keeping

Health care agencies are also businesses. Proper record keeping is required to ensure that patients are billed accurately, that new supplies are ordered, and that insurance companies receive verification of the care given to their clients. Failure to process information accurately and promptly can inconvenience your coworkers and pose serious problems for patients.

The chief reason for keeping accurate, pertinent medical records is to provide data about the patient's progress and current status for other health team members. This prevents the need for repetitious diagnostic examinations by various professionals, and it encourages a systematic approach to therapeutic care, allowing for longitudinal comparisons that facilitate a more comprehensive approach to extended health care. Well-kept records also serve as a resource for research investigations.

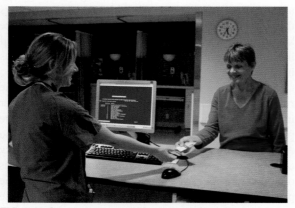

FIG 5-2 Computers simplify clerical functions in imaging departments.

Accountability is an essential term when referring to the medicolegal aspects of patient care. We cannot overemphasize the importance of correct record keeping. It is also crucial for medical records to be objective. For example, do not chart "patient is confused," because this does not demonstrate how you came to this conclusion. "Patient appears unable to relate why he is in hospital and who or what brought him here," is a clearer statement. Objectivity is particularly important when handling situations that have a strong potential for legal action, such as motor vehicle crashes. "Too drunk to climb on x-ray table" is not a validated clinical judgment. "Appeared uncoordinated, staggered severely, and was unable to climb on x-ray table without assistance; strong odor of alcohol on breath and clothing," is an objective statement.

Poorly kept medical records are often a major contributing factor when a defensible court case is lost. They may also play a significant role in cases of inappropriate billing or lack of financial reimbursement. Charting should be complete, objective, consistent, and accurate.

Paper charts require care to ensure they are legible. The following list alerts you to some rules for avoiding the mistakes frequently found when paper charts are audited:

- To delete an entry, simply draw a line through it; do not erase or use correction fluid.
- Always initial and date corrections.
- Never leave blanks on forms. Insert "NA" or "0."
- Never insert loose or gummed slips of paper.
- Always include all four digits of the year when writing a patient's date of birth. Your facility may require you to include all four digits of the year on all entries.
- Date and sign entries that you make, and include your title.

Remember that all information in patient records is considered permanent and confidential. The chart is a legal document that can substantiate or refute charges of negligence or malpractice and can also serve as a record of behavior, which may set a precedent. The course of treatment and quality of care are reflected in the chart.

The Chart as a Resource

For a radiographer's purposes, information on a patient may be found in multiple locations, and it is difficult to definitively predict where that may be from hospital to hospital. The chart is frequently your most accessible resource.

Patient medical records can be in paper or electronic format (e-charts), or both. Many organizations are transitioning from one system to another with the intent that all records will eventually be computerized. E-charts are advantageous because they are more legible than handwriting, more easily stored, and accessible from multiple locations both within and without the health care facility.

Although the organization of paper charts may vary, certain elements are consistent. Often there is a brief "at a glance" card (Figure 5-3) located near the front of the chart that lists basic patient medical information, such as the DNR/DNI status, room location, allergies, and other alerts. Allergic sensitivities are also indicated in red on the chart cover and stated in the history. The diagnosis or impression is found at the conclusion of the history. The patient's current status is found in the physicians' notes and nurses' notes, or in the joint progress notes. When a patient is admitted to the hospital, the health care team will compose a limited list of pertinent problems and develop a plan of care. Based on the plan of care, the nurses document the goals and outcomes of patient care. Usually the medication record and orders for diagnostic studies will be found in the orders section of the chart. Laboratory reports, radiology reports, and results of other studies are found in a separate section. The recording of pulse, blood pressure, and temperature in a graph format allows for a longitudinal comparison. E-charts have menus or tabs for quick access to the sections of the record (Figure 5-4). Much of the information recorded in e-charts is in the form of checking items on printed lists.

To reduce the time involved in the charting process, as well as the volume of hospital records, charting is a somewhat streamlined form of written communication. Many frequently used words are abbreviated, and comments are made in the form of brief phrases rather than complete sentences. Some practice is needed for beginners to translate this jargon accurately. The lists of abbreviations and terms in Appendix C are helpful to students learning to use medical charts.

Medical Recording by Radiographers

How you record data will depend on the system in place in your facility. E-charts can be used independently or in conjunction with other computer information or ordering systems. It is your duty to understand the proper documentation procedure.

Some facilities will have e-charts that are separate from the imaging-specific documentation or recording system.

```
┌─────────────────────────────────────────────────────────────────────────────────┐
│  ┌─────────────────────────────┐                                                  │
│  │     AT A GLANCE             │                                                  │
│  │  PATIENT INFORMATION CARD   │      PATIENT IDENTIFICATION                      │
│  └─────────────────────────────┘                                                  │
```

AT A GLANCE PATIENT INFORMATION CARD

PATIENT IDENTIFICATION

Date/Time: _____

Situation (diagnosis): _____

Background: **Mode of Transportation for tests:** ☐ Wheelchair ☐ Stretcher ☐ Bed

| **Allergies:** ☐ No   ☐ Latex Sensitivity
☐ Yes—If yes, see Admission Home Medication Report
red clip on arm band | **Code Status:**   ☐ DNR—purple clip on arm band
Height: _____   Admit Weight: _____ kg |

Special Care:

☐ Seizure Precautions ☐ Fall Risk—yellow clip on arm band **Isolation** ☐ Airborne ☐ Contact ☐ Enteric ☐ Droplet ☐ Skin Issues—fragile skin ☐ Head of Bed ↑ 30° ☐ Flat ☐ Other:_____	☐ Blind ☐ Impaired Vision ☐ Deaf ☐ Hard of Hearing ☐ Limited English Proficient (LEP) Primary Language: _____ Able to read/write in primary language ☐ Yes ☐ No ☐ Diabetic ☐ Mental Health Advance Directive ☐ Risk to harm self or others ☐ Other _____

Obstetrics: ☐ Adoption ☐ Demise   **LOC:** ☐ Alert/Oriented ☐ Confused ☐ Other: _____

Special Equipment: ☐ O$_2$ @ _____ liters ☐ IV ☐ Telemetry ☐ Drains ☐ Foley ☐ NG

Assessment: _____

Recommendations: _____

Safety Check: ☐ RN Notified   ☐ Oxygen resumed   ☐ Bed in low position
              ☐ Monitor tech notified ☐ Call light and bedside table within reach ☐ HEV status updated

NOT A PERMANENT PART OF THE MEDICAL RECORD

FIG 5-3 Often there is a brief "at a glance" sheet located near the front of the chart that lists basic patient medical information.

In this case, imaging departments have their own **radiology information management system (RIMS)** that allows the technologist access to pertinent and limited information about a patient. It is here that one can learn about a patient's room number, allergies, laboratory values, and a listing of imaging procedures performed, along with their associated radiology reports of imaging and other diagnostic tests. The RIMS also allows for ordering and billing of imaging examinations. However, no other information about a patient's health history or plan of care is available in the RIMS; for this, the technologist must reference the patient's complete e-chart or paper chart, which may also be the location to check the physician's order and the document completion of an examination.

Other facilities will have an all-encompassing e-chart that shows relatively the same view for both the radiographer and physician and the nursing staff members. All staff members have access to the same information, and any imaging examination performed is documented within this system.

Requisitions and reports are forms of particular importance to radiographers. A paper x-ray requisition can serve as the order for a diagnostic procedure. It includes patient data, a brief medical history, and specific instructions. In some situations, it may be part of a multiple-copy form that is eventually used to record the radiologist's report. Both the requisition and the report are medicolegal records and may be filed with the images or separately. Most often, they are scanned into the picture archiving and communication system (PACS) with the correlating images. All inpatient reports become part of a patient chart. Most hospitals have either computed or digital radiography with PACS, and the radiologists' reports are often likewise dictated and transcribed electronically. The report for an examination can be made available on PACS and within the patient's e-chart or RIMS, or all three.

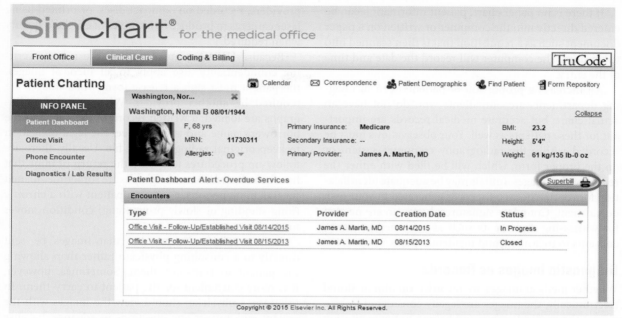

FIG 5-4 E-charts have menus or tabs for quick access to the sections of the record. (From Elsevier: Practice Management for the Medical Office Powered by SimChart for the Medical Office, St. Louis, 2016, Elsevier.)

Copies of the radiologist's report can be printed for the ordering physician or the patient, or they can be kept in the paper chart for reference.

Although radiographers are not responsible for initiating these records, they rely on requisitions for specific information about each examination they perform. They may also refer to previous reports for information about the patient's problem or the radiologist's recommendations for further studies. Any examination-specific information that needs to be communicated to the radiologist can be recorded on the requisition and then scanned into the computer system.

Documenting certain information about a patient's care in the medical record may be the radiographer's responsibility. This documentation could include the administration of contrast media or medications, changes in patient status, and reactions to contrast or medications, as well as any treatment received in the radiology department. Examples of such treatment include oxygen given to a patient who becomes short of breath or cold packs applied to the site when an intravenous line has infiltrated.

When paper charts are used, inpatient charts usually accompany patients to the imaging department. This chart is where you would record changes in status, medications, and treatments. In your hospital, the information to be recorded may be placed in chart pages titled *Nurses' Notes, Progress Notes,* or *Medication Records.* In some hospitals, completion of the procedure is routinely charted by the radiographer in the nurses' notes or on the order for the examination, or both. The information you chart should include the date, the time (using the 24-hour clock; for example, 2:15 PM is charted as 14:15), a specific statement of what occurred, and your signature. When charting observations or treatments on behalf of the radiologist, include the radiologist's name followed by a slash mark and your signature. Although nurses often use only initials to identify their entries, they are part of a small group repeatedly using the chart, and their initials with their full names are recorded elsewhere on a signature page in the chart for legal verification. When radiographers chart, they should use a full signature and a designation of their department or position so that identification is clear.

If there is no paper chart, patient information can be entered directly into the computer or written on a paper document such as a requisition that is then scanned into the system. The computer will record the date and time of the entry.

An increasing proportion of patients seen in imaging departments are outpatients who do not have an actual chart, but accurate medical records are important for these patients as well. Your observations must be recorded within the radiography computer system or on the proper form, which will be filed with either the report or the images. Initials may be adequate identification for routine notes on records generated in your own department. Complete signatures, however, are needed for witnessing documents such as informed consents, consents to treatment, and incident reports.

Diagnostic Images as Records

Whether medical images are recorded on film or stored electronically, the images are legally considered to be a part of the medical record and belong to the institution in which they are made. Patients often assume that the images belong to them because they have paid for the examination. Tact is required when explaining that the charges cover the expense of the procedure and that every effort will be made to ensure that the images are available when and wherever they may be needed to assist in the patient's care.

State laws vary on the length of time images must legally be kept on file. Usually the retention period is 5 to 7 years, with the additional requirement that images of minors be kept 5 to 7 years after the patient reaches majority or legal age (18 to 21 years, depending on the state).

Because charts can be photocopied easily, original documents are never allowed to leave the health care facility. Radiographs are more difficult to duplicate, however, and the quality of a duplicate is never equal to that of the original. For this reason, it is often helpful for original films to be made available for comparison or consultation outside the institution of origin. Many hospitals are undergoing digitization of plain films to facilitate their storage and provide easier reproducibility. Digital images from computed radiography, direct digital imaging systems, or computer-assisted modalities—including computed tomography (CT), magnetic resonance imaging (MRI), positron emission tomography, and ultrasound—can be sent electronically to other

providers, recorded on compact discs, or printed using laser cameras to produce hard copies of excellent quality when required.

Because HIPAA regulations and the rules governing confidentiality also apply to all medical images, the patient must sign a release form when images are required by another provider. When original radiographs are loaned, a written record of the date and the borrower's name and address meet the legal obligation to keep original radiographs on file. Usually, there are follow-up procedures to ensure the return of films that have been loaned, but radiographs are sometimes loaned for indefinite periods, as when a patient with a **chronic** (long-standing or slowly progressing) condition moves to another state.

It is usually recommended that images be sent directly to a consulting physician rather than allowing the patient to transport them. Sometimes, however, it is more convenient for the patient to carry them. In this case, a physician should view the images with the patient and answer any questions in advance, because the patient's curiosity may result in an attempt to interpret the images. This can lead to unnecessary confusion and anxiety. For example, patients have been known to assume that a heart shadow is a lung tumor or that a gas bubble in the stomach indicates a serious disease.

ACCIDENTS AND INCIDENT REPORTS

Any fall, accident, or occurrence that results in injury or potential harm must be reported immediately to the departmental supervisor or radiologist, or both. As soon as the victim has been properly attended to, complete an incident report (sometimes called an *unusual occurrence form*). Reporting incidents is essential whether the victim is a patient, visitor, or member of the hospital staff. Do not hesitate to report incidents in which you are injured, even if the injury may seem minor at the time. If the injured person is a patient, the details of the incident must also be recorded in the patient's chart. Do not mention the chart entry in the incident report.

Incident reports are crucial to the institution's risk management program. The reports assist in establishing or limiting institutional liability for any injury and in documenting the need for changes that may improve safety practices in the future. Appendix D provides an example of a hospital incident report form.

Occasionally, a very minor incident might not seem to require the formal procedures of an incident report. It is always a good idea to keep a record of any unusual occurrence in case it should later prove to be of greater consequence than was originally apparent. Making a note of such events in the patient's chart or on the requisition form provides an important record if questions or consequences develop with respect to the event.

Deciding whether a particular occurrence merits an incident report is a judgment call. For example, while a simple sneeze should not prompt an incident report, a severe asthmatic attack is a reportable occurrence. A mild asthmatic episode that is successfully self-treated by an outpatient with his/her own medication is an example of a situation in which judgment will vary from individual to individual. The ability to make these kinds of judgment calls develops with experience. The student radiographer should consult a supervisor when such questions arise. When in doubt, err on the side of caution by filing a report. Remember to keep the report details concise, clear, and objective.

MALPRACTICE PREVENTION

Lawsuits can result in conflict, expense, professional embarrassment, and loss of the public's confidence, even when the plaintiff is denied any award. As a result, there is a great need for caution, both in the interests of patient care and to avoid possible malpractice claims.

Research indicates that lawsuits are likely when patients feel alienated from the people providing their care. When a trusting professional relationship is established, lawsuits are less likely to occur. With this in mind, you can minimize the risk of medicolegal problems by remembering and applying the seven Cs of malpractice prevention listed in Box 5-3.

Proper patient identification (see Chapter 12), accuracy in medication administration (see Chapter 14), and compliance with patient safety requirements (see Chapters 10 and 12) are other positive steps the radiographer can take to avoid malpractice suits. Harm can result from contrast media administered without the proper precautions (see Chapter 19) or when reactions are not immediately identified and appropriately treated (see Chapter 16). Poor image quality poses a potential for misdiagnosis that can have serious consequences for both the patient and the radiographer. Because the possibility for harmful error is often greatest in stressful

---

BOX 5-3 The Seven *Cs* of Malpractice Prevention

Competence. Knowing and adhering to professional standards and maintaining professional competence reduce liability exposure.

Compliance. The compliance by health professionals with the policies and procedures in the medical office and hospital avoids patient injuries and litigation.

Charting. Charting completely, consistently, and objectively can be the best defense against a malpractice claim.

Communication. Patient injuries and resulting malpractice cases can be avoided by improving communications among health care professionals.

Confidentiality. Protecting the confidentiality of medical information is the legal and ethical responsibility of health professionals.

Courtesy. A courteous attitude and demeanor can improve patient rapport and lessen the likelihood of lawsuits.

Caution. Personal injuries can occur unexpectedly on the premises and may lead to lawsuits. (See Chapter 10.)

Reprinted with the permission of David Karp, loss prevention manager for the Medical Insurance Exchange of California.

---

situations, appropriate responses in an emergency help to minimize risk.

> **!** An appropriate response to an urgent situation depends on your level of experience and education, so do not hesitate to ask questions and receive help when necessary.

You can also help to protect the patient and the institution by reporting illegal or unethical professional activities to the proper authorities. In such a situation, you must be neither too zealous nor too hesitant. A simple, written statement that includes the facts (dates, times, names, and places), but avoids any judgments or conclusions, should be prepared as soon as possible after the occurrence. This statement should be submitted to the appropriate person, usually your immediate supervisor unless he or she was also involved in the incident. The supervisor receiving such a report is responsible for ensuring that it is given to the proper authority, who must then follow up with an investigation. A single report may not produce any change, but it can add strength to other reports or lead to increased supervision where needed.

SUMMARY

- Job satisfaction is a product of a good professional attitude coupled with conscientious self-care, an empathetic response to patients, and precautions to avoid burnout. Participation in professional activities is expected; it promotes professional growth, assists colleagues, supports the profession, and helps to maintain interest in our work.

- Professional behavior involves moral, legal, and ethical implications for our actions. Morals are right actions dictated by conscience; *ethics* are defined as the systematic application of moral principles; and laws are the means used by government to enforce commonly accepted moral standards in the interests of society. The ethical standards of a profession are defined by its published code of ethics.

- The ASRT, together with the ARRT, has developed and published the *Standards of Ethics for the Profession of Radiologic Technology.* These standards include the *Code of Ethics,* which is an aspirational document, and the *Rules of Ethics,* which are mandatory, enforceable minimum standards of conduct.

- Ethical analysis is a means of solving ethical dilemmas that involves four basic steps: identifying the problem, considering possible solutions, selecting the best solution, and defending the chosen solution. The moral agent is the person designated to implement the ethical solution.

- Patients have many rights guaranteed by law, such as the right to privacy and confidentiality, and the right to access information contained in their records. They also have other rights that are a matter of ethics and moral decency, such as the right to considerate and respectful care. The American Hospital Association has developed a comprehensive Patient Care Partnership statement (formerly called the *Patient Rights Statement*), and others also exist.

- Informed consent is the process through which a patient receives an explanation of the risks and benefits of a procedure and agrees in writing to participate in it. The process produces a legal document that is required for any procedures that involve substantial risk. Patients can revoke their permission at any time before or during the procedure. Radiographers must be aware of the procedures they perform that require informed consent, and be certain that the necessary documents are in order before beginning the procedure.

- It is generally considered that patients have a right to die with dignity when they can no longer sustain life. DNR orders may be issued by a physician in consultation with the patient or the patient's family when there is little hope that the patient will recover to resume a normal life. Patients may execute an advance directive or appoint a power of attorney for health care to ensure that their wishes will be carried out if they are unable to communicate them at a future date.

- Criminal law deals with felonies and misdemeanors, crimes against the state punishable by fines or imprisonment. Theft, fraud, and some drug-related crimes are examples of felonies. Misdemeanors are lesser crimes, such as misrepresentation of information or practicing outside the scope of ones credentials; these are usually punished by fines.

- Torts are violations of civil law, intentional misconduct, or negligence that cause harm to another person. The types of intentional misconduct that may be related to providing health care include assault, battery, false imprisonment, invasion of privacy, libel, and slander.

- Negligence is the neglect or omission of reasonable care or caution based on the standard of the reasonably prudent person.

- The patient chart is an important resource for patient information and a record of the quality of care. All written medical records must be accurate, pertinent, and legible. Computerized charting is common and requires standard procedures for the correct use of the system, and to preserve confidentiality.

- Diagnostic images form part of the medical record and are subject to requirements for retention and confidentiality as are other medical records.

- When an unusual occurrence results in harm or potential harm to a patient, health care worker, or visitor, provide assistance to the victim, notify your supervisor, and complete an incident report form to assist the institution in risk management. If the victim is a patient, record the event in the chart as well.

- Radiographers should be aware of the potential for acts of negligence and take care to limit legal liability by ensuring that no harm comes to the patient. Following established procedures and documenting your actions will limit risk and assist in defense if there is a suit. Lawsuits are rare when there is a trusting relationship between the patient and those providing the care.

REVIEW QUESTIONS

1. A moral agent is one who:
   A. behaves correctly
   B. is responsible for implementing an ethical decision
   C. judges the morality of others
   D. analyzes ethical dilemmas
2. "A response in which understanding and compassion are accompanied by an objective detachment that enables you to act appropriately." This phrase describes the characteristic of:
   A. aggressiveness
   B. assertiveness
   C. empathy
   D. sympathy
3. Which of the following is not a component of ethical analysis?
   A. Identifying the problem
   B. Determining who is at fault
   C. Developing alternative solutions
   D. Defending your selection
4. The neglect or omission of reasonable care or caution in the context of a professional relationship is termed:
   A. malfeasance
   B. malpractice
   C. misdemeanor
   D. malapropism
5. Which of the following statements about diagnostic images is true?
   A. They do not need to be kept confidential because they do not contain written information.
   B. They belong to the patient when they have been paid for by the patient or his or her insurance company.
   C. They are part of the legal medical record.

D. They may be discarded or deleted as soon as the report has been sent to the patient's physician.
6. Arm and leg restraints applied without either the patient's permission or a physician's order could result in charges of:
   A. false imprisonment
   B. negligence
   C. invasion of privacy
   D. battery
7. Standards of correct behavior by professional groups are called:
   A. morals
   B. Codes of Ethics
   C. torts
   D. regulations
8. A patient has the right to revoke consent with regard to a risky procedure:
   A. before the procedure begins
   B. during the procedure
   C. after the procedure ends
   D. both A and B
9. Health care providers may disclose a patient's protected health information without the patient's consent to:
   A. another physician providing care to the patient
   B. the patient's employer
   C. the patient's family
   D. the news media
10. In which state is there a law protecting a patient's right to die with dignity?
    A. Texas
    B. Alaska
    C. Oregon
    D. Wyoming

Answers can be found in the Answer Key on pages 429-431.

CRITICAL THINKING EXERCISES

1. Jon Russell, age 64, was brought to the hospital emergency department on Sunday afternoon for problems with his right ankle. Several days before admission, he stepped in a hole while carrying a heavy box, and the swelling had not gone down with frequent applications of ice and the use of a firm support bandage. Carol, the radiographer on duty, was reassuring, even though a busy schedule caused her to delay her lunch break once more. After positioning the ankle and completing and processing the images, she sent them to the emergency department physician on call and went to lunch. Dr. Coal, the emergency department physician, looked at the images and said to Mr. Russell, "Well, these images are less than perfect

■ CRITICAL THINKING EXERCISES—cont'd

but I do not see a fracture. You should stay off the ankle as much as possible, continue to use ice and your support bandage, and elevate your leg as often as you can." On Monday, the radiologist decided that the images were not diagnostic and Mr. Russell was asked to return for additional radiographs. The final diagnosis was that Mr. Russell had suffered an avulsion fracture of the distal tibia. Although Mr. Russell only suffered some inconvenience and no litigation was ever involved, do you think Carol was guilty of negligence? What do you think she should have done?

2. At lunchtime, the cafeteria was full of employees and visitors. Sandy, a new radiographer, saw her friend, Janet, and sat down to eat and chat. "Wow, did we have a mouthy patient just before lunch!" she said. "Do you remember that Laura Moss who runs the dress shop downtown? She was so drunk she apparently fell down and broke her leg! I could hear her in the next room; and when I looked in on them, they were giving her some kind of stuff to calm her down." A chair at the next table was pushed back abruptly. "That is completely untrue! My wife was not drunk. She tripped and fell on the stairs. The medication was glucose because she was having an insulin reaction." A formal complaint was subsequently filed with the hospital administration. Were Sandy's comments wrong? If so, what was her offense? Was she merely rude, or is there possible cause for litigation?

3. Jenny Peterson has a history of Crohn's disease, an inflammatory condition of the colon. She is a frequent patient in your imaging department and has returned today for another barium enema. She is extremely apprehensive about the outcome of this procedure. She shares with you that her physician will want her to have her entire colon removed if the barium enema reveals new areas of involvement. Because you have developed a relationship with this patient, she asks you what you think about her physician's decision. She also asks whether you think she should get another opinion if her physician recommends surgery. How should you respond to her questions? What issues should you consider when developing possible solutions and selecting the best one to handle this dilemma?

4. Jack Roberts is concerned that the afternoon supervisor is complacent about the poor performance of another radiographer in the department. The radiographer, Gene Smith, comes to work each afternoon heavily medicated because of chronic back problems. His skills and judgment are adversely affected because of the medication. Jack knows that this radiographer has a high repeat rate, fails to follow department protocols, is rude to patients, and just recently x-rayed the wrong patient. The supervisor is aware of Mr. Smith's deficiencies, but takes no action because Mr. Smith and he have been friends for many years. Mr. Roberts would like to discuss this with the radiology manager, but is concerned about how it will affect his relationship with the supervisor. List at least four possible solutions to Mr. Smith's dilemma. From your list, identify the most appropriate solution and the one that is least appropriate.

5. Joyce Easton, a former classmate, tells to you that although she passed the ARRT examination, she has not yet obtained her state license because the cost is more than $100 and she cannot spare that much money. She is working as a technologist in a local medical office. She confides that her employer knows that she does not have a license, but he has told her he is satisfied that she is adequately qualified, and that if she gets into trouble about the license, it is her problem. Ms. Easton's employer is not aware that he can be legally penalized under his state law for allowing a nonlicensed radiographer to use ionizing radiation on human beings. List at least five possible responses to hearing this information. One possible response would be for you to take no action at all. From this list, identify the most appropriate action and the one that is least appropriate.

6. While you are helping Ella Christopherson into a wheelchair, she puts her weight on the footrest causing the chair to bump her leg. Mrs. Christopherson says, "Ouch!" and rubs her leg; but when you ask whether she is all right, she smiles and insists that she is fine. Should you file an incident report? Why or why not? How could this incident have been prevented?

7. What are the possible consequences to the patient and to the radiographer when a radiographer fails to be objective and accountable in record keeping?

6

Professional Attitudes and Communications

OBJECTIVES

At the conclusion of this chapter, the student will be able to:

- List examples of how members of diverse groups may approach health care.
- Understand how cultural diversity may influence or affect the communication process and how to communicate effectively with patients whose cultural background is different from your own.
- Meet legal and clinical requirements when communicating with patients whose ability to communicate is impaired and those who do not speak English.
- Communicate effectively when using an interpreter for foreign language speakers or for the deaf.
- Describe the significance of nonverbal communication and demonstrate five examples.
- Establish rapport with patients in the process of greeting them and obtaining information.
- Compare assertive and aggressive behavior.
- Discriminate between assumed and validated statements.

- Discriminate between therapeutic and nontherapeutic communication strategies.
- Define the term *valid choice* and give an example that might be typical of a patient care situation in radiology.
- Describe age-specific approaches for infants, children, adults, and the elderly in the radiology department.
- Compare approaches for dealing with deaf patients to those that apply to patients with moderate hearing loss.
- List the two most important points to be remembered when dealing with patients in an altered state of consciousness.
- List the stages of grief and describe successful approaches for dealing with those who are grieving.
- Communicate effectively in stressful situations and respond appropriately to individuals who are hostile or threatening.
- State how communication skills learned in this chapter can be used to improve relationships with patients' families and with coworkers.

OUTLINE

Issues of Cultural Diversity
    The Scope of Diversity
    Culturally Significant Attitudes that Can Affect
      Communication
    How Cultural Issues Can Affect Care
    Professional Responsibility and Ethics
      in Relation to Diversity
Communication Skills
    Nonverbal Communication
    Listening Skills
    Verbal Skills
    Attitude
    Validation of Communication
    Communication under Stress
Communication with Patients
    Therapeutic Communication
    Addressing the Patient
    Valid Choices
    Avoiding Assumptions
    Assessment through Communication
Special Circumstances that Affect Communication
    Patients Who Do Not Speak English
    The Hearing Impaired

    Deafness
    Impaired Vision
    Inability to Speak
    Impaired Mental Function
    Altered States of Consciousness
Age-Specific Communication
    Neonate and Infant (Birth to 1 Year)
    Toddler (1–2 Years)
    Preschooler (3–5 Years)
    School Age (6–12 Years)
    Adolescent (13–18 Years)
    Young Adult (19–45 Years)
    Middle Adult (46–64 Years)
    Late Adult (65–79 Years) and Old Adult
      (80 Years and Older)
Patient Education
Communication with Patients' Families
Dealing with Death and Loss
Communication with Coworkers

KEY TERMS

ageism
aggressiveness
aphasia
assertiveness
autonomy
chronic

diagnosis
electrolarynx
ethnic
hospice
oncology
palliative

prognosis
regimen
therapeutic communication
valid choice

Communication skills, manners, and professional attitudes can have a powerful effect on your environment, your mood and efficiency, and the responses of those around you. In this context, to communicate means to convey information accurately, to express oneself clearly, and to have an interchange of ideas and information with others. **Attitude** is a state of mind, an opinion, or a feeling often revealed by body position, tone of voice, or other nonverbal signals. **Manners** are customs that express respect and are sometimes referred to as the oil that makes daily contacts run smoothly.

Accurate communication among health care workers is essential for patient care. The ability to give instructions depends on the speaker being clear and precise. The listener, however, is equally responsible for attentive and receptive behavior. The rapport we establish with patients and coworkers by listening attentively and responding in a meaningful way can be overlooked under the pressures of a busy schedule. Stress in the workplace can accelerate rapidly when interpersonal communication breaks down and good manners are neglected.

Because culture has profound effects on our attitudes and on the ways in which we perceive others and communicate with them, this chapter addresses issues of cultural diversity before discussing the communication process. When cultural differences are not recognized and respected, relationships suffer and communication becomes much less effective.

Until recently, much of the direct health care in the United States was administered by providers of Anglo-European descent. There was little sensitivity to the importance of differences between cultures. Businesses and industries, and especially the health care industry, now appreciate the advantages of cultural diversity in the workforce and of cultural awareness in providing the best possible service to clients.

ISSUES OF CULTURAL DIVERSITY

A century ago, most communities in the United States could be described as culturally homogeneous. In 1900, only one in eight Americans was of a nonwhite race. The culture of the majority prevailed, and those who were "different" were expected to "fit in." This was especially true in rural areas and small towns. In cities, immigrants gathered in neighborhoods where their own languages and cultures prevailed and did their best to conform to the majority culture in the workplace. American society today, both urban and rural, is far more culturally diverse than in our great grandparents' day. Data from the U.S. Census Bureau indicate that, today, the ratio of nonwhites to whites is one in four, and by 2070 half of all Americans will be African American, Hispanic, Native American, Asian, or Pacific Islander. Although this diversity poses certain social problems, it also creates a vast richness and creative potential.

Cultural diversity is a global health care issue. Research suggests that there are differences in the outcomes of health care treatments that are related to race and ethnicity. Lawmakers have introduced legislation to address cultural inequities in health care.* The American Hospital Association supports the growing national focus on the elimination of racial and ethnic disparities in health care treatment and outcomes, and to this end also supports diversity in health management. Your hospital or health care facility must plan for excellence in transcultural care and expect staff members to develop

*The Healthcare Equality and Accountability Act–Family Care Act of 2005 (S. 1580/H.R. 3561) and The Fair Care Act of 2005 (S. 1929).

the attitudes and the knowledge required to help implement these plans.

The Scope of Diversity

The subject of ethnic and cultural diversity is complex and fills many textbooks. Within the scope of this book, it is impossible to anticipate the many diverse ethnic and cultural situations you will encounter as a radiographer. We hope that the limited examples in the discussion that follows will help to raise your awareness of those situations in which sensitivity is needed.

The racial and **ethnic** (national) characteristics of individuals were originally identified by specific areas of the globe. Africans came from Africa, Chinese from China, and so forth. In many cases, racial characteristics such as skin color, hair texture, and the shapes of facial features were identified with specific cultures as well as with ethnic origins.

Culture is determined by language and by the customs commonly observed. As opportunities for emigration and travel increased, it became more difficult to identify the national origin of a specific individual. For example, not all patients with Asian features speak an Asian language. The physical appearance of an individual may have no relation to how extensively he or she has integrated culturally into the mainstream of American life. A person who has recently arrived from Eastern Europe wearing the latest athletic shoes, a baseball cap, and blue jeans may speak little or no English, whereas a patient wearing a turban and a dashiki may have been born in Chicago and have ancestors who have lived there for generations.

> It can be misleading to generalize about the cultural attitudes and practices of any ethnic group, because individual variations within a group depend on many factors.

When cultural diversity is mentioned, customs relating to nationality may be the first things that come to mind. Our society consists of many different groups in addition to ethnic groups, however, and each has unique characteristics that can affect the values and perceptions of individuals within the group. Examples of such cultural groups include the following:

- Gender groups: Male or female
- Racial groups: Distinguished by skin color and other physical characteristics

- Generational groups: Generation Y (millennials), generation X, baby boomers, and the elderly
- Geographic groups: North or south; east coast or west coast; native cultures in Hawaii, Alaska, and on and around reservations, plus areas where ethnic culture endures because large numbers of immigrants from a certain country have settled there, such as Mexican influences along the southern borders of Texas and California and the Scandinavian heritage in Minnesota
- Sexual preference groups: Heterosexual, gay, lesbian, bisexual, and transgender
- Religious groups
- Groups based on nonracial physical characteristics: Blind, deaf, disabled, and/or obese
- Socioeconomic groups: Low income (unemployed, welfare recipients, uninsured, underinsured), middle income, or affluent
- Groups with various types of family structure: Singles, unmarried couples with and without children, traditional nuclear families, single mother or single father heads of households, parents with children and grandchildren, and large, close-knit extended families

Historically, certain groups have been subjected to discriminatory treatment, causing some individuals to have a high level of sensitivity about their group identity.

Culturally Significant Attitudes that Can Affect Communication

The relationship between culture and communication is an integral part of our everyday life. Our reactions and habits are learned from our parents, are passed down to our children, and largely govern the way we conduct our daily activities. Each society develops unwritten rules regarding such ordinary things as how close we stand when talking to another, where we touch another person in public, and other reflections of courtesy to those around us.

For example, it is important in many Asian societies to avoid placing another person in an embarrassing position. Harmony is to be promoted, and loud or aggressive behavior is considered a sign of poor manners. Asian patients may respond more positively to a soft, quiet tone of voice than to the brisk, assertive commands so easily adopted by many Americans when in a hurry. When apprehensive or nervous, Asian patients can become reticent and unsociable, which can hinder communication.

The cultural differences in nonverbal behaviors are also highly significant. For example, a Vietnamese patient may smile to cover up disturbed feelings. Repeated head nods may indicate respect for the individual speaking rather than agreement with the subject being discussed. Gestures, eye contact, and touch may have unintended meanings when perceived by someone from a culture that assigns different meanings to the same signals. For example, many Native Americans avoid direct eye contact, considering it a mark of disrespect. Many Asian societies make no eye contact during verbal communication and may resent direct eye contact, perceiving it as being impolite and an invasion of personal space. In countries with a high-density population, eye contact and touch are less acceptable among adults than in the United States. Pointing directly at an individual can be considered insulting in many cultural groups, including our own, but it can be especially offensive to Native Americans and certain Asian groups. Beckoning with the index finger is insulting to Filipinos and to Koreans.

In Hispanic culture, embracing, touching, and close proximity are easily accepted from familiar people. This may seem to contrast with a strong sense of modesty that can be demonstrated during physical examinations, so it is important to provide both men and women with ample gowns and covering during examinations in the imaging department.

To Native Americans, personal space is highly important, and although patients may embrace or touch others with whom they feel close, touching in a professional setting should be confined to that needed to provide health care.

An old superstition of Mediterranean origin is occasionally seen among Hispanic clients. The "evil eye" or *mal ojo* is thought to bring bad luck or illness if children are praised or admired without also being touched. When praising a child, it is wise to give a touch or pat while expressing admiration. Although the parents may no longer express belief in the evil eye, the ability of individuals to cause illness in a child by looking admiringly without touching is a strong superstition.

The best way to understand people of another culture is to get to know them personally. If your geographic area has a significant number of individuals from another culture, you can enrich your life and provide better care by learning as much as possible about ethnic groups with which you come into frequent contact. We hope that this discussion will heighten your awareness, not only of differences in ethnic backgrounds, but also of diversity within your own cultural group. The more sensitive you become to the reactions of all your patients, the more comfortable your interpersonal contacts will be.

How Cultural Issues Can Affect Care

Although this discussion is limited in scope, it should help to increase your awareness of the diversity of needs, expectations, and fears that may influence your patients in the health care setting. Box 6-1 provides some examples of how various ethnic cultural groups approach both communication and health care and how their cultural status can affect the outcome of their contacts with health care organizations. This listing is not comprehensive for all health care, but it offers insight into the cultural issues that can affect patient care in imaging departments. For example, family structure may determine who makes decisions, who expects to receive information, and who usually signs documents. Although specific practices are described here in association with specific cultural groups, it is important that you understand these descriptions as broad generalizations and do not use them in any way that would stereotype individuals.

Some ethnic cultures have a high level of sensitivity surrounding modesty and physical contact in health care. This may apply to any situation, but is most often an issue when the patient and the health care provider are not of the same gender, especially if the patient is female and the health care professional is male. These attitudes are particularly prevalent in both Hispanic and Islamic cultures, but are certainly not limited to these groups.

Research shows that women perceive health care more favorably than men do. In general, women are better informed about health care issues and more willing to talk about their health problems. Because men are less aware of health issues, they may fail to seek health care promptly when needed, hoping to avoid confronting what they do not understand. They may perceive the need for treatment as a sign of weakness or vulnerability. Touching while providing health care is also perceived more positively by women than by men. Women find it reassuring and comforting, whereas men find personal touch less positive.

Our elders can remember lives lost to infections, polio, whooping cough, and diphtheria before the days of antibiotics and vaccines. Having observed these advances in medicine, the majority of those over the age of 75 years came to think of medicine as miraculous and doctors as all powerful. This generation has faith in the medical establishment and is unlikely to question the need for any test, prescription, or intervention that doctors may recommend. However, members of the baby boom generation came of age at a formative stage in the late 1960s or in the 1970s. One of the catch phrases of that time was "Don't trust anyone over 30!" This attitude is reflected in a more conservative and questioning approach to the medical establishment. Generation X has taken this approach even further, as demonstrated by an increased willingness to seek alternative health care options.

Geographic differences in population size also affect health care. The availability of sophisticated health care services in cities has generally resulted in a higher level of expectation in urban areas. Even those in lower socioeconomic strata are likely to receive adequate health care through publicly funded facilities. In a rural setting, however, patients are less likely to have access to subsidized health care. In addition, the limited selection of available services and the constraints of distance often limit options and contribute to health care problems. Consider the plight of a middle-aged woman with rheumatoid arthritis who lives on a remote ranch. The nearest rheumatologist may be many miles away, and traveling to visit this specialist will be time-consuming, costly, and painful.

Although it cannot be said that there is universal tolerance for gay, lesbian, bisexual, and transgender groups, there is more public discussion and acceptance today than was apparent during the 20th century. Homosexual patients need to feel confident that disclosing their sexual preference will not compromise their health care or their insurability.

Religion can also be a significant factor in health care. Religion is almost synonymous with culture in some countries. For example, the religion of Islam predominates in the Middle East, Roman Catholicism is prevalent in Latin America, and Hinduism influences the culture of India, but all these regions have some religious diversity as well; for this reason it can be misleading to make assumptions about religion based on national origin.

BOX 6-1   Suggestions for Improving Communication and Care with Specific Ethnic Groups

Note that these are broad generalizations that might not apply to all members of a culture.

Anglo-American
- Patients expect to know and understand details of their conditions and treatments.
- Direct eye contact is expected; avoid excessive direct eye contact with members of the opposite sex to avoid any hint of sexual connotation.
- Emotional control is expected. Privacy is important and must be respected. Caregivers are usually welcome and expected to provide psychosocial care in addition to physical care.
- Decisions are made by individuals for themselves and may be made by either parent for a child.
- Independence is valued, and self-care concepts are generally accepted.
- Patients tend to be stoic when in pain, but may also feel comfortable requesting pain medication when needed.
- Patients may prefer to be left alone when they do not feel well.
- An aggressive biomedical treatment of illness is generally preferred, but complementary and alternative medicine may also be used. Germs are understood to be the cause of many illnesses, and antibiotic treatment may be expected.

African American
- Because of a history of slavery and discrimination, African American patients may not trust "white institutions" such as hospitals, and may be easily upset by what they perceive to be discrimination. Be especially sensitive to this issue.
- Do not refer to a man as a "boy" or a woman as a "gal." These terms are often perceived as insulting. Address individuals using their titles and last names.
- Family structure may be nuclear, extended, or matriarchal. Close friends may be a significant part of the support system. The father or eldest male may be the spokesperson or primary decision maker, although this authority often lies with the eldest female in a matriarchal family.
- They may believe that disease is caused by improper diet, exposure to cold or wind, punishment by God for sin, or voodoo spells. Cultural lore prescribes appropriate treatments for these causes. There is a rich African-American tradition of herbal and home remedies.
- Many have a present time orientation that can impede the implementation of preventive medicine and follow-up care.
- Blood or organ donation may not be acceptable except to meet the needs of family members.

Asian
- The patient may indicate agreement with no intention to follow through; therefore, it is important to explain reasons for compliance with instructions and to ask open-ended questions instead of those that can be satisfied with a "yes" or "no" answer.
- Avoid direct eye contact and hand gestures.
- Because there are no pronouns in most Asian languages, references to "he" or "she" may be confused.
- Wives may defer to husbands in decision making.
- Tremendous respect is accorded to the elderly.
- Patients may be reluctant to admit pain.
- Traditional healing methods include coining, cupping, the use of herbs, and changes in temperature.
- Stigma is associated with mental illness, and emotional problems are not discussed with strangers. Mental or emotional problems can manifest as physical illness.

East Indian
This group includes Hindus and Muslims (followers of Islam) from India, Pakistan, Bangladesh, Sri Lanka, and Nepal.
- Direct eye contact may be perceived as rude or disrespectful, especially among the elderly.
- Silence may indicate acceptance or approval.
- Head movements may confuse those from Western cultures. A side-to-side head motion may indicate agreement or uncertainty, while an up-and-down nod may indicate that the listener acknowledges what the speaker is saying but does not agree.
- Husbands may answer questions addressed to their wives.
- Men should avoid shaking hands with East Indian women unless the woman extends her hand first.
- The father or eldest son usually has decision-making power after other family members have been consulted. Patients might not wish to participate in health care decisions, considering health care professionals to be the authorities in these matters. This may affect their willingness to sign consent forms.
- Same-sex caregivers may be preferred for reasons of modesty.
- Patients may be either stoic or expressive when in pain. Muslim patients may not want pain medication except under extreme circumstances.

Hispanic
- Because of the emphasis on personal relationships, it is helpful to ask about a patient's family and interests before focusing on health issues.
- Family members are likely to want to stay with patients and assist them with activities of daily living rather than

BOX 6-1 Suggestions for Improving Communication and Care with Specific Ethnic Groups—cont'd

allowing these tasks to be done by professional care givers.

- Modesty is extremely important, especially to older women.
- Traditional wives will defer to their husbands for decisions that involve care for themselves or their children.
- Many have a present time orientation that can impede the implementation of preventive medicine and follow-up care.
- Patients may respond to pain with loud outcries, depending on the audience. Men may be more expressive around family members than with health professionals.
- Patients may refuse certain foods or medications that they believe will upset the body's hot-cold balance. Avoid ice water unless requested. A high fat content in food may be perceived as healthy.

Middle Eastern

- Islam is a dominant force in the lives of most Middle Easterners. Devout Muslims pray several times a day facing Mecca (east) and appreciate privacy for this practice. They may have a fatalistic attitude about life, death, and health, believing that these matters are in the hands of Allah and that health-related practices are of little consequence.
- There is a tendency to be loud and expressive, especially during childbirth, when someone has died, and when in pain.
- Family members may feel responsible for ensuring the best care possible, and so may make emphatic demands of health care personnel.
- Sexual segregation is extremely important; therefore, same-sex caregivers should be assigned whenever possible. Every effort must be made to maintain a woman's modesty at all times. Women do not wish to remove their headscarves (hijabs), especially in the presence of men.
- Women tend to defer to their husbands for decision-making involving their own and their children's health care. Husbands may answer questions addressed to their wives. When important information is sought or provided, it is considered appropriate to speak first with the family spokesperson.
- Organ donation or autopsy may not be permitted for religious reasons.
- Dampness, cold drafts, and strong emotions are sometimes thought to cause illness. The evil eye of envy may also be thought to cause illness or misfortune,

and amulets may be worn to prevent this; the amulet should not be removed.
- Muslims do not eat pork.

Native American

- Stories and metaphors may be used to communicate ideas. For example, a story about a neighbor who is ill may be a patient's way of describing his own symptoms.
- Long pauses in a conversation usually indicate that careful consideration is being given to a question. Do not rush the patient.
- Direct eye contact should be avoided, both as a show of respect and because some may believe that this threatens the loss or theft of their soul.
- Loud or aggressive behavior is considered offensive and should be avoided.
- Historical mistreatment of Native Americans groups by white people, and especially the misuse of signed documents in this regard, may cause Native Americans to be leery of documents or to be unwilling to sign informed consents or advance directives.
- Illness of one member is a concern to all members of the family, and the extended family is highly important. Patients usually make decisions for themselves, but this can vary with tribal and kinship structures. Hopi, Navajo, and Zuni tribes are matrilineal; in these groups, descent is reckoned through the female line, and women or their brothers make the important decisions.
- Orientation to time may be based on activities rather than the clock.
- Stoicism is valued, and patients might not express their pain other than to say they do not feel well. When a patient complains of discomfort and is not given relief, the complaint may never be repeated.
- Before cutting or shaving hair, check to see whether the patient or the family wants to keep it. In some tribes, cutting hair is associated with mourning.
- A medicine bag may be worn. Do not treat this casually or remove it without the patient's permission. If it must be removed, allow a family member to do so, keep it close to the patient, and return it as soon as possible.
- Native foods tend to be high in fat content. Foods that have been blessed (according to a traditional religion or Christianity) are believed to be free from harm.
- Traditional healing may be combined with the use of Western medicine. Allow traditional healers to perform rituals when possible and do not touch or casually admire their ritual objects.

Continued

BOX 6-1   Suggestions for Improving Communication and Care with Specific Ethnic Groups—Cont'd

Russian

- Family members will be anxious about patients and will expect frequent updates about progress, treatments, and tests.
- A warm, caring attitude on the part of caregivers is especially welcome.
- Loud, abrasive demands for attention may be a reflection of the fact that this attitude was necessary to meet one's needs in the Russian health care system.
- Direct eye contact and a firm, respectful attitude are comfortable. Address patients using titles and last names. Hand gestures and facial expression may be

used by patients, especially when not proficient in English. Gestures and facial expressions may also supplement understanding when used by caregivers.

- The gender of the caregiver is not usually an issue, but it may be desirable to have a family member of the same gender present when performing personal care.
- There is a tendency to have a high tolerance for pain and to be stoic in this regard.
- Many, especially the elderly, believe that illness results from cold; therefore, keep patients covered, close windows, keep the room warm, and avoid iced drinks.

Some religious groups dictate or prohibit specific health care practices. For example, some religions do not condone blood transfusions, some prohibit any practice that punctures the skin, and others oppose the practice of vaccination. Prayer and other religious healing practices may need to be accommodated in combination with medical treatments. Religious practices may influence the acceptability of certain diets or treatments and may dictate specific actions regarding matters of life and death. Religious dietary requirements, such as kosher meals for orthodox Jews, can affect a patient's choice of medical facilities and may affect compliance with the medical **regimen** (a system designed to provide benefit).

For patients with physical disabilities or with conditions such as sexually transmitted diseases or obesity, the major deterrent in seeking health care may have little to do with their condition, but may be powerfully influenced by the attitudes of insensitive health care providers. The young woman with cerebral palsy who is frowned on when seeking birth control, the deaf patient who feels ignored, the AIDS patient who is shunned, and the obese patient who is scolded rather than advised—all feel diminished and are likely to develop negative attitudes toward health care providers.

The inability to pay for health insurance prevents many people of lower socioeconomic status from planning and implementing a health care program. Even when these patients have access to a physician, they may be unable to purchase the prescriptions, foods, or medical supplies that are prescribed. Low-income employees often have less flexibility in their work schedules; therefore, the ability to keep health care appointments may

be affected by the need to keep a job. Limited financial resources may also prompt a patient to work when it would be a better health decision to take time off for rest and healing.

Until fairly recently, the term *family* referred to a father, a mother, and children. Grandparents, aunts, or uncles were sometimes also included. Contemporary dictionaries now define a family as "a group of individuals residing under one roof." Because divorce has become more common, many single parents have been forced to cope alone with a multitude of parental responsibilities. Teaching children good health habits may fade under the pressures of work, laundry, shopping, cooking, and cleaning. Single parents may neglect their own health because of time and financial constraints. Families headed by homosexual partners and families in which grandparents are primary providers are among the nontraditional families that you are likely to encounter as they seek health care for themselves and their dependent children.

Professional Responsibility and Ethics in Relation to Diversity

You will recall from Chapter 5 that issues of cultural diversity have significant ethical dimensions. The American Society of Radiologic Technologists Code of Ethics requires radiographers to put aside all personal prejudice and emotional bias, rendering services to humanity with full respect for the dignity of mankind. Specifically, they are to conduct themselves in a professional manner, support their colleagues and associates, respond to patient needs, and deliver patient care and service unrestricted by concerns of personal attributes or the nature of the disease or illness and without discrimination on the basis of sex, race, creed, religion, or socioeconomic status.

According to Kohlberg's theory (see Chapter 5), the development of these high moral and ethical standards does not come naturally to most people and is unlikely to be attained by simply reading a code of ethics or a chapter in this or any textbook. It is a process that begins with a commitment and continues with each encounter that presents an opportunity to listen, reflect, and learn. We must open our minds to the possibility that our own perceptions are not universal and that the differing perceptions and values of others have validity and importance.

COMMUNICATION SKILLS

Nonverbal Communication

Although we perceive verbal language as our primary means of communication, nonverbal behaviors reveal a great deal about how we feel. How nonverbal communication is interpreted is largely based on cultural background. Most of us learn to respond to common cues during childhood. We perceive frowns or pursed lips as disapproval. Refusal to look directly into an individual's face while speaking conveys avoidance, submission, or rejection, whereas clenched teeth or fists suggest angry feelings under rigid control. Patients in pain may present a tight and rigid protective posture. Leaning forward while listening to another gives the appearance of intense interest in the subject being discussed. What other nonverbal behaviors do you commonly see around you (Figure 6-1)?

Eye Contact

In the United States, eye contact is considered a positive behavior. When you make direct eye contact with an individual while speaking, it is usually perceived as an expression of interest, concern, or honesty. As mentioned in the previous section on culture and communication, it is important to remember that direct eye contact is not welcome in all cultures.

Touching

Touch is also a means of communication. An abrupt or tentative touch may be perceived as distaste or reluctance to care for the individual. A positive touch is firm

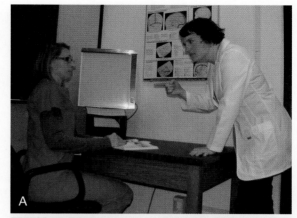
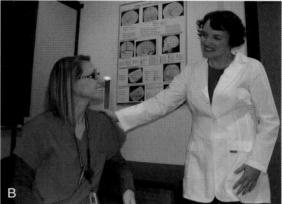

FIG 6-1 What nonverbal clues help you understand the nature of these interactions?

but gentle (Figure 6-2) and reassures the patient that you are both capable and caring. People touch one another for a variety of reasons, including:
- To provide reassurance, support, or encouragement
- To imply domination, anger, or frustration
- To form a positive connection, as in a handshake or shoulder pat
- To perform professional services, such as those provided by a doctor, hairdresser, or masseuse

Remember that the brief hug around the shoulder that is so reassuring to many Americans may be an upsetting invasion of personal space and privacy to those whose culture does not include a casual embrace. In some cultures and religions, touch by a stranger or a member of the opposite sex is unacceptable or strongly frowned upon.

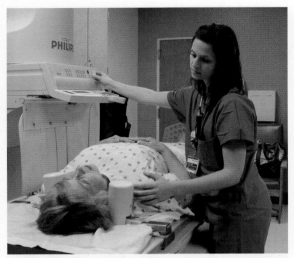

FIG 6-2 Positive touch is firm but gentle.

It is important that your touch have a professional purpose that is clear to the patient. As discussed in Chapter 5, touch should never be forced on a patient.

> When you must touch a patient, you are less likely to unintentionally offend if you tell the patient in advance what you are about to do and then use a firm, appropriate touch.

Appearance

Patients tend to place their confidence in health care workers to the degree that they feel their expectations of a professional person are being met. Everyone we meet forms an impression of us from our appearance, and whether we realize it or not, appearance is another way we communicate how we feel about our work and our patients. What does your appearance tell patients about you?

Uniforms are intended to present a simple, neat appearance and are washable and plain to make them easy to keep clean. They should fit comfortably and be worn with simple, appropriate accessories. Although fads and fashions change over time, a professional image will continue to be conservative.

The appearance of the examining room is equally important. An untidy, cluttered room is difficult to keep clean, and it shows a lack of respect for patients. It sends a nonverbal message that personnel may be too

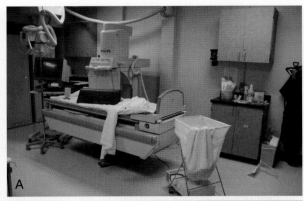

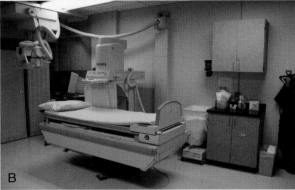

FIG 6-3 The appearance of a room affects patients' attitudes toward care. **A,** What does this room communicate to you? **B,** A clean room inspires confidence.

pressured or too uncaring to answer questions or provide reassurance (Figure 6-3).

Listening Skills

How do you feel when you are interrupted, or when the listener looks out the window while you attempt to make your point? Are you irritated when others "put words into your mouth" or change the subject without responding to what you have just said? Good communication is a two-way street, and a good listener does more than await his or her turn to speak. As a skill, listening involves the ability to give full attention to the speaker. When you focus on the speaker, you can respond to what has been said rather than making a quick switch to the next item on your mental list. In conversation, patients often give us clues about a physical problem that could be easily missed if we rush to get to the next question. This approach may seem impractical in a busy imaging department, but it can become automatic with practice. Don't you have more confidence in people who really listen to what you have to say?

Verbal Skills

Clear, distinct speech habits are always desirable, regardless of the communication circumstances. Being a good communicator also implies the ability to use language and content appropriate to your listener. This is not meant to be patronizing or demeaning. After all, you would explain a procedure differently to a retired nurse than to a certified public accountant with little knowledge of anatomy. Make it a habit to speak face to face so that the listener can see your eyes and read your expression. This habit encourages others to believe that they have your full attention and concern. Be alert to the way your listener responds to your communication, and try to modify your approach if it does not seem to elicit the desired result.

Attitude

Attitudes are revealed by nonverbal behaviors and also by tone of voice and choice of words. Listeners receive more powerful messages from our attitudes than from what we actually say. Compare the following statements. The content is similar, but the message is different:

"No! Don't do it that way!"

"Look, Martha, I think this way might work better."

Assertiveness can be a valuable strategy in communication and should not be confused with aggression. **Aggressiveness** involves anger or hostility, whereas assertiveness is the calm, firm expression of feelings or opinions. As a student, you have the right to be assertive when you require assistance in a patient care situation that is beyond your ability. Employers may be assertive when requiring employees to meet the requirements outlined in their job descriptions. When dealing with uncooperative patients, pleasant assertiveness is the most effective attitude.

Validation of Communication

Another important aspect of good communication is to validate whether you have been understood. An informal response, such as a smile, nod, or brief "okay," may be a satisfactory acknowledgment in a social situation, but when essential information is being presented, the response must be one that reflects clear understanding. This is particularly true with all instructions that involve your professional activities. As a listener, you can be sure that you have understood the message by reflecting the elements of the speaker's statement in your response:

Radiologist: "Give Mrs. Johnson 50 mL of Isovue 300, and take the first image at 60 seconds."

Radiographer: "Mrs. Johnson gets 50 mL of Isovue 300, and I'll take the first image at 60 seconds."

Radiologist: "Right."

In the communication described, the speaker's instruction is complete. The listener's response reflects complete understanding, and the instructions are validated. When the speaker receives an incomplete response, the situation changes:

Radiologist: "Give Mrs. Kirkland 50 mL Isovue 100, and take the first image at 3 minutes."

Radiographer: "Okay." (Turns to leave.)

At this point the speaker cannot be certain of having been understood, so the conversation must be continued:

Radiologist: "Wait. Tell me what you're going to do."

Radiographer: "I'll give Mrs. Kirkland 50 mL of Isovue and take the first image at 3 minutes."

Radiologist: "What strength Isovue?"

Radiographer: "Isovue 300."

Radiologist: "No. Isovue 100 this time."

Radiographer: "Oh, okay; 50 mL of Isovue 100."

Radiologist: "Right."

When presented with an incomplete message, the listener's responsibility is to obtain clarification:

Radiologist: "Give him 50 mL of Isovue."

Radiographer: "That's 50 mL of Isovue 300 for Mr. Enriques and the first image at 60 seconds, as usual?"

Radiologist: "Right."

If the listener's assumption was incorrect, the speaker must then state the intended message more accurately:

Radiologist: "No, no. I was talking about Mr. Jamison. He should have 50 mL of Isovue 100 because of his decreased renal function, then start the imaging at 3 minutes for the same reason."

Radiographer: "Okay; 50 mL of Isovue 100 for Mr. Jamison and image at 3 minutes."

Radiologist: "Right."

When the speaker did not provide some essential information, both parties might have assumed that they were referring to the same patient and that the usual dose of Isovue and routine timing would be used for the examination. When these points are not clear, the potential for error is great. The lesson for speakers and listeners is that messages must be clear and complete and that understanding must be validated or confirmed.

> Without validation, neither party can be certain that all elements of a message have been correctly understood.

Communication under Stress

Any situation that disturbs our everyday activities imposes stress. The hospital environment often proves stressful to patients and families, as well as to the health care workers responsible for their care. This is especially true in crisis situations, when speed is a factor, or when a complex situation causes disagreement about conflicting priorities.

Stress interferes with our ability to process information accurately and appropriately. You may have heard accounts about victims of a house fire who fled with an object close at hand, such as a rubber plant, rather than important papers or treasured family possessions. In a stressful situation, accurate communication can be difficult. The principles of communication already discussed are always important, but these additional suggestions can improve your effectiveness in a crisis situation:

- Lower your voice, and speak slowly and clearly when a situation is highly emotional.
- Be nonjudgmental in both verbal and nonverbal communication.
- Do not allow an upset individual's inappropriate actions or speech to goad you into a similar response.
- When you are uncertain whether the listener has understood you, request an answer. For example, "Did you read the consent form? What did it say?"

Extremely stressful situations can evoke hostile or even violent responses. If you express distaste or hostility, this can escalate the level of tension. Occasionally a patient who is recovering consciousness will become combative, or an elderly patient who is disoriented may threaten violent action. Most potentially violent situations occur in the emergency department. Hostile individuals, such as an inebriated patient involved in a motor vehicle crash or a group brought in after an unresolved gang fight, can be extremely threatening. The essential points to remember in such situations are the following:

- Do not attempt to handle the situation alone. Get help before the problem escalates, and leave the room if physical violence is threatened.
- Be pleasantly firm while explaining that your role is to provide health care only.
- Never let a combative individual get between you and the door.
- Review such situations with your supervisor and coworkers, and learn how to handle threatening events before they arise.

COMMUNICATION WITH PATIENTS

Therapeutic Communication

Therapeutic communication is a process in which the health care professional consciously influences a client or helps the client to a better understanding through verbal or nonverbal communication. Therapeutic communication involves the use of specific strategies that convey acceptance and respect and that encourage the patient to express feelings and ideas. These strategies were originally developed through the experiences of mental health professionals and have been adapted for use in nursing. Although many aspects of this approach are more specifically applicable to longer-term patient relationships, some of them can be used to enhance communication in any interaction. Table 6-1 lists therapeutic communication strategies that are useful to radiographers and gives examples. You will note other examples of these same principles elsewhere in this chapter and throughout the text where illustrations of effective communication are given.

Just as certain approaches to communication tend to be more therapeutic, it follows that certain other approaches may be nontherapeutic, actually hindering the communication and recovery processes. For example, refusal to consider a patient's idea by using a statement such as, "Let's not discuss…" indicates rejection of the patient's thoughts and may cut off all communication. Table 6-2 provides other examples of deterrents to therapeutic communication.

TABLE 6-1 **Therapeutic Communication Techniques**

Techniques	Examples
Using silence	Silence is socially uncomfortable. It may increase the client's willingness to talk.
Accepting	"Yes." "I follow what you said." "I see."
Giving recognition	"Good morning, Mrs. G..." "I notice you're sitting up today."
Using general leads (using neutral expressions to encourage continued talking by the client)	"Go on...I am listening." "Tell me about it."
Placing the event in time or sequence	"Was this before or after...?" "What seemed to lead up to...?"
Making observations	"You appear upset." "I notice you are clenching your fists."
Encouraging description of perceptions	"What do you think is happening to you right now?"
Restating	Patient: "I can't sleep. I stay awake all night." Radiographer: "You have difficulty sleeping."
Reflecting	Patient: "Do you think I should tell the doctor?" Radiographer: "Do you think you should tell the doctor?"
Focusing	"This point seems worth looking at more closely." "You said something earlier that I want you to go back to."
Exploring	"Would you describe that more fully?"
Giving information	"My name is...I am a radiographer."
Seeking clarification	"What would you say is the main point of what you said?"
Presenting reality	"Your mother is not here...I am a radiographer."
Voicing doubt	"That's hard to believe." "Really?"
Attempting to translate into feelings	"From what you say, I suspect you are feeling relieved."
Suggested collaboration	"Let's see if we can figure this out."
Summarizing	"Let's see, so far you have said..."

Addressing the Patient

The first contact with a patient is usually an introduction. In many social situations today, given names are used as soon as introductions are made. Although this may seem to project an air of friendliness and informality, it also poses certain problems. For many people, the stress of hospitalization is reflected in a strong feeling of helplessness or loss of **autonomy** (self-determination). Patients are told where and when to lie down, what to eat, when to take medications, and so on. This, in combination with anxiety over the need to seek treatment and the inability to comprehend much of the hospital jargon, magnifies the individual's need to maintain a sense of identity.

"Good morning, Mr. Torres. I'm Lynn Smith, the radiographer," is more than an example of good manners. It shows respect and concern and allows the patient to choose how he or she wishes to be addressed. In an effort to show friendliness, some staff may address

TABLE 6-2   Deterrents to Therapeutic Communication

Techniques	Examples
Rejecting	"I don't want to hear about..."
Disapproving	"That's not a good thing to do." "I wish you'd stop that."
Disagreeing	"I don't agree with..." "That can't be right."
Advising	"I think you should..." "Why don't you just..."
Requesting an explanation	"Why do you think so?" "Why do you feel that way?"
Indicating the existence of an external source	"What made you do that?" "Who told you that?"
Belittling feelings	Client: "I'm so miserable. I wish I could die." Radiographer: "Everyone gets the blues sometimes."
Denial	Patient: "I don't think I'll ever get well." Radiographer: "Don't be silly."
Changing the subject	Patient: "I feel incredibly lonely here." Radiographer: "Snow is predicted for this afternoon."

! The Joint Commission, which accredits health care organizations, requires that health care personnel use two patient identifiers to validate identity before proceeding with patient care or services. This is usually accomplished by asking the patient to state his or her full name and date of birth and by checking the patient's identification band.

Valid Choices

One way you can help patients to participate in their care is by giving them opportunities to make choices. This process of self-determination promotes confidence and a sense of autonomy. Avoid the false sort of choice expressed by such statements as, "Would you like to come down for your x-ray now?" When the patient is scheduled for 10:00 AM, little choice is involved. **Valid choices** are alternatives, all of which are acceptable to you. Valid choices require a little more thought, but the rewards in terms of patient satisfaction are well worth the effort. Effective valid choices may be very simple. Questions such as, "Would you like a blanket over your knees?" and "Would you prefer to sit where you can see down the hall or over by the window?" are reassuring to the patient who would like to feel capable of making decisions and having a share in his or her own care. Treating patients as individuals, allowing them to make valid choices, and using good nonverbal communication can help to alleviate fear while encouraging cooperation and self-care on the part of our patients.

📌 Valid choices are acceptable alternatives that help patients feel competent and involved in their care.

Avoiding Assumptions

In determining why patients fail to follow instructions, a factor frequently encountered is the assumption that the patient has understood the procedure. To make an assumption is to make a guess. For example, we could assume that because you are reading this text, you are a student in a radiologic technology program. This might be true, or you might be an instructor, a nurse, or the proofreader for this book. Making assumptions about patients implies that you might also guess about their physical status and abilities, as well as their willingness to cooperate. Can you assume that Mr. White, who may have broken his ankle, can be positioned flat on the radiographic table? No. He may also have emphysema,

adults as "honey" or "sweetie" instead of calling them by name. Others, who are focused on the work routine, may refer to "the left hip in room 2" or "that barium enema in the hall." Talking down to adults or treating them impersonally diminishes their self-esteem and raises feelings of resentment. Such feelings diminish patients' ability to understand and follow directions, prevent the retention of information, and can hinder recovery.

It is important to note that some facilities prefer the use of first names when calling patients from the waiting room or other public area. This enables the patient to maintain some degree of anonymity in public and may be part of your hospital's Health Insurance Portability and Accountability Act compliance program for maintaining patient confidentiality. Out of the public area, you can ask the patient how he or she would prefer to be addressed. In private, verify each patient's full name and date of birth.

which would interfere with his ability to breathe in a supine position.

Avoiding assumptions becomes critical when outpatients are scheduled for procedures that demand advance preparation. For example, if Ms. Elwood is scheduled for a barium enema examination, an inquiry such as, "Did you follow the prep?" may not be an effective way to find out what Ms. Elwood actually did. It implies that she was given a preparation kit, received clear instructions, and understood the question. If you rephrase the query and ask her to explain exactly how she complied with the preparation instructions, you will get a more complete picture of how well she was able to cooperate. Reviewing the printed instructions with the patient may be helpful.

Assessment through Communication

Conversing with patients allows you to use your powers of observation. Is the patient alert or confused? How well does the patient hear? Is English comprehension a problem? From observation, you can often make a tentative assessment of the patient's ability to get on and off of the examination table, walk unassisted to the bathroom, and cope with other activities. In Chapter 11, we discuss patient assessment in depth, but you should learn from this chapter that good communication with patients can help you to establish a spirit of trust and cooperation that will assist in patient care.

SPECIAL CIRCUMSTANCES THAT AFFECT COMMUNICATION

Patients Who Do Not Speak English

Federal legislation guarantees the patient's right to communicate effectively in health care situations, regardless of language barriers. Most large hospitals now have a service that will arrange for an interpreter when necessary. In areas where languages other than English are typically used, the admitting and emergency areas must post signs in the most common languages advising patients of the availability of interpreters. In some cases, certified interpreters are on call and come immediately when needed. When a large percentage of the population speaks a single foreign language, full-time interpreters may be part of the hospital staff. When an outpatient procedure is scheduled in advance, an interpreter may be scheduled at the same time.

It is becoming quite common for hospitals to use tele-interpreter services. Laptop computers on rolling carts are connected online with an interpreter of any language

selected, thus greatly reducing the need to for interpreters to be on call. Using a webcam and a microphone, interpreters are able to see and hear the patient. Difficulties can arise when the patient does not speak clearly or when limitations in laptop volume make it hard for the patient to hear the interpreter. Translation services are also available over the telephone, including unusual languages and obscure dialects. One such service called *Language Line* is provided by AT&T. Telephone translation is usually most efficient when a conference call format is used, but translators are patient if the telephone must be transferred from client to health care worker in the course of the conversation.

Your duty may be to arrange for an interpreter or translation service when appropriate, even though a "family translator" may be present. Although waiting for a professional translator can delay routine procedures, the benefits often outweigh the disruption of your schedule. With professional translation, interpersonal relationships will not interfere, and the parties to the conversation can be certain that the translations are accurate. The interpreter will explain to the patient that all information is confidential and that interpretation is a part of the medical service that is provided at no charge. If your hospital subscribes to a translation service, you will receive specific instructions about its use. These methods can be highly effective for obtaining a medical history or informed consent.

The difference between a certified interpreter and a friend or family member who assumes this role may be significant. The interpreter is trained to translate only what has been said, both by the patient and to the patient, and not to explain what is implied. Family members and friends tend to add extraneous information or to edit the conversation in an effort to be cooperative or to save time. For example, a complete explanation of positioning and breathing instructions may be abbreviated in translation to, "It's okay, Mama. Just hold still." Family members may hesitate to reveal information about the patient that they believe is private or embarrassing, and the patient may hesitate to reveal personal information through family or friends. Family members whose command of English is limited may have good intentions but may be unable to provide adequate translation of complex information.

The services of a trained interpreter provide a professional bridge in difficult communication situations. Certified interpreters must be used when:
- Obtaining the patient's medical history
- Obtaining informed consent or permission for treatment

- Giving a diagnosis
- The patient is conscious during treatment or surgery
- Confronting an emergency
- Explaining medication instructions, side effects, and dosages
- Physicians or medical staff are giving instructions
- The patient is being discharged

When using an interpreter, look directly at the patient and speak as though the patient were able to understand you. The interpreter will translate as you speak or as soon as you have finished a sentence. Speaking to the interpreter directly tends to make the patient feel left out or talked about rather than involved in the process.

> When using an interpreter, look directly at the patient and speak as though the patient were able to understand you.

Several hospitals maintain files of helpful words and phrases in languages that are in common local use, including phrases such as, "Please hold your breath," "Point to where it hurts," and other statements or questions that can be especially helpful in imaging departments. If a translator is unavailable, use demonstrations or pencil sketches to validate whether the individual understands, and make extensive use of nonverbal encouragement. A friendly smile and a warm touch can be worth many words. Appendix E provides a list of helpful phrases with guides for pronunciation in Spanish that might help you to greet Hispanic patients and assist them in situations in which only the simplest communication is required. Be cautious, however, about communicating in the patient's language if your language skills are limited. Although you can express simple ideas clearly, you may be unable to interpret patient responses accurately.

The Hearing Impaired

Many health care providers tend to treat deaf patients and those with some hearing loss essentially the same. In reality, the problems of communication are quite different. Patients with a hearing loss may display levels of impairment that vary from the need to use a high-intensity hearing aid to only a mild difficulty with hearing voices in a high or low register. Certain rules are helpful in communicating with individuals who have hearing loss:

- Talk to, not about, these persons.
- Get the patient's attention before starting to speak.

- Face the person, preferably with light on your face.
- Hearing loss is frequently in the upper register, so speak lower as well as louder.
- Speak clearly and at a moderate pace. Do not shout.
- Avoid noisy background situations.
- Rephrase when you are not understood.
- Be patient.

When in doubt, ask the person for suggestions to improve communication. Avoid potential misunderstandings by using open-ended questions and asking patients to repeat instructions. Allow the patient who wears a hearing aid to retain it as long as possible, and give all instructions before the aid is placed in a safe location. Because visual clues become much more essential when hearing is impaired, try not to remove the patient's glasses until necessary.

Deafness

The deaf patient presents a challenge unlike that of a patient with hearing loss. Many totally deaf individuals live in a cultural setting that has its own social structure, language, and even inside jokes. Certain cues help in differentiating between the patient with a hearing loss and the deaf patient, especially in an emergency. You may become aware that a seemingly alert patient is totally deaf when he and/or she:

- Does not respond to noises or words spoken out of the range of vision
- Uses lip movements without making a sound or speaks in a flat monotone
- Points to the ears and mouth while shaking the head in a negative motion
- Uses gestures or writing motions to express the need for paper and pencil

Some deaf people are adept at lip reading and are able to speak, at least to a limited degree. More often the deaf are educated in American Sign Language (ASL), which is the most common sign language in the United States. It is distinctly different from English and has unique grammar, syntax, and rules. Learning a few basic signs can aid in establishing rapport with deaf patients. A card showing the alphabet and some common useful signs in ASL should be available through your nursing service department.

As with patients who do not speak English, a certified interpreter is essential in any situation that requires complex instruction or an exchange of important information. Interpreters for deaf clients use the same ethical guidelines as foreign language translators, and the process of interpretation is essentially the same for all involved. Friends and relatives of a deaf patient should not ordinarily be used to interpret medical or treatment information, because they may add their own interpretation to the translation, changing its meaning. This could also compromise patient confidentiality and cause the patient to omit or edit information that could have a direct bearing on diagnosis and treatment.

When a totally deaf patient is admitted for care, the chart should be flagged with this information. The deaf person has the right to request a specific interpreter, if available, and to have an interpreter replaced if communication is not proceeding well. Patients also have the right to choose the most preferred method of communication, which might be pencil and paper. Be sure that writing materials are available and that the patient's writing arm is free.

The medical setting can seem especially overwhelming to a deaf child. If possible, allow the child and parents to tour the area before the examination begins. Take time to fully explain the procedures and activities to the parents so they can help the child understand what to expect. If the child is distressed, you might consider allowing a parent to stay in sight or near the child while following radiation safety precautions.

Impaired Vision

Most of us depend greatly on our eyes to sense our surroundings and ensure our safety as we move about. Vision enables us to recognize individuals and perform the activities of daily living. The ability of blind persons to accomplish these same tasks without vision can seem astounding. They rely on hearing, touch, and memory to a much greater extent than do sighted persons. With the aid of a cane or guide dog, many blind persons lead independent lives. Having learned to work outside the home, use public transportation, and maintain their own households, these patients may be insulted by attitudes that are too solicitous. However, they may welcome some special help in a strange environment. Some patients prefer to follow you by listening to your footsteps and using a cane, whereas others may wish to place a hand on your shoulder or elbow. Those who are more infirm may prefer your arm around their waist while you reassure and direct them verbally. None of these approaches applies to all blind persons. Good communication is the key to determining which form of help is acceptable and appropriate.

The person with recently failing vision and good hearing may need much verbal explanation and reassurance.

Other visually impaired individuals are capable of proceeding confidently after a quick description of a room and the obstacles in it. You might say, "This is a square room, Mrs. Daley. The x-ray table is about 5 feet in front of you and a chair is at 7 o'clock. After you're on the table, I'll be in a booth to your left."

Patients with failing vision often see better in bright light. They may be able to recognize faces, but you should offer to read written material to them without waiting for a request for assistance.

Inability to Speak

Aphasia is defined as a defect or loss of language function in which comprehension or expression of words is impaired as a result of injury to language centers in the brain. Brain lesions large enough to damage language function will often produce multiple effects. A patient who has experienced a stroke and is unable to speak may also be unable to write. For this reason, it is often helpful to ask the nursing staff how they have been able to communicate with the patient. Some patients are able to write. Many can indicate by a nod or shake of the head whether they understand your directions.

Many patients who have suffered the loss of speech because of throat cancer or an accident may choose to communicate using one of several different types of artificial speech. One tool for those who cannot otherwise talk is the handheld electrolarynx. This device is placed on the external throat wall and operates by amplifying vibrations transmitted through the tissues of the neck. Although an electrolarynx can certainly aid communication, it has an extremely metallic tone and is not always easy to understand. Esophageal speech, in which the patient swallows air and then regurgitates it, is easily understandable but is low in volume and requires extensive practice as well as a fair amount of physical effort. Some patients who cannot speak can take advantage of recent advances in artificial speech aids involving transesophageal puncture (TEP), in which a prosthesis is placed within the neck through a stoma. There are several variations. One is a semipermanent installation in which the prosthetic device remains within the stoma and is cleaned in place by the patient. Another is a removable aid that is inserted and removed by the patient for cleaning and maintenance. TEP devices also operate on a vibratory principle, but they are more easily understood than the external handheld electrolarynx.

Remember that the loss of the ability to see, hear, or speak is a communication impairment and not a reflection of the individual's ability to think. Patients with sensory deprivation or impaired ability to communicate challenge us to be more flexible and innovative in the ways we offer explanations, reassurance, and care.

> ✎ Loss of the ability to see, hear, or speak is a communication impairment and not a reflection of the individual's ability to think.

Impaired Mental Function

Special sensitivity is needed when caring for adult patients who are intellectually or emotionally challenged. Such patients may include those with congenital defects such as trisomy 21 (Down syndrome), accident victims, those with illnesses affecting the brain, and those with severe emotional disorders that affect comprehension. As with children, you must assess the patient's ability to understand and follow instructions, because this ability may vary from a near infantile response to a functional capability close to normal. In general, the same clear, simple, and direct instructions offered to children are appropriate. You may need to repeat instructions if the attention span is short. It is not appropriate to talk to these patients as if they were toddlers. Use the adult form of address, and treat them with the respect and dignity due anyone their age.

Altered States of Consciousness

Another challenge to communication arises with patients who have an altered state of consciousness. This change in the ability to respond, react, and cooperate can result from injury, illness, medication, alcohol, or drugs. The impairment can range from a state of drowsiness, in which the individual can cooperate when aroused, to total unconsciousness. You must remember two points in communicating with patients who are drowsy or in a stupor:

1. They cannot be relied upon to remember instructions.
2. They are not responsible for their actions or answers.

An individual who has loss of consciousness may seem to respond appropriately when regaining consciousness, but may also attempt to sit up and get down from the table.

> ❗ Any patient with decreased level of consciousness must be kept under constant and close observation.

An important factor that is frequently overlooked in hospitals is the ability of many patients to hear and remember conversations that occurred while they were apparently unconscious. Patients who are unconscious because of anesthesia, trauma, or illness may be completely unable to respond while still retaining the ability to hear and remember what is said. A safe rule to follow is not to make any statements within hearing range of unconscious patients that you would not make if they were conscious. As a corollary, it is important to refer to unconscious patients by name and to reassure them about your actions. The medical literature gives many examples of patients who have regained consciousness after prolonged periods and who have credited their recovery to health professionals who continued to call them by name and treat them as human beings with an identity uniquely their own.

AGE-SPECIFIC COMMUNICATION

Individuals grow and develop physically, psychosocially, and cognitively in stages that are related to their age. Individuals share certain qualities at each of these stages. Understanding them will enable you to provide individual care to patients at every stage of life.

Neonate and Infant (Birth to 1 Year)

The neonatal period includes the first month of life (Figure 6-4). During this stage, infant behavior is mostly reflexive and is influenced by your voice and touch; therefore it is important to be aware of your tone of voice and facial expression when you approach a neonate. Because neonates are at risk for heat loss, keep them tightly wrapped in a blanket, except when they must be uncovered for imaging.

Beginning in the first month of life, a strong bond is established between parent and infant, so involve the

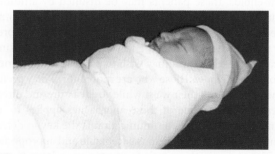

FIG 6-4 Neonates feel most secure when wrapped snugly.

parents in the examination and keep them in the infant's line of vision as much as possible. When parents cannot be present during the examination, remember that infants feel most secure when being held, so hold and cuddle the child to meet this need.

The period from 1 month to 1 year of age is characterized by rapid physical growth and development. There is a progression from reflexive to more purposeful behavior. Two- and 3-month-old infants smile because it elicits a response from others. Sucking, chewing, and vocalizing are important oral activities. By 8 months of age (Figure 6-5), infants begin to differentiate themselves from others. They recognize familiar persons, such as their parents, and they fear strangers and unfamiliar situations. At 9 months, infants experience separation anxiety. Keep the infant and parents together as much as possible, limit the number of staff members, and provide familiar objects, such as a blanket, toy, or pacifier, to reduce the stress the infant is experiencing. Using familiar objects and incorporating play will also serve to distract the infant during the examination.

Always provide a safe environment. Never leave an infant on a flat surface unattended. Keep the crib rails up at all times, and immobilize the infant during the examination whenever it is necessary (see Chapter 10 for immobilization techniques for infants).

Toddler (1–2 Years)

The fear and lack of comprehension that we often see in adults can be greatly magnified in children. By age 2 (Figure 6-6), toddlers are beginning to communicate using two- and three-word sentences. They like to explore and manipulate their environment. They are greatly attached to their parents, but are also beginning to assert their independence because they are mobile and can do more for themselves. Resistance to control by parents or health care workers can result in negative behaviors such as temper tantrums. Respond to these behaviors using a friendly but firm approach, and by setting clear limits. Allow the toddler choices when possible, and when necessary, explain to parents that immobilization techniques will need to be used to obtain the child's radiographic images. Try to find out what the toddler is called at home, and use the familiar name. If you are calm, cheerful, and unhurried, the toddler is much less likely to respond negatively to the strange surroundings and machines. Allowing the toddler to take a favorite blanket or toy to the radiology department may help promote a feeling of security. Talk to toddlers and play with them to distract them during the examination and reduce their stress. Even if they do not understand all you say, a cheerful voice is reassuring. Prepare the toddler shortly before the procedure and use

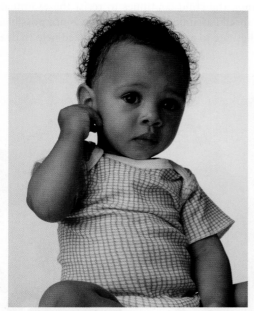

FIG 6-5 Infants begin to differentiate themselves from others at about 8 months of age.

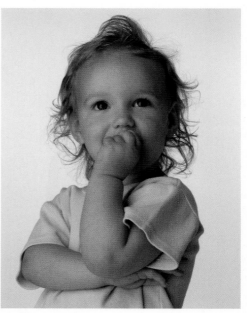

FIG 6-6 Toddlers like to explore and manipulate their environment.

demonstration rather than spoken instructions. When spoken directions are given, keep them short and simple, giving one direction at a time. Strange adults are often intimidating to children because of their stature, so try to speak to children at their own eye level. You will find that this is especially helpful when you approach the child to "make friends" before entering the x-ray room.

Preschooler (3–5 Years)

Children at this age (Figure 6-7) require somewhat different approaches to care and communication. They are demonstrating increasing independence; they are conversational and able to share information with you; and they can cooperate more fully, but they also fear a loss of self-control and need to make valid choices even more than do adults. "Would you like to climb up on the table by yourself, or would you like me to help you?" is an example. Although children have no choice about submitting to the examination, they should be encouraged to cooperate as much as possible. Apprehensive children are not reassured by such statements as "This won't hurt a bit." Frequently the only word they assimilate is "hurt," and they become even more frightened. "Have you ever had your picture taken by x-ray?" allows you to add whatever simple explanation is necessary. "We're going to take a picture of your leg with this special big camera" is understandable to most children. Because most preschoolers do not understand cause-and-effect relationships, they might not understand the reason for taking a picture of their leg., perceiving it instead as punishment for their crying. It might help to add that the reason you are taking the picture of their leg is to find out why it hurts. This age group also has a short attention span, and a demonstration is often more effective than verbal instruction. Show the child how to position the hand for a finger examination or how to hold a deep breath for a chest radiograph. Children at this age frequently ask "why" questions; if questions are asked, try to answer them simply. Never force information on children, because they can become more apprehensive if they do not understand everything that is said. It is better to treat the entire procedure in a matter-of-fact manner. Keep directions and explanations simple, direct, and honest (Figure 6-8), such as "We need to take five or six pictures, Johnny. We'll be as fast as we can."

How do you cope with the child who appears determined to be disruptive or refuses to follow directions? You set limits in clear terms, saying, "You must lie still," or "You may not get down." Above all, use praise and rewards for good behavior and cooperation. Children at this age are motivated by avoiding punishment and earning rewards. If, after a patient and reasonable attempt, the child continues to resist the examination, you should assume that cooperation is not possible. Do not hesitate to ask for more experienced help in dealing

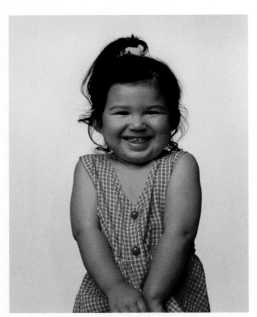

FIG 6-7 Preschool children demonstrate increasing independence.

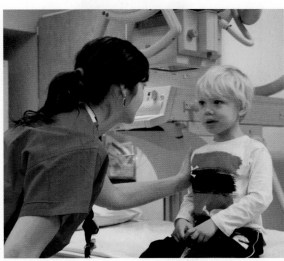

FIG 6-8 Keep explanations simple, direct, and honest.

with a difficult situation. Following department protocol, immobilize the child firmly but gently and complete the examination as quickly as you can (see Chapter 10 for immobilization techniques for children).

Remember that muscular activity is a natural response to anxiety in a small child. When the situation seems unbearable, kicking and squirming are normal. Crying also is normal for a frightened child. An order to stop crying only increases the anxiety, and trying to raise your voice over a child's screams is almost never effective. Sometimes, however, a whisper will capture a distressed child's curiosity and attention.

School Age (6–12 Years)

Children in this age group can think logically about anything that can be touched and seen. Give concrete information about the examination; be specific about the body areas or parts that will be affected. Be honest and let them know whether they will experience any pain or discomfort. Although they have an increased attention span and reasoning skills, continue to use demonstration or models to explain the examination and allow them to assist whenever possible.

Adolescent (13–18 Years)

Special sensitivity is required to deal with the emotional needs of younger adolescents (Figure 6-9). Although they may act much like adults under normal circumstances, they can become frightened and confused and may revert to childlike behavior when ill or in stressful situations.

Show empathy if the adolescent loses control of his or her emotions. Teenagers fear threats to their physical appearance and loss of control and independence. Avoid using an authoritarian approach and involve them in as much decision making as possible. Modesty and privacy are of paramount importance, and x-ray images may be feared as the "all-seeing eye," ready to unveil the patient's innermost secrets. Respect their concern for modesty and fear of embarrassment. You can establish rapport and reduce their fears and anxiety about the procedure and diagnosis by asking them about their hobbies, favorite sports, school, or friends before beginning the examination. Prepare the adolescent for the procedure away from parents and peers, if possible. If parents are present, involve them, but do not talk to parents "about" the adolescent, and include the adolescent in all discussions. This age group has moved past the physical or concrete properties of a situation and is capable of understanding abstract principles. Provide thorough explanations and the rationale for procedures, and use proper medical terminology in your explanations.

A professional approach, coupled with warm reassurance, promotes a more positive attitude in both children and adolescents. Many of the poor attitudes toward health care displayed by adults can be traced to a lack of sensitivity in the care given by health professionals during their formative years.

Young Adult (19–45 Years)

Young adults are searching for and finding their place in society (Figure 6-10). They may be struggling with

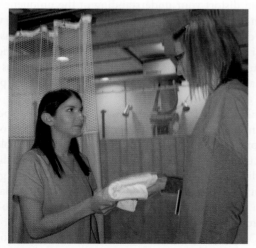

FIG 6-9 Modesty is especially important in early adolescence.

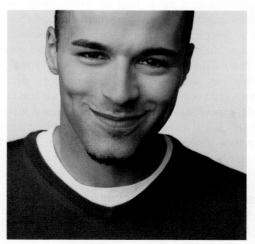

FIG 6-10 A young adult.

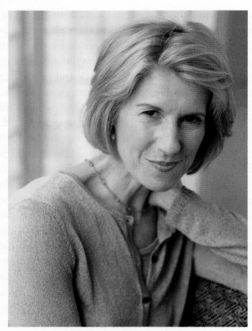

FIG 6-11 A middle adult.

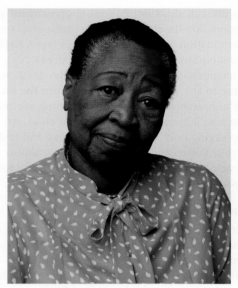

FIG 6-12 An elderly adult.

moving from dependency to roles of responsibility with higher education, the start of a career, marriage, children, and the care of aging parents. Involve them and their significant others in the procedure and any decision making. Tailor your instructions and explanations about the procedure to their level of understanding.

Middle Adult (46–64 Years)

The middle-aged adult may be experiencing lifestyle changes and changes that affect them physically and cognitively (Figure 6-11). The onset of many chronic (persistent or lasting) conditions occurs during this period in life. Toward the end of this stage, there may be vision and hearing loss, decreased short-term memory, decreased balance and coordination, loss of bone mass and skeletal height, loss of skin elasticity, and a decreased metabolic rate, which will make them less tolerant of heat and cold. Keep these changes in mind as you provide instructions and perform the examination. Allow them to make choices and involve them as much as possible in the examination.

Late Adult (65–79 Years) and Old Adult (80 Years and Older)

The health care field in the United States continues to be challenged by the increasing age of the population.

The oldest baby boomers reached age 65 in 2011. The number of elderly is expected to increase to 70 million by 2030. The increase is caused by an extension in average life span, the aging of baby boomers, and the increase in the population segment older than 85 years.

It is important not to stereotype the elderly adult. Ageism is a discriminatory attitude toward the elderly that includes a belief that all elderly are ill, disabled, worthless, and unattractive. Ageism often results in discrimination against people because of increasing age. It can distort your understanding of the uniqueness of each individual and can affect the way you interact with the elderly and care for them. It is important to assess your own attitudes toward older adults. Working to acquire specialized knowledge of the aging process can enhance your understanding and result in a more positive attitude.

Elderly patients (Figure 6-12) may require special attention because of the sensory deficits that often accompany aging. The visual and hearing problems discussed earlier in this chapter may have a direct application to many of these patients. Providing good lighting and checking to ensure the patient has glasses or a hearing aid available will help both of you to feel more comfortable.

Occasionally, you will see older people who, to varying degrees, have lost the ability to understand why they find themselves in unfamiliar surroundings.

This can be caused by Alzheimer disease or organic brain syndrome or can occur as a direct result of medication, illness, or injury. A decrease in mental acuity may make it necessary to present one idea at a time, emphasize concrete rather than abstract ideas, keep distractions to a minimum, use tactile cues, and ask for feedback to ensure understanding. Older patients who appear confused respond best to familiar situations. In these cases especially, use an individual's full name. During conversation, it helps to ask patients where they were born, whether they are from a large family, and other questions about the past. Distant memory is often clear to those who cannot remember what was served for breakfast. Keep instructions simple and give one instruction at a time. Using valid choices and treating older patients with the respect due any adult helps them to maintain their sense of identity.

We emphasize that relatively few older patients have these conditions, and it is important to evaluate the needs and abilities of each older patient on an individual basis.

PATIENT EDUCATION

The opportunities for health teaching in a radiology department are limited by the busy schedules of both the patients and the department. Under these circumstances, the most important opportunities for patient teaching include the following:
- During the explanation of procedures
- While responding to patient concerns
- As part of the instructions needed to prepare for a procedure
- During instruction for follow-up care

When you are responsible for direct patient teaching, include the patient in the plan whenever possible. After the teaching period, set aside a question-and-answer session and ask the patient to explain or demonstrate the principles to you. This validation of instructions makes patients feel involved in their care, promotes their sense of autonomy, and increases compliance with their medical regimen.

Explanation of the current procedure is essential for all patients. Patients will relax and cooperate much more readily when they know what to expect. Try to keep explanations simple, and avoid technical details unless the patient expresses an interest. Use good listening skills to respond effectively to patient concerns. Patients

frequently express apprehension about exposure to radiation. Reassure them that the risk is extremely small and is far outweighed by the benefits of the procedure. When the patient expresses any concerns, try to focus your response on both the subject and the level of anxiety. Avoid standard explanations that sound as though they were prerecorded. Such "canned" responses are impersonal and can make the patient believe the question was unimportant. If you are unsure about the answer to a question, refer the patient to a knowledgeable coworker or physician.

When patient teaching involves preparation for a procedure:
- Use prepared written materials.
- Review each step with the patient.
- Validate that the patient understands by using open-ended questions and having the patient explain the preparation back to you.
- Use your best communication skills, even in these brief patient contacts. Listen carefully, be patient, and avoid a hurried appearance, which could discourage patients from asking questions.

COMMUNICATION WITH PATIENTS' FAMILIES

When we are sick or injured, the presence of those who care about us is reassuring and may be essential to our ability to cope. It is natural that family members accompany patients to their appointments, rush to the emergency department after an accident, and visit patients during hospital admissions. You will often have to deal with family members who want to hold the patient's hand during a radiographic examination or who eagerly await the results of a diagnostic procedure. When you are busy and the patient is your primary concern, family members may appear as obstacles to your work. Dealing sensitively with families is often necessary and helps your patient in ways that may not be apparent.

Your communication with families often involves the transfer of practical information. Those waiting for a patient want to know how long the procedure will take, and they appreciate an update from you when a delay occurs. When the wait is prolonged, your attention to the waiting family's comfort might include directions to needed services, such as the restrooms, cafeteria, or telephone.

If the patient is a minor, is incompetent, or is sedated, you may need to provide instructions to a family member regarding preparations or follow-up care. Be sure that you are speaking to the person who will actually assist the patient, because information can be lost when it is passed from person to person.

Questions often arise regarding the immediate presence of family members during a procedure. The family must usually stay outside the room, preferably in a waiting area or lobby that is out of hearing range. This is done for reasons of radiation safety, but also because it allows the staff members to proceed without interruptions from concerned family members who may not understand what is happening and may require excessive explanation and reassurance.

Procedures that involve patient discomfort or some blood loss may be unsettling to loved ones. If families are waiting near the procedure room, you should be aware of this and avoid making statements within hearing range that might alarm them or betray a professional confidence.

Occasionally a family member may need to stay with the patient in the procedure room, such as with a deaf child, as mentioned earlier. In these situations, only one family member should be selected, and this person should receive a clear explanation before the procedure. You should answer questions at this point and clarify the role of the selected family member. A lead apron or other radiation shielding should be provided as necessary.

Dealing with families can sometimes be difficult. In an emotionally charged situation, we all use different means to cope with our anxiety. Some of us become dependent and wait for others to make decisions and give us instructions. Others maintain self-control by withdrawing or denying the importance of the situation. Anxiety can cause some individuals to be aggressive when asking personnel for information about patients dear to them. Families of patients in emergency situations naturally experience fear and anxiety, which can be directed toward the closest professional person, possibly you. "Watch what you're doing!" "You can't move him, he's hurt." "Are you in charge?" "Do you know what you're doing?" Such statements can elicit a negative reaction unless you recognize their hidden message. Fear frequently engenders anger. If you can understand aggressive demands for service and attention as an expression of fear, you can concentrate on providing reassurance rather than reacting to such comments as personal attacks.

Necessary activities, such as filling out forms and calling other family members, may serve to bridge the waiting period. Let families know when the patient will be moved and where the patient will be going. Although you should always refer inquiries about diagnosis (identification of condition) or prognosis (prediction of outcome) directly to the physician in charge, an expression of concern can demonstrate empathy. "I know you are worried about Barbara, Mr. Rudd. I've let the doctor know you're waiting for the results."

If families do not respond to your attempts to calm them and are preventing you from doing your work, you need help from someone who is in a better position to provide assistance. The social services department may send a counselor or chaplain to assist those who are grief stricken or in a state of panic. As a last resort, or if you feel at risk, security personnel may be summoned to intervene with hostile or belligerent relatives.

DEALING WITH DEATH AND LOSS

There may be an occasion in the future when you are present during a disaster involving fatal injuries, or even a situation involving sudden death within the imaging department. In an acute care hospital, patients sometimes die despite the most sophisticated care. The medical and nursing staff have developed specific procedures to follow in the case of death, and these responsibilities do not normally include the radiographer. The physician notifies the family while the nursing staff prepares the body for transport to the morgue.

Your role might be to provide support for the family while awaiting word from the physician. If so, do not volunteer information or discuss the staff members' actions. Your observations and opinions must not be discussed at this time. When the family reaches the anger phase of their grieving process, they may want to place blame on someone for an unavoidable death. Spontaneous comments made by caregivers under stress are sometimes quoted by families in court actions to support accusations of malpractice. If you have any question about the appropriateness of the staff members' actions surrounding a patient's death, this should be discussed later, in private, with your supervisor.

Once death has been pronounced on a candidate for organ donation, radiographs may be needed to determine correct placement of the various lines needed to support the integrity of the organs to be donated.

You may hear the term *brain dead* used, but the determination of death is based on more than a flat brain wave recorded on an electroencephalogram. The criteria can vary slightly from state to state, but when organ donation is involved, there must be agreement among several physicians that death has occurred. The need to take radiographs of a dead body that is being maintained on oxygen and that does not appear to be deceased can be emotionally upsetting. Try to keep in mind that the organ donor is providing an opportunity for several other individuals to achieve an improved quality of life.

Victims of some forms of abuse and certain types of homicide are also sometimes subjects for postmortem radiographic examinations. It can be difficult to maintain your professional composure under such circumstances. On these occasions, or when a patient dies unexpectedly during a procedure, the tension and the immediate activity may carry you through the actual event. How you cope with your feelings during the period that follows is important to your mental health, so talk about the events with a supportive person. Health professionals often see themselves as rescuers and may have unrealistic expectations that can lead to feelings of inadequacy and depression when nothing can be done for a patient. Do not be afraid to express emotion. All human beings are unique, and the death of any one of us diminishes humankind.

At some time in your professional or your private life, you will need to deal with someone who is grief stricken. The grieving process is experienced by anyone who suffers serious loss, and this includes patients who become disabled or disfigured. Terminally ill patients and their families often experience anticipatory grief. A great deal has been written on this subject. Early work by Dr. Elisabeth Kübler-Ross has greatly changed the way members of the helping professions view the dying process. Terminally ill patients and their families are now perceived as needing time to work through the grief process and achieve some measure of healing. Kübler-Ross pointed out that grief is an emotional readjustment to a new way of experiencing life and cannot be accomplished all at once. She identified five phases of the grieving process. They can occur in any order, and not all people experience all five stages, which are as follows:

1. Denial. At this stage, the grieving person refuses to accept the truth and may refuse to discuss the possibility of loss or death.
2. Anger. As denial is overcome, the person experiences the frustration of helplessness and a feeling of outrage at the apparent injustice of the loss. Rage may be vented on family, friends, and health care workers. This may be beyond the individual's control.
3. Bargaining. At this stage, the person seems to be attempting to earn forgiveness or mitigation of the loss by being "very good." Patients in this phase of grief are conscientious about following physicians' orders, are considerate of others, and seldom complain, even when suffering.
4. Depression. The depressed person is often acquiescent, quiet, and withdrawn, and may cry easily.
5. Acceptance. At the conclusion of the grieving process, the person accepts the loss or impending death and deals with life and relationships on a more realistic, day-to-day basis. Those who accept their loss are often comfortable talking about it and generally display attitudes that are appropriate to their immediate circumstances.

Although the grieving process is facilitated by supportive acceptance at each stage of grief, the time required to pass from one phase to the next varies with individuals and cannot be hurried.

In dealing with the grieving patient, the radiographer may be presented with statements or questions that require a sensitive response. The patient may say, "I wish it was all over," "How long do you think I have to live?" or "Don't you think I'm much better today?" when there has been no change. In such circumstances, you may feel a strong tendency to respond with the language of denial. A typical denial statement might be "Don't talk like that. You're going to be fine." Such responses tend to block communication and may be insulting to patients who have passed the denial phase of grief. Remember that the patient is not necessarily seeking a direct response. What is needed is a friendly, supportive listener.

Rephrasing the patient's remark encourages the patient to talk and conveys a message of acceptance. Examples of such responses to the previous remarks might be, "I'm sorry you're feeling tired of living." "You think it would help to know how long you have to live?" or "You're feeling better today?" Do not be afraid to be involved or to show that you care. Be lavish with touch and comfort measures if the patient seems responsive to this type of attention.

Terminally ill patients have the right to receive care in the facility of their choice. Although some prefer the acute care setting, an increasing number choose to die at home. In the 1970s, a movement that emphasized home care for terminal patients gained acceptance. Instead of placing an emphasis on cure, care is focused on the pain relief and comfort measures that allow patients to die with dignity in familiar surroundings. This movement was called *hospice* from the Greek term *hos,* meaning "a place of shelter." Today, hospice is a service rather than a place. When the physician determines that the patient is unlikely to live for longer than 6 months and a decision is made with the patient not to pursue further treatment of the underlying disease, a conference with the hospice staff members determines whether the family is able to assume the responsibility of providing the major portion of care. The team of physicians, nurses, home health aides, psychologists, and social workers helps to provide the patient with as much quality of life as possible during the short time that remains. Some communities have inpatient hospice facilities, but care is often given in the patient's home. The patient's home may be with family or in an assisted living or skilled nursing facility. Comfort measures and other palliative treatments (care that provides relief but is not intended to cure) are provided on call, 24 hours a day. Respite care can be offered to permit the family caregiver time to rest and regroup. After the death of the patient, the hospice team may provide counseling to the bereaved that can help them with grief and healing.

This subject is often not included in the curriculum or texts on patient care. Few professionals are totally comfortable in the presence of death, and most of us find it difficult to objectively face our own mortality and eventual death. Those who work in an acute care setting need to learn to accept death as yet one more aspect of life. We strongly urge you to expand your awareness by reading about and discussing this sensitive subject. Seek support and counseling for situations that are personally difficult to handle. Familiarize yourself with facility policies and protocols. Further education is advised for those working in situations such as radiation oncology (cancer treatment), where death is a likely occurrence (see Chapter 5 regarding the patient's right to die and do not resuscitate orders).

COMMUNICATION WITH COWORKERS

Teamwork is defined as the cooperative effort by the members of a group to achieve a common goal. The pressures in a busy imaging department can sometimes make this concept hard to apply. Our goal is the best patient care possible, and this is easier to accomplish when we work cooperatively with others on the health care team.

The ability to relay information to other health professionals is essential in the multidisciplinary situation that exists in modern hospitals. Many problems we encounter when dealing with patients are also met when communicating with professional workers. The pressures of time and patient load can cause or compound the personality conflicts encountered in any group. Good interpersonal relationships are built on the ability to make others feel good about themselves.

The nonverbal behaviors that we use with patients, such as touch and appearance, are equally effective with coworkers. Use praise and appreciation as positive reinforcements when work is well done or when others go out of their way to offer assistance. Be a good listener, and demonstrate your respect for your coworkers as individuals by avoiding cliques and gossip. Teamwork is a two-way street, and if you appreciate help when your workload is heavy, you should also assist your coworkers in similar situations. Being patient and considerate, avoiding assumptions, validating communication, and maintaining a positive attitude are all habits that will generally result in a positive response. Because good communication with your coworkers is important no matter where you work, we urge you to review the principles presented earlier in this chapter and to practice them in all your professional encounters. Many troublesome situations can be avoided by maintaining a pleasant working relationship that allows you to solve small problems before they grow. Before recurring problems become monumental, follow the chain of command discussed in Chapter 4 to seek a solution.

One aspect of your interpersonal relationships with coworkers can have legal implications. The pressure of work within the department often makes it difficult to take the time to exchange general information. For this reason, break periods or lunchtimes are often used to catch up on recent developments and share information about difficult situations. Never discuss patients in a public setting. It is acceptable to talk about changes in schedules, the hospital picnic, or the new computer system, but discussions of interesting cases, important personages, or possible treatment errors could result in damaging litigation, because such conversations are invasions of the personal rights and privacy of patients.

In today's world, a great amount of technical information is exchanged. Although much of this information is conveyed using charts and forms, informal messages can be equally important. Attention to detail, such as adding your name and the date to telephone message forms, keeps information retrieval more accurate.

Here are some guidelines for avoiding problems with telephone communications:

- Be familiar with your telephone system, including forwarding and hold functions.
- Identify yourself and your department when calling or answering a call.
- Keep paper handy, and make notes during the call to avoid losing details.
- Use a pleasant, receptive tone of voice.
- Validate the message before concluding the call.
- Be sure that messages are relayed promptly to the proper person or department.

Any written communication is valuable only if the recipient receives it in good time. Whether this is a telephone message, a personal note, or a change in schedule, be sure that important messages are placed directly in the individual's hand or posted in plain sight in a predetermined spot. Be sure to identify yourself, your department, and the time sent or received; if a reply is needed, include the address and/or phone number.

Fax transmissions and voice mail also facilitate the transmission of information and instructions between hospitals and other health care facilities. Confidential information should not be communicated in a voice mail message, because there is no way of controlling who will receive the message. Lengthy voice mail messages, even when not confidential, are usually not effective. It is better simply to leave your name and telephone number and a general statement of the purpose of the call.

Fax transmission can be a convenient and efficient way for physicians and other health care personnel to exchange information quickly and accurately. Immediate, direct written communication of orders and scheduling requests may help to prevent errors and improve service. The ability to print multiple copies of new orders makes fax transmission an especially useful tool. If you are responsible for faxing information to another institution, remember to fill out the cover sheet first. Confusion about where the information is needed or who is to receive it can cause needless delays in patient care. When sensitive, confidential information regarding a patient is to be sent by fax, it should be preceded by a phone call to alert the recipient. Confidentiality is difficult to preserve at best, and such information should be treated in a responsible manner.

SUMMARY

- American culture is becoming more diverse, and cultural diversity is a global issue in health care. Research indicates that cultural inequities affect the outcomes of health care.
- The scope of diversity encompasses ethnic, racial, and religious variations, as well as differences in gender, sexual preference, age, geographic location, economic status, physical status, and family structure.
- Cultural traditions affect both verbal and nonverbal communication and are important in establishing the rapport needed for effective health care.
- Cultural and religious differences affect attitudes and expectations with respect to health care. These differences can affect many aspects of care, including the acceptability of certain treatments and practices, adherence to standards of modesty, dietary requirements, and accommodation of religious practices.
- It is important not to stereotype individuals based on national origin because there are many variations among individuals within cultures.

- Radiographers and all health care professionals are ethically required to do all they can to meet the needs of all patients, including being aware of cultural differences and providing care that is consistent with these varying needs.
- A high percentage of the communication humans receive is by means of nonverbal signals such as posture, facial expressions, gestures, eye contact, and tone of voice. These nonverbal signals are not perceived similarly in all cultures.
- To avoid giving offense with touch, touch only as necessary to provide care, tell the patient what you are going to do and why, and use a touch that is both firm and gentle.
- Be a good listener by focusing your attention on the speaker and responding appropriately to what is being said.
- Communicate effectively by using clear, distinct speech and using language appropriate to your listener.
- Communication is most effective when approached with an attitude of respect and consideration.

Assertiveness is the calm, firm expression of feelings or opinions and is highly effective, whereas aggressiveness lends a connotation of hostility and is not well-received.

- Validation of communication is essential to be certain that there is an accurate exchange of information. A validated communication is clear and complete, and the information has been reflected back to the speaker accurately by the listener.

- Stress interferes with communication, which can make a difficult situation worse. In stressful situations, lower your voice, speak slowly, be nonjudgmental, and avoid inappropriate reactions. To be certain that you have been understood, obtain validation by asking an open-ended question.

- Therapeutic communication strategies are used to assist patients in communicating and understanding their situations more effectively. These strategies include open-ended questions and comments that recognize and accept the individual. Nontherapeutic approaches, including denial, disagreement, and criticism, are counterproductive to patient communication.

- Communicate effectively with patients by addressing them by name and showing friendliness and concern. Allow them to make valid choices, avoid assumptions, and take advantage of conversation to aid in patient assessment.

- Patients have a legal right to understand health care communication, even if they do not speak English. The use of qualified interpreters is preferable to using family translators to communicate with patients who do not speak English. When using an interpreter, look at the patient as though he or she could understand you. Trained interpreters will translate all of what is said and only what is said, and they will maintain confidentiality. Arrange for an interpreter whenever an accurate exchange of medical information is essential. Computer interpreter services and telephone translators are available and may be used by your facility.

- The hearing impaired have needs that differ from those of patients who are deaf. To communicate with individuals who have hearing loss, get their attention, face them with light on your face, speak lower and somewhat louder than usual, speak clearly at a moderate pace, and avoid noisy background situations.

- Deaf patients cannot hear at all. They may read lips and may be able to speak, but they are more likely to use ASL. They have a right to an interpreter, and the process is similar to that for other language interpreters. Some deaf persons prefer to communicate in writing.

- The ability of blind persons to make their way in the world and accomplish many tasks is greater than most sighted persons realize. Even so, they may appreciate guidance and explanations in unfamiliar surroundings. Ask what kind of help would be useful and respect their independent abilities.

- Patients who are unable to speak may have aphasia, which is damage to the speech centers of the brain. Those who are unable to speak because of injury or cancer involving the larynx may be capable of artificial speech using special devices, or by means of esophageal speech.

- When attempting to communicate with adults who have impaired mental function, use words and methods that work with children of similar mental age, but maintain the respect and dignity appropriate for adults.

- Patients with a decreased level of consciousness caused by illness, injury, or medication cannot be relied upon to remember instructions and are not responsible for their actions or answers. Protect them from injury, and speak to them as though they can hear and understand.

- Individuals develop physically, psychosocially, and cognitively in age-related stages. Grouping them according to these stages and understanding their age-specific competencies will enable you to communicate more effectively and meet their needs for care during imaging procedures.

- You may need to teach patients in order to help them understand imaging procedures, prepare for a procedure, or adhere to instructions for follow-up care. It is helpful to allow adequate time, listen to the patient's concerns, use printed materials, review each step, and validate understanding.

- It is important to patients' well-being to deal sensitively with their families and respond to their needs and concerns. Understand that families may be emotionally upset because of their loved ones' condition, and try to be tolerant of negative attitudes.

- Radiographers do not often confront death in the workplace, but they may sometimes be called upon to perform imaging procedures on patients who have expired and are being maintained on life support as organ donors, or on the bodies of those who are victims of crimes. Radiographers will also encounter patients and families dealing with grief related to death or other loss. It is important to understand and support the grieving process and to seek wise counsel when encounters with death raise disturbing emotions.

- Good teamwork requires cooperation and good communication with coworkers; therefore the communication skills learned in this chapter should be applied with teammates. Take care that communication with coworkers does not violate patients' rights to confidentiality.

- Be conscientious in communicating written and telephone messages and transmitting faxes to be certain that details are complete and accurate and received in a timely way, taking care to preserve confidentiality.

REVIEW QUESTIONS

1. Which of the following terms best describes assertive behavior?
   A. Forceful
   B. Persuasive
   C. Firm
   D. Argumentative

2. When instructions are given to a non-English-speaking patient, it is best to:
   A. speak English slowly and firmly
   B. use a sympathetic family member who speaks English
   C. draw detailed pictures
   D. use a trained interpreter

3. Deaf patients and hearing impaired patients differ in that the deaf patients:
   A. will not respond to sounds outside their field of vision
   B. may use ASL as their primary means of communication
   C. often move socially within a deaf community
   D. all of the above

4. When dealing with a hostile patient it is important to:
   A. gain control of the situation with a loud, firm voice
   B. use nonverbal behavior to show disapproval
   C. limit confusion by dealing with the situation alone
   D. ask for help before the situation escalates

5. Which of the following statements is true with respect to individuals with decreased levels of consciousness?
   A. They are not responsible for their actions or answers
   B. They are likely to be violent when regaining consciousness
   C. They cannot hear while unconscious
   D. They do not need help going to the bathroom

6. When dealing with preschool children, it is important to:
   A. calm them by giving them many choices
   B. let them know who is in charge
   C. keep directions simple, direct, and honest
   D. tell a crying child, "Stop that, or we can't take all the pictures!"

7. Grief caused by death or loss may be characterized by expressions of:
   A. Anger
   B. Denial
   C. Depression
   D. All of the above

8. Cultural differences can result in differing perceptions of which of the following behaviors?
   A. Eye contact
   B. A casual hug
   C. A loud, firm voice
   D. All of the above

9. The onset of chronic conditions is most common during which of the following life stages?
   A. Adolescence
   B. Young adult
   C. Middle adult
   D. Old adult

10. Which of the following characteristics is not typical of adolescents?
    A. They tend to move at a slower pace
    B. They fear threats to their physical appearance
    C. Modesty and privacy are of paramount importance
    D. They are capable of understanding abstract concepts

Answers can be found in the Answer Key on pages 429-431.

CRITICAL THINKING EXERCISES

1. Adam, age 4, has been brought in for radiography of an injured hand and is extremely frightened. How can you communicate successfully to Adam that he is in a safe place so that he will cooperate? What kinds of nonverbal signals can you use to support your verbal message? How would you validate the effectiveness of your communication?

2. Allison Jones, age 3, has swallowed a quarter, and the emergency department physician has ordered chest and abdomen radiographs. Both Allison and her mother are upset and worried. What can you do to calm Mrs. Jones and enlist her help in obtaining Allison's radiographs?

3. Suggest strategies for determining the ethnic background of an adult patient and learning how culture might be a factor in the patient's examination and care.

4. Contrast the special needs of deaf patients with those of patients who are hard of hearing.

7

Safety

OBJECTIVES

At the conclusion of this chapter, the student will be able to:

- List the National Patient Safety Goals for Hospitals and discuss their implementation by technologists in medical imaging departments.
- List in sequence the steps to be taken if you discover a fire in or near your work area.
- Select the appropriate type of fire extinguisher for any fire and demonstrate appropriate use of a fire extinguisher.
- List four important electrical safety precautions.

- List three common infractions of fire safety rules in hospitals.
- Discuss hazards caused by obstructions and spills and describe methods for preventing or dealing with these hazards.
- Identify and describe the types of work injuries most common among imaging technologists and suggest appropriate strategies to prevent such injuries.
- Demonstrate the practice of good body mechanics when lifting and moving heavy objects.

OUTLINE

Fire Safety
Fire Prevention
Oxygen and Fire Hazards
Be Prepared
In Case of Fire
Other Common Hazards
Electric Shock

Falls and Collisions
Chemicals and Spills
Eye Splashes
Workplace Safety
Ergonomics
Body Mechanics

KEY TERMS

base of support
body mechanics
center of gravity

ergonomics
line of gravity
nitrile

Occupational Safety and Health
   Administration (OSHA)
spontaneous combustion

This chapter focuses on safety, both in the radiology department and in the hospital setting as a whole. Here you will learn precautions to minimize risks and the procedures to follow in situations that may be hazardous. Patient safety is a primary concern for all radiographers, but note that this chapter also provides information to help ensure your own safety as you care for patients.

In 2006, recognizing the need for greater safety in the health care setting, the **Institute for Healthcare Improvement (HI)**, a nonprofit organization, launched a campaign aimed at saving 100,000 lives by reducing fatalities in health care institutions. The 3100 hospitals that participated in this initiative achieved a remarkable goal. Through their work on the campaign's interventions, combined with the goals of The Joint Commission listed in Table 7-1 and other national and local improvement efforts, these facilities saved an estimated 122,000 lives in 18 months. As a result, new standards of care began to emerge, and a new campaign was launched. The **5 Million Lives Campaign** was a national initiative to protect patients from five million potential medical harm incidents in U.S. hospitals between December 2006 and December 2008. If your clinical institution is part of the large network of health care organizations that participated in this campaign, the goals and interventions listed in Box 7-1 will be familiar to you because these goals and interventions are still emphasized to provide a sharp focus on patient safety. Specific procedures and precautions related to these goals that involve the work of radiographers are found throughout the text. For example, they will be found in the sections on emergency response in Chapters 15 and 16, in the medication precautions in Chapter 14, in the discussion of infection control

TABLE 7-1	2015 National Patient Safety Goals for Hospitals
The purpose of the National Patient Safety Goals is to improve patient safety. The Goals focus on problems in health care safety and how to solve them.	
Identify patients correctly	Use at least two methods to identify patients. For example, use the patient's name and date of birth. This is done to make sure that all patients get the medicine and treatment meant for them.
	Make sure that the correct patient gets the correct blood type when they receive a blood transfusion.
Improve staff communication	Quickly get important test results to the right staff person.
Use medicines safely	Label all medicines that are not already labeled, for example: medicines in syringes, cups, and basins.
	Take extra care with patients who take medicines to thin their blood
	Record and pass along correct information about a patient's medicines. Find out what medicines each patient is taking and compare those medicines to new medicines given to the patient. Make sure patients know which medicines to take when they get home. Instruct patients to bring their up-to-date medication lists every time they visit the doctor.
Use alarms safely	Ensure alarms on medical equipment are heard and responded to promptly.
Prevent infection	Use the hand-cleaning guidelines from the Centers for Disease Control and Prevention or the World Health Organization.
	Use proven guidelines to prevent infections that are difficult to treat.
	Use proven guidelines to prevent infection of the blood from central lines and of the urinary tract from catheters.
	Use safe practices to treat the areas surrounding surgical incisions.
Prevent mistakes in surgery	Make sure the correct surgery is done on the correct patient and at the correct place on the patient's body.
	Mark the correct surgical site on the patient's body.
	Pause before the surgery to verify correct information about the surgery.
Identify patient safety risks	Learn which patients are at risk of trying to commit suicide.

This is an easy-to-read document. It has been created for the public. The exact language of the Goals can be found at http://www.jointcommission.org/hap_2015_npsgs.

in Chapters 8 and 9, and among the precautions for prevention of pressure ulcers in Chapter 10.

Health care facilities are required to have written policies and procedures to ensure patient safety. The **Occupational Safety and Health Administration (OSHA)**, a federal agency governing safety in the workplace, provides guidelines to ensure a high level of safety for hospital workers, and these guidelines are a required part of the safety procedures in all hospitals.

BOX 7-1   Recommendations from the Institute for Healthcare Improvement 5 Million Lives Campaign

- Deploy Rapid Response Teams …at the first sign of patient decline.
- Deliver Reliable, Evidence-Based Care for Acute Myocardial Infarction …to prevent deaths from heart attack.
- Prevent Adverse Drug Events (ADEs) …by implementing medication reconciliation.
- Prevent Central Line Infections …by implementing a series of interdependent, scientifically grounded steps.
- Prevent Surgical Site Infections …by reliably delivering the correct perioperative antibiotics at the proper time.
- Prevent Ventilator-Associated Pneumonia …by implementing a series of interdependent, scientifically grounded steps.

New Interventions Targeted at Harm

- Prevent Harm from High-Alert Medications …starting with a focus on anticoagulants, sedatives, narcotics, and insulin.
- Reduce Surgical Complications …by reliably implementing all the changes in care recommended by SCIP, the Surgical Care Improvement Project (http://www.medqic.org/scip).
- Prevent Pressure Ulcers …by reliably using science-based guidelines for their prevention.
- Reduce Methicillin-Resistant *Staphylococcus aureus* (MRSA) infection …by reliably implementing scientifically proven infection control practices.
- Deliver Reliable, Evidence-Based Care for Congestive Heart Failure …to avoid readmissions.
- Get Boards on Board …by defining and spreading the best-known leveraged processes for hospital boards of directors, so that they can become far more effective in accelerating organizational progress toward safe care.

> **!** It is your duty to be familiar with the established safety procedures for your employment situation.

FIRE SAFETY

Fire Prevention

Nothing induces more terror in the hospital setting than the word *fire*. Our first discussion of safety practices is centered on fire prevention, which is certainly preferable to coping with an active fire. An awareness of potential hazards is the first step toward prevention.

Three components must be present for a fire to burn: a flammable substance (fuel), oxygen, and heat (Figure 7-1). Fire can be avoided by ensuring that these three elements never occur in the same place at the same time. Once started, a fire can be stopped if one of the elements is removed from the situation. This principle is used to fight a fire by adding water (lowering the temperature) or by smothering it (removing oxygen), such as when wrapping a blanket around a person whose clothing has ignited. Most hospital fires can be traced to one of four causes:

- Spontaneous combustion
- Open flames
- Cigarette smokers
- Electricity

Spontaneous Combustion

Spontaneous combustion occurs when a chemical reaction in or near a flammable material causes sufficient heat to generate a fire. This is a relatively uncommon cause of hospital fires, because hospital safety standards, as well as state and local safety regulations, restrict and control the use of flammable chemicals and cleaning products. Spontaneous combustion can occur during renovations or when paint products, solvents, and cleaning rags are stored in a closed environment or too close to a heat source. Oily or paint-soaked waste should be placed in tightly covered containers and stored near the maintenance department.

Open Flames

Open flames that burn out of control are a common source of fires in homes, but relatively few hospital fires begin in this way. Those that occur usually do so in kitchens or laboratories where open burners are used.

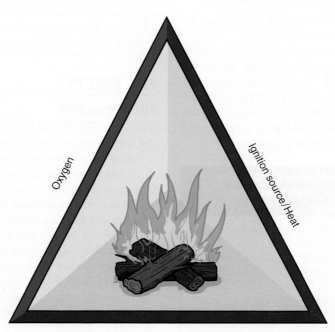

FIG 7-1 Chemistry of fire. (From Phillips N: *Berry & Kohn's operating room technique*, ed 12, St Louis, 2013, Mosby.)

Observe the following precautions to prevent fires caused by open flames:

- Keep flammable substances a safe distance from the flame.
- Use strict standards of cleanliness in kitchen areas.
- Never leave open flames unattended.
- Never burn candles.

Smoking

As health care providers, hospitals promote positive health habits by prohibiting smoking and are designated as non-smoking facilities; thus, smoking is seldom a potential cause of fires. Although this practice reduces the incidence of this type of fire, danger still exists from covert smoking. Smokers may be tempted to cope with the stress of hospitalization by smoking, but hospitals no longer accommodate them indoors, and they must be directed to a designated smoking area, which is usually located outside the building. Physicians sometimes prescribe nonsmoking aids for smokers who crave tobacco while hospitalized.

Electrical Fires

Electricity is a potential source of fire hazard and is of special concern in radiology departments where there is much electrical equipment. For this reason, we emphasize avoiding electrical hazards and preventing electrical fires (Box 7-2). The same principles apply in any area where electrical equipment is used, especially in the emergency department and the intensive care unit.

A short circuit in an x-ray control panel, especially in an older unit, can result in fire. This is usually preceded by smoldering wire insulation, which causes smoke and an unpleasant odor that is readily detectable before an actual fire.

If you suspect a fire hazard from an electrical malfunction:

- Turn off the electricity at the main power source.
- Call for qualified assistance.
- Stand by with the proper fire extinguisher.

> **!** All radiographers should be aware of the locations of fire extinguishers and instructed in their use.

During your education as a radiographer, you will learn to use a wide variety of complex electrical equipment. Do not let your familiarity with electrical items create a false sense of security.

Oxygen and Fire Hazards

Oxygen by itself does not burn, but it does support combustion. Because the presence of oxygen greatly increases the fire hazard, it is important to exercise extreme care when it is in use. There should be no smoking, no open flames, and no ungrounded appliances. Any electrical equipment that could cause a spark must not be used in the presence of oxygen use. Such equipment is required to be conspicuously marked as hazardous in situations where oxygen is in use. In most hospitals, only certain approved persons may turn off the oxygen at the main shut-off valve (see Figure 7-2). This might include someone from the facilities or engineering department, or even the incident commander.

Be Prepared

Hospitals are required to observe certain fire safety precautions to maintain their accreditation. In most hospitals, the head of the maintenance department or the chief engineer is responsible for initiating fire safety programs. These programs include clearly defined plans for staff action in the event of a fire, fire drills every calendar quarter, and frequent in-service classes on fire-fighting procedures and equipment. You must be familiar with the fire plan for the hospital, especially for the imaging department. Be sure that you know the evacuation route from your area and at least one alternate route. Maps of evacuation routes must be posted in each area. In addition, you should have at least a general knowledge of your facility's floor plan,

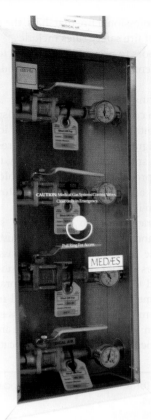

FIG 7-2 Oxygen shut-off valve.

and take special note of the locations of fire alarms, fire extinguishers, and fire doors.

A coded communication is usually used in the event of a fire to notify the staff without alarming the patients. This may be a code name announced over the paging system giving the type of emergency and its location: "Attention all staff, code red, third floor, east wing, room 321." This same code is also used for fire drills. Some hospitals may use a special message, such as "Dr. Redfern, report to Third Floor East," although most hospitals have migrated to a universal set of safety communication codes that are easily identifiable to all employees, regardless of where their training took place. This is discussed further in Chapter 15.

Fire drills must be taken seriously. Take full advantage of fire drills and in-service classes to gain confidence in evacuation procedures and the use of fire extinguishers. If you are well-prepared for a fire, your self-confidence will allow you to function effectively and will reassure those around you.

According to professional fire marshals, the most frequent infractions of fire safety rules include:

- Blocking fire doors to prevent them from closing.
- Storing equipment in corridors, which hinders evacuation.
- Improperly storing flammable items.
- Using extension cords not approved for hospital use.

Fire doors in hospitals are marked for easy identification. They are designed and constructed to restrict the spread of a fire to a small area. For this reason, fire doors should never be propped open. They should remain closed unless they are designed to close automatically when the fire alarm is activated.

Because radiographers often use mobile stretchers, wheelchairs, carts, and x-ray machines, care must be taken to ensure that these items do not obstruct passages and doorways. Corridors should not be used to store equipment; if items need to be placed there temporarily, keep them all on the same side of the hallway, and make sure there is enough room for a hospital bed to pass easily. Ask yourself the question: "If we had to evacuate the area, would this piece of equipment be a problem in this location?"

! Be prepared for a fire by knowing the locations of the following items:
- Evacuation route maps
- Fire doors
- Fire alarms
- Fire extinguishers
- Main electrical power shut-off for your area

In Case of Fire

If you discover a fire, your primary responsibility is to evacuate everyone in the immediate area to a safe location beyond at least two intervening fire doors. Second, report the fire and location using the prescribed code procedure. A small wastebasket blaze can be extinguished with a nearby pitcher of water or smothered with a pillow, but do not waste precious minutes in futile attempts. Report the fire as soon as the immediate area is evacuated so that hospital personnel trained in firefighting can assess the situation and direct an appropriate course of action.

A way to help you quickly recall the correct response in the event of a fire is the acronym **RACE**, which stands for **r**escue, **a**larm, **c**ontain, and **e**xtinguish and evacuate. Box 7-3 lists the steps to follow in case of fire using the RACE concept.

BOX 7-3 In Case of Fire

Remain calm and remember the acronym RACE.

R—Rescue
- Coordinate with nursing staff and remove patients from danger by moving them past at least two fire doors within the facility. For larger fires, follow the instructions of coordinating personnel.

A—Alarm
- Activate the alarm system directly or use the hospital call code for fire.
- Make sure that all personnel in the area are aware of the fire, being careful not to alarm patients.

C—Contain
- Close any open doors to limit the oxygen supply to the fire and to prevent the spread of smoke and heat.
- Ensure that electrical circuit breakers are turned off.
- Close the doors to patient rooms. If a patient is still in a room, place the room's trashcan in front of the door.

E—Extinguish/Evacuate
- For small fires, use the available fire extinguisher to put out the fire or smother the fire with a blanket.
- For larger fires, evacuate the area and wait for fire personnel.

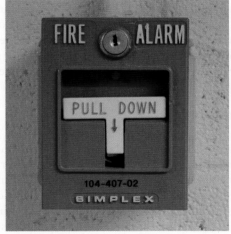

FIG 7-3 Know the location of the fire alarm closest to your working area.

During evacuation, it is especially important to remain calm and to reassure patients. Use a low voice and try to avoid using the word *fire*. Instead, you might

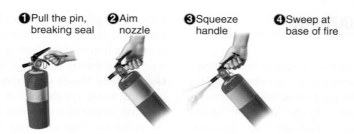

❶ Pull the pin, breaking seal   ❷ Aim nozzle   ❸ Squeeze handle   ❹ Sweep at base of fire

FIG 7-4 Fire extinguisher mechanism. (From Yoost BL, Crawford LR: *Fundamentals of nursing,* St Louis, 2016, Elsevier.)

say: "Mrs. Jensen, there is a little smoke in one of the rooms and we are going to move you outside until we can see how serious it is."

Again, there is no substitute for knowing the locations of the fire extinguishers, fire alarms (Figure 7-3), and fire doors. You must also be aware of oxygen shut-off valves and the master controls for electrical systems in your area. Although this information should be included in your hospital orientation, familiarity with these locations is your personal responsibility. Thorough knowledge of the prescribed procedure for reporting a fire is also essential.

Fire Extinguishers

Fires are classified according to the type of fuel involved:
- Class A fires involve solid common combustibles, such as paper or wood.
- Class B fires involve flammable liquids or gases.
- Class C fires involve electrical equipment or wiring.
- Class D fires involve certain combustible solids, such as metal alloys.
- Class K fires involve cooking media, for example oils and animal fats.

Fire extinguishers are marked to indicate the class or classes of fire for which their use is appropriate. A multipurpose, dry chemical extinguisher is suitable for Classes A, B, and C, and is the type most often found in hospitals and other public buildings.

Figure 7-4 shows a close-up view of a typical fire extinguisher mechanism. To use the fire extinguisher correctly, remember the acronym **PASS:**
- **P**ull the pin.
- **A**im the nozzle at the base of the fire.
- **S**queeze the handle.
- **S**weep. Use a sweeping motion from side to side to prevent the fire from spreading.

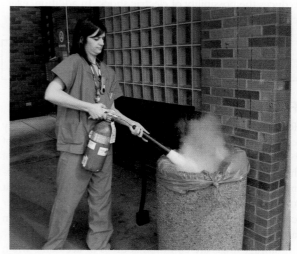

FIG 7-5 Use the fire extinguisher in a sweeping motion from side to side at the base of the flame. Stand back at a safe distance.

Do not aim the fire extinguisher steadily at the flame. A sweeping motion is more effective and covers a wider area, decreasing the likelihood that the fire will spread. Stand back so as not to endanger yourself; fire extinguishers have considerable force and are effective at a safe distance from the fire (Figure 7-5).

Fire extinguishers must be inspected regularly and recharged periodically. A tag attached to the unit should indicate the dates of the last inspection and the last recharge. The last inspection should be no longer than one year ago.

> When a fire extinguisher has been used, it must be replaced immediately with a fresh unit and then sent to the maintenance department to be recharged.

OTHER COMMON HAZARDS

Electric Shock

Electric shock can pose a serious hazard to both patients and personnel if safety precautions are not observed. This is especially true with x-ray equipment, which carries an electrical potential in excess of 100,000 volts. The hazard of lesser circuits should not be underestimated, however, because shocks from standard 120-volt outlets can prove fatal under certain circumstances. The rules for electrical safety are listed in Box 7-2. Adherence to these rules greatly reduces the possibility of electric shock. In addition, exercise extreme caution when using electricity around water.

> **!** Never stand on a wet floor or use wet hands to perform tasks involving the use of electricity.

Falls and Collisions

Reducing the risk of falls and collisions is a major safety concern in hospitals. Take precautions for the safety of both patients and personnel. Be especially conscious of hazards when moving stretchers and other mobile equipment, and do not store or park this equipment where it might cause a problem. Equipment too close to a corner can be an unseen obstruction to someone hurrying from an intersecting hallway or carrying a bulky object.

Storage areas are common sources of accidents when items are not placed properly or secured when necessary. Heavy items stored on high shelves are an invitation to an accident; they should be placed near the floor. Do not stack items precariously. Any item that could cause harm should be situated so that it will not shift unexpectedly.

Do not string electrical cords across doorways or other traffic patterns, and try to position equipment as close as possible to a suitable outlet. If a cord must cross a traffic path temporarily, secure it to the floor with tape to minimize the possibility of someone tripping over it. If you observe that hazardous, makeshift electrical connections are a common problem, use the chain of command to suggest a safe, permanent remedy.

Precautions for avoiding patient falls are addressed in detail under the topic of *Patient Transfer* in Chapter 12.

Chemicals and Spills

Spills

Spills deserve the special attention of the safety-conscious radiographer. Depending on the nature of the substance, spills may pose a chemical hazard in addition to the risk of injury from falls. Chemicals can be as simple as household cleaning agents or as complex as radioactive testing materials. Familiar substances such as household bleach or concentrated darkroom chemicals can cause eye damage or skin burns. Appropriate cleaning measures are needed to avoid potentially serious problems. Your work area should have a spill kit that includes a container of kitty litter, heavy plastic bags, a broom, a dustpan, and gloves made of **nitrile**, a special material that is impervious to many hazardous chemicals. The litter absorbs spilled liquid, turning it into a solid that can be safely swept and placed in plastic bags for disposal.

Your hospital has written policies and procedures to follow in determining appropriate action in the event of a chemical spill. OSHA requires that all chemicals be properly labeled and that **Material Safety Data Sheets (MSDSs)** for all hazardous materials be on file and easily accessible to personnel. The MSDS for any chemical will indicate the required equipment and procedure for safe handling in the event of a spill. The following steps help to ensure safety when a spill occurs:

- Limit access to the area.
- Evaluate the risks involved.
- Determine whether you have both the equipment and the expertise to clean up the spill safely.
- If you can proceed safely, clean up the spill immediately.
- If you lack the necessary skill or equipment, call your supervisor or the appropriate department.

Darkroom Chemicals

The developer and fixer solutions used to process radiographic film are classified by OSHA as hazardous materials. OSHA requires that personnel wear protective aprons, splash-proof goggles, and nitrile gloves when pouring or cleaning up film processing solutions. Splash-proof goggles fit snugly against the face to provide greater eye safety than common industrial safety goggles, which are designed only for protection from airborne debris. Nitrile gloves are required for working with darkroom chemicals; common latex gloves are not considered to provide adequate protection.

The **Environmental Protection Agency (EPA)** is the federal agency concerned with the safe disposal of hazardous waste. Together with state and local officials responsible for landfill and sewage treatment facilities, the EPA sets standards for waste disposal that protect the environment. If your imaging system requires chemical film processing, you must be aware that used fixer solution contains silver and is not permitted in the sewage system. Environmental standards require that used fixer be processed for silver removal before disposal. If your department does not reclaim the silver from used fixer, it must be drained into suitable heavy plastic containers and picked up for recycling. This service is commonly provided by companies that supply the chemicals.

Eye Splashes

Prompt treatment is essential for chemical splashes in the eyes. When a chemical eye splash occurs, flood the eye with running water for a full five minutes. If discomfort or impairment of vision persists following eyewash, see an ophthalmologist immediately.

An eyewash station is a first aid station for chemical eye splashes that sprays water into the eye from a convenient height. Some eyewash stations are activated by a foot pedal, leaving the hands free to hold the eye open. If a chemical eye splash occurs in the vicinity of an eyewash station, this is obviously the best approach. However, immediate treatment is essential, so do not waste time and endanger your eyesight by searching for an eyewash station when a splash occurs. Become familiar with the location and operation of eyewash stations in your facility before the need arises. OSHA requires that eyewash stations be immediately accessible in areas where corrosive or hazardous chemicals are frequently handled, but if an eyewash station is not convenient, any running water is satisfactory.

WORKPLACE SAFETY

Ergonomics

Ergonomics is the study of the human body in relation to the working environment. Ergonomic awareness and education in the workplace have reduced job injuries in recent years, but there is still cause for concern. The U.S. Bureau of Labor Statistics reports that workplace injury rates for hospital workers are similar to those for industrial workers. The most common injuries reported by health care workers are **musculoskeletal disorders (MSDs)**. Subcategories of MSDs as classified by OSHA include **repetitive motion injuries (RMIs)**, **repetitive strain injuries (RSIs)**, and **cumulative trauma disorders (CTDs)**. RMIs and RSIs, as their names suggest, are the result of performing repeated motions or applying pressure extensively. Stress caused by repetitive motion, overreaching, or maintaining the same positions for long periods causes microtrauma to muscle tissue. This microtrauma is the basis of cumulative trauma disorder that may produce chronic discomfort and lead to more significant musculoskeletal injury. The symptoms of CTDs include pain, numbness, tingling, clumsiness, swelling (especially in the hand and wrist), weakness, loss of function, and overdevelopment of muscle groups.

All health care workers are at risk for MSDs caused by back strain from lifting and moving patients and equipment. In addition, radiographers often experience neck and shoulder strains and rotator cuff tears from reaching overhead to move the x-ray tube. Technologists who operate computerized modalities are more likely to experience spinal stress from sitting at a console for long periods and RSIs from intensive keyboard work. Keyboard RSIs affect the hands and wrists with CTDs such as tendinitis, ganglion cysts, and carpal tunnel syndrome. Imaging technologists whose work involves extended periods of viewing cathode ray tube monitors may also be subject to vision problems.

While ergonomic awareness is important for all workers, it is particularly important for sonographers (sonographic imaging is discussed in Chapter 22). Eighty percent of sonographers experience some form of work-related injury, usually in the form of RMIs and RSIs affecting the shoulder, arm, or wrist. The causes of these problems include equipment design, poor posture, sustained pressure and force on the transducer, awkward movements, inadequate work breaks, and overall job stress. Upper extremity injuries in sonography have increased in recent years because of changes in equipment design and in the nature of the work. The older transducers were heavier, but they were attached to a stable arm on the scanner that was aligned to the patient and that supported the weight of the transducer. The new transducers are smaller and lighter, but pressure is applied by the sonographer, and finer motor skill is required.

In addition, digital systems have eliminated the need to change cassettes and process films, reducing the variety of activities. More time in each shift is spent imaging, and specialization further increases the similarity and repetition of activities. More examinations are being performed; as techniques have evolved, many examinations have become longer, more difficult, and more repetitive. OSHA is working with hospitals and equipment manufacturers to improve the ergonomics of sonography, and education programs now emphasize the importance of posture, position change, and work breaks for sonographers.

Work injury is minimized when proper equipment is available and is used correctly, and when workers help one another. Frequent break periods and changes in position help minimize both positional and repetitive stress. Studies indicate that ongoing education programs and appropriate responses by employers to the ergonomic concerns of their workers is the right approach.

Body Mechanics

The principles of proper body alignment, movement, and balance are referred to as body mechanics. The application of these principles minimizes the energy required to sit, stand, and walk. When you use these principles to perform tasks that require stooping, lifting, pushing, pulling, and carrying, your effective strength is increased, and you are less likely to injure yourself. Severe strains may require hospitalization and long-term therapy involving considerable pain, inconvenience, and expense. Applying principles of body mechanics can prevent the muscle strains that are common among hospital workers, including many types of work injuries reported by radiographers.

Three concepts are essential to understanding the principles of body mechanics (see Figure 7-6):

1. **Base of Support**—This is the portion of the body in contact with the floor or other horizontal surface. It may be represented by a horizontal line linking the points of contact, such as between the feet when the body is erect. A broad base of support provides stability for body position and movement.

2. **Center of Gravity** (**Center of Body Weight**)—This is the point around which body weight is balanced. It is usually located in the midportion of the pelvis or lower abdomen, but the location can vary

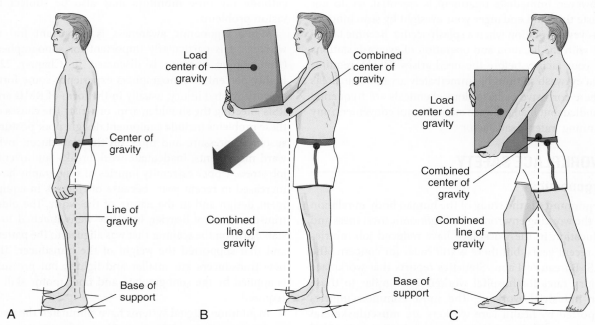

FIG 7-6 Body mechanics. **A,** With good posture, the line of gravity bisects the base of support. **B,** When the load is held away from the body, the line of gravity does not bisect the base of support. **C,** A wide stance with the load held close to the body allows the combined line of gravity to bisect the base of support.

somewhat depending on build. Any object you hold adds to the weight on the base of support; therefore, the size and position of a load affect the location of your center of gravity. The body is most stable when the center of gravity is nearest the center of the base of support.

3. **Line of Gravity**—This is an imaginary vertical line passing through the center of gravity. The body is most stable when the line of gravity bisects the base of support.

Using these concepts, the principles of body mechanics can be stated in the five simple rules listed in Box 7-4. Memorizing them is easy. Smooth performance requires practice.

Bending and twisting the back while lifting is a common cause of back strain (see Figure 7-7). A broad and stable base of support can be achieved by standing with feet apart and one foot slightly advanced. Remember that your thigh muscles are among the strongest in your body. Good body mechanics apply the combined strength of your legs, arms, and abdomen to protect the shorter, more vulnerable back muscles. Think ahead when anticipating a task that can cause muscle strain and use the resources available to you. These resources include adjusting the height of your work surface, using a cart to move a heavy load, or obtaining help to lift heavy objects. When moving heavy objects on wheels, it is much safer to push them than to pull them (Figure 7-8). Be sure to remember the proper use of body mechanics as you study patient transfer in Chapter 12.

When you injure yourself on the job, you place a greater burden on the other team members. If you injure yourself while lifting a patient, you may injure the patient as well.

BOX 7-4 Rules of Body Mechanics

- Provide a broad base of support.
- Work at a comfortable height.
- When lifting, bend your knees and keep your back straight (see Figure 7-7, *B*).
- Keep your load well-balanced and close to your body (see Figure 7-6, *C*).
- Roll or push a heavy object. Avoid pulling or lifting.

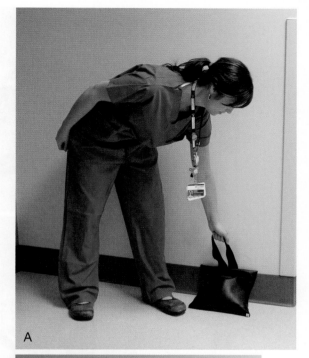
A

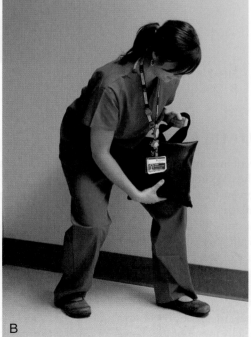
B

FIG 7-7 Using good body mechanics helps to avoid fatigue and prevent back strain. **A,** WRONG. The back is bent and twisted. **B,** CORRECT. The knees are flexed, and the back is straight.

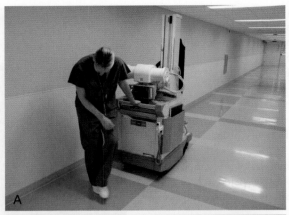

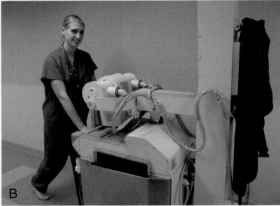

FIG 7-8 A, WRONG. Don't pull a heavy object, as it places more strain on muscle groups. **B,** CORRECT. Pushing heavy objects is more ergonomically sound for your body.

SUMMARY

- Prevent fires by ensuring that fuel, oxygen, and excessive heat do not exist together.
- Be prepared for fires by knowing the locations of fire alarms, fire extinguishers, fire doors, and electrical shut-off valves; be familiar with procedures for reporting fires and with evacuation routes.
- In case of fire, evacuate the area, report the fire, reassure patients, and, if appropriate, take steps to fight the fire, such as using a fire extinguisher.
- Electrical safety precautions are essential for avoiding the hazards of electrical fires and electric shock; be especially aware of the danger of using electricity in the vicinity of water.
- Keep passageways and corridors clear of obstruction and tripping hazards to avoid falls and collision accidents.

- When a spill occurs, limit access to the area and evaluate the spill. If you are qualified and equipped to clean it up, proceed with cleaning; otherwise, report the spill to the appropriate personnel.
- Ergonomics is the study of workplace injury prevention. The most common occupational injuries to health care personnel are MSDs caused from lifting and moving patients or equipment, or from repetitive movements or strains that cause microtrauma to muscles.
- The proper use of body mechanics increases strength and effectiveness when you perform physical tasks and decreases the likelihood of physical injury.

REVIEW QUESTIONS

1. The most likely cause of a fire in an imaging department is:
   A. spontaneous combustion
   B. open flames
   C. cigarette smoking
   D. an electrical problem
2. The federal agency governing workplace safety in the United States is:
   A. OSHA
   B. ARRT
   C. FDA
   D. CCD
3. Which of the following is not a typical component of a spill kit?
   A. nitrile gloves
   B. mop
   C. kitty litter
   D. plastic bags
4. Which of the following is not a responsibility of the radiographer in case of fire?
   A. Assess the situation and direct the activities of others.
   B. Evacuate the immediate area.
   C. Report the fire using the proper procedure.
   D. Reassure patients so that they do not become alarmed.
5. The most common types of workplace disabilities reported by health care workers are:
   A. vision problems
   B. respiratory disorders
   C. musculoskeletal disorders
   D. allergies
6. MSDS documents are likely to be needed in the event of:
   A. a fall
   B. a fire
   C. a chemical spill
   D. an electrical problem
7. The study of workplace injury prevention is called:
   A. body mechanics
   B. ergonomics
   C. environmental protection
   D. material data safety
8. Fires start when three elements occur in the same place at the same time. These three elements are oxygen, excessive heat, and:
   A. electricity
   B. water
   C. fuel
   D. smoke
9. Eighty percent of imaging technologists experience some form of work-related injury, usually in the form of RMIs and RSIs affecting the shoulder, arm, or wrist, if their area of specialization is:
   A. sonography
   B. radiography
   C. computed tomography
   D. magnetic resonance imaging
10. Stress due to repetitive motion, overreaching, or maintaining the same positions for long periods causes:
   A. back strain
   B. vision problems
   C. carpal tunnel syndrome
   D. microtrauma to muscle tissue

Answers can be found in the Answer Key on pages 429-431.

CRITICAL THINKING EXERCISES

1. If your employee orientation does not include all the information necessary to respond appropriately in the event of a fire, what should you do? Who is ultimately responsible for ensuring that you are informed?
2. List ways that you can use principles of good body mechanics recommended at work to increase your safety at home.
3. While preparing to clean a spill of darkroom fixer solution, you unconsciously wipe your face, getting fixer in your eye. What should you do?
4. When there is a chemical spill in your work area, what should you do first? What else should you do?

8

Infection Control Concepts

OBJECTIVES

At the conclusion of this chapter, the student will be able to:

- List the classifications of microorganisms, compare their physical structures, and give examples of each.
- Explain why viral diseases are particularly difficult to treat medically.
- List six factors involved in the cycle of infection.
- Define opportunistic infection, list conditions under which these infections may occur, and give examples.
- Define virulence factors and explain how these factors affect the differences between pathogenic organisms and normal flora.

- List four possible reservoirs of infection.
- List three common portals of entry and three portals of exit for pathogenic organisms.
- List and describe six main routes of infection transmission and name a disease that is transmitted by each route.
- Discuss and contrast the three basic ways in which the human body is protected from invasion by microorganisms.

OUTLINE

Microorganisms
  Bacteria
  Rickettsiae
  Viruses
  Fungi
  Prions
  Protozoa
Cycle of Infection
  Infectious Organisms
  Reservoir of Infection
  Portal of Exit
  Susceptible Host
  Portal of Entry

Transmission of Disease
  Direct contact
  Fomites
  Vectors
  Vehicles
  Droplet Contamination
  Airborne transmission
The Body's Defense Against Infection
  Natural Resistance
  Acquired Immunity
  Passive Immunity

KEY TERMS

acquired immunity
acquired resistance
airborne transmission
antibodies
antigens

bacterium (*pl.* bacteria)
direct contact
droplet contamination
endospore
fomite

fungus (*pl.* fungi)
motile
natural resistance
normal flora
nosocomial infection

As hospitals are gathering places for the sick, they are also focal points for the transmission of disease. Anyone with a health problem is more susceptible to infection, and infection control is therefore of critical importance in patient care.

As a member of the health care team, it is your professional duty to follow established infection control policies. This will promote the safety of patients, yourself, and other members of the health care team. The emergence of new diseases, the return of old ones, and the development of hospital-acquired, multidrug-resistant infections make it even more important for these policies to be followed and for everyone to play a role in preventing the spread of infection.

MICROORGANISMS

Microorganisms are living organisms that are too small to be seen with the naked eye. They include bacteria, viruses, protozoa, prions, and fungi. Most microorganisms do not cause infection or disease and are essential for our well-being. Microorganisms that live on or inside the body without causing infections or diseases are referred to as **normal flora**. They aid in skin preservation and digestion and protect us from harmful organisms that can cause infections or diseases. Microorganisms that cause infections and diseases are called **pathogens**, and their harmful effects will be discussed later in this chapter (see the section on infectious organisms).

> Microorganisms within the human body may be classified as one of two types: normal flora and pathogens. Normal flora do not usually cause disease and may be beneficial. Pathogens are disease-causing organisms.

Bacteria

Bacteria are very small, single-celled organisms with a cell wall and an atypical nucleus that lacks a membrane (Figure 8-1). The cell wall is essential for survival of the bacterium, making it the target for destruction by some antibiotics.

Bacteria grow independently and can replicate without a host cell. Most bacteria have one of three distinct shapes: spherical, called **cocci;** rod-shaped, called *bacilli;* or spiral, classified as either *spirilla* or *spirochetes* (Figure 8-2). Cocci may be further classified based on how the cells are grouped. They may exist singly, in groups of two, in long chains, or in clusters. Bacilli occur as single cells, in pairs, or in chains.

By using staining processes, bacteria can be subclassified as gram-positive or gram-negative, and as acid-fast or nonacid-fast. Following the Gram-stain process, bacteria are identified as gram-positive if they retain the dye when treated with alcohol. If the alcohol washes out the dye, they are called gram-negative. To determine whether bacteria are acid-fast, a different staining process is used. The bacteria are stained, heated, and treated with acid-alcohol to remove the color. If the bacterium resists decolorization, it is classified as acid-fast positive, indicating that acid-fast bacteria are present. If decolorization occurs, the bacterium is acid-fast negative. *Streptococci* and *Staphylococci* are gram-positive. *Escherichia coli,* a bacillus, is gram-negative, and *Mycobacterium tuberculosis,* a bacillus, is acid-fast positive, often simply called "acid-fast." There are additional staining techniques used to more specifically identify certain bacteria, such as the spirochete *Treponema palladium.* These techniques can be researched in a microbiology text.

Bacteria are also grouped by their oxygen requirements. Some require oxygen to grow and are called *obligate aerobes,* whereas others will not grow in the presence of oxygen and are called *anaerobes.* Bacteria that can adapt and grow under either aerobic or anaerobic conditions are called *facultative organisms.*

There are many classifications and subclassifications by which bacteria may be identified. Bacteria are often referred to simply by the name of their class or subclass. For example, a report might state that gram-negative

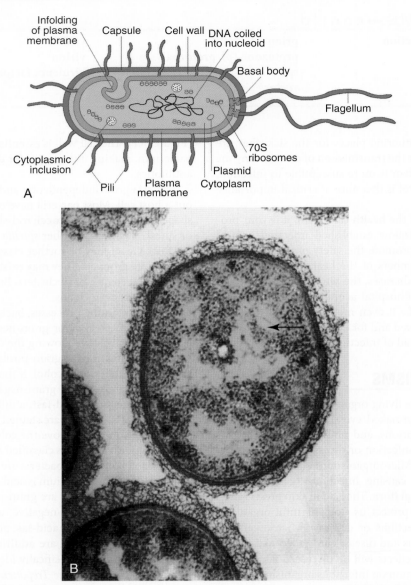

FIG 8-1 Typical bacterium. **A,** Diagram of structure. **B,** Photomicrograph. Note the absence of a nuclear membrane *(arrow)*. (A From Goering R et al. *Mims' medical microbiology*, ed 4, Philadelphia, 2007, Mosby; B from Atlas RM. *Principles of microbiology*, St Louis, 1995, Mosby.)

bacilli are present, indicating the presence of *M. tuberculosis* bacteria. It is helpful to be familiar with these classifications so that they can be immediately identified with the bacteria and diseases with which they are associated.

Some types of bacteria can generate endospores, a resistant form of the bacterium that is produced within the cell when environmental conditions are unfavorable.

Most endospore-forming bacteria live in the soil, but they can reside almost anywhere. Endospores are resistant to destruction and can remain viable for many years, often being carried through the atmosphere on virtually invisible dust particles. When conditions improve, endospores can germinate, revitalizing the bacteria.

Bacteria are able to adapt to new conditions and mutate, changing into slightly different genetic forms

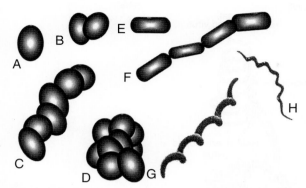

FIG 8-2 Bacterial forms. Cocci: **A**, Single coccus; **B**, Diplococcus; **C**, Chain formation *(Streptococcus);* and **D**, Cluster *(Staphylococcus).* Bacilli: **E**, Single bacillus and **F**, Chain. Spiral bacteria: **G**, Spirillum and **H**, Spirochete.

that allow them to resist and survive in the presence of antimicrobial drugs.

Significant diseases caused by bacteria include tuberculosis (caused by *M. tuberculosis*); streptococcal pharyngitis (strep throat) and necrotizing fasciitis (flesh-eating bacteria), both of which are caused by streptococcal Group A; and infectious diarrhea and hemolytic uremic syndrome, both of which are caused by *E. coli* 0157:H7.

Rickettsiae

Although rickettsiae are considered bacteria, they are discussed separately because they are atypical. They are smaller than most bacteria and are just barely visible in an ordinary light microscope. Their most significant identifying feature is that they only grow inside animal cells (for example, in rabbits and rats). Rickettsiae do not survive in the environment; they are transmitted among animals when they are bitten by infected arthropods, such as ticks, lice, fleas, and mites. Humans are only accidental hosts. Rickettsiae are causative agents for Rocky Mountain spotted fever and typhus fever.

Viruses

Viruses are subcellular organisms and are among the smallest known disease-causing organisms. Because of their small size, they must be viewed with an electron microscope. A fully developed viral particle, called a **virion**, is made up of genetic material, either deoxyribonucleic acid (DNA) or ribonucleic acid (RNA), which is protected by an outer protein coating called the *capsid*. The capsid may be covered by a lipoprotein envelope that has projecting spikes (Figure 8-3). Enveloped

viruses, such as influenza, human immunodeficiency virus (HIV), and hepatitis B, use these spikes to attach to host cells. Some viruses, such as the rhinoviruses that cause the common cold, lack both the envelope and spikes, so the capsid assists these viruses in attaching to host cells.

Viruses cannot survive independently. A virus invades a host cell for which it has specificity and stimulates it to participate in the formation of additional virus particles. For example, the hepatitis virus attaches to receptor sites on liver cells. Because viruses reside in and use the host cell to replicate, it has been difficult to create antiviral drugs that are not also harmful to the host cell. Only a few antiviral agents exist, and these are useful against only a limited number of viruses. Viruses can mutate quite rapidly, becoming resistant to drugs that were originally effective against them.

Other common viruses include the Epstein-Barr virus, which causes infectious mononucleosis, and varicella, which causes chicken pox and herpes zoster (shingles).

Fungi

Fungi (*sing.,* **fungus**) occur as single-celled yeasts or as long, branched, filament-like structures called **molds** that are composed of many cells (Figure 8-4). Some fungi can exist in either form, depending on the environment. Yeasts reproduce by forming buds, whereas molds reproduce by spore formation. There are more than 100,000 diverse species of fungi, many of which serve useful purposes. They are a key ingredient in the production of alcoholic beverages, are responsible for the flavor of cheese, give bread its lightness, and produce the antibiotic penicillin. Fungi are also important in nature because they help decompose dead plants and animals, making their components available for plant growth.

Some species of fungi are destructive to natural materials like wood and leather, whereas others cause diseases in plants, animals, or humans. In humans, fungi cause skin infections, such as athlete's foot and ringworm; respiratory infections, such as histoplasmosis and coccidioidomycosis; and **opportunistic infections** (infections caused by usually nonpathogenic organisms), such as *Pneumocystis carinii* pneumonia (PCP) and pharyngeal and esophageal candidiasis in individuals with compromised immune systems.

Prions

The smallest and least understood of all pathogens is the **prion**, which was discovered in 1983. Scientists believe

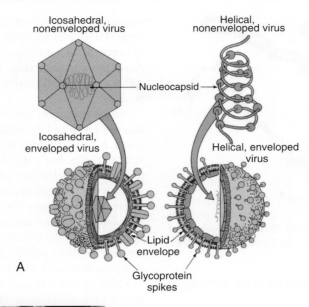

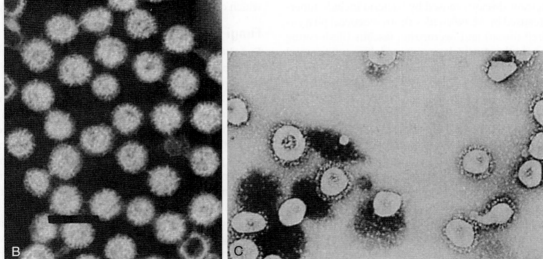

FIG 8-3 Typical viral structure. **A,** Diagrams of nonenveloped and enveloped viruses. **B,** Photomicrograph, nonenveloped virus. **C,** Photomicrograph, enveloped virus. (A modified from Murray PR, Drew WL, Kobayashi GS, et al., editors. *Medical microbiology,* St Louis, 1990, Mosby; B and C from Tille PM. *Bailey and Scott's diagnostic microbiology,* ed 13, St Louis, 2014, Mosby.)

that prions may be infectious proteins. Their method of replication is not completely understood. Prions do not have DNA or RNA, but they are capable of automatically transforming healthy proteins in nerve cells into more prions. Prions are resistant to the body's natural defenses and can continue to multiply unchecked, causing irreversible neurologic damage. They were first identified as the cause of scrapie, a degenerative disease affecting the nervous systems of sheep. It is thought that prions are the cause of bovine spongiform encephalopathy (mad cow disease) and both classic and variant Creutzfeldt-Jakob disease in humans. The classic form of Creutzfeldt-Jakob disease is rare and occurs either for no known reason or as a result of inheriting the abnormal protein (prion).

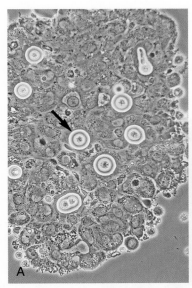
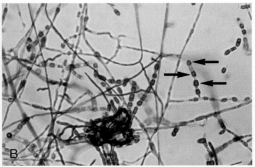

FIG 8-4 **Fungi. A,** Single-cell yeasts. **B,** Molds are multicellular fungi. (From Tille PM. *Bailey and Scott's diagnostic microbiology,* ed 13, St Louis, 2014, Mosby.)

The variant form is infectious and is related to mad cow disease; it occurs when someone is exposed to contaminated products, such as corneal transplants from infected donors or consumption of infected meat. Both forms cause sponge-like changes in the brain, leading to progressive dementia. Creutzfeldt-Jakob disease may be related to other conditions characterized by slow deterioration of the nervous system. Further study of prions may help researchers understand the cause of Alzheimer disease.

Protozoa

Protozoa (*sing.,* **protozoon**) are complex single-celled animals that generally exist as free-living organisms. However, a few protozoa are parasitic and live within the human body. They may be classified as **motile** (moving) or *nonmotile*. If motile, they are further classified by their method of motility. Some move by changing their shape to form pseudopods (false "feet"), whereas others move using flagella (whip-like formations) or cilia (fine, hair-like projections) (see Figure 8-5). Most parasitic protozoa produce some type of resistant form, such as a cyst, to survive in the environment outside the host. Other protozoa have complex life cycles involving alternate residence in the human body and an insect vector. This is true of the protozoan that causes malaria, which lives alternately in mosquitoes and humans. Protozoa can infect the gastrointestinal, genitourinary, respiratory, and circulatory systems. Common protozoal diseases include:

- Amebiasis and giardiasis, both of which affect the gastrointestinal tract and cause diarrhea.
- Trichomoniasis, a sexually transmitted disease affecting the male and female genitourinary tracts; it causes a greenish-yellow discharge from the male urethra and from the vagina in females.
- Toxoplasmosis, which is contracted from contact with cat feces or eating undercooked meat containing the protozoan. Toxoplasmosis affects the blood and lymphatic vessels and can cause congenital infection in a fetus or neurologic impairment in the immunocompromised.

CYCLE OF INFECTION

The factors involved in the spread of disease are sometimes called the **cycle of infection** (Figure 8-6). For infections to be transmitted, there must be an infectious organism, a reservoir of infection, a portal of exit, a susceptible host, a portal of entry, and a means of transporting the organism from the reservoir to the susceptible individual.

Infectious Organisms

Microorganisms capable of causing disease are called **pathogenic organisms** or **pathogens**. They possess

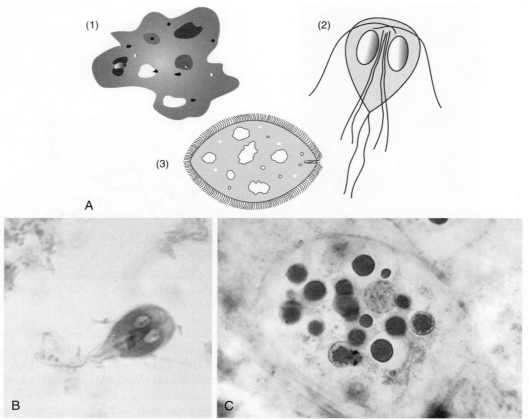

FIG 8-5 A, Motile protozoa: ameba *(1)*, flagellate *(2)*, ciliate *(3)*. **B,** Photomicrograph of *Giardia lamblia,* a flagellate. **C,** Photomicrograph of *Entamoeba histolytica,* an ameba. (B and C from Tille PM. *Bailey and Scott's diagnostic microbiology,* ed 13, St Louis, 2014, Mosby.)

certain properties called **virulence factors** that distinguish them from nonpathogenic organisms or normal flora. These factors enable bacteria to destroy or damage host cells and resist destruction by the host's cellular defenses. Each bacterial pathogen has an affinity for a certain type of cell in the body. They attach to these cells and excrete protein substances called *toxins* that can kill or injure the host cells. They can destroy red and white blood cells and activate enzymes in the host cell that enable them to spread through tissues. Virulence factors assist the pathogen to avoid recognition by the host cell and resist destruction by white blood cells. Their destructiveness and resistance allow them to grow and cause the signs and symptoms of disease. The pathogens that cause diphtheria, pertussis, typhoid fever, and dysentery have these virulence factors. Table 8-1 provides other examples of pathogens.

Normal flora are capable of causing disease when they are not confined to their usual environment, when an individual's resistance is weakened, or when broad-spectrum antibiotics disrupt the ecological balance of the resident flora. For example, *E. coli,* normal flora of the gastrointestinal tract, can become pathogenic if it enters the bladder. This occurs more often in females because of the shorter urethra. *Candida albicans* may be found in the throat or gastrointestinal tract of many healthy persons, yet this same organism can assume a pathogenic role, causing vaginal yeast infections in females when competing bacteria are destroyed by antibiotic treatment. *Candida* is an opportunistic organism that proliferates when immunity is compromised, causing both esophagitis and respiratory infections in patients with acquired immunodeficiency syndrome (AIDS).

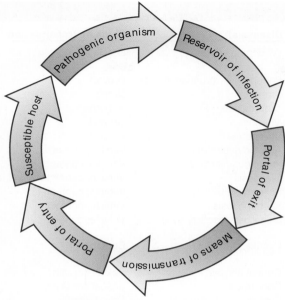

FIG 8-6 Cycle of infection.

> Normal flora can cause infections when they are located outside their usual environment or when the host's immune system is compromised. Such infections are called *opportunistic infections.*

Reservoir of Infection

The reservoir or source of infection may be any place where pathogens can thrive in sufficient numbers to pose a threat. Such an environment must provide moisture, nutrients, and a suitable temperature, all of which are found in the human body. A reservoir of infection might be a patient with hepatitis, a radiographer with an upper respiratory infection, or a visitor with staphylococcal boils.

Because some pathogens live in the bodies of healthy individuals without causing apparent disease, a person may be the reservoir for an infectious organism without realizing it. These individuals are called carriers. Many of us have throat cultures that are positive for *Staphylococcus aureus,* but do not have a sore throat. A susceptible patient with an open wound could contract a life-threatening infection if sufficiently contaminated with this organism. The classic example of a carrier of infection is "Typhoid Mary," who was a "healthy" food handler. Many cases of typhoid fever were attributed to contamination of the meals she helped to prepare. Better

sanitation and food-handling education have reduced the incidence of foodborne diseases. An example of a carrier of infection today is the asymptomatic individual infected with HIV who spreads the disease through sexual intercourse or by sharing contaminated needles with intravenous drug users.

Although the human body is the most common reservoir of infection, any habitat that will support the growth of microorganisms has the potential to be a secondary source, such as a damp, warm place that is not cleaned regularly. Other examples of nonhuman reservoirs include:

- Animals, the reservoir for *Salmonella*
- Soil, the reservoir for *Tetanus*
- Food, the reservoir for *Botulinum*
- Water, the reservoir for typhus and Legionnaires' disease

Portal of Exit

The portal of exit from the human body may be any route through which blood, body fluids, excretions, or secretions leave the body. Examples include the respiratory, urinary, and gastrointestinal tracts; an infected wound; and the bloodstream.

Susceptible Host

Susceptible hosts frequently are patients who have a reduced natural resistance to infection. In addition to the primary problem that caused their hospitalization, they may develop a **nosocomial infection** (hospital-acquired infection or health care-associated infection). Examples of nosocomial infections are discussed in Chapter 9 under *Infectious Diseases.*

Hospital infections also pose a threat to health care workers. When contracted by health care workers, these infections are called **occupationally acquired infections** rather than nosocomial infections. Hepatitis B and C viruses are the biggest concerns, because both are spread by blood and blood products. For a discussion of these and other important occupationally acquired infections, see the section on *Infectious Diseases* in Chapter 9.

Hospital workers are exposed to many pathogens. In a single day, a radiographer may care for ambulatory outpatients, hospital patients in isolation, and emergency trauma patients with "dirty" wounds. The radiographer who must work when resistance is low because of fatigue, stress, or a low-grade infection has increased susceptibility to contagious diseases. A healthy, well-rested body is your best protection.

TABLE 8-1 **Examples of Pathogens**

Body System	Name	Classification	Disease(s)	Mode of Transmission
Respiratory tract	Bordetella pertussis	Bacterium	Whooping cough	Droplet
	Candida albicans	Fungus	Pneumonia, thrush in infants	Droplet
	Corynebacterium diphtheriae	Bacterium	Diphtheria	Droplet
	Mycobacterium tuberculosis	Bacterium	Tuberculosis	Airborne
	Mumps virus	Virus	Mumps	Droplet
	Streptococcus pyogenes	Bacterium	Strep throat	Droplet
	Entamoeba histolytica	Protozoan	Amebic dysentery	Vehicle, contact
	Escherichia coli O157:H7	Bacterium	Infectious diarrhea	Vehicle, contact
	Giardia lamblia	Protozoan	Giardiasis	Vehicle, contact
	Poliomyelitis virus	Virus	Poliomyelitis	Vehicle, contact
	Salmonella species	Bacterium	Salmonellosis	Vehicle, contact
	Shigella species	Bacterium	Shigellosis (bacillary dysentery)	Vehicle, contact
Genitourinary tract	Escherichia coli	Bacterium	Cystitis, nephritis	Contact
	Herpes simplex, type 2	Virus	Genital herpes	Sexual contact
	Neisseria gonorrhoea	Bacterium	Gonorrhea	Sexual contact
	Treponema pallidum	Bacterium	Syphilis	Sexual contact
Skin	Varicella	Virus	Chicken pox, disseminated herpes zoster, shingles	Contact, airborne
	Herpes simplex, type 1	Virus	Fever blisters	Contact (and predisposition)
	Measles virus (rubeola)	Virus	Measles	Airborne
	Nonhemolytic Streptococcus (Enterococcus)	Bacterium	Surgical wound infection	Contact
	Staphylococcus aureus	Bacterium	Boils, wound infection	Contact
	Tinea capitis, Tinea pedis	Fungus	Ringworm, athlete's foot	Contact (and predisposition)
Blood	Plasmodium species	Protozoan	Malaria	Vectors (mosquitoes)
	Salmonella typhi	Bacterium	Typhoid fever	Vehicle, contact

Infections acquired in hospitals or health care facilities are termed *nosocomial infections* or *health care-associated infections* when they affect patients; when they affect health care workers, they are called *occupationally acquired infections*.

Portal of Entry

The portal of entry is the route by which microorganisms gain access into the susceptible host. Examples include the respiratory, urinary, and gastrointestinal tracts; an open wound or break in the skin; the mucous membranes of the eyes, nose, or mouth; and the bloodstream.

TRANSMISSION OF DISEASE

The most direct way to intervene in the cycle of infection is to prevent transmission of the infectious organism from the reservoir to the susceptible host. To accomplish this, you must understand the six main routes of transmission, which include: (1) direct contact, and indirect routes that involve transport of organisms by way of (2) fomites, (3) vectors, (4) vehicles, (5) airborne means, and (6) droplet contamination.

Direct Contact

The first route is **direct contact**. This transmission mode requires that the host is touched by an infected person and that the organisms are placed in direct contact with susceptible tissue. For example, syphilis and HIV infections may be contracted when infectious organisms from the mucous membrane of one individual are placed in direct contact with the mucous membrane of a susceptible host. Also, skin infections often occur among hospital workers because of the frequent contact with patients who have staphylococcal and streptococcal diseases.

Fomites

An object that has been in contact with pathogenic organisms is called a fomite. A contaminated urinary catheter is a typical example. Other fomites in the radiology department might include the x-ray table, vertical bucky, image receptors, positioning sponges contaminated with infectious body fluids, or perhaps contaminated gloves.

Vectors

A vector is an arthropod in whose body an infectious organism develops or multiplies before becoming infectious to a new host. Bites by infected insects can transmit diseases to humans. Some examples of vectors are mosquitoes that transmit malaria or dengue fever, fleas that carry bubonic plague, and ticks that spread Lyme disease or Rocky Mountain spotted fever.

Vehicles

A vehicle is any medium that transports microorganisms. Examples include contaminated food, water, drugs, or blood.

Droplet Contamination

Droplet contamination often occurs when an infectious individual coughs, sneezes, speaks, or sings in the vicinity of a susceptible host. Droplet transmission involves contact of the mucous membranes of the eyes, nose, or mouth of a susceptible person with large droplets containing microorganisms and measuring more than 5 μm (microns, micrometers, 0.001 mm) in diameter. These particles do not remain suspended in the air and travel only short distances, usually 3 feet or less. Influenza, meningitis, diphtheria, pertussis, and streptococcal pneumonia are examples of respiratory illnesses that spread by means of droplet contamination.

Airborne Transmission

Airborne transmission occurs from dust that contains spores or droplet nuclei. **Droplet nuclei** are defined as particles of evaporated droplets containing microorganisms and measuring 5 μm or smaller in diameter. They can remain suspended in the air for long periods. These particles may be dispersed by air currents and may be inhaled by a susceptible host. Special air handling and ventilation are required to prevent airborne transmission of these infected particles. *M. tuberculosis,* rubeola, and the varicella viruses are examples of airborne infections. Varicella can also be contracted through contact with the vesicles that form on the skin of patients infected with these viruses.

Although many pathogenic organisms are fragile, requiring continuous warmth, moisture, and nutrients to exist, the endospores formed by some bacteria are resistant to heat, cold, and drying and can live without nourishment. Endospores can float through the air and lurk in dusty corners waiting for the opportunity to invade a susceptible host. Spore-forming bacterial organisms are responsible for serious but relatively uncommon diseases such as tetanus, anthrax, and botulism. The spores are transmitted to a host through inhalation, ingestion, or contact. The host provides the moisture, warmth, and nutrients that enable the endospore to germinate into a bacterial cell.

Epidemiological studies have shown that some viruses can resist drying for weeks at a time. An example of this is the virus that causes herpes (both oral and genital). The need for cleanliness as a defense against infection from both spores and viruses cannot be overstated.

> Environmental cleanliness is an important aspect of preventing disease transmission because certain viruses and spore-forming bacteria and fungi can survive on surfaces in the clinical area for long periods.

THE BODY'S DEFENSE AGAINST INFECTION

The human body is protected from the invasion of microorganisms in three ways: natural resistance and defenses, acquired resistance (also known as *active immunity*), and short-term passive immunity.

Natural Resistance

Mechanical barriers such as intact skin and mucous membranes provide natural resistance. Injuries such as severe burns, cuts, and abrasions can disrupt this protective skin barrier and allow microorganisms to pass into tissues and proliferate, increasing the risk of infection.

The mucous membranes of the respiratory, urinary, gastrointestinal, and reproductive systems secrete mucus, which traps foreign particles. Additionally, the respiratory tract is lined with cilia that transport mucus containing dust and microorganisms out of the body. The urinary tract is protected from ascending infections by the composition and outward flow of urine.

Chemicals, such as lysozyme in human tears and acids produced by the stomach, vagina, and skin, also help destroy invading microorganisms. The pH, salt content, and dryness of the skin limit the number of bacteria that can reside there, and beneficial normal flora prevent the overgrowth of undesirable organisms.

In spite of these barriers, microorganisms do gain access into the body. This occurs as a result of common daily activities, such as brushing one's teeth and shaving. This invasion initiates our second line of defense, the inflammatory response. Inflammation increases blood flow to the site and permits the passage of fluids and white blood cells into the tissues to engulf and destroy the invading pathogens. This process is called **phagocytosis**.

When viruses infect the body, virus-infected cells produce *interferons,* small protein molecules that protect the uninfected cells from invasion by the original virus as well as others. Interferons are species-specific and are currently being produced in laboratories for the treatment of herpes and chronic hepatitis B and C.

Acquired Immunity

Humans are born with a certain amount of immunity, but most humans become resistant to a disease by becoming infected with a specific organism. This infection may or may not manifest itself as an obvious illness. Immunity can also be conferred from vaccines made from dead or weakened strains of microorganisms for a specific infection or from an inactivated toxin.

This state of being resistant to a specific infection is called **acquired immunity**. Acquired immunity occurs because the body is able to distinguish itself from foreign protein substances that enter the body. These substances are called **antigens**. **Antibodies** are protein substances formed in response to specific antigens. They are produced by a specific white blood cell, the B-cell, which works with other white blood cells to destroy invading foreign substances and prevent reinfection by a particular antigen. Because the body forms its own antibodies to the specific antigen, acquired immunity is long term.

Passive Immunity

Passive immunity occurs following an injection of *preformed* antibodies to a particular infection. This is the case when individuals are given immunoglobulin (pooled human blood and antibodies from the general population) before and after exposure to hepatitis A. The antibodies act immediately and prevent disease but will weaken over time. Newborns are temporarily immune to infections because of the antibodies that are passed from mother to fetus *in utero.* Infants will continue to receive this passive immunity if breastfed after birth. Because the body does not produce these antibodies, passive immunity is short term.

> Active or acquired immunity occurs when individuals develop their own antibodies to a specific antigen as a result of having the disease or being immunized against it. This resistance is long term. Passive immunity occurs when individuals receive antibodies produced outside their bodies, such as those from the mother that exist in the newborn, or those produced in a laboratory for emergency immunization. This resistance is short term.

■ SUMMARY

- Microorganisms are living organisms too small to be seen with the naked eye. They include bacteria, viruses, protozoa, prions, and fungi.
- Some microorganisms benefit and protect humans and are called *normal flora;* some are harmful, causing infections and disease, and are called *pathogens.*
- Bacteria are single-celled microorganisms characterized by a cell wall and a nucleus that lacks a membrane. They occur in various shapes and groupings and are subclassified by staining processes. Gram-stain and acid-fast methods are commonly used.
- Endospores are bacterial forms that are resistant to destruction and can remain viable for many years. They may germinate when conditions are favorable.
- Rickettsiae are atypical bacteria that grow inside animal cells, particularly rodents, and are transmitted by insect vectors.

- Viruses are very small subcellular organisms that consist of genetic material protected by a protein coating called a capsid. They cannot survive independently, and each is specific to a certain type of host cell in which it replicates.
- There are many species of fungi; some occur as single-celled organisms called yeasts, and some as multicellular molds. Although many are useful, some are pathogenic.
- Prions are infectious proteins that attack the nervous system. Little is known about them.
- Protozoa are complex single-celled animals that generally exist as free-living organisms. A few are parasitic and live within the human body, causing diseases of the digestive, respiratory, genitourinary, and circulatory systems. They are classified as either motile or nonmotile.
- The factors involved in the spread of disease make up the cycle of infection and include: an infectious organism, reservoir of infection, portals of exit and entry, mode of transmission, and susceptible host.
- Virulence factors are responsible for the behavior and infectious characteristics that distinguish pathogenic organisms from nonpathogenic organisms.
- Opportunistic infections are those caused by normal flora in individuals with compromised immunity.
- The reservoir of infection is usually an infected individual in which microorganisms live and multiply. Infected animals and contaminated soil, water, and food can also serve as reservoirs of infection.
- The portal of exit is any route by which contaminated body fluids leave the body. The portal of entry may be via the respiratory tract, urinary tract,

gastrointestinal tract, blood stream, or any mucous membrane.
- A susceptible host is any vulnerable individual exposed to a sufficient number of pathogenic organisms. Hospital patients have a reduced resistance to infection because of their other health problems. A nosocomial infection is a hospital-acquired infection that affects a patient. Health care workers may also become susceptible hosts.
- There are six main routes of disease transmission: direct contact, and indirect routes that involve transport of organisms by way of fomites (contaminated objects), vectors (insects), vehicles (contaminated food, water, and soil), droplet contamination, and airborne means (dust particles containing spores and droplet nuclei).
- The human body is protected from the invasion of microorganisms in three ways: natural resistance and defenses, acquired immunity, and short-term passive immunity.
- The skin, mucous membranes, and other natural protective features of the body provide resistance to invasion by microorganisms.
- Acquired immunity is long-term resistance to a specific infection that occurs when an individual develops antibodies to a particular organism as a result of either infection or immunization.
- Passive resistance occurs when an individual receives preformed antibodies from others to provide temporary immunity. Examples include immunoglobulin injections to prevent infection after exposure to certain viruses and the immunity that is passed to infants from their mothers at birth and in breast milk.

REVIEW QUESTIONS

1. Microorganisms that live on or inside the body without causing disease are referred to as:
   A. pathogens
   B. endospores
   C. microbial flora
   D. parasites
2. Bacteria can be classified or grouped based on:
   A. staining
   B. oxygen requirements
   C. shape
   D. all of the above
3. Microorganisms classified as acid-fast are a type of:
   A. virus
   B. bacteria
   C. rickettsiae
   D. protozoa
4. Yeasts are one type of:
   A. bacteria
   B. mold
   C. fungus
   D. prion

▌REVIEW QUESTIONS—cont'd

5. Bacterial forms that are resistant to destruction and can remain viable for many years are called:
   A. endospores
   B. gram-negative
   C. cocci
   D. facultative organisms
6. Tuberculosis, strep throat, and necrotizing fasciitis are diseases caused by:
   A. fungi
   B. prions
   C. protozoa
   D. bacteria
7. The term *reservoir of infection* refers to the:
   A. place where the pathogen resides
   B. method by which the pathogen enters the body
   C. method by which the pathogen leaves the body
   D. individual with reduced natural resistance to infection
8. The term *nosocomial* applies to infections that are:
   A. caused by viruses
   B. hospital-acquired
   C. caused by normal flora in persons weakened by other diseases
   D. transmitted by droplet contamination

9. An object that has been contaminated with a pathogenic organism is called a:
   A. vehicle
   B. fomite
   C. vector
   D. prion
10. Particles of evaporated droplets containing microorganisms and measuring 5 μm or smaller are called:
    A. droplet nuclei
    B. droplet contamination
    D. vehicles
    D. fomites
11. The immunity transferred from mother to child at birth or via breast milk is classified as:
    A. natural resistance
    B. acquired resistance
    C. active immunity
    D. passive immunity

Answers can be found in the Answer Key on pages 429-431.

▌CRITICAL THINKING EXERCISES

1. Compare and contrast active immunity with passive immunity.
2. Give two examples of situations in which a radiographer might transmit an infection to a patient. Give two examples of situations in which a patient might transmit an infection to a radiographer.
3. Define *virulence factors* and explain how these factors affect the differences between pathogenic organisms and normal flora.
4. List the six common modes of disease transmission in the order of how commonly each might occur in an imaging department. Defend your conclusions.

9

Preventing Disease Transmission

OBJECTIVES

At the conclusion of this chapter, the student will be able to:

- Define *medical asepsis*, *disinfection*, and *isolation*.
- State five examples of personal hygiene that help to prevent the spread of infection.
- Demonstrate techniques for effective hand hygiene.
- Describe or demonstrate the correct method of linen disposal using medical asepsis principles.
- Name the agent and state the dilution used for disinfecting radiographic equipment, as recommended by the Centers for Disease Control and Prevention (CDC).

- Demonstrate proper disposal of contaminated equipment in the clinical area.
- Contrast isolation techniques for infectious patients with those for immunodeficient patients.
- Demonstrate removal and disposal of gowns, gloves, and masks without breaking isolation principles.

OUTLINE

Infectious Diseases
Emerging Diseases
Health Care-associated Infections
Bloodborne Pathogens
Tuberculosis
Preventing Disease Transmission
Historical Perspective

Standard Precautions
OSHA Bloodborne Pathogens Standard
Medical Asepsis
Handling and Disposing of Contaminated Items and Waste
Isolation Technique

KEY TERMS

acquired immunodeficiency syndrome (AIDS)
asepsis
disinfection
epidemic
health care-associated infection (HAI)

human immunodeficiency virus (HIV)
immunosuppressant
methicillin-resistant *Staphylococcus aureus* (MRSA)
microbial dilution

pandemic
sharps container
Standard Precautions
sterilization
tuberculosis (TB)
vancomycin-resistant enterococci (VRE)

In Chapter 8, you learned about the causes of infectious diseases and the processes by which infectious organisms spread from one individual to another. In this chapter you will learn about specific contagious diseases, especially those you are likely to encounter in hospitals in the United States. You will learn the basic principles of infection control and the accepted procedures for preventing the spread of infection in a health care setting.

INFECTIOUS DISEASES

Emerging Diseases

There are many new diseases in the world, and some old diseases once thought to be under control are returning in epidemic (substantially increased) proportions after years of low-level incidence. As a worker in the health care field, you will be on the front line of exposure to both old and new diseases. The infection control department within the hospital is responsible for keeping track of these infections and developing infection control policies to protect you, other staff, and patients, based on recommendations from the Centers for Disease Control and Prevention (CDC). The CDC monitors and studies the types of infections occurring in the nation, compiles statistical data about these infections, and publishes this information in both a weekly report and an annual surveillance summary report. The World Health Organization (WHO) studies, collects, and compiles infection data from every country in the world and makes this information available worldwide.

> The CDC is the most complete source of information about infectious diseases in the United States. www.cdc.gov.

Emerging diseases include new diseases appearing in the population, existing ones that are rapidly increasing in incidence or geographic range, and resurgent or recurrent old diseases caused by an old or mutated pathogen. Disease emergence is precipitated by many factors:

- Increased human exposure to vectors in nature
- Population growth and migration to crowded cities
- Rapid international travel and transportation of goods
- Contact with new strains of dangerous pathogens

- Pathogen mutation caused by overutilization of antimicrobial agents
- Breakdowns in public health measures
- Climate change
- Bioterrorism

Inadequate public health measures in South America and Africa have resulted in cholera outbreaks due to poor sanitation and insufficient chlorine levels in water supplies. Drastic political change and the resulting deterioration of public health programs accounted for the resurgence of diphtheria in the former Soviet Union. Russian immigrants reintroduced this disease to the United States.

The outbreak of Hantavirus pulmonary syndrome (a potentially fatal respiratory disease) in the southwestern United States in 1993 was blamed on a 6-year drought followed by a mild, wet winter and spring. These conditions were favorable for a dramatic rise in the population of deer mice, which increased their contact with humans. *Hantavirus* infection is contracted by inhaling dust containing particles of droppings from these mice.

The unusually warm temperatures in Mexico and southern Texas in 1995 provided ideal conditions for mosquitoes carrying dengue fever to reproduce and transmit the flavivirus. Dengue fever, also called *breakbone fever,* is characterized by a high fever, headache, muscle and joint aches, malaise, and often a rash. The disease may range from a mild illness to a severe, sometimes fatal, condition with hemorrhage and shock.

Reforestation increases populations of deer and deer ticks, the vector for Lyme disease. When humans move closer to these forests, it is easier for the pathogen that causes Lyme disease to spread from its normal host into humans.

Human migration from isolated areas of the world to crowded cities is responsible for the spread of once-localized infections, such as human immunodeficiency virus (HIV), cholera, and dengue fever. International travel has the potential to spread many pathogens around the world.

The outbreak of anthrax in the United States in 2001 demonstrated the ease with which terrorists can spread diseases once thought to be under control. This has raised public concern about other diseases that could affect a large portion of the population.

Travelers from Asia brought the virus for severe acute respiratory syndrome (SARS) to North America in the spring of 2003. Air transport of used tires from Asia introduced the mosquitoes carrying dengue fever to the United States.

Influenza spreads rapidly across the globe as travelers meet and exchange infections. The influenza virus mutates readily, resulting in many different strains of influenza and the frequent appearance of new strains. In recent years, deadly strains of the H1N1 virus (swine flu) and the H5N1 virus (bird flu) have been in the news. Although bird flu has not moved significantly into the human population as was originally feared, swine flu reached **pandemic** (widespread epidemic) proportions in humans in 2009. Fortunately, a vaccine for this virus was quickly developed and made available, and the virus has now mutated into a less virulent form.

Although some *Escherichia coli* bacteria exist as normal flora in the digestive tract, some strains of this organism can cause serious illness. Ingestion of food contaminated with *E. coli* O157:H7 causes diarrhea and hemorrhagic uremic syndrome. This strain of *E. coli,* which can cause severe illness and death, has been linked to the consumption of undercooked hamburger meat, unpasteurized apple juice, dried venison, contaminated spinach, and other foods. Another deadly strain of *E. coli,* identified as 104:H4, caused the deaths of dozens of people in Germany and many serious illnesses in France in May of 2011. In June of 2011, the first death due to 104:H4 was reported in the United States. At first the outbreak was traced by scientists to bean sprouts grown on a German farm, but the bacterium was then identified in other types of edible sprouts as well, and is believed to have originated from fenugreek seed grown in Egypt and mixed with other seeds when packaged by a firm in the United Kingdom. This demonstrates how rapidly emerging diseases can spread and how difficult it may be to identify the source. This particular bacterium has two traits that may be responsible for it causing the deadliest *E. coli* outbreak in recent history. One trait is the production of a toxin called *Shiga toxin* that causes severe illness, including bloody diarrhea and kidney failure. The second trait is that the bacteria aggregate on the surface of the intestine to form a dense pattern that enhances the ability of the bacteria to pump the toxin into the body. Unlike other strains, this one tends to attack young and middle-aged women.

The most recent multi-country outbreak is that of the Ebola virus, which reached historic proportions in 2014 in West Africa. Originally identified in 1976 near the Ebola River, there are five strains of *Ebolavirus,* four of which affect humans. Ebola spreads quickly through direct contact with 1) blood and body fluids from an infected person, 2) objects contaminated with the virus, and 3) infected fruit bats or primates. Typical flu-like signs and symptoms of this infection appear 2-21 days after exposure, and include fatigue, headache, weakness, diarrhea, abdominal pain, vomiting, fever and hemorrhage. Statistics provided by the CDC over a 1-year period in 2014 indicate that there were more than 21,400 cases and approximately 8,500 deaths across nine countries, with roughly 99.8% of those cases occurring in Sierra Leone, Guinea, and Liberia. The rapid transmission and delayed onset of symptoms have induced many countries, including the United States, to set forth strict nationwide Ebola health care preparedness and isolation procedures. There is no vaccine approved by the U.S. Food and Drug Administration for use against Ebola, although experimental vaccines are under development. Basic interventions used to treat symptoms and complications increase the chance of survival. Proper use of personal protective equipment (PPE) and disinfection protocols are the most effective ways to prevent contracting this virus.

Health Care-associated Infections

Hospital-acquired infections, also called *nosocomial infections,* are defined as those that occur more than 48 hours after being admitted to the hospital. A more recent term for these conditions is **health care-associated infections (HAIs).** Approximately 722,000 patients admitted to hospitals each year acquire HAIs, and although many of these infections are not life-threatening, the CDC estimates that 75,000 patients die each year of hospital-acquired infections. HAIs are one of the 10 leading causes of death in the U.S., account for $28-34 billion in health care costs, and notably, most of them are preventable.

Medical settings provide an ideal environment for the development and transmission of HAIs. Typical sources of these infections include:
- Contaminated hands of health care providers
- Contaminated instruments
- Urinary catheters, ventilators, central lines, and surgical sites, which can allow microbes to gain easy entrance into the body

Invasive procedures permit pathogens to enter the bloodstream and overcome the defense mechanisms of immunocompromised patients. The wide and inappropriate use of broad-spectrum antibiotics has led to the development of drug-resistant infections in hospitals as well as in the community. Some of these infections are untreatable because they are resistant to the available drugs. Development of a new drug takes time, is costly, and does not seem to be a lasting solution to this complex problem.

There are several HAIs that greatly concern health care providers and their hospitalized patients because they are multidrug-resistant. This means the infectious agents are resistant to more than one antibiotic. Methicillin-resistant *Staphylococcus aureus* (MRSA) and vancomycin-resistant enterococci (VRE) both contribute to surgical wound, urinary tract, and bloodstream infections. MRSA can also cause respiratory infections. Penicillin-resistant *Streptococcus* and *Pseudomonas aeruginosa* cause respiratory infections. The overuse of antimicrobial agents and poor infection control practices have been implicated in the emergence and spread of these multidrug-resistant infections. These pathogens are very difficult to treat, and intensive infection control is required to limit their spread.

MRSA has been recognized as a problem in the health care setting for the past 20 years. More recently, MRSA has also become a problem in the community, and is referred to as *community-associated* or *CA-MRSA*. According to the CDC, this variant has been associated with recent antibiotic use, sharing contaminated personal items, living in crowded settings, and poor hygiene. This form of MRSA is associated with skin and soft tissue infections that are treatable with alternate antibiotics. The following groups have been affected: injection drug users, men who have sex with men, prison inmates, military recruits, children in childcare facilities, and athletes. Even today, other organisms are adapting to the drugs used to treat them and will soon emerge to present new infection control threats in health care facilities and possibly in our communities.

Another type of HAI that is very common in the hospital environment is *Clostridium difficile* colitis, a gastrointestinal infection that causes diarrhea. *C. difficile* is a gram-positive bacillus that is especially difficult to control because it is a spore-forming bacterium that is not eliminated by routine asepsis methods. Patients receiving antibiotic therapy are particularly susceptible to developing this infection because antibiotics tend to upset the normal balance of intestinal flora. About 20% of hospital patients receiving antibiotics develop

C. difficile infections. Treatment is usually quite successful, but about 20% of treated patients relapse, sometimes developing a chronically recurring disease.

Bloodborne Pathogens
HIV and AIDS

You are no doubt familiar with the abbreviations HIV and AIDS. HIV, which stands for human immunodeficiency virus, is so named because infection with this virus results in the destruction of an individual's immune system. In the early 1980s, HIV was identified as the cause of acquired immunodeficiency syndrome (AIDS). AIDS is called stage 3 HIV infection for reporting purposes. Two major types of HIV have been found to infect humans: HIV Type 1 (HIV-1), the predominant type throughout the world, and HIV Type 2 (HIV-2), found primarily in heterosexual populations in West Africa.

HIV is an RNA retrovirus. RNA viruses are called *retroviruses* because they replicate in a "backward" manner, converting from RNA to DNA after they invade a host cell. HIV can infect a number of different cells in the body, including cells of the central nervous system, but it is the adverse effect on immune system cells that produces the immunosuppression and manifestations of AIDS. The virus has specificity for the receptors on CD4 lymphocytes, attaching to and invading these cells and becoming a permanent part of their genetic material. Cell replication produces infected CD4 cells and additional HIV.

 HIV is the bloodborne virus that causes AIDS.

An HIV-infected individual can transmit the virus to others a few days after infection. Without therapy, this individual will pass through several phases of infection over a span of months to years, before exhibiting the immunosuppression of full-blown AIDS. In the early stages of the infection, there is usually a brief period of flu-like symptoms, often followed by years without symptoms. During the asymptomatic phase, the virus is silently replicating in the body and decreasing the number of CD4 lymphocytes. At the end of the asymptomatic period, before the full development of AIDS, the individual will experience night sweats, oral infections, weight loss, persistently enlarged lymph nodes, and low-grade fever. The appearance of AIDS is characterized by a low

CD4 count and the occurrence of multiple opportunistic infections and malignant diseases. The most common opportunistic infection observed is *Pneumocystis carinii* pneumonia. Others include mucocutaneous *Candida,* disseminated herpes, and cytomegalovirus. There is also increased risk of contracting tuberculosis and developing active disease. Kaposi's sarcoma, a malignancy of pigmented skin cells, is the most common form of cancer affecting AIDS patients.

Although no cure exists, antiretroviral drugs that first became available in 1996 have significantly prolonged the time required for HIV infection to progress to AIDS. With early diagnosis and appropriate treatment, it appears that progression to AIDS may be delayed indefinitely for some individuals. The latest hemodynamic research has hinted at the groundbreaking possibility of successful treatment by utilizing stem-cell transplants to functionally cure HIV-positive patients.

Fortunately, the AIDS virus is not acquired by casual contact. Touching or shaking hands, eating food prepared by an infected person, and contact with drinking fountains, telephones, toilets, or other surfaces does not result in transmission of HIV. The routes of transmission are through sexual contact, contaminated blood or needles, fluids containing blood, or from mother to fetus via the placenta. Infection can also be transmitted to infants through breast milk.

 HIV is transmitted by means of:
- Sexual contact
- Contaminated blood or needles
- Fluids containing blood
- Placental communication from mother to fetus
- Mothers' milk

According to the CDC, more than 1.2 million people in the United States are living with HIV infection, and approximately 14% of these infections are undiagnosed. The global annual mortality rate is 1.5 million, and the worldwide cumulative death toll is over 39 million people since the pandemic began. The incidence of AIDS has dropped significantly since the mid-1990s, due largely to prevention efforts; the survival rate has increased as a result of medical treatment and early diagnosis. In spite of these factors, the total number of HIV patients continues to rise. This is attributable not only to new cases, but also to the increasing number of

HIV-infected individuals who have used antiretroviral drugs and thus avoided converting to AIDS. Despite the improving statistics, the spread of HIV and AIDS is very troubling.* Public health concern is particularly focused on the number of new HIV infections occurring nationwide. Males who have sex with males account for the largest number of cases of AIDS in this country, followed by intravenous drug users and individuals engaged in high-risk heterosexual contact (unprotected contact with a person known to have or be at high risk for having HIV). The incidence of AIDS is increasing at a faster rate than the incidence of HIV within the following groups: non-Hispanic blacks, Hispanics, and women. The higher rate of AIDS in these groups has been attributed to poor access to health care, which has improved in the last few years, and/or failure to follow prescribed drug regimens. The continued decline in AIDS diagnoses and deaths will depend upon better access to health care, simpler drug regimens, and the continued development of effective antiretroviral drugs or other therapies.

As a health care worker in today's world, you must expect to encounter unidentified or undiagnosed cases of AIDS and other bloodborne diseases. The patient's right to confidentiality regarding the AIDS diagnosis within the hospital setting prevents health care workers from being informed about diagnosed cases, and additional undiagnosed cases may be encountered as well. For this reason, anxiety about HIV infections is typical and understandable among health care workers, but the occupational risk is not great. The vast majority of health care workers infected with HIV were exposed as a result of activities unrelated to their work. The most common occupational exposure is the needlestick, but according to the CDC, the probability of infection following a needlestick injury with blood containing HIV is only 3 out of 1000 exposures (0.3%). The risk of infection from exposure to mucous membranes is 0.09%, and other less common types of exposure carry even less risk. Thousands of needlesticks have been reported over the years, but as of December 2001 (the most recent report of this type available), only 57 health care workers with no other identified risk factors had been diagnosed as HIV-positive. Of these 57 cases, 26 developed AIDS. If current statistics were available, the number of diagnosed cases in health care workers would, of course, be

---

*http://www.cdc.gov/nchhstp/newsroom/docs/2012/HIV-Infections-2007-2010.pdf.

greater, but the ratio of needlesticks to infections would be similar. The implications here are obvious. Although prevention at work is essential, self-care in terms of safe sexual practice and the avoidance of other high-risk activities is equally crucial.

Hepatitis

In the 1990s, there was some evidence that new forms of hepatitis existed, but researchers have since found that some of these other viruses do not cause hepatitis or any human illness. Only the five common forms of hepatitis are addressed here. They are classified as A through E. Hepatitis A and E are transmitted through food and water contaminated with feces. Hepatitis B, C, and D are bloodborne. Hepatitis E is uncommon in the United States, and hepatitis D appears only as a co-infection with hepatitis B. Hepatitis B can be spread through contact with blood or blood products; contact with body fluids such as saliva, semen, and vaginal secretions; and through maternal-fetal contact. Hepatitis C is primarily spread by contact with blood or blood products. The risk for contracting this virus is greatest for persons with large or repeated percutaneous exposures to blood, such as intravenous drug users, whose risk is 60%. The risk is lowest for those who are subject to sporadic percutaneous exposures, such as health care workers, whose risk following a needlestick is 1% to 2%. The risk is 15% to 20% for sexual transmission and 5% to 6% for maternal-fetal transmission.

Hepatitis B is more infectious than hepatitis C. Although a needlestick injury is the most efficient method of transmitting the hepatitis B virus (HBV), another mode of transmission is through nonintact skin contact with infected blood on environmental surfaces. HBV and HCV (hepatitis C virus) have been demonstrated to survive in dried blood on environmental surfaces for at least a week. This means you can contract either disease if you have an open wound and touch a contaminated surface.

The manifestations of all forms of hepatitis are similar: jaundice, fatigue, abdominal pain, loss of appetite, nausea, vomiting, and diarrhea. Hepatitis C is a more silent infection, and may not cause symptoms or awareness of the infection until there is liver damage. Both hepatitis B and hepatitis C have the potential to develop into chronic infections and cirrhosis, although the risk is greater with hepatitis C. Following infection with hepatitis C, about 85% of individuals develop chronic infection,

approximately 70% develop liver disease, 10% to 20% develop cirrhosis, and 1% to 5% develop liver cancer. These sequellae take place over a 10- to 20-year period.

In December 1991, the Occupational Safety and Health Administration (OSHA) published regulations that require health care employers to provide the following: 1) HBV immunizations to employees, and 2) procedures and equipment to prevent the transmission of HIV and other bloodborne diseases to which employees may be exposed. The HBV vaccine is administered in a series of three injections. The second dose is given 1 to 2 months after the first, and the third is given 4 to 6 months after the first or at least 2 months after the second dose. One to two months after the third injection, employees must have their blood tested for antibodies. If sufficient antibodies are present, the employee has a positive titer. If antibodies are not found or are found in insufficient numbers, the series should be repeated. The hepatitis B vaccine usually provides immunity for 10 or more years; health care workers who have a positive titer following the initial series do not need to be tested for antibodies again in the future. There is currently no proven effective vaccine for hepatitis C, despite researchers' best efforts, as the virus varies greatly among strains and mutates quickly.

The number of new cases of hepatitis B and C has decreased because of immunizations for hepatitis B, less needle sharing among intravenous drug users, and required blood donor screening for both the B and C viruses. However, there are periodic increases in the incidence of hepatitis A. Large outbreaks of hepatitis A occur infrequently, with the last such multistate outbreak in 2014 originating from pomegranate seeds imported from Turkey. Small outbreaks are more common and involve fewer than 100 people. Hepatitis A remains the most common form of the disease and is best controlled by practicing good personal hygiene, especially hand hygiene.

There is also a vaccine for hepatitis A, but it is indicated only in certain situations: for individuals with medical, behavioral, or occupational risks, or other indications, such as for travelers to developing countries.

> There is only a vaccine for hepatitis A and B; none for C. Protection from all forms of hepatitis is best achieved by following the established pathogen infection control practices at your institution.

Management of Occupational Exposures to Bloodborne Pathogens

If an accidental needlestick occurs, or the skin is broken by a contaminated object, allow the wound to bleed under cold water and wash it with soap. If your eyes, nose, or mouth are splashed with a patient's bodily fluids, rinse these mucous membranes with water. An incident report must be filed, even though the injury or incident might seem insignificant.

Follow the personnel health policies of your institution regarding what actions to take after exposure. Most hospitals now ask that a baseline blood sample be drawn to help rule out infection acquired before the occupational exposure. Blood is drawn from the staff member and from the patient to whose body fluids you were exposed, if known. There are forms to complete to get approval for these tests. The process is usually handled through the emergency department, the employee health department, or the office tasked with employee health oversight. Follow-up testing will be conducted as needed to determine whether an infection develops. Because HIV infection may not be immediately apparent in the blood, another sample is tested for HIV at 3-6 months. The latest testing methods are able to detect HIV infection as early as 9 days post-exposure.

You will also be advised by the medical provider about post-exposure prophylaxis (PEP) therapy following a puncture with a contaminated needle. If treatment is recommended, it should be administered within 2 hours of the blood exposure. For most HIV exposures that warrant PEP, a 4-week, two-drug regimen is recommended, and several drug options are available. At the same time you are tested for HIV, you will also be tested for hepatitis B and C. If you have not had the hepatitis B vaccine series, it will be initiated along with hepatitis B immunoglobulin for immediate immunity. There is no effective prophylactic therapy for hepatitis C at this time, so if testing reveals that you were exposed to an HCV-positive source, follow-up HCV testing will be necessary to see if an infection develops.

Tuberculosis

Tuberculosis (TB) is a contagious, airborne lung disease caused by the acid-fast bacillus *Mycobacterium tuberculosis,* also referred to as *tubercle bacillus.* Historically, this disease was called *consumption* because of the victim's tendency to lose weight steadily and "waste away." In the past, the incidence of TB in the United States was spread across all economic groups. Today, the highest rate of active cases is seen among the homeless, recent immigrants, and immunosuppressed individuals. Although the incidence of cases in this country is much lower now than it was before 1950, the appearance of drug-resistant strains of the bacteria has raised grave concern.

Pulmonary TB is spread through airborne droplet nuclei that are generated when an infected person coughs or speaks. These particles are 1 to 5 μm in size, have a protective waxy coat, and are able to remain suspended in the air for several hours, thus making them easily transmitted. The probability that a susceptible person will be infected depends upon the concentration of the infectious droplet nuclei in the air. The waxy coat allows the nuclei to live longer on surfaces than any other pathogen—perhaps even for years!

A great majority of those infected with the tubercle bacillus will not develop a clinical disease and become infectious. Within 2 to 10 weeks following infection, the body, aided by its immune system, begins walling off the infection, preventing its multiplication and spread. When walled off, the disease is inactive or dormant, but it can be reactivated at any time. Reactivation may occur when an individual's immune response is weakened as it is in old age, illness, or malnutrition, or with **immunosuppressant** therapy involving drugs that decrease the body's normal immune response.

An individual with a weakened immune system is more likely to progress to active TB. Symptoms of active disease include productive or prolonged cough, fever, chills, loss of appetite, weight loss, fatigue, and night sweats. As the bacilli multiply, they cause tissue necrosis that results in lung cavities, as illustrated in Figure 9-1. These spaces are major reservoirs for the infection that can then be spread by coughing. Severe cases can be fatal.

Extrapulmonary TB, which infects bone or organs other than the lung, accounts for a small percentage of TB infections. Patients with extrapulmonary infection and no active pulmonary disease do not require airborne precautions.

The simplest and most common method of testing for TB infection is the tuberculin skin test (TST), also called a PPD test (PPD stands for *purified protein derivative,* which is obtained from killed tubercle bacilli). This test is administered to health care workers in parts of the United States where TB is prevalent to establish a baseline, as well as to workers exposed to individuals with infectious TB. The test involves an intradermal

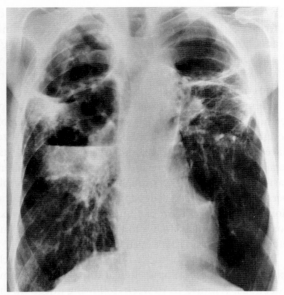

FIG 9-1 Chest radiograph demonstrates advanced tuberculosis with many large cavities exhibiting air-fluid levels. Note also chronic fibrous changes and upward retraction of the hila. (From Eisenberg RL, Johnson NM. *Comprehensive radiographic pathology,* ed 6, St Louis, 2016, Mosby.)

injection on the anterior forearm. The induration (palpable swelling) that is produced is measured 48 to 72 hours later by a trained health care worker to determine whether the individual has been infected. A negative baseline test usually indicates that the person has never been infected with TB. If a new employee has not had a baseline skin test in the last 12 months, the initial test may be falsely negative. Most institutions will administer a second skin test 1 to 3 weeks after the initial test to boost the immune system. A negative test the second time confirms that the person has never been infected. A positive result indicates that a person has at one time been infected and has developed antibodies to the organism. Because few people develop clinical symptoms or become infectious, many people have a positive skin test without having active disease. If a health care worker is known to have been exposed to TB in the work setting, a TST or blood test may be administered immediately following the exposure and again 8 to 10 weeks later, because it takes up to 8 weeks from the time of exposure for a person to react to tuberculin.

Even if no symptoms are present, therapy may be recommended when a skin test is newly recognized as positive, depending on an individual's risk factors. This therapy usually consists of isoniazid administration for a period of 6 to 9 months to prevent active disease. If symptoms are present, a chest radiograph is ordered to rule out active disease. When there are symptoms and signs of active disease on the chest radiograph, sputum smears and cultures are tested for acid-fast bacilli. Positive results are definitive proof of active disease and are an indication to begin treatment.

Screening is often mandatory for those who work in contact with vulnerable or high-risk populations. For example, schoolteachers, corrections officers, and health care workers are often required to have pre-employment TSTs.

In 2013, the CDC reported approximately 9500 new cases of TB diagnosed in the United States. This is the lowest number of reported cases since national reporting began in 1953, when over 84,300 cases were documented. Although TB rates have declined in both American-born and immigrant populations, this decline has been substantially lower among foreign-born populations. The continued decline in the number of reported cases since 1992 reflects improvements in TB prevention and control programs by state and local health departments, but falls short of the national goal the CDC has set to eventually eliminate this disease from our population.

Although we have seen a decline in the number of new cases in the United States, TB is still a worldwide problem. One third of the world's population is infected with TB, and TB is the infectious disease with the second highest number of cases in the world (with HIV/AIDS being the first). According to the WHO, there were 9 million new cases reported globally in 2013; 1.1 million of these cases occurred in individuals with HIV, and 480,000 cases are identified as multi-drug resistant TB (MDR-TB). TB tends to be a disease of poverty, affecting mostly young adults in their reproductive years. The vast majority of deaths are in the developing world; 1.5 million such deaths were attributed to TB in 2013. Since 2002, the number of foreign-born persons with TB in the United States has exceeded the number of TB cases in American-born persons. Foreign-born cases in the United States will continue to increase and outnumber the United States-born cases if global TB control is not achieved. This means that this disease may never be eliminated from the United States, and radiographers will continue to x-ray and care for patients with this disease for a long time.

Early identification, isolation, and treatment are required to minimize transmission of TB. Health care workers are at risk of contracting this disease if the patient is exhibiting signs and symptoms of active TB. The diagnosed patient will be isolated in a room with negative pressure (air flows from the hallway into the room) and more than six air exchanges per hour. Personnel and visitors must wear special masks and follow all precautions and procedures designated by the institution for the care of patients with airborne infections (see page 159).

According to OSHA's standard on TB, infection control experts within the health care facility are to assess the actual risk for TB transmission in inpatient and outpatient settings. If the findings reveal risk, they are to develop TB infection control interventions. These include free TB skin or blood tests, the provision of personal respirator equipment, the operation of one or more isolation rooms with negative air pressure and special ventilation or circulation, annual employee training about the disease, and implementation of effective work practices. OSHA estimates that the average lifetime occupational risk of TB infection may be as high as 386 infections per 1000 workers exposed to TB on the job. The average lifetime occupational risk of developing active TB disease ranges from 3 to 39 cases per 1000 exposed workers.

PREVENTING DISEASE TRANSMISSION

Historical Perspective

When infectious disease was rampant, those infected were often *quarantined,* meaning all members of the household were prevented from leaving the home or allowing others to enter. This practice helped to confine the infection to one family. Although quarantine is no longer commonly used, the United States Public Health Service still has the legal authority to detain and quarantine individuals when necessary to prevent the spread of certain serious infections. Diseases for which quarantine is currently authorized include cholera, diphtheria, infectious TB, plague, smallpox, yellow fever, SARS, and viral hemorrhagic fevers such as Ebola.

Decades ago, hospitals developed policies that involved separating patients admitted with infectious diseases from other patients. Contact with other persons was rigidly controlled. This isolation was a logical outgrowth of the practice of quarantine, and these techniques provided for specialized methods of asepsis when the danger of disease transmission was exceptionally great. Although isolation techniques were effective when used correctly, no mechanism existed for the prevention of serious diseases carried by asymptomatic individuals such as those with HBV or HIV. The following paragraphs describe the systems of precautions that were used before the current system, **Standard Precautions**. These systems were introduced to protect health care workers from contracting infections from all patients, regardless of diagnosis, by preventing contact with their blood and body fluids.

Universal Precautions (1985)

In acknowledgment that many patients with bloodborne infections are not recognized, the CDC introduced a system in 1985 known as Universal Precautions (UP). Under this system, all patients are treated as potential reservoirs of infection. The system is based on the use of barriers for all contacts with blood and certain body fluids known to carry bloodborne pathogens, rather than focusing on the isolation of a patient with a diagnosed bloodborne disease. The need to use barriers, such as gloves and masks, depends on the nature of the interaction with the patient rather than on the specific diagnosis. Emphasis is placed on blood and certain body fluids as potential sources of infection, regardless of diagnosis.

Body Substance Precautions (1987)

Because UP placed emphasis on bloodborne infections and did not include precautions for contamination by feces, nasal secretions, sputum, sweat, tears, urine, and vomitus (unless contaminated with visible blood), a new system was introduced in 1987 called Body Substance Precautions (BSP). This system focused on the use of barriers for all moist and potentially infectious body substances from all patients. The system was developed to protect health care workers from acquiring and transmitting infections from all pathogens.

Standard Precautions

In 1996, the CDC recommended a new system that combined the features of UP and BSP. This is the current system, and it is called *Standard Precautions*. In recent years, some documents refer to Standard Precautions as Universal Precautions. To avoid misunderstanding, this text continues to refer to the current system as Standard Precautions. Standard Precautions refers to an infection control system designed to reduce the risk of transmission of infections from unrecognized sources of bloodborne diseases and from other pathogens in health care institutions.

  Standard Precautions apply to:
- Blood
- All body fluids
- Secretions and excretions (except sweat), regardless of whether they contain visible blood
- Nonintact skin
- Mucous membranes

Standard Precautions also reduce the risk of transmission from recognized sources of infection by including precautions for three modes of transmission: airborne, droplet, and contact. These transmission-based precautions are discussed later in this chapter in the section on isolation techniques.

✸ You must decide when to take the extra time to protect both yourself and your patients. How you assess these risks and respond to them will vary with the setting and your level of experience. As a beginning student, your level of precautions should be very high. Although you may observe more experienced workers taking fewer precautions, do not think that you must follow their example. At this stage in your education, it is far better to take too much precaution than to use too little.

📌 Remember that the key to effective protection using Standard Precautions is using a consistent approach to *all* contact with *all* body substances of *all* patients at *all* times.

OSHA Bloodborne Pathogens Standard

OSHA published the *Occupational Exposure to Bloodborne Pathogens* standard in 1991 to protect workers exposed to blood and other potentially infectious materials. As a result of this standard, employers are required to develop an exposure control plan for the work site describing employee protection measures. The plan must include how an employer will use a combination of engineering and work practice controls, ensure the use of personal protective clothing and equipment, provide signs and labels to identify biohazard materials, and take other measures to protect workers. Employers must also provide annual bloodborne pathogen training, hepatitis B vaccinations, and medical care in the event of an occupational exposure.

Congress passed the Needlestick Safety and Prevention Act in November 2000 in response to the high number of skin punctures occurring with contaminated sharps. OSHA continued to revise this bloodborne pathogen standard and expanded the definition of engineering controls. The revision defines engineering controls as use of effective and safer medical devices, such as sharps with engineered sharps injury protections and needleless systems. This revision became effective in 2001. Some of these devices are illustrated and discussed in Chapter 14. As part of this policy, employers must document the process used for consideration and selection of these safer devices and involve employees in this process.

Medical Asepsis

Medical asepsis deals with reducing the probability of infectious organisms being transmitted to a susceptible individual. The healthy human body has the ability to overcome a limited number of infectious organisms, but this resistance can be overwhelmed by a massive exposure. On the other hand, reduced resistance caused by disease, cancer chemotherapy, immunosuppressants, or extremes in age may result in infection after only minimal exposure. The fewer organisms to which a patient is exposed, the more likely it is that he or she will resist infection. The process of reducing the total number of organisms is called microbial dilution and can be accomplished at several levels.

First, simple cleanliness measures, such as proper cleaning, dusting, linen handling, and hand hygiene techniques, can reduce the transmission of microorganisms. The second level is disinfection and involves the destruction of pathogens by using chemical materials. The third level is surgical asepsis, or sterilization. This involves treating items with heat, gas, or chemicals to make them germ-free. The sterile items are then stored in a manner that prevents contamination. Surgical asepsis and sterilization techniques are discussed in Chapter 18.

Armed with the knowledge of disease transmission, how can you fight the spread of infection?

- Stay home when you are ill, if possible. If you *must* work, avoid contact with immunocompromised patients.
- Use a tissue to cover your mouth when you sneeze, and wear a mask if you are coughing. If a tissue or mask is not available, sneeze or cough into your elbow so as not to contaminate your hands.
- Wear a clean uniform or hospital scrubs daily, and remove them before leaving the hospital or clinic. The best option is to wear hospital scrubs so they can be laundered by the hospital.
- Perform hand hygiene frequently, especially after touching your face or blowing your nose.
- Use established precautions when handling patients, linens, or items contaminated with body substances.
- Change or remove contaminated gloves after handling a patient or before touching other objects or equipment in the room.
- Practice good housekeeping techniques in your work area.
- When in doubt about the cleanliness of any object, do not use it.
- Dispose immediately of linens, instruments, or other items that touch the floor. The floor is always considered contaminated.
- Ask patients who are coughing or sneezing to cover their mouths and noses with tissues or masks.

Hand Hygiene

The first three principles in the preceding list are simple and self-explanatory. Handwashing may also seem obvious, but it is frequently overlooked in many hospital settings. Unfortunately, evidence shows that most physicians, nurses, and other health care workers do not wash their hands often enough or well enough. There are several reasons that contribute to poor adherence to regular handwashing in health care facilities: inaccessibility to sinks, lack of time in between patients, lack of role models, and the concern that handwashing is irritating to the skin and causes dryness. Medically aseptic handwashing is illustrated in Procedure 9-1.

> Medically aseptic handwashing is an easy and effective method to control the transmission of infections.

As previously stated, the CDC estimates that each year nearly 722,000 patients in the United States get an infection in the hospital, and about 75,000 patients die as a result. In an effort to address this adverse outcome, the CDC issued a revised hand hygiene guideline in 2002. An important part of the guideline is the recommended use of an alcohol-based hand rub (a preparation in the form of a gel, rinse, or foam containing 60% to 95% isopropanol or ethanol alcohol). Alcohol-based hand rubs have some benefits that the CDC believes will improve compliance with hand hygiene. Use of an alcohol-based hand rub requires about 15 seconds of time versus about a minute to walk to a sink and another 30 to 60 seconds to complete the handwashing procedure. An alcohol-based hand rub is more accessible than a sink because dispensers are located throughout the health care facility and can be installed with less expense in a smaller space than a sink (Figure 9-2). Additionally, hand rubs have been found to be more efficacious than soap and water in reducing the incidence of nosocomial infections. They are also less irritating to the skin, especially when skin-conditioning agents are added to the formulation. They are very effective against many microorganisms (gram-negative, gram-positive, *M. tuberculosis*, fungi, and some viruses), including multidrug-resistant organisms. However, hand rubs cannot destroy bacterial spores such as those of *C. difficile* and *Bacillus anthracis*. Handwashing with soap and water is still recommended to physically remove spores from the surface of contaminated hands.

Alcohol-based hand rubs should not replace handwashing with soap and water when hands are visibly soiled or contaminated with blood or body secretions or excretions. Gloves should always be worn to prevent contact with the patient's blood or other body fluids. Following the removal of gloves, the hands should be decontaminated through use of an antiseptic hand rub or antiseptic hand wash to reduce bacterial counts.

Studies reveal that health care workers who wear artificial nails are more likely than those who have natural nails to harbor bacteria at the fingertips below the nails, both before and after hand hygiene. Therefore, many health care institutions do not permit health care workers to wear artificial nails. According to the CDC, artificial fingernails or extenders should not be worn by health care workers who have direct contact with patients at high risk, such as those in the intensive care unit and in the operating room. Additionally, the tips of natural nails should be kept less than 1/4 inch long. Most facilities also have rules regarding nail polish; it must have been applied within 4 days and must not be chipped.

Throughout this text, you will find reminders to perform hand hygiene. *Hand hygiene* refers to the

PROCEDURE 9-1   ASEPTIC HANDWASHING TECHNIQUE

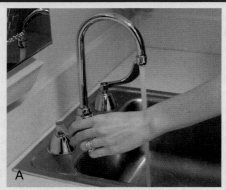

A, Turn on water and adjust temperature.

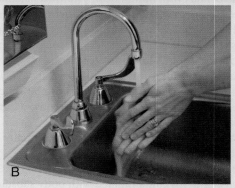

B, Wet hands thoroughly. Keep hands lower than elbows so water will drain from clean area (forearms) to most contaminated area (fingers).

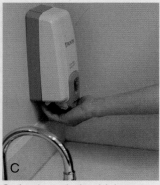

C, Apply antimicrobial soap.

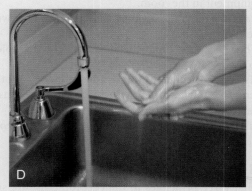

D, Lather well. Rub hands and fingers together with firm rotary motion for 20 seconds. Friction is more effective than soap in removing microorganisms from skin. Rub palms, backs of hands, and areas between fingers.

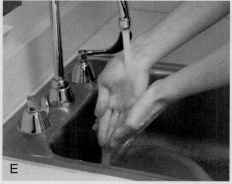

E, Rinse, allowing water to run down over hands.

PROCEDURE 9-1 ASEPTIC HANDWASHING TECHNIQUE—cont'd

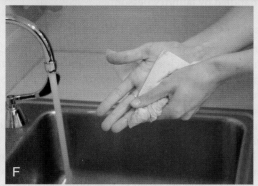

F, Use a paper towel to dry thoroughly from fingertips to elbows.

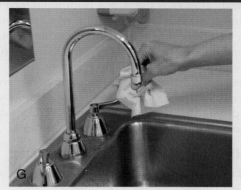

G, Turn off the water with a paper towel to avoid contaminating hands.

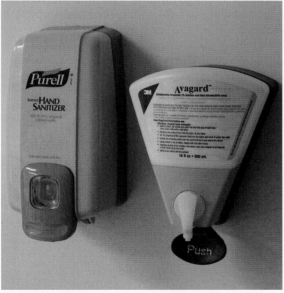

FIG 9-2 Examples of alcohol-based hand rub dispensers. These should be placed at a consistent height throughout the hospital to promote use through muscle-memory.

decontamination of the hands using soap and water, an antiseptic hand wash, or an alcohol-based hand rub. Box 9-1 lists the CDC recommendations for the use of alcohol-based hand rubs in the clinical setting.

Housekeeping

Good housekeeping in the workplace reduces the incidence of airborne infections and the transfer of

BOX 9-1 CDC Guidelines for the Use of Alcohol-based Hand Rubs in the Clinical Setting

When to use:
1. Use before and after patient contact as long as the hands are not visibly soiled or contaminated.
2. Before donning gloves.
3. After removal of gloves.
4. After contact with inanimate objects (including medical equipment) in the immediate vicinity of the patient.

How to use:
Apply product to palm of hand and rub hands together, covering all surfaces of hands and fingers, until they are dry. Follow the manufacturer's recommendations regarding the volume of product to use.

(From the Centers for Disease Control and Prevention, *Morbidity and Mortality Weekly Report* [MMWR, October 25, 2002; 51/RR-16:1–44]. Available from www.cdc.gov/handhygiene.)

pathogens by fomites. A clean, dry environment discourages the growth of all microorganisms. Much of the cleaning in the radiology department may be done at night by the housekeeping staff, but the radiographer is responsible for inspecting the work area regularly and maintaining high standards of medical asepsis.

Several general principles apply whenever cleaning is required:
- Always clean from the least contaminated area toward the more contaminated area and from the top down.
- Avoid raising dust.
- Do not contaminate yourself or clean areas.

- Clean all equipment that comes into contact with patients after each use. Use a cloth moistened with disinfectant such as Sani-Cloths or Clorox wipes. The CDC recommends sodium hypochlorite bleach (Clorox) as an inexpensive, effective disinfectant for preventing the spread of HIV.

Hospitals have detailed written procedures concerning preferred cleansing agents and the extent of responsibility for disinfecting rooms (see Appendix F). Consult the infection control procedure for your clinical area.

Handling and Disposing of Contaminated Items and Waste

Handling Linens

Objects or linens soiled with body secretions or excretions are considered contaminated and may serve as fomites even when no stains are apparent. Any linen used by patients should be handled as little as possible. To prevent airborne contamination, fold the edges of linens to the middle without shaking or flapping, and immediately place loosely balled linens in the hamper. Never use any linen for more than one patient.

Most institutions today handle all linen the same way, regardless of the degree of contamination. The linen is placed in plastic bags, and laundry handlers follow established precautions to prevent infection transmission. Many hospitals provide laundry bags that dissolve in hot water, reducing the number of times linen must be handled by laundry personnel.

Disposing of Contaminated Waste

A modern hospital uses many disposable items, from simple objects such as paper cups and tissues to more complex items such as catheterization sets. Disposable items are designed to be used only once and then discarded. The only exception to this rule involves the immediate reuse of an unsterile item (for example, an emesis basin) by the same patient.

Each hospital has a protocol for discarding disposable items. Some separate glass, plastic, and paper into covered containers, while others place everything together. Follow the procedure for your institution. Regulations demand that objects contaminated with enough blood or body fluids to cause dripping when the material is squeezed must be discarded in a suitable container and marked with the biohazard symbol (Figure 9-3). Small amounts of dried blood or body fluids do not require this precaution. Good judgment is needed to avoid unnecessary usage of biohazard bins, which are expensive to provide and to dispose of.

Used needles and syringes are placed in a special container called a **sharps container** that is designed to receive the syringe without recapping it (Figure 9-4).

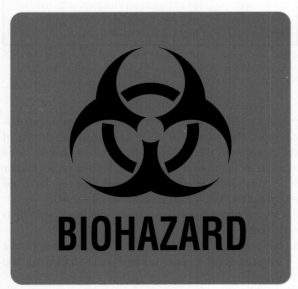

FIG 9-3 Biohazard symbol. (Courtesy of United Ad Label, Brea, CA.)

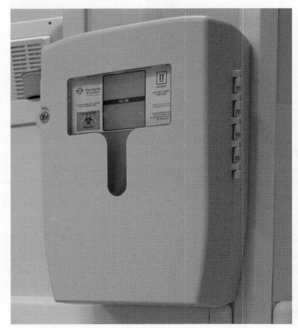

FIG 9-4 Sharps container. Safe disposal practices prevent the rehandling of needles and syringes.

OSHA's requirement for safer medical devices reduces the high number of needlesticks that previously occurred when workers had greater contact with unprotected sharps. A broad array of these safer medical devices is available. Some provide a sheath that slides forward to shield the contaminated needle. Others have a retractable needle that the health care worker can draw back into the syringe after removing it from the vein. It is important to use these safety features to prevent accidental needlesticks. A needleless system provides the greatest protection from needlesticks and should be used to introduce medications and contrast media after initial venous access is established (see Chapter 14).

Before sending specimens to the laboratory, place them in clean containers with secure caps and slip them inside a plastic bag labeled with a biohazard symbol (Figure 9-5).

Always wear gloves when assisting patients with bedpans or urinals. Be sure to empty these immediately unless a specimen is needed (see Chapter 10). Rinse them well over the hopper or toilet and discard them, or put them in the proper place to be sterilized, unless they are to be reused immediately by the same patient.

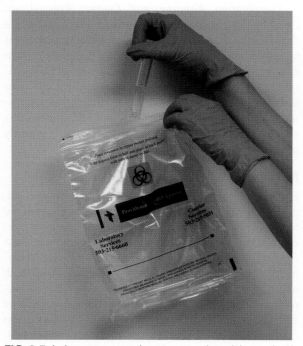

FIG 9-5 Laboratory specimens are placed in a plastic bag labeled with a biohazard symbol.

Isolation Technique

Diagnosis or suspicion of a communicable disease was the reason for placing patients in isolation before the development of UP. When it was recognized that *all* patients were potentially infectious, UP, and later BSP, were established (see page 169). Hospitals began using these new precautions in combination with their isolation policies, which consisted of one of two systems: a category-specific system with seven different types of isolation or a disease-specific system. The CDC later added isolation procedures to BSP when forming the guidelines for Standard Precautions. The current guidelines replace both of the older systems. Part of the CDC document *Guidelines for Isolation Precautions: Preventing Transmission of Infectious Agents in Healthcare Settings* is reprinted in Appendix G.

Transmission-Based Precautions

The CDC now recommends isolating patients using transmission-based precautions as part of Standard Precautions instead of the category- and disease-specific precautions. These isolation guidelines are designed to reduce the risk of airborne, droplet, and contact transmission. They may be used separately or in combination for diseases with multiple routes of transmission, and *must* be used with Standard Precautions. Refer to Figure 9-6 for examples of precaution cards used with this system.

> Transmission-based precautions are the CDC's latest recommendation for isolating patients with contagious diseases. These precautions MUST be used with Standard Precautions to ensure effectiveness.

Airborne Precautions. Airborne precautions are designed to reduce the risk of transmitting dust particles containing the infectious organism or airborne droplet nuclei (5 µm or smaller) to a susceptible person. Airborne precautions are used to prevent diseases such as TB and measles (rubeola). Health care workers and visitors entering the room of an infectious person must wear particulate respirators approved by the National Institute for Occupational Safety and Health (NIOSH). These masks must be capable of filtering particles 1 micron in size, have 95% efficiency, and should be fit-tested to ensure safety. The most commonly seen particulate respirator in the hospital is the orange, flat-fold N-95 "duck-bill" mask (Figure 9-7). An improvement on these masks is the powered air purifying respirator (PAPR) shown in Figure 9-8. These

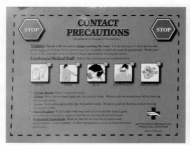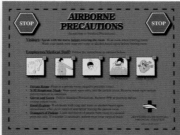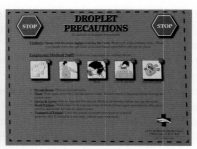

FIG 9-6 Precautions signs serve as reminders for staff and visitors that patients are under contact, airborne, or droplet precautions. (Copyright © Elsevier Collections.)

respirators are motorized systems that use a filter to clean the air before it is delivered to the breathing zone of the user. The system typically includes a blower, battery, headpiece and breathing tube. Some PAPR systems provide a higher level of respiratory protection than non-powered air-filtering respirators. The constant flow of air helps provide a feeling of coolness and greater comfort for the wearer. Loose-fitting headgear options provide respiratory protection without the need for a tight face seal or fit testing. The battery-powered blower pulls the air through the filter, resulting in no additional breathing resistance to the wearer. Patients under airborne precautions are placed in rooms with negative airflow and special air circulation with more than six air exchanges per hour to the outdoors or through high-efficiency particulate air filters. The doors to these rooms must always remain closed.

Droplet Precautions. Droplet precautions are designed to reduce the contact of large-particle droplets (greater than 5 μm) with the conjunctivae or with mucous membranes of the nose and mouth of a susceptible person. Droplet precautions are used to prevent the transmission of diseases such as diphtheria, pneumonia, and influenza. Health care workers and visitors coming in close contact with these patients must wear surgical masks, but no special air circulation is required in these rooms. If contact with secretions is likely, gowns and gloves are required as well.

Contact Precautions. Contact precautions are designed to reduce the risk of transmitting pathogens by direct contact with skin or mucous membranes, or indirect contact with a contaminated object. Contact precautions are used to prevent transmission of diseases such as multidrug-resistant wound infections caused by MRSA and VRE, the strains of *E. coli* (O157:H7 and 104:H4) that cause renal problems, and various skin infections, such as impetigo. Health care workers who come in close contact with

infected patients must wear gloves and a gown. Shared equipment should be decontaminated with disinfectant wipes.

Contact Precautions – Enteric. *Clostridium difficile, Norovirus, Rotavirus,* and *Adenovirus* are types of diarrheal illnesses and require disinfection procedures that differ from regular contact precautions. Similarly, health care workers who come in contact with infected patients must wear gloves and a gown. Alcohol-based sanitizer and disinfectants do not kill these pathogens, so shared equipment needs to be cleansed with Clorox bleach wipes, and health care workers are to wash hands with soap and water.

Combination Airborne and Contact Precautions. Combination airborne and contact precautions are designed to reduce the risk of transmitting pathogens by both airborne droplet nuclei and direct skin-to-skin contact. These precautions are used to prevent transmission of the virus that causes SARS and the varicella virus that causes chicken pox and disseminated herpes zoster. Health care workers who have not had chicken pox should avoid contact with infected patients. Previously infected personnel need not wear masks.

Radiography of Isolation Patients

Radiography of the isolation patient requires two people, preferably two radiographers. The "dirty" member of the team positions the patient, and the "clean" member handles the equipment. Although both radiographers must follow all designated isolation precautions, the "clean" member has no direct contact with the patient, the bed, or any items the patient may have touched. This radiographer is the only one who handles the x-ray machine and the uncovered image receptors (IRs). This team method minimizes contamination of x-ray equipment, which is difficult to disinfect completely.

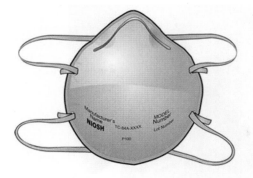
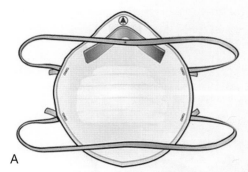
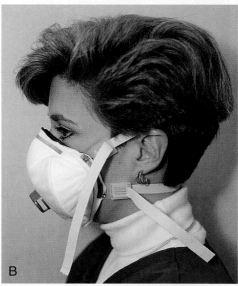

Example of Exterior Markings

Manufacturer Business ← Approval holder business name, a
Name or Private Label registered trademark or an easily
understood abbreviation. If private
labeled, the private label name or
logo is here instead of the approval
holder business name.

NIOSA ← NIOSH name in block letters
or NIOSH logo

TC-84A-XXXX ← TC - approval nuber

Filter Designation ← NIOSH filter series followed by
(Alphanumeric Rating) user efficiency leval (P100)

Model # XXXX ← Model number

Lot # XXXX ← Lot number (recommended)

Example of Interior Markings

(↑) UP ← Generic orientation marking (recommended)
Location is per manufacturer

A

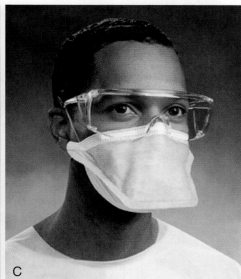

B   C

FIG 9-7 Disposable particulate respirators provide defense against airborne infections. **A,** Features of disposable particulate respirator approved by the National Institute for Occupational Safety and Health (NIOSH), a branch of the CDC. **B,** Disposable particulate respirator in use. **C,** Commonly used N-95 "duck-bill" disposable health care particulate respirator. (B from Potter PA, Perry AG, Stockert PA, Hall A. *Essentials for nursing practice,* ed 8, St Louis, 2015, Mosby; C courtesy of Kimberly-Clark Healthcare, Roswell, GA.)

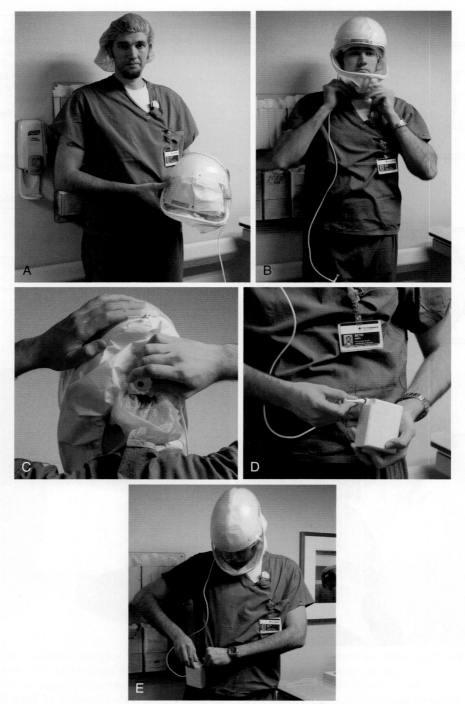

FIG 9-8 Powered Air Purifying Respirator (PAPR). **A,** To use the respirator, begin with the PAPR hood. **B,** Adjust hood. **C,** Attach hood connector. **D,** Plug hood into battery pack. **E,** Attach battery pack to belt.

Before you and your teammate enter the isolation room, prepare the necessary IRs by placing each one in a smooth-fitting plastic bag or pillowcase, and don your lead apron. Remove your jewelry and watch and place them in your pocket or pin them to your uniform. At the door, you will find the necessary supplies for the required precautionary measures (for example, disposable gloves, gowns, and masks). Use the posted isolation guidelines for the designated type of isolation, don protective clothing (Procedure 9-2), and enclose the IR in a protective cover (Figure 9-9). If the room was designed well for isolation, this procedure may take place in a vestibule adjoining the patient area.

Now you are ready to approach the bedside. Greet the patient, make introductions, and explain the procedure. Patients placed in isolation often tend to feel rejected and "untouchable." You can help alleviate these feelings by expressing a friendly interest in the patient and by avoiding any display of fear or revulsion as you perform your duties.

The dirty member of the team places the IR appropriately, making certain that the exposure side is toward the x-ray tube (Figure 9-10). The clean teammate positions the machine, sets the controls, and makes the exposure. As each exposure is completed, the IR is retrieved and the protective cover partially removed. It is then offered to the clean teammate with the edge exposed (Figure 9-11). The contaminated cover is placed in the proper container, and the IR is stored in the machine compartment.

When the examination is complete, make certain that the patient is comfortable and secure before removing your isolation attire. The correct method for removing contaminated isolation attire is illustrated in Procedure 9-3. Try to remove the gown and gloves as one unit,

PROCEDURE 9-2 PREPARATION FOR EXAMINATION IN ISOLATION

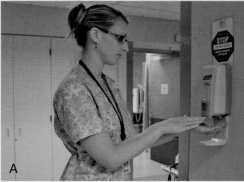

A, Perform hand hygiene.

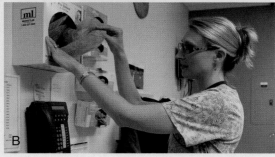

B, Don cap or hood.

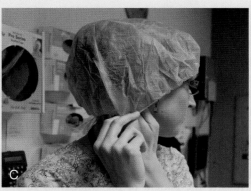

C, Make sure that all hair is covered.

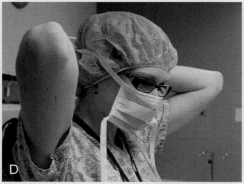

D, Don mask, making certain that nose and mouth are completely covered and nose piece fits snugly.

Continued

PROCEDURE 9-2 PREPARATION FOR EXAMINATION IN ISOLATION—cont'd

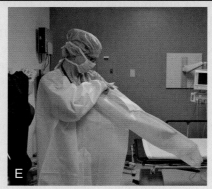

E, Put on gown.

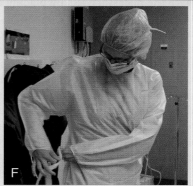

F, Fasten gown securely, making sure that uniform is completely covered.

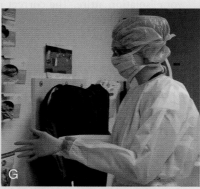

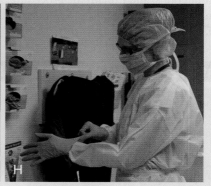

G and H, Don protective gloves.

so that you never have contact with the contaminated outer surface. First, remove your gown and gloves by firmly pulling the gown away from the front of your body to detach the neck strings and waist belt. Take care to hold it away from you as you fold the contaminated sides together and place it in the trash. Then untie the mask strings and remove the mask without touching the contaminated face portion. Hold it by the strings or rubber band, and place it in the container provided. Next, repeat hand hygiene.

Clean the mobile x-ray unit thoroughly before taking it back to the radiology department (Figure 9-12). If additional images might be needed, you may leave the mobile unit in a safe location just inside the isolation area and postpone cleaning until the images have been processed and evaluated. When no further

exposures are needed, push the unit into the corridor for cleaning.

Isolation Patients in the Radiology Department

If it is necessary to transport an infectious patient to the radiology department, the first step is to identify the isolation category involved and prepare for the examination accordingly. Cover the stretcher or wheelchair with a sheet, then with another sheet or cotton blanket. Depending on the isolation category involved, you may need to protect yourself and your uniform by wearing a gown, mask, and gloves. The patient with respiratory disease should wear a mask while being transported (Figure 9-13).

Transfer the patient to the wheelchair or stretcher, folding the inner cover around the patient, then the

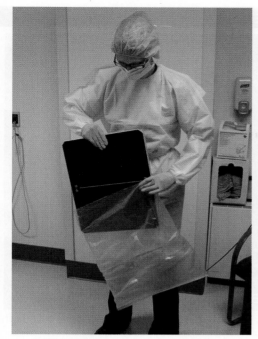

FIG 9-9 Place IR in protective cover.

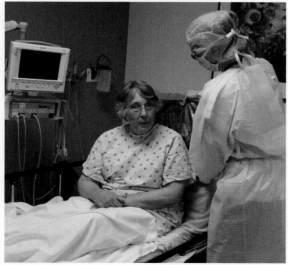

FIG 9-10 Place covered IR as required for radiographic examination.

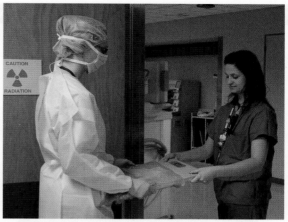

FIG 9-11 Following exposure, pull back contaminated cover without touching IR, offering "clean" IR to teammate.

outer cover, and tucking them both in securely. Once the patient is ready to travel, you may be required to remove all PPE until you have arrived at your destination. This prevents contamination of the surfaces you touch while transporting the patient.

When you arrive at the radiology department, take the patient directly into the x-ray room if possible. Protect the table with a sheet. Work with a partner so that one radiographer handles the patient and the other handles the equipment and controls, as previously described. Position the patient and make your exposures as efficiently as possible. Return the patient to the wheelchair or stretcher, rewrapping the sheet and blanket. Place the sheet from the table and any other contaminated linen in the linen bag. Place tissues, caps, and other disposable contaminated materials in the proper container. Disposable contaminated materials that are not soaked with blood or body fluids can be placed in the regular trash. Anything wet and contaminated with blood or body fluids must be placed in a red bag or a special container marked with a biohazard symbol.

After returning the patient to the bed, remove your gown and gloves and perform hand hygiene, as previously described. Clean the wheelchair or stretcher, repeat hand hygiene, and return to the radiology department. During this period, your partner should finish cleaning any other equipment used, including the table, and should then complete the task with hand hygiene.

Protective Precautions

Protective precautions are designed to prevent the spread of infections to compromised patients. A compromised patient has very limited immunity and requires special

PROCEDURE 9-3 REMOVING ISOLATION ATTIRE

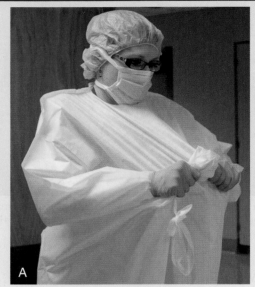

A, Pull and tear gown to remove.

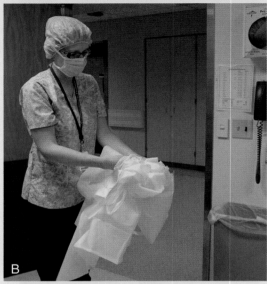

B, Remove gloves as gown sleeves are pulled off. Fold contaminated surface inward.

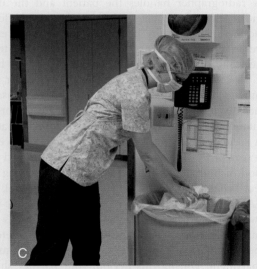

C, Discard gown and gloves.

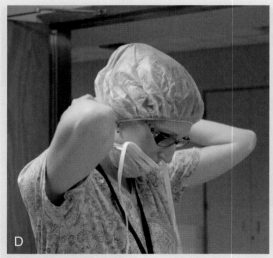

D, Remove mask.

PROCEDURE 9-3 REMOVING ISOLATION ATTIRE—cont'd

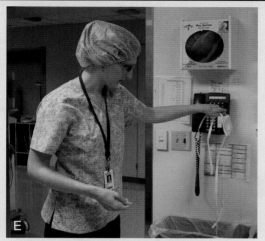

E, Mask is contaminated. Handle by ties only; discard.

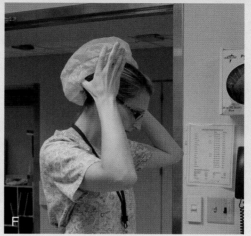

F, Remove cap or hood.

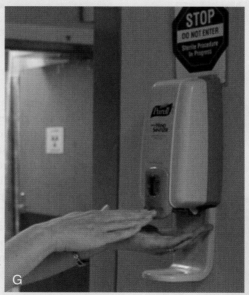

G, Repeat hand hygiene.

precautions to avoid exposure to potential infection. These patients may have undergone organ transplants and may be taking immunosuppressant medications. Burn patients and neonates at risk may also require these precautions. Protective precautions are sometimes used for patients receiving chemotherapy, which reduces their resistance.

These precautions were once referred to as *reverse isolation* or *protective isolation*. Federal isolation guidelines published in 1983 eliminated the category of protective isolation, largely because the purpose and procedure are the opposite of those for other isolation categories. The basic principles are unchanged, and you may find that these terms are still used in the clinical setting. The

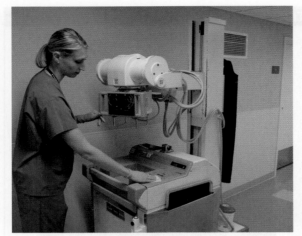

FIG 9-12 Disinfect mobile x-ray unit when procedure is complete.

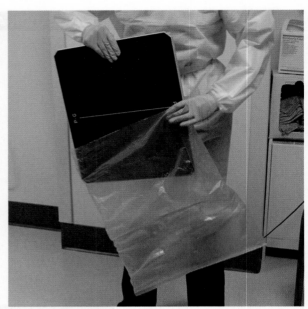

FIG 9-14 Place IR in clean cover for protection of patient with compromised resistance.

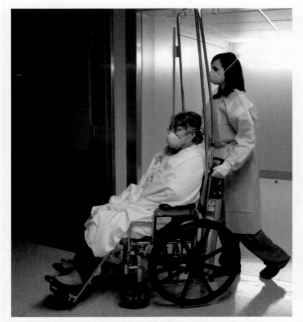

FIG 9-13 Patient under respiratory isolation is transported to imaging department.

correct terminology should be *protective precautions* or *neutropenic precautions*.

Precautions for the compromised patient require that the equipment be cleaned *before* entering the patient's room. Hand hygiene is required before touching the

patient, the bed, or articles handled by the patient. Masks, caps, gowns, and gloves may provide additional protection for the patient at risk. In extreme cases, sterile gowns and gloves may be worn in the same manner used for a surgical procedure (see Chapter 18), or a modification of surgical asepsis may be indicated. The modified technique results in a very high degree of asepsis without requiring the rigorous protocol of sterile technique. Specific precautions are posted outside the patient's room.

Under the system of protective precautions, the radiographer who positions the patient is the "clean" member of the team. Wearing the proper protective clothing, this radiographer avoids contact with uncovered IRs, the x-ray machine, and other potentially contaminated articles. To cover the IR properly, this radiographer folds back the edges of the sterile cassette cover and holds it open while the second radiographer places the IR inside. Care must be taken to not contaminate the outside of the cover (Figure 9-14). The "clean" radiographer touches only the patient, the bed, the covered IR, and "clean" or sterile items, whereas the dirty radiographer touches only the equipment. These roles are the exact opposites of those for isolation technique.

SUMMARY

- Emerging diseases include new diseases, preexisting diseases that are rapidly increasing in incidence or geographic range, and recurrent old diseases caused by old or mutated pathogens. A variety of factors can precipitate emerging diseases, including increased exposure to vectors, population growth, migration to crowded cities, international travel, overutilization of antimicrobial agents, a breakdown in public health measures, and bioterrorism.

- HIV and AIDS are a significant public health concern in the United States and worldwide. Males who have sex with males and intravenous drug users make up the greatest number of cases in the United States. The routes of transmission are through sexual contact; contact with contaminated blood; needles, or body fluids containing blood; from mother to fetus via the placenta; and to infants from breast milk. HIV is a bloodborne pathogen that has a very low risk of transmission to the health care worker.

- There are five types of hepatitis; hepatitis B and C are the greatest concern to health care workers because both are bloodborne. There is a vaccine and preventive therapy for hepatitis B, but neither is available for hepatitis C. Health care workers have a lower risk of contracting hepatitis C, but if you do become infected, there is a higher risk of developing chronic infection and liver cirrhosis. Hepatitis A and E are transmitted through food and water contaminated with feces. There is a limited-use vaccine available for hepatitis A, which is the most common form of the disease.

- Health care workers must follow the established post-exposure procedures in place at their health care institution in the event of a needlestick with a contaminated needle, or when their eyes, nose, or mouth are splashed with a patient's body fluids.

- TB is primarily a lung disease caused by *M. tuberculosis* and is transmitted through airborne contamination. The highest incidence of TB in the United States is among foreign-born residents. The simplest method of testing for TB infection is through administration of the tuberculin skin test. Hospitals that have an actual risk for TB transmission must have interventions in place, such as tuberculin skin testing or blood testing for employees, personal respirators, and one or more isolation rooms with negative air pressure and special ventilation.

- Medical asepsis deals with reducing the probability of infectious organisms being transmitted to a susceptible individual. Performing frequent hand hygiene is the best medical aseptic practice. Hand hygiene includes handwashing with soap and water and the use of alcohol foams or gels when the hands are not visibly soiled with blood or body secretions or excretions. Good housekeeping reduces the incidence of airborne infections and transfer of pathogens by fomites. Dusting, disinfecting, proper handling of linens and disposal of dry and wet waste, and the use of sharps containers are examples of how medical asepsis may be carried out.

- Current isolation and infection control policies have evolved from the practice of quarantining ill family members in the home to include caring for patients infected with all contagious illnesses, including bloodborne pathogens. Standard Precautions practiced when caring for all patients involve protective barriers and hand hygiene based on the level of contact with the patient. Transmission-based precautions are designated for patients diagnosed with contagious illnesses. Health care workers must don protective attire regardless of the level of contact with the patient. The precaution categories, designed to reduce the risk of airborne, droplet, and contact transmission, may be used separately or in combination.

- Radiography of the isolation patient requires two people: (1) the "clean" radiographer positions the x-ray equipment, and (2) the "dirty" radiographer places the covered image receptor and positions the infectious patient. Cross-contamination is minimized when both radiographers remember their roles. Both radiographers don the attire necessary to enter the isolation room and perform the examination. Upon completion of the examination, the radiographers carefully remove the contaminated isolation attire, disinfect the equipment and IR, and perform hand hygiene.

- Isolation patients may need to be transported to the radiology department for imaging studies. All imaging studies are best performed with two radiographers who don the protective attire and work as a team to complete the exam: one to position the patient and the other to position the equipment and controls. The stretcher or wheelchair must be covered with a sheet and disinfected after transport of the patient. The x-ray room must also be disinfected; linen and contaminated wet and dry waste should be disposed of appropriately.

- Compromised patients such as those with weakened immune systems due to immunosuppressant drugs, those with uninfected burns, and neonates, require

protective, or neutropenic, precautions. Two radiographers work as a team with the roles reversed: the "clean" radiographer positions the patient, and the "dirty" radiographer handles the equipment. The protective measures can vary from simply using hand hygiene, to wearing a clean gown, gloves, and mask, to donning complete sterile attire.

REVIEW QUESTIONS

1. HAI stands for an infection that was formerly referred to as:
   A. multi-drug resistant
   B. nosocomial
   C. epidemic
   D. bloodborne
2. The most complete source of information about infectious diseases in the United States is the:
   A. CDC
   B. WHO
   C. OSHA
   D. MRSA
3. A gastrointestinal HAI that causes diarrhea and is caused by a gram-positive spore-forming bacillus is:
   A. tuberculosis
   B. hepatitis A
   C. *Pseudomonas aeruginosa*
   D. *Clostridium difficile*
4. Mucocutaneous *Candida*, disseminated herpes, cytomegalovirus, and *Pneumocystis carinii* pneumonia are all examples of:
   A. HAIs
   B. multi-drug resistant infections
   C. opportunistic infections associated with AIDS
   D. airborne diseases
5. The risk of contracting HIV from a needlestick injury is:
   A. 100% unless promptly treated
   B. approximately 50%
   C. 10% to 20%
   D. less than 1%

6. Which of the following diseases can be prevented by vaccination?
   A. Hepatitis B
   B. Hepatitis C
   C. HIV/AIDS
   D. *C. Difficile*
7. A particulate respirator is essential for protection from exposure to which of the following diseases?
   A. Hepatitis A
   B. Tuberculosis
   C. HIV
   D. Anthrax
8. Under the system of protective or neutropenic precautions, the "dirty" technologist touches the:
   A. x-ray equipment
   B. patient
   C. covered image receptor
   D. A and C
9. Which of the following forms of hepatitis has no vaccine?
   A. Type A
   B. Type B
   C. Type C
   D. Type D
10. What is the most likely mode of transmission for hepatitis A?
   A. Airborne contamination
   B. Droplet contamination
   C. Vehicle or direct contact
   D. Vector

Answers can be found in the Answer Key on pages 429-431.

CRITICAL THINKING QUESTIONS

1. Billie Cross was recently diagnosed with leukemia and requires a mobile chest x-ray. Upon arrival, you find a sign on his door with a warning: "Do not enter—Protective Precautions." Outline the procedure you would follow to complete his examination, and identify the attire you may need to don before entering his room. Apply this to your clinical setting, following the policy in place at your institution.

2. Mr. Newton is in isolation with bacterial pneumonia, and you have been asked to transport him to the x-ray department. What will you need to do before you enter his room, and how will you prepare Mr. Newton to be transported? What procedure will be followed when you arrive in the x-ray department?

3. Mr. Mowrey was admitted through the emergency department with a staphylococcal infection resulting from leg trauma. List some persons who might become contaminated with microorganisms from this patient if proper precautions are not followed.

4. Name the type of isolation necessary for Mr. Mowrey, and list the protective attire that should be worn by those who care for him.

10

Response to Patients' Personal and Physical Needs

OBJECTIVES

At the conclusion of this chapter, the student will be able to:

- Demonstrate how to drain and measure the output from a urinary collection bag.
- List three personal comfort needs common to most patients.
- List five common body positions used in the health care setting, and place a fellow student correctly in each position.
- List four complications that may arise from improper patient positioning.
- Demonstrate the correct use of pillows and positioning blocks to ensure patient comfort on the x-ray table.

- List three situations in which the patient's head should be elevated.
- State the purpose of physical restraints and the conditions in which they should be applied.
- Demonstrate immobilization techniques utilizing sponges, sandbags, stockinet, and the mummy wrap technique.
- Demonstrate infant immobilization using the commercial device(s) available in your clinical facility.
- List and identify signs of possible physical abuse or neglect in infants, the elderly, or other vulnerable adults.

OUTLINE

Personal Concerns of Patients
Physiological Needs
  Water
  Elimination
Positioning for Safety and Comfort
  Body Positions
  Support and Padding

Considerations for Elderly and Debilitated Patients
Restraints and Immobilization
  Restraints
  Immobilization
Observation for Signs of Abuse
  Child Abuse
  Elder Abuse

KEY TERMS

battered child syndrome
catheter
colostomy
debilitated
decubitus ulcer
elder abuse
emesis
Fowler's position

ileostomy
immobilization
incontinence
kyphosis
lordosis
nonaccidental trauma (NAT)
nothing by mouth (NPO)
orthopnea

prone
recumbent
restraints
Sims' position
stoma
supine
Trendelenburg position

PERSONAL CONCERNS OF PATIENTS

Uncertainty about an upcoming procedure, fear of a possible diagnosis, or concern about the effect of illness on family members can cause varying reactions in patients. Sometimes these concerns are expressed as anger and demonstrated by inappropriate speech or rude behavior toward personnel. Other expressions of anxiety may include a need to talk constantly, or conversely, becoming quiet and withdrawn. You may observe fidgeting or other nervous mannerisms. Anxiety can also be caused by a concern over modesty, especially when enemas, catheterizations, or urinary procedures are expected. Reassure patients by providing ample covers, an explanation of the procedure, and a matter-of-fact attitude.

Your presence is comforting to the anxious patient. Touch patients reassuringly, and tell them what to expect. Let them know when you leave the area and when you expect to return. Escort ambulatory patients to the bathroom or back to their waiting area. It can be very distressing to patients if they must wander about in a hospital gown, wondering where to go. During a procedure, try to remain near the patient. If possible, postpone your lunch or break until the procedure is complete. If you must leave and have another radiographer take your place, introduce your replacement and excuse yourself rather than simply vanishing. If patients must wait in an x-ray room or dressing room, let them know that you are within hearing distance and that they may call on you for help. A call button is available in most patient bathrooms. Show patients how to use it, and assure them that someone will assist them promptly if they call.

Physical discomfort adds to tension as well. Remember that most patients will find it hard to remain still on a hard surface during a long procedure. This is especially difficult for a thin patient or an elderly person with **kyphosis** (convex curvature of the upper back). Lying flat on the table may cause obese patients and those with cardiac or respiratory impairment to have difficulty breathing. As you move briskly around the room, the temperature may seem warm enough to you, but patients who are inactive and ill often feel chilly. Note skin temperature when you touch the patient, and inquire whether a warm blanket is needed. Tuck blankets around the patient to provide both additional warmth and a sense of security. If the patient is coughing or sneezing, offer tissues and position a waste container

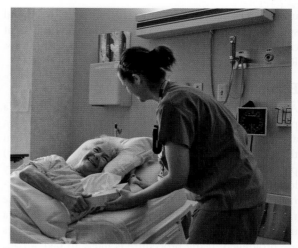

FIG 10-1 Small comfort measures are greatly appreciated.

within reach for their disposal (Figure 10-1). When responding to the physical needs of patients, be alert to the need for preventing the spread of infection and wear gloves whenever there is potential for contaminating your hands.

If dentures must be removed, place them in a safe and visible location in a suitable disposable container. When you return dentures, rinse them for the patient or direct the patient to a sink, as dentures slide in much more easily when wet. Glasses and hearing aids also require responsible care. These items are essential for daily living and are difficult and expensive to replace or repair. A plastic box with a lid, labeled with the patient's information, is a useful container for these items. Choose a safe location in view of the patient, use the same place consistently, and point out the location to the patient. This is especially important for outpatients who have not been provided with a locker to secure valuables such as a watch or wallet.

PHYSIOLOGICAL NEEDS

Water

Medication or anxiety can cause a dry mouth. If an inpatient requests water, first check the chart and note whether oral fluids are permitted. Many patients receiving intravenous therapy are allowed **nothing by mouth**. The abbreviation for this order is NPO (for the Latin *nil per os*, meaning *nothing by mouth*). This means no food or liquid, not even ice chips or small sips of water, until the physician orders otherwise. Often, a damp oral sponge will help alleviate a dry mouth. If the patient cannot sit up and water is permitted, offer it with a straw. Remember to record the amount taken in the chart.

Elimination

An urgent need to void can be very bothersome to a patient. A full bladder may cause discomfort, irritability, and difficulty remaining still during a procedure. When this need is ignored, an older or **debilitated** (feeble) patient may experience **incontinence.** This involuntary loss of bladder or bowel control can cause acute embarrassment for the patient and cleanup problems for the radiographer. Be especially sensitive to the need for a urinal, bedpan, or bathroom facilities when procedures are prolonged. If the procedure is likely to take a considerable amount of time, you might point this out and ask if the patient would like to visit the bathroom before getting onto the table.

> A patient's immediate and pressing needs must take precedence over the requirements of the imaging procedure. Practice observing and inquiring about patient needs before and during radiologic examinations.

When a urine specimen is needed, provide the proper container, cleansing supplies, and instructions for obtaining a clean-catch midstream specimen. These instructions are included in Appendix H and are often printed on signs posted in patient restrooms.

When a patient needs to defecate or urinate and is unable to walk or be taken to the bathroom in a wheelchair, a bedpan or urinal is needed. Placing a patient on the bedpan or offering the urinal is not a complex task. If you are unfamiliar with this procedure, the chief obstacle to overcome is embarrassment. Learn the location of the equipment needed and practice these procedures before you need to use them in a clinical situation.

There are two types of bedpans. A fracture pan (Figure 10-2) has a flat lip in the front that makes it easy to slide under a patient who has problems lifting the pelvis for bedpan placement (such as a patient in a cast). The regular bedpan is somewhat larger and deeper with a rounded lip designed to support the buttocks. Single-use bedpans and urinals made of disposable materials are now available in many emergency departments

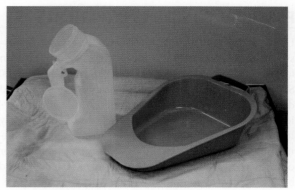

FIG 10-2 Urinal and fracture type bedpan.

and short-stay hospital departments. Special disposal units accept both container and contents, which minimizes handling. To assist a patient with a bedpan, assemble the supplies you will need, don nonsterile gloves, and follow the procedure outlined in Box 10-1.

Be sure the patient is adequately covered for privacy. When a female patient is placed on the bedpan, the upper torso needs to be slightly elevated to prevent urine from running up her back. When a patient has restricted mobility, two people may be needed to assist the patient onto the bedpan. If the patient is lying on the x-ray table, one person should stand on each side of the table to prevent the patient from falling. Patients may find it difficult to use the bedpan if they feel they are being watched, so remain out of their line of sight if possible while staying close enough to meet safety requirements.

When the patient has finished, you may have to assist with wiping. Wear gloves and have toilet tissue, a wet washcloth, and a dry towel conveniently placed. Assist the patient in lifting the hips or rolling away from you onto one side while you steady and remove the pan. Place it safely aside and help the patient by wiping from front to back with paper first, and then with a wet cloth before drying. Offer the patient a disposable moist towelette or a clean wet cloth and towel to cleanse the hands.

Male patients may need to use a urinal. If he is unable to use it himself, don nonsterile gloves and spread the patient's legs; lift the sheet with one hand and slide the penis into the urinal with the other. It may be advisable to hold the urinal in position until the patient is finished.

Check the chart *before* emptying bedpans or urinals to see if the patient needs to have a urine or feces specimen collected, or if intake and output (I&O) need to

BOX 10-1   Assisting the Patient with a Bedpan

1. Assemble your equipment: bedpan with cover; toilet tissue and/or perineal wipes; washcloth and towel or disposable hand wipes; and a sheet or blanket.
2. Perform hand hygiene and don disposable gloves.
3. Close the drapes and/or door to provide privacy.
4. If the patient is on the x-ray table, elevate the torso with pillows or angle sponges.
5. Cover the patient.
6. Ask the patient to bend at the knees and raise the hips.
7. Assist the patient by lifting with one hand under the small of the back while you slide the bedpan under the buttocks with the other hand.
8. Ask the patient to call when finished. Elevate the side rails of the bed or stretcher.
9. When the patient is finished, provide toilet tissue or perineal wipes, then a wet washcloth and towel or disposable wipe for the patient's hands.
10. Ask the patient to raise the hips, then remove the bedpan.
11. Cover the bedpan and put it aside until the patient is settled and secure. *Do not place the bedpan on the floor.*
12. Dispose of the bedpan contents in the toilet or hopper; remove gloves, and repeat hand hygiene.
13. Record the elimination in the patient's chart.

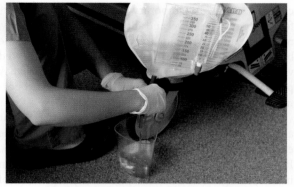

FIG 10-3 Measuring urinary output.

be measured and recorded. The nursing staff should call this to your attention. Make sure the correct container is available, and ask the nursing staff for instructions if you are unfamiliar with the procedure. The exact procedure for specimen collection will vary somewhat with the institution. Patients sometimes require a quantitative urine test that demands that all specimens be saved; failure to comply may invalidate an entire 24-hour collection. If such a test is needed, a special container should be provided.

If no tests requiring specimens are ordered, measure and discard the urine and record the amount. Most urinals are marked in milliliters for easy measurement, but urine in a bedpan must be emptied into a graduated container for measurement. If stool is present, observe it for obvious blood or diarrhea, and record any such observations. Empty the bedpan or urinal carefully into the hopper or toilet to avoid splashing. Rinse all containers

and place them in the correct location for disposal or sterilization. Remember to perform hand hygiene after removing your gloves.

Urinary Catheters and Collection Bags

Some patients will have a urinary **catheter** (tube). These tubes are inserted through the urethra into the bladder, allowing urine to be continuously emptied into an attached collection bag. The most common type is called a Foley catheter. It has a small balloon at the tip that can be inflated with water to hold the tip securely within the bladder. When these patients are transferred from the wheelchair or stretcher to the radiographic table, hold urine collection bags below the level of the patient's bladder to prevent urine in the tube or bag from being siphoned back into the bladder, causing discomfort and potentially allowing bacteria access into the bladder.

If the bag is full, empty it, measuring the urine if necessary. Some collection bags consist of a rigid measuring container within a flexible plastic reservoir. Urine flows first into the graduated section, and tipping the unit empties the measured urine into the reservoir. Most collection bags have a drainage outlet at the bottom. Wearing nonsterile gloves, open the clamp and allow the bag to empty into a suitable waste container or a graduated pitcher (Figure 10-3). Reclose the clamp! Because most patients with urinary catheters require I&O measurement, be sure to record the amount.

Colostomy Care

Occasionally you will encounter a patient who has a **colostomy** or **ileostomy**. These are surgically formed passages from the large or small bowel through the abdominal wall that terminate in an external opening called a **stoma.** A temporary colostomy may be performed to rest the bowel and allow it to heal after surgery, massive trauma, infection, or chronic disease. After the bowel is healed, the healthy portions are reconnected via anastomosis, and the temporary opening is closed. A permanent colostomy is one in which the diseased portion of the bowel is removed.

Patients with colostomies or ileostomies wear an external bag to collect fecal material and may be extremely sensitive about wearing this apparatus. Patients with a recent colostomy may find the alteration in body image difficult to accept, and any expression of revulsion on your part may be perceived as disgust and rejection. If you have never seen a colostomy, your first encounter should be as an assistant to an experienced radiographer. More detailed information about colostomies and their care can be found in Chapter 17.

These patients almost invariably carry supplies with them. When outpatients are scheduled for procedures that require removing a colostomy bag, remind them to bring their own supplies because brands of colostomy bags vary in size and shape of the opening.

Most patients with colostomies have their own supplies and are able to perform their own colostomy care. By studying and observing experienced coworkers, you will be prepared to help those who require assistance.

If it is necessary to empty a colostomy bag, the patient may prefer to complete this procedure in private. You may need to provide a sealable bag for the used supplies, and facilities for hand hygiene. If you must empty the bag, don gloves and empty the bag into the toilet. If the empty bag is disposable, seal it inside a plastic bag and place it in the container for contaminated waste disposal. Because some patients rely on reusable colostomy bags, check before you dispose of the used bag. If the patient does not have a clean bag, rinse the used one with cold water and allow the patient to reattach it. Otherwise, empty the reusable bag, rinse it, seal it in a plastic bag, and return it to the patient. Be sure to perform hand hygiene after removing your gloves.

If the patient is unable to perform his or her own colostomy care, you may need to apply or assist with the application of a fresh colostomy bag. Procedure 10-1 demonstrates the basic procedure when performed by a

competent patient. When assisting the patient, be sure to wear protective gloves. The unit includes two principal parts. A base portion surrounds the stoma and attaches to the body by means of a special adhesive. It protects the skin surrounding the stoma and has a rigid flange that forms a secure connection with the second part of the system, the disposable pouch. Products vary to meet individual patient needs and manufacturers' standards. Product inserts contain complete application instructions.

Sanitary Supplies

Occasionally a patient requires a sanitary napkin, so be sure that you know where these are kept. If a soiled napkin is to be removed, direct the patient to a bathroom or place a paper bag within reach. Place the bag with the soiled napkin in the appropriate container.

Patients who suffer from poor urinary control or stress incontinence may use urinary pads to protect their clothing. These supplies are similar to sanitary napkins, are usually stored in the same location, and are disposed of in a similar manner. If a replacement is necessary, urinary pads are preferable, but a sanitary napkin may serve as a temporary substitute.

POSITIONING FOR SAFETY AND COMFORT

Body Positions

Common body positions have names. It is easier to communicate with other members of the health care team and to follow physicians' orders if you are familiar with these terms (Figure 10-4).

The term **recumbent** refers to any position in which the patient is lying down. **Supine** (see Figure 10-4, *A*) defines the position in which the patient is lying on his or her back. This is the usual position for stretcher transfers and is also a common radiographic position. When lying face down, the patient is said to be **prone** (see Figure 10-4, *B*). Lateral recumbent denotes that the patient is lying on one side. This term may be modified by adding *right* or *left* to indicate which side is in contact with the bed or table. The patient in Figure 10-4, *C* is in the left lateral recumbent position. The **Sims' position** (see Figure 10-4, *D*) is a comfortable position that is sometimes used for rectal examination and for taking a rectal temperature; it is the best position for enema administration. **Fowler's position** (see Figure 10-4, *E*) is a

PROCEDURE 10-1   APPLYING A CLEAN DISPOSABLE COLOSTOMY BAG

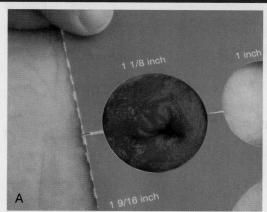

A, Begin by measuring the stoma. (Courtesy Coloplast, Minneapolis, MN.)

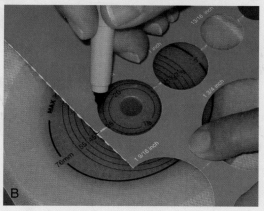

B, Trace the measurement onto the skin barrier. (Courtesy Coloplast, Minneapolis, MN.)

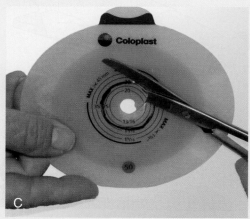

C, Cut the opening into the wafer. (Courtesy Coloplast, Minneapolis, MN.)

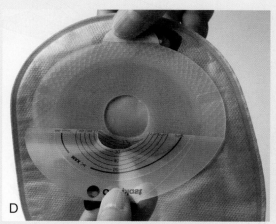

D, Remove the protective backing. (Courtesy Coloplast, Minneapolis, MN.)

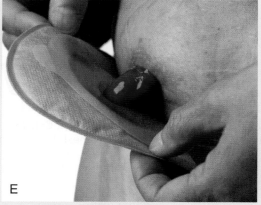

E, Apply the pouch over the stoma. (Courtesy Coloplast, Minneapolis, MN.)

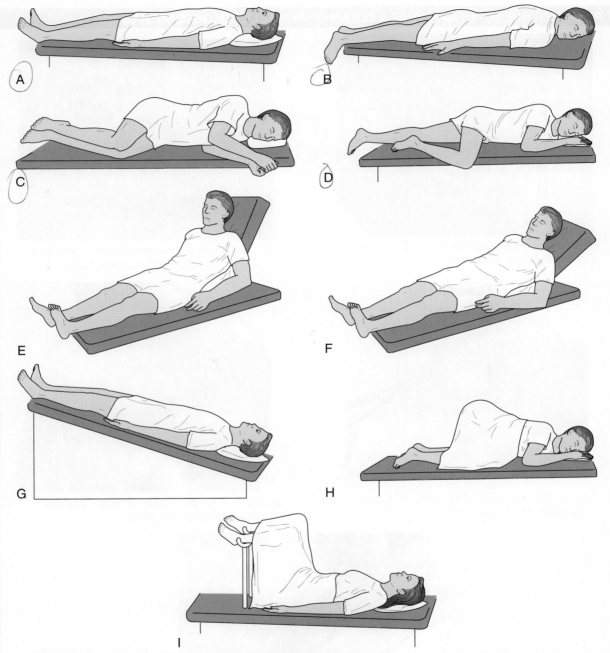

FIG 10-4 Identification of body positions. **A,** Supine. **B,** Prone. **C,** Lateral recumbent. **D,** Sims'. **E,** Fowler's. **F,** Semi-Fowler's. **G,** Trendelenburg. **H,** Knee-chest. **I,** Lithotomy.

modification of the supine position in which the patient's upper body is elevated. The semi-Fowler's position (see Figure 10-4, *F*) is a modification of the Fowler's position in which the upper body is only partially elevated. In the **Trendelenburg position** (see Figure 10-4, *G*), the patient's head is lower than the feet. Usually the table is tilted approximately 15 degrees. This position is used during some radiographic and fluoroscopic procedures and is helpful in treating patients suffering from shock. The knee-chest position (see Figure 10-4, *H*) and the lithotomy position (see Figure 10-4, *I*) are not commonly used by radiographers, but are standard positions used by physicians and nurses in diagnostic examinations and therapeutic procedures.

Support and Padding

When lying on a hard surface such as a radiographic table, patients are more comfortable with radiolucent sponges or cushions strategically placed for support. Sets of radiolucent sponges in various shapes and sizes are available in the radiology department for this purpose (Figure 10-5).

If a cushion or pillow under the head will not be a hindrance to the examination, it can enable the patient to see what is occurring and thus help relieve apprehension. Elevation of the patient's head also relieves neck strain, allows easier breathing, and helps avoid the uncomfortable sensation that the head is lower than the feet.

A bolster under the knees of a supine patient relieves lumbosacral stress by straightening **lordosis,** the lordotic or concave lumbar curve (Figure 10-6). This is especially comforting to patients with **kyphosis** (those with a pronounced convex curvature in the upper back),

to those with arthritis, and to most elderly persons. Bolsters are essential for patients with spine injuries and those who have recently undergone spinal or abdominal surgery. Patients with abdominal pain should have the head elevated and a bolster placed under the knees to relieve strain on the abdomen.

The measures used to promote comfort are frequently the same interventions designed to prevent complications. When the body is supine, the weight of the abdominal contents pushes the diaphragm up into the thoracic cavity, making it more difficult to take a deep breath. This is no problem for most of us, but if patients become short of breath when supine, you must help them to sit up immediately. The term for difficulty breathing when lying down is **orthopnea;** this condition may be caused by asthma, lung disease, or heart conditions.

Patients who are nauseated also need to have their heads elevated, because this position helps control nausea and prevents aspiration of **emesis** if the patient vomits. Patients who become nauseated and cannot be assisted into the Fowler's position should be rolled into a lateral recumbent position.

> Patients who experience difficulty breathing, nausea, or abdominal pain need to be positioned with their heads elevated.

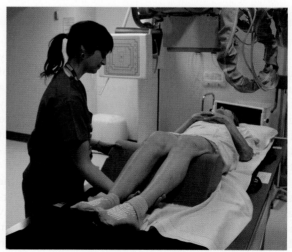

FIG 10-6 A bolster under the knees eases lumbosacral stress and helps alleviate abdominal pain.

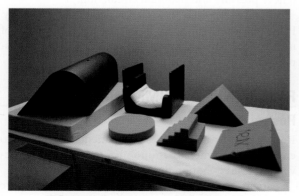

FIG 10-5 Radiolucent positioning aids.

Padding placed under body prominences, such as the sacrum, heels, or midthoracic curvature, is often essential for comfort on a hard surface. When patients are reasonably comfortable, they are better able to maintain the positions needed for an effective examination. If a patient will be in one position on the x-ray table for longer than 10 minutes, a full-size radiolucent pad should be used. This is an important consideration for patients undergoing extended studies such as small bowel series or excretory urograms. Older or debilitated patients can develop ulcerated areas over prominent bony structures when pressure is exerted for even a short period of time. These lesions are referred to as **decubitus ulcers** or bedsores and are discussed further in the following section on considerations for elderly and debilitated patients.

Empathy for patients is enhanced by experiencing what they feel during a radiographic examination. Practice positioning with your classmates until positioning and ensuring comfort are part of the same action.

CONSIDERATIONS FOR ELDERLY AND DEBILITATED PATIENTS

Age does not automatically determine a person's health status. Many older patients are quite active and healthy. The condition of an elderly patient may fall anywhere along a spectrum that ranges from vibrantly healthy and alert to seriously confused and/or debilitated.

> Assessment of an elderly person's physical and mental abilities will help you determine the level of care and assistance that is required.

Normal, healthy elderly patients will usually display certain characteristics that are typical of advanced age. For example, one attribute of aging is a tendency to proceed at one's own pace, both mentally and physically. Older patients do not respond well to feeling pushed or hurried, so take your time, assist them as needed, and always provide a safe, uncluttered environment.

Age is also accompanied by physical changes in the skin and in the circulatory system. A decreased tolerance to changes in temperature is common, so you may need to provide extra blankets during the examination. Loss of the sense of balance and lack of depth perception may increase the likelihood of falls, so you may need to assist the elderly during ambulation. Do not leave them unattended on the x-ray table if your assessment leads you to be concerned about falls.

Precautions must be taken to protect the skin while moving and positioning older patients. Rough handling or sliding against the table surface may injure the skin of elderly or debilitated patients. A subcutaneous fat layer cushions the skin of young persons, but this underlying padding decreases with age and may be nonexistent in the elderly. When the subcutaneous fat layer is lost, any shear pressure can cause the skin to tear and bleed.

The skin of the feet and legs is especially delicate on patients whose circulation is compromised; you must pay special attention to avoid bumping this skin. Do not wear jewelry on hands or wrists that could injure a patient during the process of moving or positioning. Even minor contusions or abrasions may increase the likelihood of decubitus ulcer formation.

The cause of decubitus ulcers is simple to understand and important to remember. Pressure on a limited area of tissue inhibits circulation, depriving the cells of oxygen and nutrition. The cells in the middle of the area are affected first. If the pressure is not relieved and circulation restored within a few minutes, the cells in the central portion die, and an ulcer forms. Weak or debilitated patients may be in a poor nutritional state and have impaired circulation. In such cases, the ulcers do not heal well and may even require skin grafting.

A circle or "doughnut" ring is an ineffective type of padding to use. Although it does prevent pressure on a specific bony prominence, it restricts circulation to the central area by placing the pressure all around it. It is preferable to distribute weight over as large an area as possible.

If a debilitated patient must be left on the table or on a stretcher for an extended time, the radiographer should assist the patient in changing positions periodically to relieve pressure and maintain circulation.

It is also important to keep the patient clean and dry. Patients who perspire heavily or who are incontinent of urine or feces may develop skin irritations that predispose them to ulcer formation.

RESTRAINTS AND IMMOBILIZATION

Restraints

Restraints are used to restrict patient movement to ensure safety, whereas **immobilization** methods prevent undesired motion during imaging procedures.

Patients who are active and disoriented may require physical restraints. These may consist of wrist and ankle bands and/or a vest with straps tied to the bed or stretcher. Restraints are used to prevent patients from injuring themselves or from disengaging therapeutic devices such as intravenous lines or oxygen masks. *The application of these physical restraints on an adult patient requires a physician's order.* Although restraints may be annoying to patients, they are neither painful nor harmful when properly used. Restraints are usually fitted before the patient comes to the radiology department. The same restraints used by the nursing service may be employed by the radiographer. If you remove restraints for transport or to meet the requirements of an imaging procedure, be sure to replace them as soon as possible.

> Remember that the application of physical restraints on an adult patient requires a physician's order. A charge of false imprisonment may result from the unauthorized use of restraints.

Safety straps or side rails must be used consistently on beds and stretchers to prevent falls when patients are asleep, weak, disoriented, or sedated. *A physician's order is not needed to apply these types of safety devices.* Safety straps or compression bands may be used on the x-ray table during waiting periods as a precaution against falling. Patients whose motion is restricted by safety devices must be monitored carefully. Never leave a patient unattended who is unable to change position. Difficulty breathing, or the need to cough or vomit, may require an immediate position change. The patient's inability to respond to this need may pose a serious hazard; if you must leave the room, another qualified person must remain with the patient. When patients are coherent and cooperative and are neither sedated nor in distress, deciding whether to leave them alone for a brief period must be based on existing hospital or departmental policy.

> **!** Do not leave patients alone when restrained in any way that prevents them from changing position. They may be endangered if unable to sit up or turn to the side when they have difficulty breathing or need to vomit.

Immobilization

Immobilization refers to the use of various devices to keep patients from moving during imaging procedures.

These applications are not categorized as restraints and do not require a physician's order. Several methods may be used to aid in the immobilization of adults who have difficulty remaining still.

When tremors complicate the procedure, support the patient as comfortably as possible. Place a compression band across the abdomen or the knees and/or a sandbag across an extremity proximal to the area of interest to provide stabilization during radiography. If tremors can be controlled in the hands and arms, this often stills tremors throughout the body. One way to do this when the patient is supine is to place the hands and wrists under the buttocks, if this position will not interfere with the examination.

Although it is preferable to win the confidence of small children and have them submit willingly to examination, occasionally you must immobilize children for their safety or to meet technical procedure requirements. The weight of a sandbag or of lead protective devices can be used to help maintain position. Sheets of translucent plastic are useful for holding a tiny extremity in position against an image receptor (IR). Tape can also be used to maintain a position. Tape can be used to hold a tiny finger in position on an IR or to strap a small patient's hips to maintain a supine position on the x-ray table. Be certain that cloth or a tissue protects the skin from the adhesive surface of the tape, or twist the tape so that the nonadhesive side is against the patient. Stockinet can be used to immobilize the legs or applied to keep the patient's arms above the head (Figure 10-7).

Figure 10-8 demonstrates the mummy wrap method used to immobilize an infant or a small child. Fold

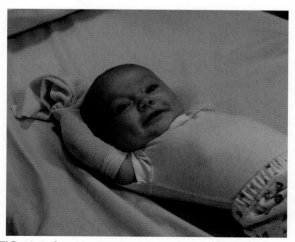

FIG 10-7 Stockinet may be used to immobilize arms or legs.

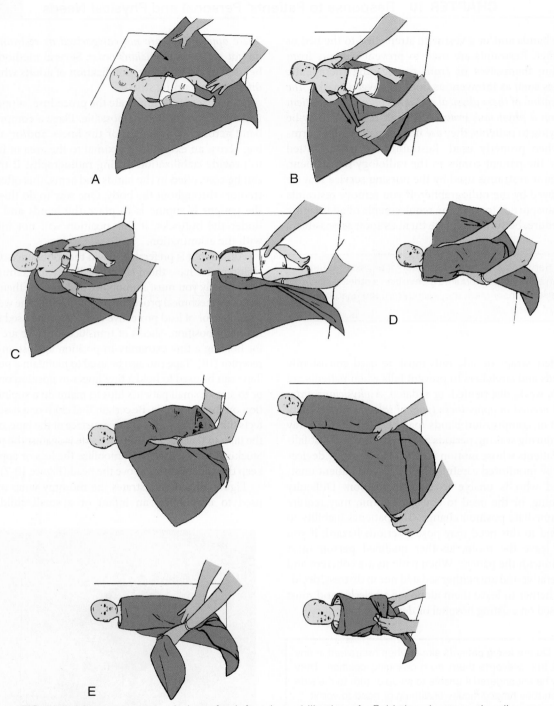

FIG 10-8 Mummy wrap technique for infant immobilization. **A,** Fold the sheet on the diagonal to make a triangle; place the child supine with the shoulders just below the center of the fold. **B,** Wrap one corner up over an arm, tuck it under the body, and pull it through to the other side. **C,** Wrap the first corner across the chest and around the second arm, and tuck it under the body. **D,** Wrap the second corner over the chest and secure it under the body. **E,** Complete the mummy wrap by securing the second corner around the child. (From Long BW, Frank ED, Ehrlich RA: *Radiography essentials for limited practice*, ed 4, St. Louis, 2013, Saunders.

down the top edge of a small sheet or lightweight blanket to form an inverted triangle. Place the child supine with shoulders just below the fold. Pull one point of the sheet across one arm, tuck it behind the back, and pull it through to the opposite side. Wrap this same point across the child's chest and around the second arm and tuck it securely under the patient. Then grasp the second point and wrap it across the chest, and tuck it behind the back.

Immobilization equipment, such as circumcision boards and other specialty devices, is commercially available to help immobilize children simply and effectively. Figure 10-9 shows two of these devices: the Papoose Board, a radiolucent board with Velcro wraps and straps available in several sizes, and the Octostop positioning device that rotates to place the patient into any of eight positions. The Pigg-O-Stat infant chair (Figure 10-10) holds infants and toddlers firmly in the correct upright position for chest radiography. This device incorporates a cassette holder and gonad shielding.

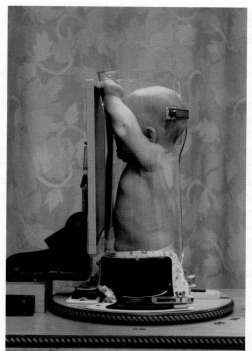

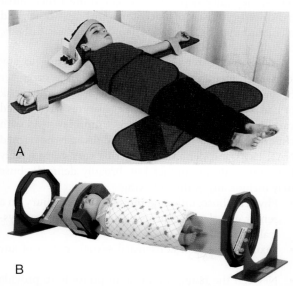

FIG 10-9 Commercially available devices for immobilizing infants and children for medical procedures, including imaging. **A,** Papoose Board provides selective restraints by means of sturdy wraps with Velcro closures attached to a rigid radiolucent board. Papoose Boards are available in several sizes to accommodate infants, children, and adults. **B,** Octostop positioning device rotates to change patient position. (A courtesy of Natus Medical Incorporated, Seattle, WA; B from Long B, Frank E, Ehrlich RA. *Radiography essentials for limited practice,* ed 3, St Louis, 2010, Saunders.)

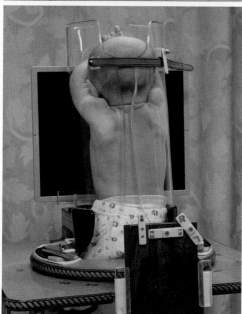

FIG 10-10 Pigg-O-Stat infant chair for upright chest radiography.

OBSERVATION FOR SIGNS OF ABUSE

Child Abuse

Whenever an injured child is brought for treatment, physicians and other health care personnel should be alert for indications of **battered child syndrome**, or characteristics of physical abuse, also referred to as **nonaccidental trauma (NAT)**.

The incidence of child abuse is remarkably high. The total abuse rate is estimated to be as high as one case in every 10 children. The majority of these cases are attributable to neglect, but these statistics also include sexual, emotional, and physical abuse, with considerable overlap between the categories. Approximately one-fourth of abused children suffer physical abuse or battering. Any of the following signs should raise concern about this possibility:

- Multiple injuries
- Evidence of chronic or repeated injury with no other explanation
- Injuries that are not consistent with the parents' report of the trauma
- Failure to seek prompt treatment for serious injury
- Bruise marks shaped like hands, fingers, or objects (such as a belt)
- Specific patterns of scalding (seen when a child is immersed in hot water)
- Burns from an electric stove, radiator, heater, or other hot objects on the child's hands or buttocks
- Cigarette burns on exposed areas or the genitals
- Black eyes in an infant
- Human bite marks
- Lash marks
- Choke marks around neck
- Circular marks around wrists or ankles (twisting)
- Separated skull sutures or bulging fontanel in an infant
- Unexplained unconsciousness in an infant

The last two items on this list are evidence of possible brain injury. Because of the difference in size and strength between adults and children, the abused child can be severely injured or killed unintentionally. Shaking an infant, for example, can cause bleeding over the brain (subdural hematoma), which can cause permanent brain damage or death. This condition is called shaken baby syndrome.

Figure 10-11 illustrates a classic case of battered child syndrome. The radiographs of the lower legs show periosteal reaction from repeated bruising of the bone. This type of injury is sometimes referred to as classic metaphyseal lesion (CML). Because abuse was suspected, a skeletal survey was done; that is, radiographs were taken of the skull, extremities, and thorax. The chest and rib study showed highly suspicious fractures of five ribs, which had partially healed. Four months after the skeletal survey, the child was again treated, this time for a fracture of the forearm. The parent stated that this injury had occurred on the previous day, but the radiographs showed evidence of healing at the fracture site, indicating that this injury had been present for a longer time. CML was also noted at the wrist. In this case, the diagnosis of battered child syndrome is undeniable.

Elder Abuse

Each year hundreds of thousands of older persons are abused, neglected, and exploited. Many victims are people who are frail, vulnerable, and cannot help themselves; they must depend on others to meet their most basic needs. Abusers of older adults are both women and men, and may be caregivers, family members, friends, or "trusted others."

In general, **elder abuse** is a term referring to any knowing, intentional, or negligent act by a caregiver or any other person that causes harm or serious risk of harm to a vulnerable adult. Legislatures have passed various forms of elder abuse prevention laws. As with children, physical abuse in older adults may be termed NAT. Laws and definitions of terms vary considerably from one state to another but, broadly defined, abuse may include any of the following:

- Physical abuse: inflicting physical pain or injury on a senior, e.g., slapping, bruising, or restraining by physical or chemical means
- Sexual abuse: non-consensual sexual contact of any kind
- Neglect: the failure by those responsible to provide food, shelter, health care, or protection for a vulnerable elder
- Exploitation: the illegal taking, misuse, or concealment of funds, property, or assets of a senior for someone else's benefit
- Emotional abuse: inflicting mental pain, anguish, or distress on an elder person through verbal or nonverbal acts, for example: humiliating, intimidating, or threatening a person

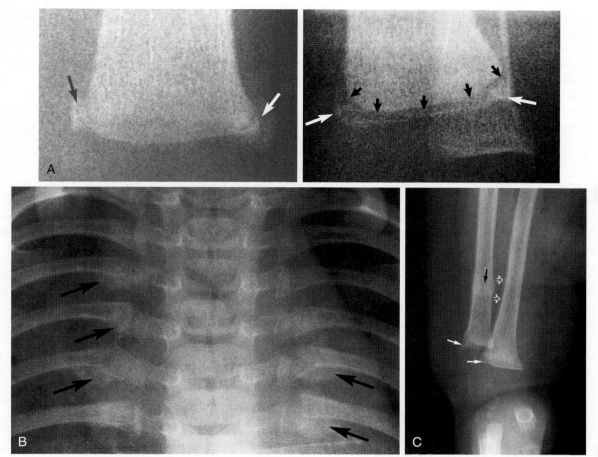

FIG 10-11 Nonaccidental trauma. **A,** Distal tibias revealed periosteal reaction from repeated bruising of the bone (*Black arrows,* periosteal reaction; *white arrows,* avulsion fractures). **B,** Skeletal survey revealed five healing rib fractures *(black arrows).* **C,** Four months later, the patient was treated for fracture of the forearm. Radiographs revealed evidence conflicting with the parent's report of the trauma; *white arrows* show periosteal reaction, *black arrow* shows healing fracture. (From Kleinman PK. *Diagnostic imaging of child abuse,* St Louis, 1998, Mosby.)

- Abandonment: desertion of a vulnerable elder by anyone who has assumed the responsibility for care or custody of that person
- Self-neglect: the failure of a person to perform essential, self-care tasks, threatening his/her own health or safety

As you learned earlier in this chapter, elders tend to bruise easily, their skin is easily damaged, and if there is dementia, their reports may be confused or inaccurate. For these reasons, it may be difficult to determine whether injuries are evidence of abuse, and whether an individual's complaints or reports are true.

Although one sign does not necessarily indicate abuse, there are some telltale signs that there could be a problem, as follows:

- Bruises, pressure marks, broken bones, abrasions, and burns may be an indication of physical abuse, neglect, or mistreatment.
- Unexplained withdrawal from normal activities, a sudden change in alertness, and unusual depression may be indicators of emotional abuse.
- Bruises around the breasts or genital area can occur from sexual abuse.

- Sudden changes in financial situations may be the result of exploitation.
- Decubitus ulcers, unattended medical needs, poor hygiene, and unusual weight loss are indicators of possible neglect.
- Behavior such as belittling, threats, and other uses of power and control by spouses or adult children are indicators of verbal or emotional abuse.
- Strained or tense relationships, or frequent arguments between the caregiver and elderly person are also signs.

Although your contact with patients is often brief and not ongoing, you may be in a position to recognize signs of physical abuse or neglect. When you do, notify your supervisor while the patient is still in the imaging department.

> It is your role to be observant and to alert others when you observe signs that raise suspicions of abuse. It is not your responsibility to verify that abuse is occurring.

SUMMARY

- When a patient requests water or needs to use a bedpan or urinal, first check the chart to determine if water is permitted or if specimens are needed. Record intake and output, if ordered, by recording fluid intake and by measuring and recording the amount of urine emptied from a urinary collection bag.
- Be prepared to assist with colostomy care and to provide sanitary supplies or urinary pads when needed.
- Be familiar with the names and appropriate uses of body positions such as prone, supine, recumbent, Fowler's, Sims', knee-chest, and lithotomy.
- Elderly and debilitated patients are especially likely to sustain skin injuries or suffer from circulatory compromise that may cause decubitus ulcers. Avoid

bumping or damaging the skin, keep the skin clean and dry, and use radiolucent sponges to provide padding under bony prominences.
- Patients who are active and disoriented may require restraints for their safety; physical restraints may be legally applied to adults only on the order of the patient's physician.
- Use straps, side rails, compression bands, and sand bags to stabilize patient positions and provide safety. Special devices and techniques are available to immobilize and position pediatric patients for imaging procedures.
- Be alert for signs of NAT in infants, children, and elders. Report suspicious cases to your supervisor.

REVIEW QUESTIONS

1. It is important to check the patient chart for I&O orders when patients:
   A. arrive in the imaging department
   B. are ready to leave the imaging department
   C. request a drink of water
   D. are receiving intravenous fluids
2. When emptying a urinary collection bag, it is important to:
   A. wear protective gloves
   B. measure the quantity emptied
   C. record the quantity in the chart
   D. all of the above
3. Which of the following positions is considered safe for a patient who is nauseated and may vomit?
   A. Supine
   B. Prone
   C. Trendelenburg
   D. Lateral recumbent
4. The definition of decubitus ulcers is tissue death due to:
   A. bacteria on the skin
   B. failure to keep warm
   C. lack of adequate circulation
   D. improper use of restraints
5. What is the name of the position in which the patient is lying supine with the head lower than the feet?
   A. Sims'
   B. Trendelenburg
   C. Fowler's
   D. recumbent
6. The term for loss of bladder or bowel control is:
   A. debilitation
   B. lordosis
   C. incontinence
   D. orthopnea

7. It is most comfortable for a patient with abdominal pain to be positioned:
   A. in the semi-Fowler's position
   B. with a bolster under the knees
   C. prone
   D. both A and B

8. A physician's order is legally required in order to:
   A. raise the side rails on a bed or stretcher
   B. immobilize a child for chest radiography
   C. use a compression band to prevent a fall from the x-ray table
   D. use wrist and ankle straps to secure a patient to the bed

9. Periosteal reaction from repeated bruising of the bone is visible radiographically and should lead to suspicion of:
   A. nonaccidental trauma
   B. lordosis
   C. incontinence
   D. orthopnea

10. Which of the following signs should raise concern about the possibility of elder abuse?
    A. Incontinence
    B. Bruises, abrasions, or burns
    C. Forgetfulness
    D. Confusion

Answers can be found in the Answer Key on pages 429-431.

CRITICAL THINKING EXERCISES

1. Mrs. Gibbons has been brought from an extended care facility for an x-ray examination of her hip after falling from her bed. She expresses fear about returning to the care facility, and you notice that there are a number of bruises on her arms and legs. What should you do?

2. Under what circumstances would you check the chart for I&O orders? If this order is present, how would it affect your patient care duties?

3. Carrie Weldon is 10 months old and is scheduled for a chest x-ray. What equipment might you use to obtain an upright radiograph without the need for someone to hold the child?

4. Taylor Connors is active, disoriented, and very strong. His physician has ordered wrist, ankle, and vest restraints to keep Taylor from injuring himself. Explain how you would transport Taylor to the imaging department and obtain the necessary images.

11

Patient Assessment

OBJECTIVES

At the conclusion of this chapter, the student will be able to:

- State four reasons for learning good assessment skills.
- List the AIDET technique for communicating with patients during an examination.
- Demonstrate how to take a history appropriate to a specific procedure.
- Find the admitting diagnosis in the patient's chart.
- Measure and record temperature, pulse rate, respiration rate.
- Use terms such as *dyspneic, diaphoretic,* and *tachycardia* accurately to describe patients' physical status.

- Describe the difference between a carotid pulse and an apical pulse.
- State the normal values for temperature, pulse, respiration, and blood pressure.
- Obtain and record blood pressure readings.
- List common laboratory tests used for patient assessment and identify the purpose of each.
- Identify common cardiac arrhythmias on an ECG tracing.

OUTLINE

Patient Assessment, an Essential Skill
Taking a History
    Questioning Techniques
    Elements of a History
Assessing Current Physical Status
    Checking the Chart
    Physical Assessment
    Vital Signs
Common Laboratory Tests for Patient Assessment
    Complete Blood Count

Erythrocyte Sedimentation Rate
Blood Clotting Assessments
Blood Chemistry Tests
Electronic Patient Monitoring
    Pulse Oximeter
    Electrocardiograph Monitors
    Arterial Catheters
Electroencephalography

KEY TERMS

AIDET
apex
apical
asystole
bradycardia
bradypnea
cardioversion
catheter
cyanotic
dehydration

diaphoretic
diastolic
dyspnea
electrocardiogram (ECG, EKG)
embolus (pl. emboli)
emphysema
fibrillation
hypertension
hypotension
level of consciousness (LOC)

metabolism
orthopnea
shock
sinus rhythm
sphygmomanometer
systolic
tachycardia
tachypnea
thrombus (pl. thrombi)

Observation, assessment, and evaluation are critical thinking skills so woven into our lives that we take them for granted. Every day we note changes in our environment without making a conscious effort. The house next door has a fresh coat of paint, new shrubs have been planted in the hospital parking area, and so on. We observe a new product at the store that promises increased effectiveness at slightly higher cost. We buy it, assess whether it meets our expectations, and then evaluate whether the difference in performance is worth the price. These same skills, when consciously practiced in the clinical area, will increase your value as a radiographer and help you become more sensitive to the conditions of your patients.

PATIENT ASSESSMENT, AN ESSENTIAL SKILL

> The ability to perform basic patient assessment is an essential skill for all who may be responsible for the care of patients who are ill or injured.

In the imaging suite, the radiographer is sometimes the only person present to recognize a patient's need for a medical response. Being alert to adverse changes in a patient's condition will allow earlier intervention and may help to avoid a life-threatening emergency.

Patient assessment is important when setting priorities. Radiographers are frequently responsible for scheduling the operation of a specific room and may need to determine how to sequence patients effectively. Good assessment and evaluation skills will allow you to be both comfortable and flexible while arranging schedules to meet the needs of patients who are acutely ill, obviously in pain, or presenting with valid emergencies.

Another aspect of your role as a radiographer is the responsibility for relaying information to the radiologist. Your ability to take a relevant history and report pertinent observations will assist the radiologist in making decisions about diagnosis and treatment.

TAKING A HISTORY

Radiologists depend on radiographers to assist them by obtaining accurate information about the patient's history and current condition. The answers you receive from the patient may influence how the examination is conducted. The history also helps the radiologist to focus the interpretation to meet the referring physician's needs. This is not a detailed medical history, but rather a thoughtful determination of why this particular radiographic study is being done and can be as simple as indicating the site of injury.

Patients sometimes complain that they feel like products on an assembly line. The process of taking a history presents an opportunity for you to give the patient some individual attention and build rapport. Your ability to gain the patient's confidence will also influence the amount of relevant information you obtain. Remember to introduce yourself, address the patient by name, and deal with any immediate patient concerns as soon as possible. Many facilities implement the AIDET communication tool to help facilitate communication between patients and care givers. AIDET stands for:

- **Acknowledge:** warmly greet the patient by name.
- **Introduce:** tell the patient who you are (name, title, length of time in the profession) and what you will be doing for them.
- **Duration:** explain how long the exam will take, and frequently update the patient of any delays.
- **Explanation:** describe the exam the patient will be undergoing. This is the opportunity to collect pertinent history.
- **Thanks:** express gratitude to the patient for choosing your facility for his/her care, for exhibiting patience, for being positive throughout the exam, and so forth.

Questioning Techniques

To improve data-gathering when obtaining a history, employ the following questioning techniques to encourage communication and prevent the patient from wandering off the subject:

- Open-ended questions
- Facilitation
- Silence
- Reflection or reiteration
- Clarification or probing
- Summarization

Histories should begin with open-ended questions to encourage patients to provide a narrative, share information about their condition, and explain why they are having a specific imaging study performed. Closed or direct questions may be used after patients provide their narrative and can be used to obtain missing information.

These questions will elicit a short "yes" or "no" response. As patients tell you about their conditions, you should nod or say "yes" to facilitate or encourage them to continue with the story. Using silence gives patients time to think and organize their thoughts without interruption from you. Reflection or reiteration gives you an opportunity to restate what the patient has said and enables you to determine whether you are listening carefully and recording the information accurately. You will want to use clarification or probing questions to elicit more information from the patient. For example, when a patient tells you that the reason for the x-ray examination is stomach pain, ask the patient to tell or show you the exact location. Use terminology that is understandable to the patient when asking probing questions. When the patient has finished giving you all the information, summarize the history to ensure you have not missed an important point and that everything has been recorded accurately. Ask for anything else that they may have forgotten to mention.

Elements of a History

Employing the therapeutic communication skills learned in Chapter 6 and the questioning techniques listed previously, you may begin the history by asking a general question about the nature of the problem, such as, "Do you know why Dr. Chen wants you to have an x-ray image of your chest?" Be realistic in the scope of your questions, and focus on expanding the information provided on the imaging requisition form by using probing questions. This is especially important when the request or order does not give the rationale for ordering the procedure. Most departments have policies stating that such information must be provided, but in practice, the only recorded information received is often the admitting diagnosis, which may seem irrelevant without further explanation. The information you obtain is most useful when recorded on the forms used by your institution. This may be the paper requisition form itself or another form specific to your setting. You may also be required to enter the information directly into the hospital information retrieval (computer) system.

Certain examinations require very specific histories, and the exact information required varies among radiologists. For example, if an intravenous (IV) iodine contrast agent is to be given, your history should include allergy information and any available data on the patient's renal function (see Chapter 19). Patients may

be asked to complete a questionnaire before a study is started. Table 11-1 provides some appropriate history questions and observations pertinent to many patient complaints. You can use it to become familiar with the types of information that are most useful in specific situations.

Examinations for patients with chronic conditions, or those receiving posttreatment follow-up, may require a comparison with previous diagnostic examinations. If these are not part of the current file, your history should contain information on previous relevant examinations, including when and where they were done. Information on other tests may also be important. For example, has the patient had blood drawn for laboratory tests, or been examined by a specialist for a specific problem?

In the event that a detailed history is required, the following standard format is frequently used to determine and describe the chief complaint. Using this outline will allow you to elicit the greatest amount of data in the least amount of time and help you to avoid missing relevant information.

- **Onset:** How did it start? What happened? When did it first trouble you? Was it sudden or a complaint that gradually got worse?
- **Duration/chronology:** Have you ever had it before? Has it been continuous? Does it bother you all the time? How long has this attack been bothering you?
- **Specific location:** Where does it hurt (or where is the problem)? Can you put your finger on where it hurts the most? Does it hurt anywhere else?
- **Quality of symptoms:** What does it feel like? Sharp, stabbing pain? Dull ache? Throbbing pain?
- **Severity of pain:** How severe is it? Mild, moderate, or severe? (Some like to use a pain scale of 0 to 5 or 0 to 10, with 0 being no pain at all and the highest number representing the worst pain the patient can imagine.) Does it wake you up at night?
- **What aggravates/alleviates:** What seems to make it worse? When is it worst? Is it worse after meals? At night? When you walk? What has helped in the past? Does that still help? What seems to help now? Does the time of day (amount of rest, change in position, and so on) make a difference? Associated Manifestations: Are there any other symptoms that you are experiencing that may be related to your chief complaint?

Tact and caution are required when obtaining a history, because anxious patients may read too much into your

TABLE 11-1 Guidelines for Taking a History

Examination	Questions	Observations	Example of History
Orthopedic, acute injury	How did the injury occur? When? Can you show me exactly where it hurts?	Swelling, deformity, discoloration, laceration, abrasion	Twisting injury, L ankle, while skiing today; swelling & pain over lateral malleolus.
Neck	Did you injure your neck? How? When? Where does it hurt? Do you have any pain, numbness, or tingling of the shoulder or arm? On which side?	Range of motion	MVA 10/12/15; lower neck pain & L shoulder pain; numbness & tingling, L hand.
Spine	Did you injure your back? How? When? Do you have pain, numbness, tingling, or weakness of the hip or leg? On which side? Any bowel or bladder problems?	Gait, range of motion	Lifting injury 2 weeks ago. LBP radiating to R hip.
Head	Were you injured? When? How? Do you have pain? Where? Did you lose consciousness? For how long? Speech, orientation, gait normal?	Speech: clarity, confusion	Severe HA, blurred vision, dizziness, & general weakness, 24 hr. No known injury. Speech slurred.
Chest	Do you know why your doctor ordered this examination? Are you short of breath? Do you have a cough? Do you cough anything up? Do you cough up blood? Have you had a fever? Do you have any heart problems?	Respiration, cough	SOB, wheezing & R chest pain since resp. flu 4 weeks ago. Moderate, nonproductive cough.
Abdomen, gastrointestinal examinations	Do you know why your doctor ordered this examination? Do you have pain? Where? Do you have any nausea? Diarrhea? Have you had any other tests for this problem? (Lab tests? Ultrasound?) Do you know the results? Have you ever had abdominal surgery? When? Why?	—	LLQ pain, incr. over past mo ? of mass seen on US done here 10/21/14.
Urology	Do you know why your doctor ordered this examination? Do you have pain? Where? For how long? Do you have trouble passing urine? Pain? Urgency? Frequency? Have you ever had this problem before? Do you have high blood pressure?	—	Two prior episodes of UTI; current malaise, fever, & mid back pain.

Can you identify the common abbreviations used by radiographers, such as MVA for motor vehicle accident? See Appendix C.

questions. Information regarding such serious matters as cancer, surgery, or heart attacks is best elicited in a general way rather than through blunt questions. "Do you know why your doctor ordered this examination?" is less threatening than, "Is your doctor checking for cancer?"

At this point the process of taking a history may seem complex and confusing, but this is a skill that improves with practice. Role-playing with other students, including taking turns as a critical observer, will improve your ability to take a history with sensitivity and confidence. As you gain knowledge and experience from clinical practice, you will find that your observation and history-taking skills become increasingly accurate and pertinent.

ASSESSING CURRENT PHYSICAL STATUS

The decisions you make and the communications you initiate in the course of a radiographic procedure will be most accurate if you begin with a clear understanding of the patient's current status. In addition, the radiographer is often the first and primary observer of a significant change in the patient's current condition. To accurately assess change, you must first establish a baseline for your observations.

Checking the Chart

Before you start the procedure, it is important to review the requisition. Often the requisition will not have enough specific information, so this is an area in which your skill in history-taking will prove valuable. When you add patient history to a requisition, sign and date the addition unless your identification and the date are added automatically when the document is scanned into the computer. When the patient is an in-patient, you will have access to the chart and will be able to verify both the order for the procedure and the accuracy of the requisition. Note the admitting diagnosis and the most recent progress notes. This analysis will help you to assess the patient's current physical status and determine whether the preparation for the examination has been done successfully. Although the pressures of scheduling may make such a thorough approach seem difficult, the more familiar you become with the organization of charts and requisitions in your facility, the easier it will become to find pertinent information quickly.

Nurses' notes may also be helpful. If a recent notation reads, "Unable to stand to void," you can anticipate a need for help when transferring this patient to the x-ray table. A statement such as "emesis × 3" during the previous 24 hours should be brought to the radiologist's attention before proceeding with a barium swallow. Medication may be necessary to calm the patient's stomach long enough for the examination to take place. If such a medication has already been given, it may affect peristaltic action and therefore the interpretation the radiologist will give to a fluoroscopic study.

Some notes have special significance for the radiographer. Allergies may be noted in red on the outside of the chart holder as well as in the history. Many facilities have elected to use standardized color-coded bracelets or clips on a patient's identification band (Fig. 11-1) as a means of visually alerting caregivers to allergies (red), fall risk (yellow), or DNR status (purple). A patient with a previous history of allergies is sometimes referred to as an *"allergenic individual"* and is more likely to have an adverse reaction to contrast media. You must report a complete account of allergies to the radiologist if the patient is to receive a contrast medium for the examination. Further assessment of allergy potential is discussed in Chapter 18.

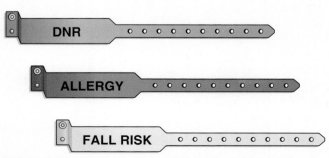

FIG 11-1 Standardized color-coded medical alert wristbands.

Physical Assessment

In the context of this chapter, assessment is an ongoing process of observation, comparison, and measurement to note and evaluate the changes in a patient's condition before, during, and after procedures in the imaging suite. How do you know when the patient's condition is worsening? What should you look for?

The most important process in patient assessment is sometimes called *eyeballing the patient.* A skilled observer compares the actions and appearance of the current patient with those of other similar patients and the appearance of this patient now with how he or she appeared earlier. Similarly, you will learn to respond to subliminal changes in the overall appearance of the patient.

Skin Color

One of the easiest signs to recognize is a change in skin color. Individual complexions vary, but when pale skin becomes cyanotic or olive skin takes on a waxen pallor, the change is usually quite apparent.

The term **cyanotic** denotes a bluish coloration in the skin and indicates a lack of sufficient oxygen in the tissues. This is most easily seen in the mucous membranes, such as the lips or the lining of the mouth. Nail beds may also show a bluish tinge. For some patients with heart or lung conditions this may be a chronic or usual state, but the patient who *becomes* cyanotic needs oxygen and immediate medical attention.

> **!** Any patient who looks pale and anxious and does not "feel well" may faint and needs to sit or lie down immediately. Do not leave the patient! A patient who loses consciousness and falls to the floor may suffer injuries far more serious than the cause of the fainting.

Skin Temperature

In Chapter 6, we discussed the importance of touch as a form of communication and reassurance. Contact with your hands also allows you to make physical observations about the ongoing status of your patients. The acutely ill patient in pain may be pale, cool, and diaphoretic, in what is frequently called a *cold sweat.* Hot, dry skin may indicate a fever, whereas warm, moist skin may only be a response to the weather or the room temperature. Acute anxiety can cause cool, moist skin with wet palms and shaking hands. Anxious patients may find it

difficult to concentrate and may need additional instruction during the radiographic procedure. They often need more precise instructions, and you should give written instructions for any follow-up care.

Level of Consciousness

A sudden change in a patient's mental acuity may indicate a critical problem that requires immediate treatment. To recognize such a change, you must first make a baseline observation of the patient's consciousness. Four levels of consciousness (LOCs) are generally recognized and may be described as follows:
1. Alert and conscious
2. Drowsy but responsive
3. Unconscious but reactive to painful stimuli
4. Comatose

To establish a baseline when eyeballing the patient, note whether the patient seems alert. Observe the patient's eyes. Are they open and focused? Does the patient look at you when you speak and respond appropriately? If your observations raise questions about the patient's alertness or awareness, ask additional questions, for example, "Do you know what day it is?" or "Do you know where you are?"

Occasionally a patient will lose consciousness for no apparent reason. The only warning may be a sudden change in expression, especially if the eyes seem unfocused. The cause of such an episode may be that the patient suffers from a seizure disorder and the loss of consciousness is precipitated by the stress of the occasion (see Chapter 16). Absence (petit mal) is a seizure disorder without convulsions that can cause a brief loss of consciousness without warning. If the patient is upright, sudden unconsciousness may be caused by a temporary decrease in oxygen to the brain, resulting in a fainting spell. For information about this condition, see the section on Syncope in Chapter 16.

> **!** Based upon your baseline observation of the patient's level of consciousness you should be able to recognize a sudden change in mental acuity and initiate medical treatment immediately.

Breathing

Changes in breathing may signal the onset of serious distress, so it is important to note how the patient is breathing. Normal breathing is quiet and calm and requires no particular attention. On the other hand, breathing that is audible, such as wheezing, gasping, or coughing, or appears to present a struggle for the patient, may require further assessment. A marked increase in the depth and rate of respiration is usually the first sign of respiratory distress.

Chronic conditions such as emphysema and cardiac insufficiency affect breathing and should be noted when assessing the patient. When patients with these complaints come to the imaging department, a chronic respiratory problem may be the presenting condition, or they may be admitted for a completely unrelated problem. For example, the emphysematous patient who needs a hernia repair or other surgery may come in for a chest radiograph before admission.

Radiographers must be alert to identify patients with emphysema, a form of chronic obstructive pulmonary disease that prevents patients from exhaling effectively, limiting their capacity for inhaling fresh air. Patients with emphysema share several characteristics. An increased anteroposterior thoracic diameter gives them a barrel-chested appearance. This is frequently associated with an elevation of the shoulder girdle and retraction of the neck muscles—all symptomatic of costal respiration. If these patients have received instruction in positive-pressure breathing, you will observe that they purse their lips when exhaling. Recognition of the emphysematous patient is a valuable skill from a technical viewpoint, because these patients may require special adjustments in exposure for chest radiography.

The anxious patient who breathes too deeply and too often (hyperventilation) may complain of feeling faint or dizzy and of tingling and numbness in the extremities. These patients have inhaled too much oxygen and exhaled too much carbon dioxide, disturbing the chemical balance of the blood. Try to persuade them to breathe more slowly or to breathe into a paper bag, which will help return their carbon dioxide level to normal.

Positioning can affect a patient's ability to breathe. For example, a patient with cardiac insufficiency will find it easier to breathe with the upper body elevated. Any sudden onset of orthopnea that is not immediately relieved in the Fowler's position may indicate a serious change in the patient's condition. Count the pulse rate and respirations as discussed in the section on vital signs in this chapter. If there has been any change in skin color or evidence of diaphoresis or pain, notify your supervisor or the radiologist immediately.

If your assessment of the patient's physical status reveals an abnormal skin color, skin temperature, level of consciousness, or ability to breathe, it is important to determine whether this is a new problem. A sudden change in any of these cardinal signs is significant and may be life-threatening. Determine the reason for this sudden change. If the patient has just received a contrast medium or a new medication, you may be observing the first signs of an allergic reaction. Regardless of whether you can identify the cause, notify your supervisor, the radiology nurse, or the radiologist immediately when there is a change in the patient's physical status. Many facilities have a *Rapid Response Team* available for assisting with a sudden change in a patient's condition (see Chapter 15). This critical care team of clinicians is paged overhead and will respond to the distressed patient's location to assess whether the patient is stable, or will likely experience a cardiac or respiratory event and thus need further care. The assessment procedures in the sections that follow may be necessary for further patient assessment when such changes occur.

Vital Signs

The following procedures used for assessment are usually referred to as the *vital signs*. They involve the measurement of temperature, pulse rate, respiratory rate, and blood pressure. Radiographers do not take vital signs on most patients; when the need does arise, it is often in response to an urgent situation. You cannot respond appropriately if you are wondering whether there is a right or wrong side to the blood pressure cuff! Sharpen your skill at taking vital signs before the need arises, and review your technique frequently. Accuracy is especially important when taking blood pressure measurements. When time allows, practice your technique with your coworkers and other volunteers so your skills will be sharp when needed in an emergency.

Most radiology departments have a drawer or box in which to keep a blood pressure cuff and gauge (sphygmomanometer), a stethoscope, and any other equipment that may be required in an emergency. Know where this equipment is stored, because even before you are proficient you may be asked to obtain it in an emergency. Table 11-2 provides a quick reference for normal vital signs according to patient age. Further discussion of normal ranges for each of the vital signs is included in the sections that follow.

TABLE 11-2   A Quick Reference to Normal Vital Signs by Age

Age	Temperature (oral)	Temperature (rectal)	Pulse	Respiration	Blood Pressure (Systolic)
Premature newborn	—	99.6° F (37.5° C)	140	< 60	50–60
Full-term newborn	—	99.6° F (37.5° C)	125	< 60	70
6 months	—	99.6° F (37.5° C)	120	24–36	90
1 year	—	99.6° F (37.5° C)	120	22–30	96
3 years	—	99.6° F (37.5° C)	110	20–26	100
5 years	98.6° F (37° C)	99.6° F (37.5° C)	100	20–24	100
6 years	98.6° F (37° C)	99.6° F (37.5° C)	100	20–24	100
8 years	98.6° F (37° C)	99.6° F (37.5° C)	90	18–22	105
12 years	98.6° F (37° C)	99.6° F (37.5° C)	85–90	16–22	115
16 years	98.6° F (37° C)	99.6° F (37.5° C)	75–80	14–20	<120
Adult female	98.6° F (37° C)	99.6° F (37.5° C)	60–100	12–20	<120
Adult male	98.6° F (37° C)	99.6° F (37.5° C)	60–100	12–20	<120

Temperature

An accurate temperature reading provides important information about the body's basic metabolic state. Although few patients will need you to take their temperature, you should be able to do so competently. In addition, this is one skill that may be useful in your own home.

Body temperatures vary during the day, being lowest in the morning and highest in the evening. Normal oral temperatures vary from 96.8° F to 99.8° F (36° to 38° C). Rectal temperatures range from 0.5° F to 1.0° F higher than oral temperatures; axillary temperatures range from 0.5° F to 1.0° F lower. In addition, normal temperatures vary slightly from person to person. A tense, "highly strung," quick-moving individual is likely to have a higher basic temperature than a placid, slow-moving person, all else being equal. What is your average temperature range?

Although the Fahrenheit scale has traditionally been used to record temperature, an increasing number of hospitals have completely converted to the metric system, which means that temperatures are recorded in Celsius units. See Box 11-1 for the formulas to convert Fahrenheit to Celsius and vice versa.

Fever (pyrexia or hyperthermia) is a sign of increased body **metabolism** (energy use), usually in response to an infectious process. For adults, fever commonly refers to any temperature of 100.4° F or above when taken orally or 101.4° F when taken rectally.

Temperatures may be obtained by the oral, rectal, axillary, tympanic, and temporal artery routes.

BOX 11-1   Fahrenheit ↔ Celsius Conversion

To convert from Fahrenheit to Celsius temperature:
$C = (F - 32) \div 1.8$
To convert from Celsius to Fahrenheit temperature:
$F = (C \times 1.8) + 32$
Examples:
1. Convert normal body temperature, 98.6° F, to the Celsius scale.
   $C = (98.6 - 32) \div 1.8 = 66.6 \div 1.8 = 37° C$
2. Convert 25° C to the Fahrenheit scale.
   $F = (25 \times 1.8) + 32 = 45 + 32 = 77° F$

Alert, cooperative patients usually prefer the familiar oral route. A long-standing belief exists that the oral method is less accurate than the rectal method, but research does not confirm this. The oral route provides an accurate measure of changes in the body's core temperature when taken correctly with the probe of the thermometer placed well under the base of the tongue.

The oral method is not appropriate when the patient has recently had a hot or cold beverage, is receiving oxygen, or is breathing through the mouth. In these situations, the rectal or axillary method may be used. The rectal temperature is accurate and faster, whereas the axillary temperature takes more time and is somewhat less accurate. The axillary method may sometimes be preferred, however, because it is less invasive. Rectal temperatures may be contraindicated in certain patients with cardiac conditions to avoid stimulating the vagus nerve, the tenth cranial nerve, which has connections to the sympathetic nervous system throughout the thoracic, abdominal, and pelvic cavities, and within the rectum. Stimulation of this nerve produces physiological changes called the *vasovagal response*: relaxation of the muscles in the walls of the blood vessels, slowing of the heart rate, lowering of blood pressure, and sometimes fainting. Radiographers are seldom required to obtain rectal temperatures. In the past, the rectal route was preferred for pediatric patients, but has been largely replaced by the use of tympanic and temporal artery thermometers. Hospitals commonly specify tympanic or temporal artery routes for children younger than 6 years of age and for anyone who is confused or unable to follow directions.

You are probably familiar with the use of glass thermometers, but these are no longer being used in clinical settings because of new Occupational Safety and Health Administration (OSHA) regulations that strictly limit the use of any devices containing mercury.

Hospital patient care units use digital electronic thermometers that consist of a handheld power unit with either an oral or a rectal probe (Fig. 11-2). Disposable sleeves are used to cover the probe, avoiding the need to disinfect the thermometer after each use. The unit emits a short beep when the highest temperature is recorded and the temperature can be read from a digital display in 1 minute or less. Some digital thermometers incorporate the power supply, probe, and digital display in a single small unit. This type is less sophisticated, less expensive, and generally not used by a nursing service, but it may be used in the radiology department, in outpatient settings, or in the home.

A general procedure for digital thermometer use with each route is found in Box 11-2. Remember to tell your patient what you are about to do. When taking an oral temperature, remind the patient not to bite down and to keep his or her lips closed. Never leave a patient alone with a rectal or axillary thermometer in place.

> While the oral method is the most common method of measuring temperature for the alert patient, tympanic, and temporal methods can be used easily on any patient.

Tympanic thermometers (Fig. 11-3) measure temperature at the tympanic membrane in the ear. The probe is placed in the external ear canal and a small

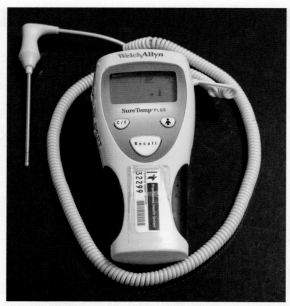

FIG 11-2 Electronic thermometer used for oral, rectal, and axillary measurements.

button is pressed to activate the sensor. A tone indicates that the reading is complete within a couple of seconds.

Temporal artery thermometers (Fig. 11-4) contain an infrared sensor that measures the temperature over the temporal artery in the region of the forehead. The gentle scan across the forehead and temporal region is easily and quickly accomplished and is not objectionable to patients. Research indicates that this method is more consistently accurate than the tympanic method.

Patients who have unstable body temperatures can now be monitored continuously by using a special probe inserted into the external ear canal that sends an electronic signal to a digital display monitor. This system is most commonly used for comatose patients in an intensive care unit and for premature or low birth-weight infants in the neonatal intensive care unit.

Pulse

A pulse is the advancing pressure wave in an artery caused by the expulsion of blood when the left ventricle of the heart contracts. Because this wave occurs with each contraction, it is an easy and effective way to measure heart rate. The heart rate is measured in beats per minute (bpm).

BOX 11-2   Taking a Patient's Temperature

Oral Route

- Implement hand hygiene.
- Cover the oral probe with a clean plastic sleeve.
- Turn on the thermometer.
- Insert the probe under patient's tongue. Instruct patient to keep lips closed.
- Remove probe when the audible tone or flashing number indicates that the maximum temperature has been reached (about 1 minute).
- Note the temperature reading.
- Remove and discard plastic sleeve.
- Repeat hand hygiene.
- Turn off the thermometer and return it to its storage place.
- Record the temperature.

Axillary Route

- Implement hand hygiene.
- Cover the probe with a clean plastic sleeve.
- Turn on the thermometer.
- Place the probe in the axilla so that the skin folds are in direct contact with the probe.
- Instruct patient to hold upper arm firmly against chest wall.
- Remove the probe when the audible tone or flashing number indicates that the maximum temperature has been reached (about 1 minute).

- Note the temperature reading.
- Remove and discard the plastic sleeve.
- Repeat hand hygiene.
- Turn off the thermometer and return it to its storage place.
- Record the temperature.

Rectal Route

- Implement hand hygiene.
- Don protective gloves.
- Cover the rectal probe with a clean plastic sleeve.
- With the patient in a lateral recumbent position, cover the patient and expose the anus by raising the top fold of the buttocks.
- Slowly insert the probe past the anal sphincter. Hold the probe in place.
- When the audible tone or flashing number indicates that the maximum temperature has been reached (about 1 minute), remove the probe slowly.
- Note the temperature reading.
- Remove and discard plastic sleeve.
- Remove and discard gloves.
- Repeat hand hygiene.
- Turn off the thermometer and return it to its storage place.
- Record the temperature.

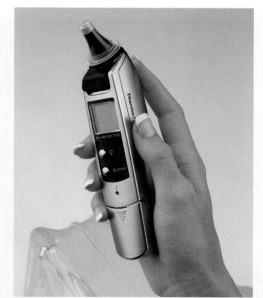

FIG 11-3 Tympanic thermometer probe is inserted into external auditory canal. (Courtesy Welch Allyn.)

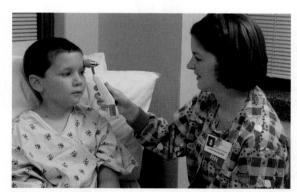

FIG 11-4 Temporal artery scanning thermometer. (From Perry AG, Potter PA, Ostendorf WR: *Nursing interventions and clinical skills,* ed 6, St Louis, 2016, Mosby.)

Common pulse points are shown in Fig. 11-5. The most common site for palpation of the pulse is the radial artery at the base of either thumb. Because your own thumb has a pulse, you cannot take an accurate pulse using your thumb. Place your fingers over the artery with your thumb on the back of the wrist and compress gently but firmly. By compressing the artery against the radius, the pulse is easy to feel, especially if the patient's wrist is held palm down (Fig. 11-6). When the radial pulse rate is taken routinely, it is common to count for 15 seconds and then multiply the result by 4. Whenever there is an irregular rate or rhythm, count for a full 60 seconds.

If the radial pulse is weak or difficult to count, you can use the carotid artery. Place your fingers just below the angle of the mandible (Fig. 11-7). This site is easily accessible and is particularly important if a patient loses consciousness. If the pulse is not palpable at this site, the heart is not beating effectively and emergency measures are necessary (see Chapter 16).

The *dorsalis pedis* or pedal pulse is taken over the instep of the foot (Fig. 11-8). This pulse may be significant

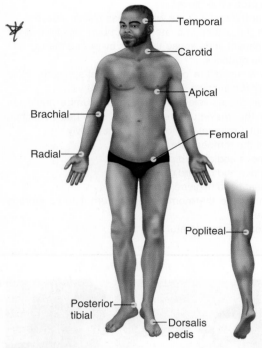

FIG 11-5 Common pulse points. (From Yoost BL, Crawford LR: *Fundamentals of nursing*, St Louis, 2016, Elsevier.)

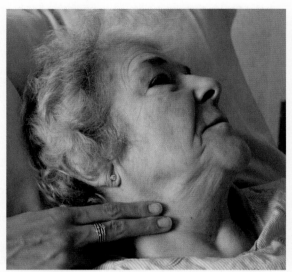

FIG 11-7 Gently palpate for carotid pulse just below angle of mandible.

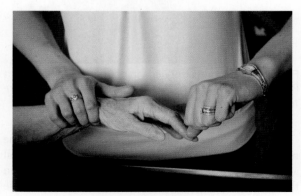

FIG 11-6 Taking a radial pulse with patient's palm down.

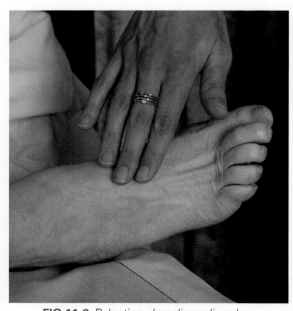

FIG 11-8 Palpating *dorsalis pedis* pulse.

when there is a question of compromise in the peripheral circulation. For example, radiographers may be requested to check the pedal pulse during or after an arteriogram involving catheterization through the femoral artery or following the application of a cast to the lower extremity. Because this pulse may be an important diagnostic sign, you must practice until you are certain you have the ability to detect it when it is present.

If the pulse is slow or irregular, you may want to take an **apical** pulse, a measurement taken by listening to the heartbeat through a stethoscope placed over the apex of the heart. Look at the stethoscope carefully, and become familiar with its use. It may have a bell as well as a diaphragm (bimodal instrument); less expensive models may have a diaphragm only. On a bimodal stethoscope, you can switch from bell to diaphragm, but for most purposes the diaphragm is preferred. Hold the earpieces of the stethoscope horizontally in front of you so that the ear tips point up slightly (Fig. 11-9). Insert the tips into your ears and then tap the diaphragm gently with your finger to be sure you can hear. Now press the diaphragm firmly over the **apex** or tip of the heart. This is normally found in the fifth anterior intercostal space at the left midclavicular line. Count the pulse for a full minute, and record the rate and any irregularities. Compare the radial rate with the apical rate, and record both rates in the chart or on the requisition. If the apical rate is faster, the heart is not beating efficiently. If the patient also shows signs of distress, you should report this to your supervisor or the radiologist.

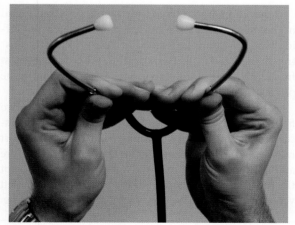

FIG 11-9 Stethoscope ear tips point up slightly. Correctly placed ear tips improve accuracy.

Tachycardia (abnormally rapid pulse) occurs when the heart rate is greater than 100 bpm. This may be temporary, as a result of exertion, nervousness, or excitability, but can also be caused by a damaged heart. A rapid pulse rate may also result from interference with oxygen supply or from a large blood loss. This occurs because the heart must beat faster to circulate the remaining blood to carry as much oxygen as possible to all the cells of the body. Average normal pulse rates in adults vary between 60 and 100 bpm. A tense, nervous individual is more likely to be in the upper range, whereas athletes tend to have a slower rate.

In addition to rate, the pulse volume or quality may vary. A weak or "thready" pulse, especially if quite rapid, may indicate that the heart is not pumping enough blood.

> **!** When a patient suddenly develops an irregular pulse, complains of feeling faint, weak, or nauseated, or has a sudden onset of pain in the chest, shoulder, or jaw, notify a physician immediately about the possible onset of a heart attack.

Respiration

When a patient shows evidence of respiratory distress, a respiratory rate will help in making an assessment. To count breaths, simply note the number of inhalations per minute. This is often done while continuing to hold the wrist after the pulse has been counted, because some patients may force a change in the respiratory rate if they are aware that a count is being made. If you are having difficulty counting breaths, place one hand lightly on the patient's back or anterior ribs at the level of the diaphragm. Compare your findings with the normal adult range of 12 to 20 breaths per minute. Slow breathing with fewer than 12 breaths per minute is called **bradypnea**, and rapid breathing in excess of 20 breaths per minute is called **tachypnea**. If a patient complains of **dyspnea** (difficulty in breathing), or exhibits an abnormal respiratory rate, you should inform the radiologist and prepare oxygen equipment for immediate use. See Chapter 15 for information on oxygen administration.

Patients in shock or with significant blood loss have a marked increase in pulse rate and in rapid, shallow breathing as the body attempts to supply oxygen to the tissues by increasing the speed of circulation. Pleurisy (inflammation of the pleura causing adhesions between the lungs and the chest wall) or abdominal pain may also cause rapid, shallow breathing because the patient attempts to avoid pain by moving the affected area as little as possible.

Blood Pressure

At any given time in the United States, about 15% of the adult population will have a significant degree of **hypertension** (abnormally high blood pressure). Of this number, approximately one fourth is unaware of their condition. Hypertension is more common in men younger than the age of 50 and in women older than age 50. In an aging population, the incidence of hypertension gradually increases until approximately 30% of individuals will show some elevation above normal. Essential (sometimes called primary) hypertension accounts for 85% to 90% of the diagnoses, with most of the remaining (secondary) incidence caused by kidney disease or damage. Hypertension contributes to the incidence of cerebrovascular accidents (strokes) and congestive heart disease.

Abnormally low blood pressure, or **hypotension**, can result in a potentially life-threatening condition called shock. The various types of shock, their causes, identification, and treatment are discussed in Chapter 16.

Blood pressure is measured using a stethoscope and a blood pressure cuff called a sphygmomanometer. There are three basic types of sphygmomanometers: mercury-gravity, aneroid, and electronic. The traditional mercury-gravity instruments have been phased out in response to the OSHA goal to remove mercury from the workplace, so small, portable aneroid instruments are now commonly used. The term *aneroid* literally means "not wet" or without liquid; thus an aneroid manometer is simply one that does not contain mercury. These devices use air pressure to obtain a measurement. Although they do not measure pressure in millimeters of mercury directly, they provide readings in the same units. There are several designs of electronic instruments, some of which measure pressure automatically at regular intervals. You may observe potentially unstable patients having their blood pressure automatically monitored with electronic sphygmomanometers that display a digital readout. This allows patients to be monitored continuously from a remote location. In the intensive care unit, you may observe nurses using a Doppler unit to measure blood pressure when patients have an extremely weak or low pressure.

BOX 11-3 Measuring Blood Pressure

- Implement hand hygiene and explain the procedure to the patient.
- The patient may be sitting or lying down, but the cuff should be at the level of the heart. Either arm may be used.
- Wrap the cuff snugly with the bottom edge above the antecubital space. Most cuffs are self-securing.
- Place the gauge where you can easily read the dial.
- Palpate the brachial artery pulse in the antecubital space.
- Place the stethoscope's ear tips in your ears, and press its diaphragm over the brachial artery.
- Close the valve on the bulb pump, and inflate the cuff rapidly to approximately 180 mm Hg.
- Open the valve on the pump and slowly release the pressure.
- Listen for the beat of the pulse while watching the gauge. Note the figure at which the pulse is first heard. This is the systolic reading.
- As the pressure is released, the sound increases in intensity and then, suddenly, becomes much softer. Note this point as the diastolic reading.
- Release the remaining pressure.
- If the situation permits, ask the patient to raise the arm and clench and release the fist. Then lower the arm and repeat the procedure to check the results.
- Remove the cuff, and record the results as systolic over diastolic (for example, 140/86).
- Clean the ear tips and diaphragm of the stethoscope with alcohol, and return the equipment to its storage place.
- Repeat hand hygiene.

Aneroid manometers are the type most often found in the imaging department. The procedure for measuring blood pressure is detailed in Box 11-3 and is illustrated in Fig. 11-10. Because this procedure is most frequently used in an emergency, it is important to be proficient before the need arises.

A blood pressure reading is usually expressed in two figures, such as 120/78. The top figure is the **systolic** pressure and is a measure of the pumping action of the heart muscle itself. The bottom figure is the **diastolic*** pressure and indicates the ability of the arterial system to accept the pulse of blood forced into the system when the left ventricle contracts. If you are angry, afraid, or exercising,

---

*A good way to remember is to think, "D is for Down."

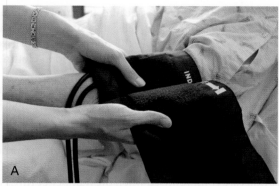
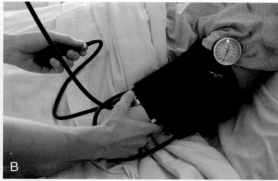

FIG 11-10 Measuring blood pressure. **A,** Wrap the cuff snugly above the antecubital space. **B,** Place the gauge for easy visibility.

the top figure greatly increases. The diastolic figure may also rise, but to a lesser degree. What is a normal blood pressure? The acceptable range of blood pressure varies depending on age, weight, and physical status. As a rule of thumb, a normal systolic pressure will measure between 95 and 119 mm Hg, while the normal diastolic pressure may vary from 60 to 79 mm Hg. A systolic pressure between 120 and 139 mm Hg and diastolic pressure between 80 and 89 mm Hg was once considered normal, but is now considered prehypertension, even if just one measure, either the systolic or diastolic, falls within this range. In stage 1 hypertension, the systolic reading ranges from 140 to 159 mm Hg, and the diastolic reading ranges between 90 and 99 mm Hg. In stage 2 hypertension, the most severe form, the systolic reading is 160 mm Hg or greater and the diastolic reading is 100 mm Hg or greater. The new normal reading is set lower because evidence supports that a blood pressure greater than 119/79 in the prehypertension range is likely to increase the risk of a heart attack or stroke if left untreated.

Hypotension is reflected by a diastolic pressure less than 50 mm Hg or a systolic pressure below 90 mm Hg. This reading may also indicate shock. Hypotension is confirmed when either reading is 20% below the patient's normal baseline.

When an outpatient is to receive intravenous contrast or systemic medication, it is recommended that a blood pressure reading be taken before the procedure begins to provide a baseline. This is best done in the same position the patient will assume for the procedure. Hospital patients will have a reading recorded in the chart, but it is advisable to check the blood pressure if it has not been taken within the past 24 hours.

Generally a baseline or average blood pressure is established for an individual by taking three readings over a period of time. In an emergency, a single reading can be reported to the physician and should be compared with previously recorded results, if available. Take an additional reading as soon as possible.

COMMON LABORATORY TESTS FOR PATIENT ASSESSMENT

Although radiographers are not usually responsible for monitoring laboratory test results, they should have a general knowledge of such values and their significance with respect to the current condition of the patient. This information is particularly relevant when anticipating injection of contrast media for special examinations (see Chapter 19). The following is a brief discussion of some of the more common tests. Normal values are shown in Table 11-3.

Complete Blood Count

A complete blood count (CBC) is frequently performed as part of a diagnostic workup or a complete physical examination. The scope of a CBC may vary, depending on the laboratory and equipment available. As many as 12 different determinations may be performed as part of a routine CBC. All CBCs include a red blood cell (RBC) count, hemoglobin concentration (Hgb), hematocrit (Hct), RBC indices, white blood cell (WBC) count, WBC differential count, and platelet count. The RBC indices include mean corpuscular volume (MCV), mean corpuscular hemoglobin (MCH), mean corpuscular hemoglobin concentration (MCHC), and

TABLE 11-3   Normal Values for Common Laboratory Tests

Laboratory Test	Gender/Age	Normal Value
Red blood cell (RBC) count	Men	4.7–6.1 million per mm³
	Women	4.2–5.4 million per mm³
	Children	4.6–4.8 million per mm³
White blood cell (WBC) count	—	4000–10,000 per mm³
Platelet count	—	150,000–450,000 per mm³
Hemoglobin (Hgb)	Men	13–18 g/dL
	Women	12–16 g/dL
Hematocrit (Hct)	Adults	38–54%
	Children	30–40%
Partial thromboplastin time (PTT)		30–45 sec
Activated partial thromboplastin time (APTT)		21–35 sec
Serum creatinine	Infants to 3 years	0.3–0.7 mg/dL
	Children, ages 3–18	0.5–1.0 mg/dL
	Adults, 18 and older	0.6–1.3 mg/dL
Blood urea nitrogen (BUN)	Children	5–18 mg/dL
	Adults	7–18 mg/dL
	Adults older than age 60	8–20 mg/dL
Serum bilirubin	Indirect	<1.1 mg/dL
	Direct	<0.5 mg/dL
	Total	0.2–1.0 mg/dL
Blood glucose	12–14 hr fasting	70–100 mg/dL
Cholesterol	Total	170–199 mg/dL
	LDL	62–160 mg/dL
	HDL	29–77 mg/dL

HDL, High-density lipoprotein; *LDL,* low-density lipoprotein.

red cell distribution width (RDW). Some laboratories also report the mean platelet volume (MPV), but the diagnostic value of this test remains uncertain in routine testing. A microscopic evaluation of a stained peripheral blood smear is performed when there are significantly abnormal results in the automated CBC. This manual differential includes evaluation of WBC, RBC, and platelet morphology.

The CBC provides specific information about the types and numbers of cells that make up the blood. These blood cells enable the body to transport oxygen and carbon dioxide and to facilitate blood clotting and immune responses.

The RBC count, Hgb value, and Hct value all relate to the red cell component of the blood. Hemoglobin is the pigment in RBCs that carries oxygen from the lungs to the tissues and is essential to sustain life. Carbon dioxide is produced when oxygen is utilized, and is transported by RBCs back to the lungs to be exhaled. These functions are compromised when the number of RBCs in the circulation is decreased. This is reflected as an abnormally low RBC count, low Hgb, and/or low Hct. This information is helpful in the diagnosis and evaluation of specific disease processes affecting the blood, such as deficiency anemias, hemolytic anemias, hypoplastic bone marrows, and chronic systemic disorders such as liver, renal, and endocrine diseases. Low RBC, Hgb, and Hct values are associated with anemia, blood loss, and abnormal hydration (fluid retention), whereas elevated values are seen with polycythemia (an abnormally high level of RBCs in the circulating blood) and **dehydration** (fluid loss). Dehydration is an undesirable condition when anticipating injection of contrast media because it is a predisposing factor for a reaction to the contrast media and contrast nephropathy. The RBC count, Hgb, and Hct are the principal indicators of RBC abnormality, and the RBC indices are helpful in identifying the specific types or causes of anemias.

WBC counts and differential counts of the various types of WBCs are taken to detect infection or inflammation and to diagnose hematoproliferative disorders, such as leukemia. These values are also helpful in monitoring treatment for cancer or immune deficiency diseases. The WBC count increases when infection or inflammation is present, providing extra cells to fight infection and perform phagocytosis. Depression of the WBC count is indicative of immunosuppression. A low WBC level is also seen in cases of excessive exposure to radiation and in patients receiving radiation therapy or chemotherapy.

Erythrocyte Sedimentation Rate

Another blood test frequently ordered is the erythrocyte sedimentation rate (ESR or *sed rate*). This test is most commonly used to determine the presence and/or extent of infectious conditions and inflammatory processes that are systemic in nature. A test that provides similar information about inflammatory conditions is the blood test for C-reactive protein (CRP).

Blood Clotting Assessments

It is important for blood to clot adequately so that the patient will not hemorrhage from minor injuries or invasive diagnostic or surgical procedures. On the other hand, when the blood clots too readily, clots may form within the blood vessels, preventing blood flow and causing tissue necrosis. A blood clot formed on the wall of a vessel is called a **thrombus** (*pl.*, thrombi). A thrombus formed in a large vessel sometimes detaches from the vessel wall, becoming a free-floating clot called an **embolus** (*pl.*, emboli). Emboli are carried in the bloodstream until they reach a vessel that is too small for them to pass through it freely. Clots lodged in cerebral vessels cause strokes; blockage of a coronary artery causes a myocardial infarction (a heart attack); pulmonary embolism (PE) results when one or more emboli lodge in the lung.

Platelets are involved in the blood clot–forming mechanism. A significant reduction in the platelet count indicates that a patient may bleed under circumstances that would normally not result in any bleeding. Several laboratory measurements are used to evaluate the blood's ability to clot: the platelet count, which is part of the CBC, a platelet function analysis test and the coagulation tests known as prothrombin time (PT) and partial thromboplastin time (PTT). The results of these tests are used to assess the risk of both hemorrhage and stroke. Sometimes additional coagulation studies are used. The Heparin Xa assay is used to monitor the anticoagulant heparin, and the D-dimer test is used to detect the presence of disseminated intravascular coagulation. The D-dimer is also used to screen for pulmonary embolism or deep vein thrombosis.

Patients at risk for stroke or heart attack may be treated with anticoagulant medication such as heparin or warfarin (Coumadin). Patients receiving heparin are monitored with either the PTT or Heparin Xa assay. Those taking Coumadin are closely monitored by PT testing, and their medication dosage is determined by the test result. The importance of accurate and reliable PT measurements for these patients, coupled with variations in testing chemicals and standards across the globe, has resulted in the establishment of a standardized reporting system for PTs called the *international normalized ratio* (INR).

The PT is reported in seconds for purposes of screening for inherited or acquired coagulation factor deficiency states. The INR is reported as a numeric ratio with a therapeutic range between 2.0 and 3.0 for patients taking oral anticoagulant medications. The PT may affect the choice of contrast media. A prolonged PT or increased INR may be a contraindication for certain invasive procedures and contrast media examinations.

Blood Chemistry Tests

Other laboratory tests measure the presence of certain biochemicals, or *analytes*, in the blood, and a great variety of these tests is available to the physician. A few common tests of particular interest to radiographers include glucose, cholesterol, urea nitrogen, creatinine, and bilirubin tests.

Glucose

Glucose is a form of sugar, so this test is commonly referred to as a *blood sugar test*, but the preferred name is either *serum glucose* or *plasma glucose*. An abnormally high glucose level is called *hyperglycemia*, and low glucose is called *hypoglycemia*. Blood glucose levels are measured to diagnose and manage patients with diabetes mellitus and a group of conditions referred to as *fasting hypoglycemia* (see Chapter 16).

Cholesterol

Because high cholesterol has been identified as a major risk factor for heart disease, cholesterol measurements have become quite common. A total serum cholesterol test is actually a measurement of the sum total of cholesterol incorporated in a family of cholesterol-containing substances called *lipoproteins*. There are two basic types of lipoproteins that are commonly assayed along with the total serum cholesterol: high-density lipoprotein (HDL) and low-density lipoprotein (LDL). LDL is sometimes called the *bad cholesterol* because elevated levels (greater than 160 mg/dL for normal individuals or greater than 100 mg/dL for those with diabetes or other heart disease risk factors) are considered to be a positive risk factor for the development of heart disease. Conversely, an elevated HDL level (greater than 60 mg/dL) is considered a negative risk factor, and HDL is often referred to as *good cholesterol*. Physicians most commonly evaluate patient risk using the total serum cholesterol, LDL, and HDL levels because total serum cholesterol testing alone may be misleading. The normal total serum cholesterol range is 100 to 199 mg/dL.

BUN and Creatinine

Serum urea nitrogen, also called *blood urea nitrogen* (BUN), is a by-product of protein metabolism, and creatinine is a metabolite associated with skeletal muscle mass. Both BUN and creatinine are nonprotein nitrogenous waste products excreted by the kidneys. When a disease process compromises kidney function, the ability of the kidneys to clear these potentially toxic substances is impaired and the serum levels increase. For this reason, the levels of both BUN and serum creatinine are measured to facilitate the assessment of renal function. Abnormally high BUN levels (called *azotemia*) may indicate impaired renal function. Elevated BUN values (greater than 20 mg/dL) are also seen in cases of acute myocardial infarction, congestive heart failure, dehydration, and excessive protein intake.

Except in individuals with significantly increased skeletal muscle mass, elevated creatinine levels (greater than 1.5 mg/dL) are rarely observed in situations other than compromised kidney function, so an elevated creatinine level is considered a more specific indication of impaired kidney function than the BUN. Creatinine assays from both serum and urine are utilized in the procedure known as *creatinine clearance testing*. This comparison of blood and urine creatinine values can be used to detect very early loss of kidney function, even before abnormal increases in serum levels of BUN or creatinine occur. Because some contrast media may cause kidney failure in patients with impaired renal function, BUN and creatinine levels are useful in screening patients for whom contrast media may have a toxic effect (see Chapter 19).

Serum Bilirubin

Serum bilirubin testing is a blood chemistry assessment that measures the amounts of waste products from the breakdown of hemoglobin. Normally, these waste products are processed by the liver into conjugated bilirubin and excreted as part of the bile through the common bile duct into the duodenum. Physiologically, bile aids in the digestion of dietary fats. Because any obstruction to the flow of bile out of the liver may result in increased amounts of conjugated bilirubin entering the peripheral circulation, increased serum levels of conjugated bilirubin may indicate early liver disease. When bilirubin levels are very high, the patient's skin and the sclera of the eyes take on a yellow color, and the patient is described as *jaundiced*. Some imaging studies of the gallbladder and biliary system rely upon the liver's uptake of the contrast agent and cannot be performed when the bilirubin level is elevated (see Chapter 19). Although radiographic examinations of the biliary system were once quite common, they have largely been replaced by ultrasound studies, nuclear medicine scans, and fiberoptic examinations.

ELECTRONIC PATIENT MONITORING

Although acutely ill patients are usually assigned to an intensive care unit, and x-ray examinations are performed using mobile units (see Chapter 20), critical patients must sometimes be moved to the imaging department for the use of specialized equipment. They are usually accompanied by staff from the critical care unit. Some of these patients will be monitored electronically. Patients may also be sent from the emergency department with monitors already in place.

Pulse Oximeter

A common monitoring device is a pulse oximeter, which is placed on a finger, toe, or earlobe. It continuously monitors both pulse rate and blood oxygen levels (Fig. 11-11). This device is often used to observe the

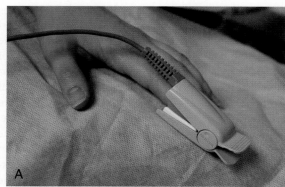

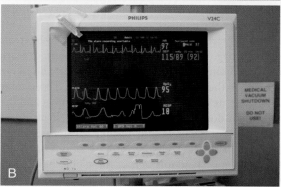

FIG 11-11 Pulse oximeter.

condition of patients who have received sedatives that may suppress respiration and is commonly used in the magnetic resonance imaging suite and in radiographic departments during endoscopic studies of the biliary and pancreatic ducts. Pulse oximeters are sometimes used to measure and record oxygen saturation levels in conjunction with the routine measurement of vital signs.

A photosensitive cell in the oximeter detects the difference between deoxygenated and oxygenated hemoglobin, and a digital readout displays the current status of the patient. Normal values range from 95% to 100%, and readings of less than 95% may indicate that tissues are receiving inadequate oxygen perfusion. Because the sensor depends on reflected light, fingernail polish may need to be removed before applying the oximeter to a finger. Patients with poor circulation because of chronic obstructive pulmonary disease, coronary problems, or vasoconstricting medications may have unreliable readings. If you are able to observe the digital readout and the value falls below the normal range, first assess the patient for any adverse changes. If the patient is not pale, diaphoretic, or exhibiting decreased respiration, check the equipment. Ensure that the pulse oximeter probe is still attached to the patient. If the patient has been prescribed oxygen, verify that the oxygen is flowing unimpeded, that the tubing is not pinched, and that the delivery device (nasal prongs or face mask) is in place. If the reading is still abnormal and the patient is in distress, have a nurse or physician check the patient before continuing with the examination.

Electrocardiograph Monitors

An electrocardiograph is a device that measures the electrical activity of the heart and displays the information graphically in the form of waves on a paper tracing or a monitor screen. The graph that is produced is called an electrocardiogram (ECG or EKG). Deviations from normal are automatically recorded and may activate an auditory alarm.

Continuous ECG monitoring is standard practice in most critical care units. Patients may be brought to the imaging department while being monitored over time to detect and record cardiac irregularities. Patients from the emergency department who suffer from various acute medical or traumatic problems may also come to the radiology department while connected to an ECG monitor. ECG monitoring may be ordered during special imaging procedures or treatments to closely watch the patient's cardiac function.

When a patient is being monitored by ECG, electrodes on the patient are attached to cables that connect to an electronic display unit (Fig. 11-12). ECG electrodes are electrical contacts that can receive tiny electrical signals produced by the patient's heart. They are incorporated into disposable adhesive patches attached to the patient's skin. It is essential that the cables and electrode patches remain secure. When a patient moves, an abnormal tracing may result, which may seem to indicate an arrhythmia. If the electrodes become loose or detached, a *flat-line* tracing may result that seems to indicate **asystole,** the cessation of cardiac activity.

> ⚠ Always check the patient and the electrodes before initiating a code.

Three electrodes are commonly used for continuous monitoring. The two primary contacts are placed on the anterior chest, one on each side of the sternum at the level of the second intercostal space. A third is attached on the side of the chest at the level of the sixth or seventh intercostal space (Fig. 11-13). These are then connected to three colored and/or labeled cables: white (RA – right atrium), black (LA – left atrium), and red (LV – left ventricle), which send the heart's electrical signal to a monitor. A common rhyme to remember which color cable to connect to which electrode is: "White on Right, Smoke over Fire." The white cable attaches to the electrode on the upper right side of the patient, the black to the electrode on the upper left side, and the red on the lower left electrode patch. If a cable is loose, reattach it by snapping or clipping it onto the button

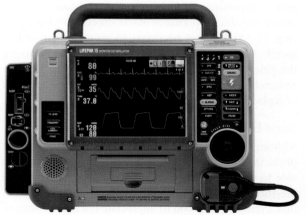

FIG 11-12 Cardiac monitor. (Courtesy Physio-Control, Inc.)

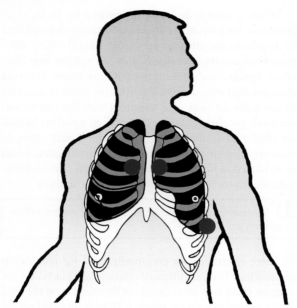

FIG 11-13 Typical electrode placement for ECG monitoring.

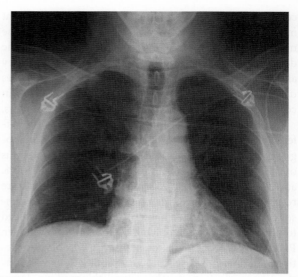

FIG 11-14 Chest radiograph with ECG electrode artifacts.

contact on the electrode patch. If the patch falls off, cleanse the skin with a gauze pad, apply a fresh electrode patch, and attach the cable to the new patch. Supplies are usually kept in drawers in the rolling cabinet that supports the monitor.

Patients who are being monitored by ECG are sometimes temporarily disconnected from monitors when going to the radiology department. In such cases, the electrode patches may be left in place on the patient's chest so that the patient can be easily reconnected to the monitor on returning to the nursing unit or emergency department. Although the patches produce minor metallic or plastic artifacts on chest radiographs (Fig. 11-14), it is not necessary to remove them unless specifically ordered to do so by a physician. Leaving the patches in place saves time if monitoring must be resumed on an emergency basis and saves the expense of replacing the patches.

Basic ECG Rhythm Recognition

Although the diagnostic interpretation of ECGs is a physician's responsibility, it is important for you to be able to recognize the configurations that may indicate life-threatening situations. An understanding of the cardiac cycle will help you to appreciate the significance of ECG rhythm patterns. You may also find it helpful to review the basic anatomy and physiology of the heart.

There are two types of myocardium (heart muscle tissue): contracting tissue and conducting tissue. Figure 11-15 illustrates the conducting muscle tissue and its position in relation to the four chambers of the heart. The cardiac impulse is a tiny electrical current that originates at the junction of the vena cava and the right atrium conducting myocardium called the sinoatrial node. It spreads in circular waves over the atrial walls, causing the atria to contract. The impulse then passes through the atrioventricular node, a second area of conducting myocardium. From this node it passes through a band of conducting muscle connecting the atria to the ventricles that is called the *bundle of His*. The bundle of His divides into the left and right bundle branches, conducting the cardiac impulse to the left and right ventricles. The bundle branches further divide into Purkinje fibers: fine strands of conducting muscle that transmit the impulse to the contracting muscles of the ventricles.

The normal cardiac cycle includes atrial contraction, ventricular contraction, and rest. The transmission of the electrical wave causing contraction of the chamber walls is called *depolarization*. Each contraction is followed by repolarization, an electrical recovery period. Following the ventricular repolarization, the heart rests for a moment in a state of polarization and then the cycle begins again. When the heart is functioning normally, this cycle is repeated 70 to 100 times per minute with a regular rhythm.

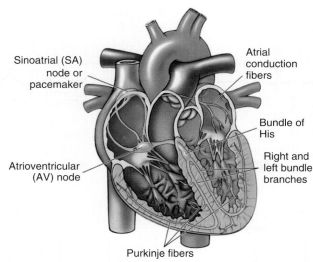

FIG 11-15 Electrical conduction system of the heart. (From Herlihy BA, Maebius NK: *The human body in health and illness,* ed 4, Philadelphia, 2010, Saunders.)

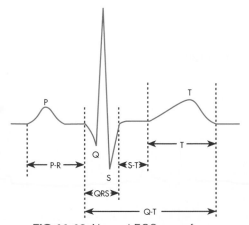

FIG 11-16 Normal ECG waveform.

The ECG graph is centered on an isoelectric line. Deflections above and below this baseline indicate specific electrical impulses. These deflections are referred to as *waves* and are labeled *P, Q, R, S,* and *T* (Fig. 11-16). Together, the Q, R, and S waves are called the *QRS complex.* The QRS complex represents ventricular contraction. The P wave indicates contraction of the atria and the beginning of depolarization. The space between the P wave and the R wave is called the *P-R interval* and represents the time from the beginning of the atrial contraction to the beginning of the ventricular contraction. The S-T segment

indicates the time between ventricular contraction and the beginning of ventricular recovery. The T wave represents ventricular recovery (repolarization). After the T wave, the tracing shows a straight line indicating the heart's resting period. On rare occasions, you may observe a small U wave following the T wave. This is an abnormal wave that indicates a low serum potassium level or other metabolic disturbance affecting the conduction of the cardiac impulse.

> Observations of the morphology (shape), amplitude (height), and duration (graph width) of each wave are considered in relation to the baseline and the other waves. Taken together, these findings demonstrate disturbances in heart rhythm and permit identification of abnormalities.

The normal waveform is called *sinus rhythm* and is demonstrated at a normal heart rate in Fig. 11-17.

Sinus tachycardia (Fig. 11-18) is a rhythm in which the tracing shows a rapid heart rate without any other deviations from normal. This ordinarily results from an increase in physical activity or from fear, excitement, or chemical stimulation, such as too much caffeine. For patients who have a preexisting heart problem, however, this rapid rate may be a precursor to a life-threatening ventricular tachycardia.

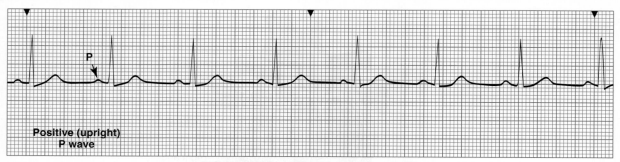

FIG 11-17 Normal sinus rhythm, rate 80.

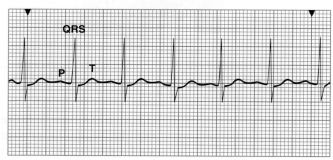

FIG 11-18 Sinus tachycardia, rate 120.

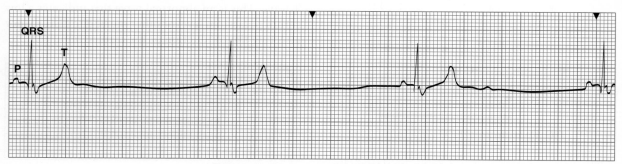

FIG 11-19 Sinus bradycardia, rate 30.

Sinus **bradycardia,** an abnormally slow heart rate (fewer than 60 bpm), is shown in Fig. 11-19. This slow heart rate may be perfectly normal for the healthy individual and is frequently seen in athletes who have developed a large cardiac output. In other patients, this slow rate is insufficient to provide adequate oxygen supply to the brain and vital organs, and a pacemaker may be needed to increase and regulate the heart rate.

Premature ventricular contractions (PVCs) are irregular, early ventricular contractions that interfere with the normal rate and rhythm of the heart (Fig. 11-20). This is demonstrated on the ECG by a wide, irregular QRS complex and a loss of the P wave, which is buried in the QRS wave. PVCs can often be felt by patients who complain that "my heart flutters" or that it feels as though the heart "flops over." Although an occasional PVC is not unusual and should not cause undue alarm,

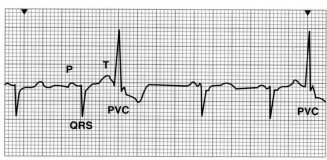

FIG 11-20 Premature ventricular contractions.

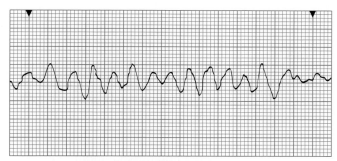

FIG 11-21 Ventricular fibrillation.

a run of PVCs can reduce the cardiac output by 12% to 15% if untreated.

If allowed to progress, PVCs may initiate ventricular **fibrillation,** where the heart quivers or fibrillates and loses the ability to contract effectively (Fig. 11-21). Ventricular fibrillation is the most common cause of sudden death. Whether or not a pulse is detected, a code must be called. If the patient has no pulse, a single shock is delivered using the defibrillator and this is followed by cardiopulmonary resuscitation. The code team will give the patient an initial administration of 1 ml of epinephrine, which causes vasoconstriction, increasing the coronary perfusion pressure and allowing more oxygenated blood to reach the heart. This enhances the contractile state of the heart and stimulates spontaneous contractions.

In ventricular tachycardia (Fig. 11-22), the heart rate may be as high as 150 to 250 bpm. Although the heart may be beating regularly, the cardiac output is too low to be effective and the patient may lose consciousness and become hypotensive. In most cases amiodarone is administered intravenously, and in some cases the patient will need to be defibrillated. If untreated, ventricular tachycardia may progress to ventricular fibrillation.

Atrial fibrillation (Fig. 11-23) results from continuous and irregular reentry of electrical impulses back into the atria. Because these impulses are so rapid and continuous, they spur a rapid and irregular ventricular response. Atrial fibrillation in a young patient may be caused by rheumatic mitral valve disease. Atrial fibrillation is more common in older patients in whom arteriosclerotic heart disease is the major cause. Palpitations, nausea, weakness, and fatigue may occur during an attack of atrial fibrillation. Sudden attacks tend to occur periodically before this condition becomes chronic. If the patient suffers from mitral stenosis or other left ventricular disease, cardiogenic shock or acute pulmonary edema may result (see Chapter 16). Treatment is initiated primarily to slow ventricular response and increase cardiac output. If the patient does not respond to medication, **cardioversion** may be performed. Cardioversion is an electrical stimulation of the heart to restore its normal rhythm.

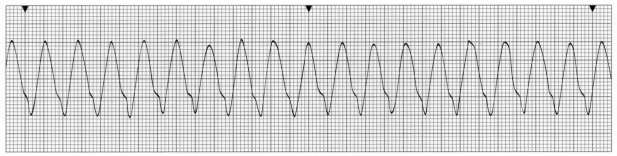

FIG 11-22 Ventricular tachycardia.

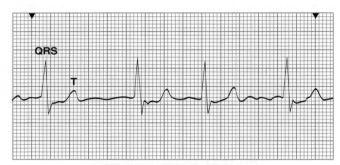

FIG 11-23 Atrial fibrillation.

Diagnostic electrocardiography is an examination commonly used to assess the nature and severity of heart disease. It is similar to ECG monitoring, but provides a more comprehensive assessment and a permanent record. The job descriptions of radiographers do not usually include these studies.

Arterial Catheters

One comprehensive way to monitor cardiac activity is to introduce a special arterial catheter into a large artery where it can provide continuous measurement of the heart rate and blood pressure. Catheter placement is a special procedure applied under sterile surgical conditions. These catheters and their placement are discussed in Chapter 20.

ELECTROENCEPHALOGRAPHY

Another physiologic monitoring and recording device is the electroencephalograph (EEG). This device is not commonly seen in the radiology department. The EEG machine is similar in function and design to the ECG unit, but the cables are attached to electrodes on the patient's scalp to record or monitor the electrical activity of the brain. This device is commonly used to evaluate patients with convulsive disorders, but it can also help the physician diagnose other conditions that affect brain activity. An EEG can show a cessation of electrical activity in the brain, providing one of the criteria used to determine legal death, especially in situations involving organ donation.

Most electronic monitoring devices are applied in a critical care setting, and special training is necessary both to apply and monitor these electronic instruments. They are useful in providing rapid and accurate information, but are also subject to error when connections become loose, are placed incorrectly, or when the patient moves. Chapter 19 provides more information about some of the highly sophisticated patient monitoring systems used in the intensive care unit.

SUMMARY

- Patient assessment is an essential skill for radiographers because it enables them to identify patient needs, set priorities, provide the radiologist with pertinent information, and identify changes in a patient's condition that may be life-threatening.
- Taking a history pertinent to the examination is an essential skill that improves with practice; a good history assists the radiologist by providing facts that relate to the diagnosis.
- A baseline assessment of a patient's current status involves checking the chart, *eyeballing* the patient, determining the level of consciousness, and noting whether or not breathing appears normal.
- Vital signs include measurements of temperature, pulse rate, respiratory rate, and blood pressure. Accurate measurement and recording of vital signs is an essential skill for radiographers. They must also have knowledge of normal values and the significance of abnormal values.
- Laboratory tests including complete blood counts, blood clotting time measurements, and blood chemistry studies assist in the assessment of the patient's status. Radiographers should be familiar with the most common studies and aware of the significance of abnormal values.
- Continuing assessment of patients at risk is accomplished with various types of monitoring equipment, including the pulse oximeter that monitors heart rate and oxygen saturation levels in the blood, arterial catheters that provide continuous assessment of the heart rate and blood pressure, and ECG monitors that provide graphic information on heart rate and rhythm. Radiographers must recognize life-threatening conditions when they are indicated by these monitors.

REVIEW QUESTIONS

1. Part of your initial assessment of a patient's status should include assessment of body temperature by:
   A. checking the temperature graph in the patient's chart
   B. evaluating skin temperature by touch
   C. taking a rectal temperature
   D. taking an axillary temperature
2. 110/78 mm Hg is a typical measurement for which of the following vital signs?
   A. Blood pressure
   B. Pulse rate
   C. Respiratory rate
   D. Body temperature
3. A serum bilirubin test is used to measure:
   A. blood oxygen levels
   B. nitrogen in blood
   C. blood glucose status when fasting
   D. conjugated hemoglobin content in blood
4. When a patient's appearance takes on a bluish color, especially in the nail beds and mucous membranes of the mouth, the patient is described as:
   A. jaundiced
   B. hypertensive
   C. cyanotic
   D. hyperventilating
5. The normal heart rate for an adult is:
   A. 12 to 20 bpm
   B. 80 to 120 bpm
   C. 60 to 100 bpm
   D. 98 to 99 bpm
6. When the heart rate is measured by placing a stethoscope on the chest directly over the heart, this is called a(n):
   A. carotid pulse
   B. apical pulse
   C. pedal pulse
   D. radial pulse
7. The term *tachycardia* refers to:
   A. high blood pressure
   B. rapid breathing
   C. rapid heart rate
   D. fever
8. Which of the following instruments is used to monitor both the pulse and the oxygen saturation of the blood?
   A. Sphygmomanometer
   B. Electrocardiograph
   C. Electroencephalograph
   D. Pulse oximeter

Answers can be found in the Answer Key on pages 429-431.

CRITICAL THINKING EXERCISES

1. Mrs. Morgan, a missionary's wife, has just returned from overseas with a fever of unknown origin and has been referred for a chest radiograph. What can you think of that may be causing Mrs. Morgan's fever? How would you use the history guidelines in this chapter to obtain relevant information for the radiologist?

2. A 16-year-old male, Larry Doyle, was hunting when he was attacked by a swarm of yellow jackets. While running away, he fell and severely twisted his ankle. He has been admitted to the emergency department to rule out a fracture of the ankle. The numerous stings have caused swelling over much of his exposed hands and arms. Would it be important to monitor Larry's vital signs? Why or why not? What problems could you encounter? How could his pulse and respiration be affected by anxiety and pain?

3. Any sudden change in vital signs can be extremely important. Hector Garcia has been given an antibiotic for a urinary tract infection. This is the second occurrence of infection in 6 weeks, and he has now been referred for an excretory urogram. While waiting for the initial image to be checked, he complains of feeling short of breath and has poorly defined discomfort in his chest. What could cause these symptoms? What should you do?

4. Margaret Nelson was transported by stretcher from the emergency department to the imaging department for lumbar spine radiographs following a motor vehicle crash. On arrival she appeared alert, but during the examination she became sleepy. When questioned, she seemed to be confused. How would you describe this change in Margaret's condition? Is it likely to be significant? What should you do?

12

Patient Transfer

OBJECTIVES

At the conclusion of this chapter, the student will be able to:

- List two steps to be taken to ensure accuracy of patient identification.
- Demonstrate safe techniques for moving and transferring patients, using the principles of good body mechanics.
- Safely assist a patient into and out of a wheelchair.
- Use a gait belt to assist a weak patient to stand and walk.
- Demonstrate the correct method for assisting patients who are weak on one side.
- List precautions to take in moving and positioning patients following a surgical hip replacement.
- Perform two-person transfer of a patient from bed to stretcher and stretcher to bed.
- Demonstrate use of draw sheets, a slider board, and a sliding mat to facilitate stretcher transfers.
- Demonstrate proper use of safety straps and side rails on stretchers.

OUTLINE

KEY TERMS

draw sheet
gait belt

orthostatic hypotension
sedation

slider board
sliding mat

PATIENT TRANSFER CONSIDERATIONS

When inpatients are moved from one place to another in a hospital, wheeled transport is required. Patients may believe that they can walk to the radiology department, but they must not be allowed to do so. If an ambulatory patient becomes weak or faints in a corridor or elevator during the trip, there is no safe way to cope. Likewise, infants and small children should not be carried to the radiology department. A change in the patient's status may require that you have both hands free to deal with the problem or to obtain help.

> ! Inpatients must not be allowed to walk to the imaging department. Likewise, infants and small children should not be carried. Wheeled transport is necessary.

The usual method of transport is a wheelchair for patients who can stand and sit with safety and comfort, and a stretcher for those who cannot. Patients who cannot stand, and those who have not stood or walked since an accident, surgery, stroke, or heart attack, should not be transported by wheelchair; stretcher transfer is a safer method. These patients must not be allowed to stand or walk in the imaging department, even if they believe they are capable of doing so. A stretcher is also the best means of transfer for patients who have had recent trauma and/or surgery to the spine.

When a patient's condition makes it extremely difficult or hazardous to move him/her onto a stretcher, the patient may be transported in the bed. Bed transfers require at least two people because the bed is heavy and cumbersome, and patients who must be transferred in their beds require careful attention to their physical status during transfer. They may also require considerable auxiliary equipment.

Active infants and toddlers are often transported in their cribs. The high sides of the crib provide greater safety than the side rails of a stretcher, and the crib provides a safe place if the child must be left unattended at any time. Premature infants may be transported in a closed incubator, an infant bed with a plastic hood that provides a closed environment for warmth, moisture, and oxygen while reducing exposure to airborne infection (see illustration in Chapter 20, Fig. 20-2).

 Transfer by stretcher is the proper method for patients who cannot stand safely and those who cannot sit comfortably or climb safely onto the radiographic table.

PREPARATION FOR TRANSFER

The steps in preparing for patient transfer are summarized in Box 12-1. Always check with the nursing station before transferring a patient to the imaging department. The nursing service must be advised because they are responsible for knowing the patient's whereabouts at all times. In addition, nurses can often provide you with helpful information about the patient's status and transfer requirements; they may also assist with the transfer if necessary. If paper charts are used, obtain the patient's chart from the nursing service at this time.

The next step in safely moving a patient is to be certain that you have the right patient. You must make use

---

BOX 12-1   Preparing for a Safe Patient Transfer

- Check with nursing service.
- Obtain the chart unless electronic medical records are used.
- Check patient identification.
- Plan what you are going to do and prepare your work area.
- Obtain equipment and check it for safety and function.
- Check the area for equipment attached to the patient. A urinary collection bag, IV fluids, and pump may need to be transferred; oxygen or suction may need to be discontinued.
- Enlist the patient's help and cooperation. Remember to tell the patient what you are doing as you proceed.
- Obtain additional help when necessary. Ensure that your assistants understand their roles in the transfer plan.

! If the patient is very ill, receiving multiple intravenous fluids, or on ECG monitoring, a nurse should monitor the patient during transport and during the procedure. If you are not comfortable transporting the patient alone, you should not hesitate to ask for assistance in transporting the patient.

---

of two patient identifiers, as required by The Joint Commission. Check the identification bracelet against the name and birth date on the x-ray requisition, or ask the patient to state both his/her name and birth date, and compare this response with the order or requisition.

 Always double-check two patient identifiers before transport.

A brief visit with the patient will help you assess how much the patient can help with the transfer, allowing you to plan for additional hands if needed to ensure a safe move. Most patients appreciate an estimate of how long the procedure will last. Decide on the safest, easiest method of moving your patient, obtain the necessary equipment, and ensure that it is functional and safe. The person transporting the patient is responsible for ensuring that the buckles on safety straps are secure, that side rails lock in the up position, and that brakes work properly. Move any furniture or obstacles that may be in the way.

Take note of any special equipment that may need to be transported with the patient, such as monitors or medication pumps. A urine collection bag may need to be detached from the bed and attached to the stretcher or wheelchair below the level of the patient's bladder. Portable oxygen equipment may be required if the patient is currently receiving oxygen from a wall outlet. Other equipment may need to be disconnected or rearranged before patient transfer, but consult the nursing service before disconnecting any equipment.

Next tell the patient what you plan to do, and explain his or her role in the transfer. Because patients can often anticipate painful errors, you should listen carefully and allow the patient to participate in the plan.

After the patient has been safely moved to the stretcher or wheelchair, check that the safety rails or straps are in place and that the patient is comfortable and adequately covered for warmth and modesty. Have you forgotten anything? An emesis basin or a small box of tissues may be handy along the way. If hard copy charts are used, transport them with the patient.

WHEELCHAIR TRANSFERS

Transferring a patient from a bed to a wheelchair may seem simple, but it is a common cause of falls and accidents. The correct technique makes this procedure safer and easier (Procedure 12-1).

Start by lowering the bed to the level of the wheelchair seat and elevating the head of the bed. Position the wheelchair parallel to the bed with wheels locked, footrests out of the way, and a sheet covering the sitting surface of the wheelchair. With the patient in the supine position, place one arm under the patient's shoulders, one under the knees, and in a single, smooth motion, raise and turn the patient to a sitting position with his or her feet dangling over the side. Patients with back pain may find it easier to sit up from a lateral recumbent position.

Take a moment to assist the patient with his/her slippers and a robe and allow time for the patient to regain a sense of balance. After long periods of rest, many patients have **orthostatic hypotension,** a mild reduction in the oxygen supply to the brain that occurs with changes in body position and may cause them to feel light-headed or faint when rising suddenly.

At this point, competent patients are able to stand and move to the wheelchair with little assistance, although a steadying hand at the patient's elbow is a good practice.

A **gait belt,** also called a *transfer belt*, should be used when assisting patients who are weak or unsteady (Fig. 12-1). These belts are heavy fabric straps with a strong buckle. When placed snugly around the patient's waist, they provide a secure handhold for you to use in helping the patient to stand and walk.

If assistance is required, stand facing the patient, grasp the gait belt or reach around the patient and place your hands firmly over the scapulae; the patient's hands may rest on your shoulders. On your signal, lift upward and help the patient rise to a standing position. Remember to use a broad base of support and keep your back straight.

> **!** If working independently, it is wise to remember that patients wearing gait belts are considered to be at risk for falling—do not assume they will be able to walk and/or bear their own weight unassisted for more than a brief moment. Consider the size of the patient in relation to yourself and determine if you need additional help should they become unsteady.

Now instruct and assist the patient to pivot a quarter turn so that the edge of the wheelchair is touching the back of the knees, then ease the patient into a sitting position in the chair. Position the foot and leg rests, and cover the patient's lap and legs with a sheet or bath blanket to provide warmth and comfort and protect modesty.

The most common type of fall associated with a wheelchair transfer occurs when the patient backs into the wheelchair to sit down. The patient may miss the edge of the seat or tip the chair by sitting too near the edge. To avoid such an accident, be sure to lock the wheels of the chair and assist the patient until he/she is seated securely.

To move the patient from the wheelchair to the x-ray table, follow the steps illustrated in Procedure 12-2. Place the wheelchair parallel to the table, lock the brakes, and move the footrests out of the way. At this point, the procedure will vary depending on whether you are fortunate enough to have an x-ray table that is adjustable in height.

If the height of the x-ray table is adjustable, lower the table to chair height. In this instance, the transfer to the x-ray table is the reverse of the transfer from the bed. Using the face-to-face assistance explained previously, help the patient to stand and pivot with the patient's back to the table. Then ease the patient into a sitting position on the edge of the table.

PROCEDURE 12-1 WHEELCHAIR TRANSFER

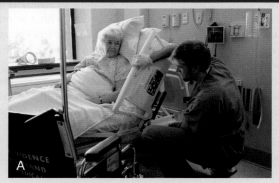

A, Lower the bed to its lowest position; then lower side rails.

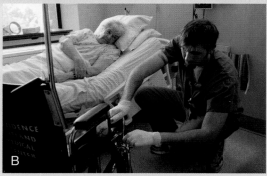

B, Position wheelchair parallel to patient's bed with wheels locked and foot-rests out of the way.

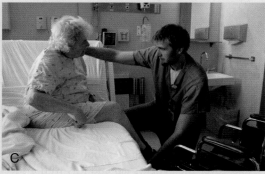

C, Lift patient to a sitting position; pivot while lifting, allowing patient's legs to clear edge of bed. Allow patient to rest briefly before standing.

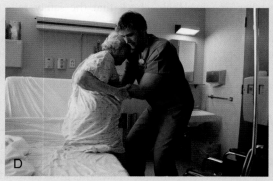

D, Use face-to-face assist to raise weak patient to standing position.

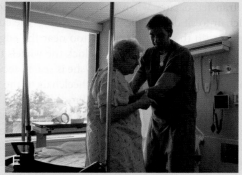

E, Help patient pivot with his/her back to wheelchair.

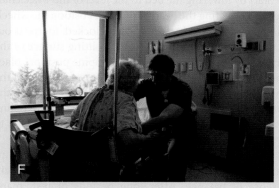

F, Ease patient to sitting position.

PROCEDURE 12-1   **WHEELCHAIR TRANSFER—cont'd**

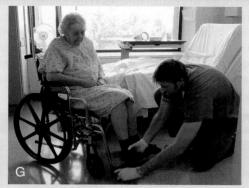

G, Adjust leg-rests and footrests.

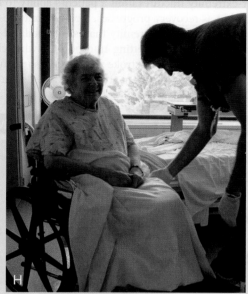

H, Cover patient's lap and legs.

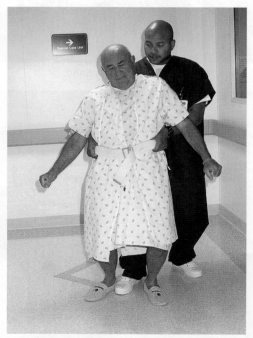

FIG 12-1 Gait belt provides a secure handhold when assisting a patient to stand and walk. (From Perry AG, Potter PA, Ostendorf WR: *Nursing interventions and clinical skills,* ed 6, St Louis, 2016, Elsevier.)

If the table height is stationary, position a step stool with a tall handle nearby. Have the patient place one hand on the stool handle, put the other arm on your shoulder, and step up onto the stool, pivoting with the back to the table. Now ease the patient to a sitting position.

When the patient is seated on the table, raise it if the height is adjustable. Then place one arm around the patient's shoulders and one under the knees. With a single, smooth motion, place the patient's legs on the table while lowering the head and shoulders into the supine position. Patients with back pain may want to lie on one side before moving into the supine position.

Special Considerations for Wheelchair Transfers

Stroke

Stroke patients typically have weakness on one side of the body. Determine which side is the patient's weak side, and position yourself on that side. Brace the patient's weak leg with your knee as the patient stands, as illustrated in part *B* of Procedure 12-2. When moving from the wheelchair to a bed or table, position the patient with the strong side adjacent to the bed or table and instruct him/her to lead with the strong leg. It is often advisable to use stretcher transport with these patients.

Fractures of the Lower Extremity

Lower-extremity fractures limit a patient's ability to bear weight, but as recovery progresses, a patient may be able to bear weight on an extremity that is immobilized in a cast or splint, thus permitting transport by wheelchair. The skills used to assist a stroke victim are also useful in this case. Support the patient from the affected side and encourage him/her to lead with the strong leg. Elevate the leg-rest of the wheelchair to support the injured leg during the transfer, and help the patient lift the leg when changing position. Take care that the fractured limb is not twisted or bumped during the transfer. Similar precautions are appropriate for the patient with an undiagnosed leg injury who is sufficiently stable to allow transfer by wheelchair.

PROCEDURE 12-2   ASSISTING PATIENT ONTO RADIOGRAPHIC TABLE

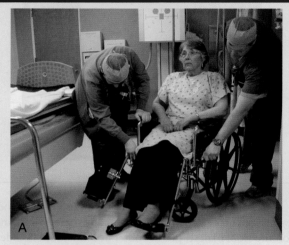

A, Lock wheelchair brakes and move footrests.

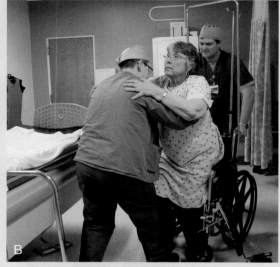

B, Assist patient to stand.

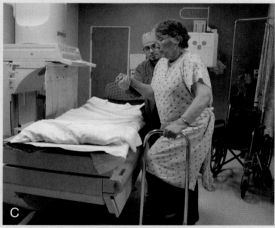

C, Assist patient with step stool, if necessary.

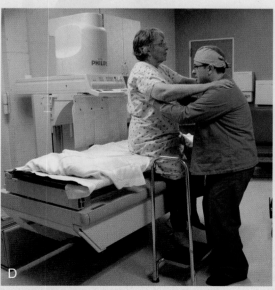

D, Assist patient to pivot and sit on table.

PROCEDURE 12-2   ASSISTING PATIENT ONTO RADIOGRAPHIC TABLE—cont'd

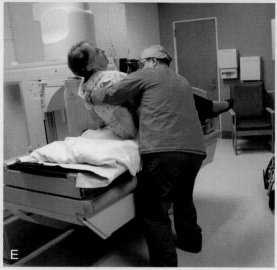

E, Support patient's shoulders while raising his/her legs onto table; ease patient to supine position.

Joint Replacements

Joint replacement surgery makes it necessary for a patient to receive special care, especially when being transferred during the recovery period. Restrictions vary in accordance with the surgical approach taken (Table 12-1). Movement must be restricted to avoid any stress on muscles that have been surgically disrupted, so always check the chart to determine the patient's limitations.

Hip Replacement. Patients who have undergone hip replacement by means of the anterior surgical approach are able to sit upright in a chair at a 90-degree angle. Do not permit the patient to adduct, abduct, or rotate the affected leg, and avoid any hyperextension, especially when walking.

Patients who have undergone hip replacement by means of the posterior approach, which is the most common, are able to tolerate abduction, but must not be allowed to cross the affected leg over the midline; both adduction and internal rotation must be avoided. Furthermore, these patients must not flex at the hip beyond 90 degrees. These restrictions prevent stress on the posterior joint capsule, which needs time to heal and strengthen after surgery. During the initial period after surgery, patients must be transported by stretcher. If they need to sit up for any reason, take care that they do not

TABLE 12-1   Precautions for Patients with Hip Replacements

Surgery via the Anterior Approach	Surgery via the Posterior Approach
May sit upright	Must not flex hip beyond 90 degrees
Weight bearing is usually tolerated (check chart)	Weight bearing is usually tolerated (check chart)
Avoid abduction	Abduction is permitted
Avoid adduction	Avoid adduction
Avoid internal or external rotation	Avoid internal rotation
Avoid hyperextension	

bend forward, because most dislocations occur when the patient bends forward past 90 degrees, such as when getting up from a low chair. Patients are at an increased risk of dislocation for up to 1 year after surgery.

Knee Replacement. Knee-replacement surgery requires similar considerations when transferring a patient. Weight bearing is usually tolerated, but a walker is needed when taking more than one or two steps. Move the patient toward the strong side and provide support under the calf and knee of the affected leg for comfort and safety.

Spinal Trauma or Spinal Surgery

Patients suffering from spinal trauma or recovering from recent spinal surgery should be transferred by stretcher. During the initial phase of injury or postoperative recovery, the patient should be accompanied by the primary caregiver who will instruct the radiology staff in safe positioning. As recovery progresses, transfer by wheelchair may be tolerable and safe. Moving from a supine position to a sitting position, or from sitting to a supine position, places considerable stress on the spine. Instead, the patient should sit from a lateral recumbent position. When lying down, the patient should lie first on one side and then turn to the supine position with the knees flexed. Provide support and assistance to the patient while extending the legs, and place a bolster or pillow under the knees for support when he/she is supine.

Patients Who Cannot Stand Safely

Inpatients that are paralyzed or unable to stand for any reason are always transported by stretcher within a hospital, but outpatients who are unable to stand may arrive at the hospital in a wheelchair. Depending on the design of the chair and the requirements of the procedure, examinations of the extremities and chest radiography may be performed with the patient seated in the wheelchair, but most procedures will require placing these patients on the radiographic table. When a patient in a wheelchair cannot stand, a hydraulic lift is required (Procedure 12-3). Do not attempt to use this equipment until you have been properly instructed in its safe use. When a patient must be lifted from a wheelchair and no mechanical lift is available, a two or three-person lift is used (see Appendix I).

> **!** Do not attempt to operate the hydraulic lift until you have been instructed in its safe use.

STRETCHER TRANSFERS

A stretcher, sometimes called a *cart* or *gurney,* should be used to transport any patient who is unable to stand safely. This is also the method of choice for patients who cannot sit comfortably for an extended period. Remember that the patient may have to wait in the imaging department before or after the examination. A weak patient who cannot stand may be under a physician's order to sit in a chair as part of the daily routine. A visit to the radiology department should not be seized as an opportunity to meet this requirement. Such patients can be moved from chair to bed more easily than from chair to x-ray table, especially if the table height cannot be adjusted. If you have any doubt about the patient's ability to transfer safely from the chair to the table, be safe and start with a stretcher.

If the patient's safety or comfort requires elevation of the head, select a stretcher that provides upper body support. The following stretcher transfer techniques may be used to move patients to the stretcher from either the bed or the radiographic table. It is not recommended to attempt a stretcher transfer by yourself except in the case of providing assistance to a patient who is capable of self-transfer. To avoid injury to yourself and the patient, it is best to obtain the help of one or more persons; additional help is essential if the patient is obese or very weak.

Respect the patient's privacy by closing the door to the hallway or drawing the curtain around the bed. Start the procedure with the patient near the edge of the bed in the supine position with both knees flexed and feet flat. Adjust the bed and the stretcher to the flat horizontal position, and adjust the height of the bed to the height of the stretcher. Position the stretcher parallel to the bed and lock the wheels. Check to ensure that oxygen lines, intravenous tubing, and urinary catheters are free and will not be pulled during the transfer.

If you must work alone, lean across the stretcher, placing one arm under the patient's shoulders and the other arm under the pelvis. On your instructions, have the patient push with feet and elbows as you lift and pull him/her toward the stretcher. Do not attempt to make the transfer in a single motion. The maneuver may be repeated several times until the transfer is complete.

When you are working with an assistant, one person supports the head, neck, and shoulders while the second person lifts at the pelvis and knees (Fig. 12-2). Both use the lift-pull or lift-push motion with the patient's assistance until he/she is safely positioned on the stretcher.

As soon as the patient is situated on the stretcher, provide a cover, secure a safety belt across the pelvic area if available, and raise the side rails. Elevate the head of the stretcher, if necessary. Before you leave the room, check to ensure you have everything you will need. Equipment may be placed at the foot of the stretcher beside the patient's feet.

To reverse this transfer, position the stretcher parallel to the bed, lock the wheels, and lower the side rails.

PROCEDURE 12-3 HYDRAULIC LIFT

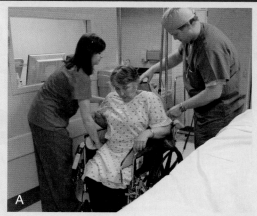

A, Lean patient forward in wheelchair, placing sling behind and around him/her.

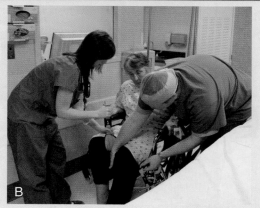

B, Pull sling's lower attachments to center, around patient's legs.

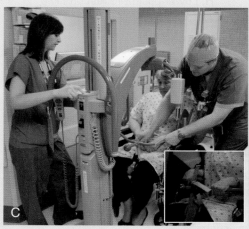

C, Connect sling attachments to the lift mechanism.

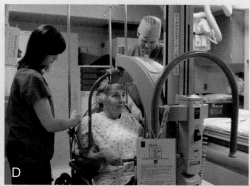

D, When attachment is complete and patient is secure, start raising lift.

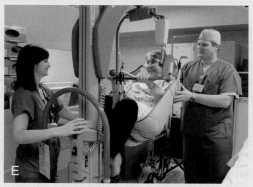

E, Do not move unit until patient has been lifted high enough to clear wheelchair.

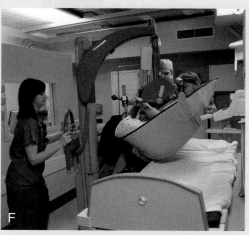

F, Slowly move unit toward table.

PROCEDURE 12-3   HYDRAULIC LIFT—cont'd

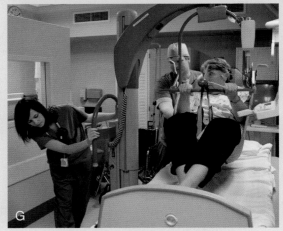

G, Position patient over table.

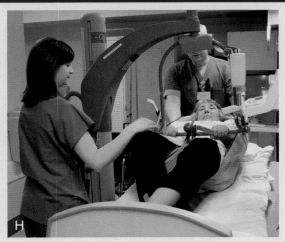

H, Lower patient to rest on table.

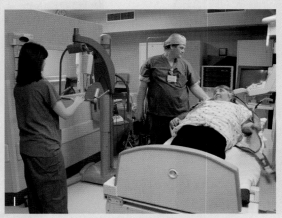

I, Detach link and remove unit.

Return the stretcher to the flat horizontal position if the head has been elevated; move any equipment out of the way. Because beds are wider than stretchers, it may be easier to work from the stretcher side. Position and support the patient as before. This time, on a signal, the patient pushes toward the bed while you assist with a lift-push movement. Repeat as required until the transfer is complete. This same method may be applied to transfers from the stretcher to the x-ray table, but it may be easier to reach across the table and pull the patient toward you.

Various techniques are used for stretcher transfers, depending on the patient's weight and ability to assist.

With problem transfers, it is best to obtain experienced help. Three methods of transfer involve the use of draw sheets, slider boards, and sliding mats. These are often useful when the patient is unable to assist with the transfer. Practice these transfers in class before attempting to use them with patients.

In addition to the methods described here, some hospitals may have Air-Assisted Lateral Patient Transfer devices. These inflatable devices facilitate transfers and repositioning of patients with paralysis or multiple lines, and especially those who are morbidly obese. This method requires at least two people and must only be done by those who have received

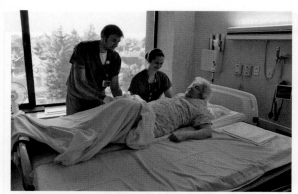

FIG 12-2 Conventional stretcher transfer. Allow patient to help as much as possible.

special training in the use of this equipment. Most facilities have trained lift teams to assist with difficult transfers.

Draw Sheet Transfers

Patients who need frequent help with moving are often placed on a draw sheet. This is a single sheet folded in half that is placed under the patient and over the middle third of the bed. When moving the patient, the edges of the draw sheet are loosened from the bed and rolled up close to the patient's body (Procedure 12-4). The rolled edge provides a handhold for lifting and pulling the patient. Care must be taken that the patient's head and feet move safely with the trunk of the body, which requires two or more persons.

Slider Board Transfers

Transfers using slider boards and sliding mats are variations of the draw sheet method. The slider board is a strong sheet of smooth plastic large enough to support the patient's body with handholds cut into the edges. The patient is rolled to one side and the board is slipped below the draw sheet and about halfway under the patient's body (Procedure 12-5). The remaining width of the board covers the space between the stretcher and the bed. With the patient's arms folded safely across the chest, two people grip the draw sheet and slide the patient safely and smoothly across the board. Where the patient is being transferred onto an exam table, the entire slider board may be transferred under the patient; otherwise, the board is simply a sliding tool to bridge the gap between the bed and stretcher.

! Flexible slider boards must not be used in place of rigid backboards for spinal immobilization.

PROCEDURE 12-4 DRAW SHEET TRANSFER

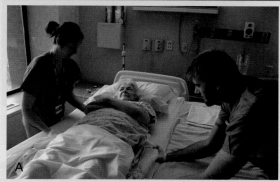

A. Roll draw sheet on each side of patient to provide handholds.

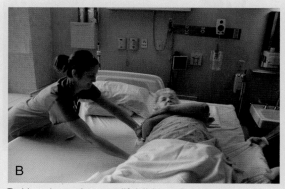

B. Use draw sheet to lift/slide patient onto stretcher.

Sliding Mat Transfers

A sliding mat is a soft, tubular sheet of flexible plastic that has a low friction surface and is used in more or less the same way as a slider board (Procedure 12-6). The sliding mat is especially helpful when transferring patients from soft mattresses, waterbeds, or other specialty mattresses. Be sure to remove the sliding mat once the patient is securely positioned on the stretcher.

Safety Side Rails

Stretchers are equipped with side rails to ensure that patients do not fall or attempt to climb off without assistance. This is especially important when the patient's

PROCEDURE 12-5   SLIDER BOARD EASES STRETCHER TRANSFER

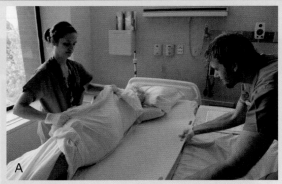

A. Using draw sheet, roll patient to one side and place slider board under patient.

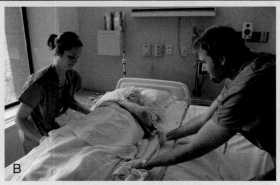

B. Use draw sheet to help slide patient across slider board onto stretcher.

PROCEDURE 12-6   SLIDING MAT TRANSFER

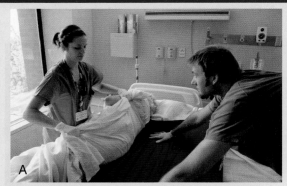

A. Using draw sheet, roll patient to one side and place sliding mat under him/her.

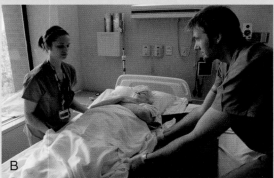

B. Slippery double surface of mat facilitates draw sheet transfer. Remove sliding mat once patient is on stretcher.

state of consciousness is impaired because of **sedation** (calming medication), intoxication, shock, or senility. Application of side rails during transport is such an important safety practice that it must be followed without exception (Fig. 12-3). Side rails must also be in the elevated position whenever a patient is left unattended on a stretcher.

> **!** Safety straps must be used if available and stretcher side rails must be in the up position except when moving patients on or off the stretcher.

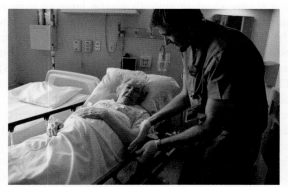

FIG 12-3 Side rails and safety straps, if available, must always be used on stretchers.

SUMMARY

- Before transporting a patient, check with the nursing service, obtain the patient's chart, check the patient's identification, plan the transfer, check the equipment, communicate effectively with the patient, and obtain help if necessary.
- Wheelchair transfers are appropriate for patients who can sit, stand, and walk safely. Set the brakes before the transfer and assist the patient until he/she is safely seated.
- Additional precautions are necessary for patients who have suffered strokes or lower extremity injuries,

and for those who have undergone joint replacement surgery.
- A patient who is unable to stand must be assisted from a wheelchair using a hydraulic lift.
- Transfer by stretcher is appropriate for patients who cannot be safely transported by wheelchair.
- When the patient is unable to assist with stretcher transfer, two people using a draw sheet, with or without a slider board or sliding mat, are necessary for a safe transfer. Use of side rails is essential.

REVIEW QUESTIONS

1. A slider board or sliding mat can be used to:
   A. evacuate the area
   B. immobilize a child
   C. facilitate a stretcher transfer
   D. provide comfort on the
      x-ray table
2. When a patient arrives by wheelchair and cannot stand to get onto the x-ray table, which of the following methods is most appropriate?
   A. Slider board transfer
   B. Hydraulic lift
   C. Face-to-face assist
   D. Draw sheet transfer
3. Patients who have not stood or walked since an accident, surgery, stroke, or heart attack should be transported by:
   A. wheelchair
   B. hydraulic lift
   C. stretcher
   D. slider board
4. When assisting a patient to sit from a supine position, or to lie down from a sitting position, you should place your arms under the shoulders and:
   A. knees
   B. head
   C. buttocks
   D. waist
5. Infants and toddlers are usually transported in:
   A. incubators
   B. cribs

C. stretchers
D. wheelchairs

6. A feeling of faintness or light-headedness that occurs with changes in body position after long periods of rest is termed:
   A. orthostatic hypertension
   B. orthostatic hypotension
   C. secondary hypertension
   D. momentary hypertension
7. When an ambulatory patient has a weak leg as a result of a stroke or other condition, it is helpful to:
   A. position the patient with the weak side against the bed or table
   B. position yourself on the patient's weak side
   C. position yourself on the patient's strong side
   D. encourage the patient to lead with the weak leg
8. Patients who have undergone which of the following procedures must not flex at the hips more than 90 degrees?
   A. Knee replacement
   B. Spinal surgery
   C. Hip replacement via the anterior approach
   D. Hip replacement via the posterior approach
9. Which of the following items is NOT useful for facilitating a stretcher transfer?
   A. Slider board
   B. Transfer belt
   C. Sliding mat
   D. Draw sheet

10. When transferring a patient who is unable to assist with transfer to or from a stretcher, you should position the patient's arms:
    A. across the chest
    B. at the sides
    C. over the head
    D. behind the body

Answers can be found in the Answer Key on pages 429-431.

CRITICAL THINKING QUESTIONS

1. Your supervisor has sent you to bring Elizabeth Nelson to the radiography department for a lower gastrointestinal series. List the considerations that would help you determine whether to transfer Ms. Nelson by wheelchair or by stretcher. How would you get the information to make this decision?

2. Ralph Barnes has undergone hip replacement surgery in the past week and been brought to the imaging department by stretcher for follow-up radiographs of his hip. How would the surgical approach (anterior or posterior) affect requirements for assisting Mr. Barnes from the wheelchair to the radiographic table? How would you know which type of surgery Mr. Barnes had undergone? Describe the precautions that are necessary following both types of surgery.

3. While you are helping Ella Christopherson into a wheelchair she puts her weight on the footrest, causing the chair to tip and bump her leg. Mrs. Christopherson says, "Ouch!" and rubs her leg; but when you ask whether she is all right, she smiles and insists that she is fine. Should you file an incident report? Why or why not? How could this incident have been prevented?

4. Curtis Drummond is to be moved from a waterbed mattress onto a stretcher and is unable to assist. What equipment would be most helpful? Describe the procedure.

13

Medication Information

OBJECTIVES

At the conclusion of this chapter, the student will be able to:

- Describe the radiographer's role in medication administration and explain why a general knowledge of medications is of value to the radiographer.
- Give an example of a trade name and a generic name of a medication typically seen in the radiology department.
- Demonstrate how to look up a medication in a comprehensive drug reference book.
- Define *efficacy, potency,* and *toxicity* as related to medications.

- List the four processes that comprise pharmacokinetics.
- Compare and contrast the following medication effects: therapeutic effects, side effects, allergic effects, and toxic effects.
- List four classes of medications commonly used in imaging departments and at least one example of each category.
- Describe precautions needed for patients taking opiate or opioid medications.
- Explain the difference between drugs that are agonists and those that are antagonists.

OUTLINE

KEY TERMS

agonist
allergen
allergic
anesthetic
antagonist
antidote
edema

efficacy
excretion
generic
idiosyncratic
metabolite
metabolize
narcotic

opiate
opioid
potency
potent
synergistic
toxic
toxicity

THE RADIOGRAPHER'S ROLE

Although a comprehensive knowledge of drugs is not essential for a radiographer, you must become familiar with the names, dosages, and routes of administration for medications used in imaging departments. If this seems intimidating, be reassured that only a limited number of drugs, and a few standard dosages of each, are used with any regularity. Knowledge of these medications greatly facilitates the task of assisting the physician and aids in determining whether departmental stocks of medications and medication supplies are adequate and up to date. It also enables the alert radiographer to prevent errors by questioning and double-checking any medication orders or records that seem unusual or inappropriate.

Any drug can produce side effects in certain patients. Radiographers use this knowledge to anticipate possible adverse drug reactions and to recognize and report signs and symptoms of adverse effects as they occur. For information on responding to drug reactions, see Chapter 16.

> **!** Medication awareness is very important because radiographers are often the first to observe the onset of medication responses that could have serious consequences.

MEDICATION NOMENCLATURE AND INFORMATION RESOURCES

The terms *drugs* and *medications* are often used interchangeably in the health care field. Medications are substances prescribed for treatment that produce therapeutically useful effects. Drugs, the more general term, denotes substances used in diagnosis, treatment, or disease prevention, or as a component of a medication. In common usage, this term is also applied to chemicals such as narcotics or hallucinogens that affect the central nervous system (CNS), causing behavioral changes and possibly addiction. Drugs can replace a missing substance in the body, such as estrogen or insulin. Some medications, such as digitalis, are made from plants; others, such as heparin, come from animal sources. Still others, such as penicillin, are produced by microorganisms. Many drugs today are manufactured from synthetic materials. Drug synthesis and the rapidly expanding application of genetic engineering promise vast possibilities for the future.

Each medication has a generic name that identifies its chemical family. If the drug consists principally of one chemical, it may also be referred to by its chemical name. For example, acetylsalicylic acid is the chemical name for the generic drug aspirin. Manufacturers give their products brand names that are also called *proprietary* or *trade names*. The same generic substance may be manufactured by several different companies and given a different trade name by each. For example, a synthetic antibacterial containing trimethoprim and sulfamethoxazole is produced by Roche under the name Bactrim and by GlaxoSmithKline as Septra. A drug often becomes recognized by the proprietary name given to it by the company that first develops and markets it, and this proprietary brand is usually more expensive than its generic equivalent. The generic and trade names of some drugs are used interchangeably. For instance, the generic term *epinephrine* is used just as frequently as the trade name Adrenalin for this common emergency drug. Because medications may be ordered by either generic or trade names, you should be familiar with both terms. When the radiologist calls for epinephrine, the knowledgeable radiographer will be aware that it may also come labeled as Adrenalin and will not need to read the small print on each container in the emergency drug box.

Setting the standards for control of drugs is part of the role of the United States Food and Drug Administration (FDA). These standards include strict rules concerning efficacy (effectiveness), purity, potency (strength), safety, and toxicity (potential for harm) of both prescriptive and nonprescriptive over-the-counter (OTC) medications.

The study of drugs is an ongoing process, because new medications are constantly added to the medical repertoire. In addition, no single textbook can provide information for all contingencies. For these reasons, you should be acquainted with other methods of obtaining medication facts on a continuing basis. One useful resource is the information sheet enclosed in each drug package. The FDA requires that all drug packages include the following data: trade name, generic name, chemical composition, chemical strength, usual dose, indications, contraindications, and reported side effects. Package inserts from frequently used drugs may be kept on file in the imaging department to avoid opening a package when this information is needed. Collect and study inserts from the drugs used most frequently to develop a useful information base for medications that are important in your clinical setting.

Another useful medication reference is the *Physicians' Desk Reference (PDR)*. This book, which is published annually, lists drugs alphabetically by their generic names, by their trade names, and according to their uses. A separate section indexes the products made by each manufacturer. In the product description, you will find information similar to that found in the package inserts. The radiology department library usually includes a current edition of the PDR or a similar reference, and the radiographer should become familiar with its use. *Clinical Pharmacology* (available at http://www.clinicalpharmacology.com) is another comprehensive medication reference. It provides instant access via the Internet to the most current medication information updates. Several companies publish drug guides especially for nurses. These references may be useful to you as well because they tend to emphasize the most common side effects and may help you recognize physical changes that might be significant. Changes in the pharmaceutical industry, including the introduction of so-called designer drugs, have increased the speed at which medications are developed, approved, and marketed. As a result, medication references quickly become outdated, so it is more important than ever that medication information sources be current. In-service classes and college courses may also provide useful medication information. This is especially important if your state law and job description permit you to administer medications and contrast media.

> Medication information is available on package inserts, in medication reference books such as the PDR, and at numerous sites on the Internet.

MEDICATION PROPERTIES

Pharmacokinetics

Pharmacokinetics is the study of the way the body processes a drug and includes how drugs are absorbed, reach their site of action, are **metabolized** (physically and chemically changed), and exit the body. These

processes are important because they affect the ways in which patients respond to medications. Individual responses can vary greatly depending on age, physical condition, gender, weight, or immune status.

Absorption

Absorption is a process involving the movement of a drug from the site of administration into the systemic circulation in order to produce a desired effect. Oral medications are absorbed through the mucosal lining of the gastrointestinal tract. Other medications are injected and absorbed through the blood vessels in the muscles, subcutaneous tissues, or dermal layers. When medications are injected directly into a vein or artery, no absorption is needed.

Distribution

Distribution is the means by which a drug travels from the bloodstream to the target tissue and site of action. This process depends on adequate circulation. Drugs act more quickly in organs with an abundant blood supply, such as the liver, heart, brain, and kidneys.

Metabolism

Metabolism is the process by which the body transforms drugs into an inactive form that can be excreted from the body. Most drug metabolism occurs in the liver, where enzymatic action transforms a drug into **metabolites** (products of metabolism) that can be excreted via the intestinal tract or the kidneys.

Excretion

Excretion refers to the elimination of drugs from the body after they have been metabolized. Drugs may be excreted by way of the kidneys, intestines, lungs, breast milk, or exocrine glands. The kidneys are the chief organs of excretion, but the route depends largely on the chemical makeup of the drug. Portions of some drugs can escape metabolism and be excreted unchanged in urine or feces. Volatile substances such as alcohol and certain anesthetics are excreted through the lungs. For this reason, postoperative patients are encouraged to cough and breathe deeply to help clear their bodies of the anesthetic agent. Other drugs are metabolized in the liver, excreted into the bile, and then routed through the intestines for elimination. The metabolites of other medications metabolized in the liver are transported by the bloodstream to the kidneys for excretion. If kidney function is impaired or the patient is dehydrated, drugs can be retained in the body and a toxic (poisonous) effect can occur. Toxic effects are more likely when patients have insufficient fluid intake.

Pharmacodynamics

Pharmacodynamics is the study of the effects of drugs on the normal physiological functions of the body. The most common mechanism of drug action is drug binding to the receptor sites on a cell. After a drug reaches its site of action, it exerts its effects on the cell's receptor sites. The drugs and receptors fit together much like a lock and key. The action of a drug on specific cells is called the *therapeutic effect,* and it results in anticipated outcomes such as diuresis, increased cardiac output, or relief from pain. When receptors and drugs lock together, the therapeutic effects occur. Each cell in the body contains specific, unique receptors. For example, the antihistamine diphenhydramine (Benadryl) blocks the receptor sites of histamine cells and reduces the itching and swelling caused by an allergic reaction. A drug that produces this type of specific action and promotes the desired result is referred to as an agonist. A drug that attaches itself to the receptor, preventing the agonist from acting, is called an antagonist.

MEDICATION EFFECTS

As stated in the previous section, medications are administered to produce a predictable physiologic response called the therapeutic effect. In addition to the desired outcome, side effects may occur, which may or may not be harmless. If the side effects are severe enough to outweigh the benefits of the medication, the physician may choose to discontinue the drug. Table 13-1 summarizes medication effects.

Toxic effects develop when a drug accumulates in the body because of inadequate excretion, impaired metabolism, overdose, or drug sensitivity. The specific drug that treats a toxic effect is called an antidote.

> Elderly patients are more likely to have poor cardiac, renal, or hepatic function, which increases the likelihood that toxic effects might occur.

An idiosyncratic reaction occurs when a patient overreacts or underreacts to a drug or has an unusual reaction. For example, some individuals become very agitated, rather than sedated, when phenobarbital is administered.

TABLE 13-1	Summary of Medication Effects		
Effect	**Definition**	**Cause**	**Examples**
Therapeutic effect	Purpose of the medication	Usually, drug binds to receptor sites on cells	Pain relief, blood pressure control, reduced inflammation
Side effect	Predictable action or effect of a drug other than that desired	Related to the chemical and therapeutic characteristics of the medication	Nausea, headache, insomnia, dry mouth
Toxic effect	Poisonous, potentially lethal	Inadequate excretion, impaired metabolism, overdose, or drug sensitivity	Respiratory depression, kidney failure
Idiosyncratic effect	Overreaction, underreaction, unusual reaction	Unknown, unique to individuals	Sedative causes anxiety, increases/decreases appetite, mild stimulant causes extreme excitation
Allergic response	Characteristic response to an allergen	Prior sensitization to an initial dose of the medication or one of its components	Hives, asthma attack, bronchospasm
Synergistic effect	Responses to combined drugs that differ from their individual effects	Chemical or physiological drug interaction	Combination of hypertension medication and diuretic drug causes weakness and fainting

An **allergic** reaction occurs when a patient has been sensitized to the initial dose of a medication and develops an allergic response to the **allergen** (substance to which a sensitivity has been established) and related drugs. Drug allergies may be slight or severe, and the extent of the reaction is unpredictable. [mild]

Knowledge of some of the more common medications helps you evaluate changes in the condition of patients in your care. Referring to the medication record in the patient's chart can help you determine whether a change in status is caused by medication or by deterioration in the patient's condition. For example, an anticholinergic medication such as atropine may cause a dry mouth. This side effect has nothing to do with the patient's state of hydration. Opiates may slow the respiratory rate, and vasodilators may cause the blood pressure to drop. Such effects are the usual consequence of the specific medication and are taken into account when the drug is prescribed.

Adverse side effects are not a normal consequence of most prescribed medications. Side effects may range from mild nausea, flushing, or diarrhea to critical situations including cardiac arrest or other life-threatening states. Hives, respiratory distress, or abrupt changes in blood pressure are all symptoms demanding a physician's immediate intervention. See Chapter 16 for information on responding to allergic reactions and other changes in a patient's condition that may occur as adverse effects of medications.

In addition to toxic effects, there are many occasions when drugs taken together have a **synergistic** (additive) effect that may go far beyond the desired outcome. For example, a patient who is taking a prescribed medication for high blood pressure and then takes an OTC diuretic may become hypotensive and feel weak and faint. Because many drugs interact when taken together, the physician who orders a new drug should have the patient's chart and should question the patient about taking nonprescription medications or drugs prescribed by other physicians.

FREQUENTLY USED MEDICATIONS

The medications listed in the text that follows are used regularly in many radiology and special imaging departments. These general descriptions illustrate how such medications are used but are not meant to be exclusive. The specific drugs used at your institution to meet the

same needs may be different. Table 13-2 provides a more extensive list of medications that you may encounter.

Medications Used to Treat Allergic Reactions

Diphenhydramine (Benadryl) is the most frequently used antihistamine. It also has sedative and anticholinergic (drying) side effects. It can be given orally before the injection of iodinated contrast media to patients who are at risk of having an allergic reaction. For adults, the usual oral dose is 25 to 50 mg; and for children weighing more than 20 pounds, the dosage is 12.5 to 25 mg. Benadryl may also be given intramuscularly (IM) or intravenously (IV) if the patient has an allergic reaction. The adult dosage is 10 to 50 mg, IV or IM, and may be increased to 100 mg as necessary. The maximum safe dosage in a 24-hour period is 400 mg IM or IV. Short-acting corticosteroids such as cortisone acetate are anti-inflammatory medications that may also be prescribed before the injection of contrast media.

For patients with an acute allergic reaction, epinephrine (Adrenalin) is administered subcutaneously (SC), IM, or IV. This drug stimulates the heart and the sympathetic nervous system. To control angioedema, shock, or respiratory distress, the physician administers a small dose of epinephrine (0.2–1 mL of a 1:1000 solution) and increases the dosage if required.

When patients with a severe or incapacitating allergic response do not appear to respond to the treatment just described, methylprednisolone (Solu-Medrol) may be administered IV. This long-acting corticosteroid acts as an anti-inflammatory agent, preventing or reducing **edema** (swelling) of the tracheobronchial tree. This treatment minimizes the possibility of respiratory arrest. Solu-Medrol is provided in a two-compartment vial with the diluting fluid and soluble powder separated by a plunger/stopper. The directions for mixing are provided, but you should become familiar with the preparation of this and all common medications before the need arises.

> Medications used to treat allergies are stocked in imaging departments because of the possibility of allergic reactions to contrast agents.

Antimicrobials

This category includes antiseptics such as alcohol and Betadine, an iodine compound commonly used in imaging departments for skin preparations before sterile

TABLE 13-2 Some Common Medications

Category	Effect	Example	Common Side Effects
Adrenergics (vasoconstrictors)	Stimulate the sympathetic nervous system, causing relaxation of smooth muscles of bronchi (bronchodilation); vasoconstriction; cardiac stimulation	Epinephrine (Adrenalin), ephedrine (Isuprell), metaraminol bitartrate (Aramine), phenylephrine hydrochloride (Neo-Synephrine), norepinephrine bitartrate (Levophed)	Dry mouth
Adrenergic blocking agents	Block the production of epinephrine in the body, causing dilation of blood vessels and decreased cardiac output; used as an antihypertensive	Methyldopa (Aldomet), clonidine (Catapres), prazosin (Minipress)	Fatigue, light-headedness
Analgesics	Relieve pain	Acetaminophen (Tylenol)	Negligible
		Aspirin, phenacetin, ibuprofen (Advil)	Anticoagulant
		Codeine, hydrocodone (Vicodin), oxycodone (Percocet), hydromorphone hydrochloride (Dilaudid), meperidine (Demerol), methadone, morphine, fentanyl (Sublimaze)	Respiratory depression
Anesthetics	Promote loss of feeling or sensation	General: thiopental sodium (Pentothal), halothane (Fluothane), nitrous oxide	Nausea
		Local: lidocaine (Xylocaine)	
Antiarrhythmics	Prevent or relieve cardiac arrhythmias (dysrhythmias)	Quinidine, verapamil, propanalol, amiodarone, lidocaine	Bradycardia, congestive heart failure
Anticholinergics	Depress the parasympathetic nervous system and act as antispasmodics of smooth muscle tissue; decrease contractions, saliva, bronchial mucus, digestive secretions, and perspiration; used as preparation for surgery and endoscopy to suppress secretions	Atropine, belladonna, propantheline bromide (Pro-Banthine), scopolamine (Hyoscine)	Dry mouth
Anticoagulants	Inhibit the clotting mechanism of the blood; used to keep IV lines and arterial catheters open during diagnostic procedures	Heparin, warfarin (Coumadin)	Bruising, spontaneous bleeding
	Prevent blood clots following heart attack or stroke	Clopidogrel bisulfate (Plavix), apixaban (Eliquis), dabigatran (Pradaxa), and rivaroxaban (Xarelto)	Bruising, spontaneous bleeding
Anticonvulsants	Inhibit convulsions	Phenytoin (Dilantin), carbamazepine (Tegretol) Lorazepam (Ativan), fosphenytoin (Cerebyx)	Rash, slurred speech Rash, itch, sun sensitivity
		Divalproex sodium (Depakote)	Sedation, dizziness, weakness, unsteadiness

Classification	Purpose	Examples	Side Effects
Antidepressants	Relieve or prevent depression	Amitriptyline (Elavil)	Drowsiness, dizziness, weight gain
		Imipramine (Tofranil), Fluoxetine (Prozac), Duloxetine hydrochloride (Cymbalta)	Nervousness, diarrhea
Antiemetics	Relieve or prevent vomiting	Trimethobenzamide hydrochloride (Tigan), prochlorperazine (Compazine), dolasetron mesylate (Anzemet)	Drowsiness, dry mouth, blurred vision
Antifungals	Treat or prevent fungal infections	Systematic: griseofulvin; topical: tolnaftate (Tinactin); mucosal: nystatin (Mycostatin)	Negligible
Antihistamines	Relieve the symptoms of allergic reactions	Diphenhydramine (Benadryl), chlorpheniramine maleate (Chlor-Trimeton)	Drowsiness
		Cetirizine hydrochloride (Zyrtec), loratadine (Claritin), fexofenadine hydrochloride (Allegra)	Negligible
Antihypertensives	Control high blood pressure	ACE inhibitors: captopril (Capoten), enalapril (Vasotec), lisinopril (Prinivil)	Drowsiness, fainting, weakness
		Beta blockers: propranolol (Inderal), metroprolol (Lopressor, Toprol XL)	Headache, depression, nausea, diarrhea, rash, nightmares
Antimicrobials	Suppress the growth of microorganisms	Internal: Penicillin, tetracyclines, sulfadiazine, erythromycin, cephalosporins (Keflex, Keflin, Rocephin, Cefazolin)	Diarrhea, yeast infections, allergic reactions
		External: Sulfonamides, thimerosol (Merthiolate), Betadine	Allergic reactions
Antiperistaltics	Slow peristalsis of the gastrointestinal tract	Tincture of opium (Paregoric), loperamide (Imodium)	Constipation
Antipsychotics	Treat psychoses, schizophrenia	Haloperidol (Haldol), fluphenazine (Prolixin), risperidone (Risperdal)	Nausea, decreased sweating, dry mouth, stiffness, constipation, shaking
Antipyretics	Reduce fever	Aspirin	Bruising
		Acetaminophen (Tylenol)	Negligible
Antitussives	Reduce coughing	Dextromethorphan (Romilar)	Negligible
		Codeine	Nausea, drowsiness
Antivirals	Prevent or treat viral diseases	Acyclovir (Zovirax), amantadine (Symadine), zidovudine (AZT)	Nausea, vomiting, diarrhea, headache
Barbiturates	Depress the CNS, respirations, and blood pressure; induce sleep	Pentobarbital sodium (Nembutal), secobarbital (Seconal), phenobarbital	Nausea, itching, constipation
Bronchodilators	Dilate smooth muscle; used to treat asthma attacks and some allergic reactions	Theophylline (Theo-Dur), aminophylline, albuterol (Proventil), albuterol inhaled (Xopenex)	Insomnia, decreased appetite, irritability, hypertension, angina, vomiting, vertigo
Cardiac depressants	Restrain or slow heart activity	Quinidine, procainamide (Pronestyl)	Nausea, diarrhea, heartburn

Continued

TABLE 13-2   Some Common Medications—cont'd

Category	Effect	Example	Common Side Effects
Cardiac stimulants	Strengthen and tone the heart; increase cardiac output	Digitalis, gitalin (Gitaligin), lanatoside C (Cedilanid)	Weakness, blurred vision
Cathartics	Stimulate peristalsis; promote defecation	Bisacodyl (Dulcolax), magnesium citrate, polyethylene-glycol (Miralax)	Dehydration, weight loss, abdominal cramping
Diuretics	Stimulate the flow of urine	Chlorothiazide (Diuril), furosemide (Lasix), acetazolamide (Diamox)	Potassium depletion, diarrhea, cramps, fatigue, metallic taste
Emetics	Induce vomiting	Ipecac	Potential dehydration
Hypoglycemics	Lower blood sugar level	Insulin, tolbutamide (Orinase), glyburide (Micronase) liraglutide (Victoza), sitagliptin (Januvia) Metformin (Glucophage)	Cold sweats, anxiety, headaches, confusion Hypoglycemia Risk of severe acidosis in cases of kidney failure. Contraindicated with iodine contrast media until normal kidney function has been validated
Opioids	Analgesic sedatives (narcotics) with a potential for addiction; classified as controlled substances under the Harrison Act	Injectable: Morphine, meperidine (Demerol), hydromorphone hydrochloride (Dilaudid), fentanyl (Sujblimaze) Oral: Hydrocodone (Vicodin), oxycodone (Percocet), codiene	Respiratory depression
Opioid antagonists	Prevent or counteract respiratory depression and depressive effects of morphine and related drugs	Naloxone hydrochloride (Narcan), nalorphine (Nalline), naltrexone (Trexan)	Nausea, vomiting, tachycardia, hypertension
Radioisotopes	Radioactive forms of elements used for diagnosis and treatment	Iodine-131, cobalt-60, technetium-99m	Negligible
Sedatives	Depress and relax the central nervous system and reduce mental activity	Barbiturates, paraldehyde, chloral hydrate	Clumsiness, dizziness, drowsiness
Skeletal muscle relaxants	Relax skeletal and striated muscle tissue	Succinylcholine chloride (Anectine), pancuronium bromide (Pavulon)	Respiratory depression
Stimulants	Stimulate the CNS	Caffeine, sodium benzoate, amphetamines (Benzedrine, Dexedrine)	Insomnia, restlessness
Tranquilizers	Reduce anxiety	Minor: diazepam (Valium), lorazepam (Ativan), chlordiazepoxide (Librium), midazolam (Versed); major: chlorpromazine (Thorazine), trifluoperazine (Stelazine)	Drowsiness, decreased coordination; slurred speech
Vasodilators	Relax the walls of blood vessels, permitting a greater flow of blood	Isosorbide dinitrate (Sorbitrate) Nitroglycerin hydralazine (Apresoline)	Dizziness, headache, flushing, tachycardia Headache, hypotension, anorexia, vomiting, diarrhea, palpitations

NOTE: Drugs are listed first by their generic names. Proprietary names appear in parentheses.

injection procedures. The antimicrobial category also includes *antibiotics,* which are medications given to treat wound infections and infectious diseases. Antibiotics can be subclassified as antibacterial, antifungal, and so on, according to the type of organisms against which they are most effective. Some antibiotics treat a very narrow range of microorganisms. Bactrim, for instance, is used to treat specific infections of the urinary tract. Others are referred to as *broad-spectrum* antibiotics and are effective against a wide variety of pathogens.

Anticonvulsants

Anticonvulsant medications are prescribed for patients with chronic seizure disorders (see Chapter 16). Preventive doses taken regularly allow seizure-prone individuals to continue the activities of daily living. When seizures are prolonged or follow closely, IV administration of medications such as diazepam (Valium) or fosphenytoin (Cerebyx) may be necessary. Diazepam, which is also used as a tranquilizer or sedative, is often available on the emergency cart or in the emergency drug box. Physicians commonly order an initial dose of 5 to 10 mg of diazepam IV. The dose may be repeated at 10- to 15-minute intervals up to a total dose of 30 mg.

Antiarrhythmics

A wide variety of medications is used to treat chronic cardiac arrhythmias. For acute attacks of ventricular tachycardia or ventricular arrhythmia, however, amiodarone (Pacerone) is often the drug of choice. It is available on the crash cart and is administered as an IV infusion. Both ventricular and atrial arrhythmias may be treated with amiodarone, lidocaine, quinidine (Quinidex), and several other drugs in this class.

Analgesics

Analgesics are drugs that can relieve pain without causing a loss of consciousness. As a group, opioids are the most effective analgesics. The term **opioid** describes any drug, natural or synthetic, that acts similarly to morphine. The opioid family, whose name derives from opium, includes morphine, codeine, and meperidine (Demerol); **opiate** is the more specific term applied only to natural opium derivatives. The term **narcotic** means "sleep-inducing" and was once used as a synonym for analgesic, but this word can no longer be used with precision because it has come to stand for too many different things. It denotes not only those analgesic CNS depressants that may lead to physical dependence, but also to cocaine, marijuana, and lysergic acid diethylamide (LSD), which are legally classed with opiates as narcotics.

Controlled substances are drugs with a high potential for abuse and misuse and therefore are kept in a locked container. Stocks of these medications must be counted daily, and when any of these medications is given it must be listed on forms that include the date, the patient's name, the dose, and the name and title of the person administering the medication. The United States Drug Enforcement Administration (DEA) monitors the use of these drugs and permits them to be prescribed only by individuals who hold a DEA license.

Opioids act by depressing the CNS, relieving pain, and producing drowsiness. Excessive doses can result in depressed respirations, coma, and possibly death. They may be injected or given orally. Common oral opioid analgesics include hydrocodone (Vicodin) and oxycodone (Percocet). Among the most frequently prescribed injectable opioids are morphine sulfate (MS), meperidine (Demerol), and hydromorphone hydrochloride (Dilaudid), at the following dosages: 10 to 30 mg of morphine, 50 to 150 mg of meperidine, or 1.3 to 2 mg of hydromorphone hydrochloride, usually injected IM. Fentanyl (Sublimaze), another highly **potent** (powerful) opioid analgesic, is given to patients who are sensitive to other analgesics or to those who are not deriving adequate pain relief from such medications. The physician determines the dosage of this medication based on age, weight, use of other drugs, and the procedure involved. The action of Sublimaze is almost immediate and lasts 30 to 60 minutes after IV administration. It is supplied at a strength of 50 µg/mL, and the usual dose is 1 to 2 mL. Respiratory depression peaks 5 to 10 minutes after injection and may last for several hours, depending on the dosage.

Patients who have received any CNS depressant must be monitored closely. Respiratory depression is a life-threatening side effect, so narcotic antagonist medication and resuscitation equipment should be immediately available. Because patients may be some distance from the radiographer, a pulse oximeter is attached to the patient's finger, toe, or earlobe. A digital readout of the pulse and blood oxygen saturation can be viewed from the control room or console area. If the oxygen saturation drops below 95%, the patient is asked to respond and take a few deep breaths and is then observed closely. If the oxygen saturation continues to drop or the patient does not respond adequately, a physician is notified immediately.

> **!** Patients receiving opioids or other medication that depresses the CNS must be carefully monitored for respiratory depression.

Analgesics may be given to help the patient cope with painful procedures or to lessen pre-existing pain during the procedure. Although the pain might be the reason for the examination, it might also be caused by an unrelated problem that produces enough discomfort to prevent compliance. For example, a patient may have painful arthritis of the cervical spine that makes it extremely difficult to lie still throughout a magnetic resonance imaging study of the abdomen.

Analgesics with a low potential for side effects, such as aspirin, ibuprofen, acetaminophen, and naproxen sodium, are classed as nonsteroidal anti-inflammatory drugs (NSAIDs) and are frequently used to alleviate discomfort. Although these drugs have analgesic properties, they are not controlled substances and are sold in moderate strengths without a prescription. Self-medication with these OTC analgesics is very common, especially in the elderly. Children should never be given OTC medications in the radiology department without a physician's order. As a rule, even at home, children should only be given analgesics other than acetaminophen (Tylenol) under the direct instruction of a physician.

Sedatives and Tranquilizers

Sedatives and tranquilizers exert a quieting effect, often inducing sleep. They are not analgesics but may provide relief from pain by promoting muscle relaxation.

Phenobarbital and other barbiturates are sedatives and were formerly used as preoperative medications. Their use for this purpose has been largely supplanted by lorazepam and diazepam. Phenobarbital is still used with other medications to treat patients with seizures.

Tranquilizers reduce anxiety and mental tension more effectively than sedatives and often provide some sedation as well. As a group, they are commonly referred to as *benzodiazepines,* a term that describes their similar chemical composition. At low doses, tranquilizers do not impair mental acuity, but as the dosage increases, patients tend to feel drowsy, and their speech may become slow and slurred. Some patients experience a brief loss of inhibition, similar to the effect of alcohol, which causes them to talk and act inappropriately. Individuals taking tranquilizers may have slowed reaction time and should not drive or operate machinery.

Lorazepam (Ativan) and diazepam (Valium) are tranquilizers that are commonly prescribed as premedication for various interventional diagnostic procedures. Lorazepam is given more commonly. These medications may be given with morphine to patients who are both anxious and in pain. The premedication IV dosage of lorazepam for an adult is usually 44 μg/kg or 2.0 mg total, whichever is smaller. A dose of 2 mg should not ordinarily be exceeded in patients over 50 years of age. IV doses in excess of 2 mg should be restricted to patients of unusually large size, in which case the physician may order a dose of 0.03 mg/kg. The adult dose of diazepam for anxiety ranges from 2 to 20 mg given IM or IV. The physician may administer larger doses as needed to achieve relaxation. Very large doses are sometimes given to control grand mal (major motor) seizures. When diazepam is injected IV, it is administered slowly, taking at least 1 minute for each 5 mg (1 mL) given. Avoid using the small veins of the hand and wrist, because this medication irritates blood vessels and may cause phlebitis and damage to the vein. When diazepam infiltrates the surrounding tissues, it can be very painful, causing both irritation and swelling.

For amnesia and sedation, midazolam (Versed) is often used because it begins acting in only 1.5 to 5 minutes, and the peak effect is almost immediate. It is sometimes given when previous administration of an analgesic or tranquilizer has not relaxed the patient or relieved pain. The initial dose of Versed in this instance is 1 mg and can be increased to a usual maximum of 10 mg at the physician's discretion.

Antagonists

The most common antagonists encountered by radiographers are those formulated to counteract the effects of sedatives and analgesics.

Ativan, Valium, and Versed are benzodiazepine drugs that may be given to produce relaxation and/or sedation, as previously described. An overdose produces respiratory depression and loss of psychomotor function as a toxic effect. Flumazenil (Romazicon) is a medication developed to counteract the effect of these drugs.

Romazicon can antagonize the sedation and the impairment of recall and psychomotor function produced by benzodiazepines. Patients who receive Romazicon should be monitored for resedation, respiratory depression, or other residual effects for up to 2 hours based on the dosage and duration of the benzodiazepine used. For the reversal of conscious sedation by benzodiazepines, the recommended initial dose of Romazicon is 0.2 mg (2 mL) administered IV over 15 seconds. If the desired level of consciousness is not obtained after waiting an additional 45 seconds, additional doses may be given to a maximum of 1 mg (10 mL) until the desired effect is achieved. To minimize the possibility of pain or inflammation, Romazicon should be administered through a freely flowing IV line into a large vein. The use of Romazicon is associated with seizures in some patients who have been taking benzodiazepines over a long period of time.

Naloxone (Narcan) counteracts the effects of opiates, such as morphine, and prevents or reverses respiratory depression, sedation, and hypotension. A rapid reversal of opiate depression can cause nausea, vomiting, tachycardia, and nervousness. Although Narcan can be administered SC or IM, the most rapid onset of action is obtained with a dilution of Narcan in saline or 5% dextrose in water administered IV. To reverse respiratory depression, 0.1 to 0.2 mg Narcan should be administered IV at 2- to 3-minute intervals until adequate ventilation is achieved.

Local Anesthetics

Lidocaine (Xylocaine) is a local anesthetic injected to eliminate sensation in a specific area before a painful procedure. You may have received such an injection before having dental work or when having stitches placed to close a wound. Xylocaine is provided in a variety of strengths and is available with or without epinephrine. The addition of epinephrine causes constriction of adjacent blood vessels and localizes the anesthetic effect to the immediate area. If your department stocks more than one type, be sure you understand which one the physician requires.

Paralytic Agents

When working in a trauma unit or emergency department, you may occasionally encounter patients who have received a paralytic agent, a skeletal muscle relaxant that may be given to facilitate insertion of an endotracheal airway or to initiate diagnostic studies and treatment for patients who are combative because of shock, fear, or intoxication. Because all muscles are temporarily paralyzed, artificial respiration is necessary, and patients must be monitored closely until the effects of the medication wear off. A nurse will accompany patients who have received a paralytic agent.

There are three basic types of paralytic agents: short-term agents such as succinylcholine chloride (Anectine) are effective for a period of 10 to 30 minutes; intermediate paralytic agents such as mivacurium (Mivacron) have a maximum duration of 35 to 45 minutes; long-acting agents such as metocurine and gallamine have a maximum duration of 2 to 3 hours. Paralytic agents do not cause unconsciousness, and the inability to respond may cause patients to be very anxious; it is important to talk to these patients and reassure them. As their paralysis dissipates, they are frequently agitated or combative.

Hypoglycemic Agents

These drugs are used to control the level of glucose in the blood, primarily as a treatment for diabetes mellitus (see Chapter 16). Type I diabetes mellitus is treated with insulin, whereas type II, or non-insulin dependent diabetes mellitus, is often treated with oral agents: sulfonylurea (Amaryl or Glucotrol), tolbutamide (Orinase), chlorpropamide (Diabinase), rosiglitazone (Avandia), metformin (Glucophage), apixaban (Eliquis), dabigatran (Pradaxa), or rivaroxaban (Xarelto). It is helpful to recognize these agents in a drug list, because they will alert you and the radiologist to the diabetes diagnosis. It may be significant to know when patients who need iodinated contrast agents are taking oral hypoglycemic agents (see Chapter 19).

Antihypertensives

There are two principal types of medications for the control of high blood pressure: angiotensin-converting enzyme (ACE) inhibitors and beta blockers. ACE is a chemical produced by the body that is part of a complex system that regulates blood pressure. This enzyme stimulates the adrenal glands to produce other enzymes that increase blood pressure. ACE inhibitors such as captopril (Capoten), enalapril (Vasotec), and lisinopril (Prinivil) lower blood pressure by interrupting this cycle. They are used primarily to treat hypertension, but are also prescribed to treat other disorders such as cardiac failure and renal disease. These medications are all quite similar in their effects, but differ in dosage and route of excretion. Common side effects include dizziness due to hypotension, headache, drowsiness, and weakness.

Beta blockers, also called *beta adrenergic blocking agents,* suppress the action of the sympathetic nervous system by blocking the activity of catecholamines (epinephrine and norepinephrine). In addition to treating hypertension, these drugs are prescribed to treat a number of cardiac conditions including irregular heart rhythm and the occurrence of angina pectoris (spasmodic chest pain, see Chapter 16). Common beta blockers include propranolol (Inderal) and metoprolol (Lopressor, Toprol XL).

General Precautions

Some of the drugs discussed in the previous sections can cause respiratory depression, and any of them could cause an allergic reaction in a sensitive individual. Know where the resuscitation equipment and oxygen are kept, and be familiar with the code routine of your institution (see Chapter 15).

This discussion has touched on some of the medications frequently encountered by radiographers in the clinical setting. You must become thoroughly familiar with the protocols of your institution. The package inserts serve as a handy resource to help you stay current in your knowledge of the dosage, actions, and side effects of these drugs.

SUMMARY

- Medications are identified by chemical names that define their composition, generic names that identify the substance, and proprietary or trade names given by the manufacturer. Radiographers should be familiar with both the generic and trade names of commonly used medications.
- Drug package inserts, medication reference books, and medication websites are good sources of information about specific medications, their various names, their effects, recommended dosages, and their common side effects.
- Pharmacokinetics is the study of the way the body processes a drug and includes how drugs are absorbed, reach their site of action, are metabolized, and are excreted. Absorption is the process by which a drug enters the systemic circulation to provide a desired effect. Distribution is the means by which a drug travels via the bloodstream to the site of action. Metabolism is the process that occurs primarily in the liver by which the body transforms drugs into an inactive form that can be excreted from the body. Excretion is the elimination of drugs from the body by way of the kidneys, intestines, lungs, breast milk, or exocrine glands.
- Pharmacodynamics is the study of the effects of drugs on the normal physiologic functions of the body. The most common mechanism of drug action is the binding of drugs to the receptor sites on a cell.
- The desired outcome of medication administration is called the therapeutic effect. Side effects are effects other than the therapeutic effect that may or may not be harmless. Toxic effects are harmful effects, usually due to excessive dose or excretion failure. An idiosyncratic effect is one that differs from what is expected, and a synergistic effect is an additive effect that can occur when more than one medication is given.
- Frequently used medications encountered by radiographers include antihistamines (such as diphenhydramine) and anti-inflammatory drugs (such as Solu-Cortef) that treat allergic reactions; sympathetic nervous system stimulants (such as epinephrine) to treat acute allergic reactions and other acute conditions; antimicrobials (such as alcohol) to prevent infections; anticonvulsants (such as diazepam) to treat seizures; antiarrhythmics (such as lidocaine or amiodarone) to treat irregular heart rhythm; analgesics (such as morphine or aspirin) to relieve pain; sedatives and tranquilizers (such as lorazepam or diazepam) to reduce anxiety; antagonists (such as flumazenil or naloxone) to reverse the effects of sedatives and some analgesics; local anesthetics (such as lidocaine) to cause numbness when a procedure may be painful; muscle relaxants (such as succinylcholine chloride) to cause temporarily paralysis; hypoglycemic agents (such as insulin and metformin) to regulate blood glucose levels; and ACE inhibitors (such as captopril, enalapril, and lisinopril) to control hypertension.

REVIEW QUESTIONS

1. A common side effect of an anticholinergic drug is:
   A. nausea
   B. dry mouth
   C. bruising or spontaneous bleeding
   D. constipation
2. Medications used to regulate blood glucose levels include insulin and metformin. These medications are classified as:
   A. antiarrhythmics
   B. anticonvulsants
   C. analgesics
   D. hypoglycemic agents
3. Opioid medications are prescribed for the purpose of:
   A. alleviating pain
   B. reversing the effects of opium
   C. regulating heart rhythm
   D. preventing infection
4. The name given to a medication by the manufacturer is called its _____ name.
   A. chemical
   B. proprietary
   C. generic
   D. common
5. Narcan is an antagonist drug that may be given in cases of an overdose of a(n) _____ medication.
   A. opiate
   B. benzodiazepine
   C. anticholinergic
   D. hypoglycemic
6. The method by which drug metabolites are eliminated from the body is called:
   A. absorption
   B. assimilation
   C. excretion
   D. distribution
7. An idiosyncratic medication reaction is one that is:
   A. additive
   B. allergic
   C. therapeutic
   D. unusual
8. A common medication that is classed as both a tranquilizer and an anticonvulsant is:
   A. meperidine
   B. diphenhydramine
   C. Betadine
   D. diazepam
9. The intended effect of succinylcholine chloride is:
   A. anesthesia
   B. muscle paralysis
   C. heart stimulation
   D. sedation
10. Diphenhydramine is classified as a(n) _____ medication.
   A. antihistamine
   B. analgesic
   C. anticholinergic
   D. ACE inhibitor

Answers can be found in the Answer Key on pages 429-431.

CRITICAL THINKING EXERCISES

1. Matt Wren, age 5, was discharged from the hospital after a short stay for treatment of burns to his arms and chest suffered in a fall into a bonfire. Today he has been sent for chest radiographs because of a persistent, severe cough. He is crying and extremely agitated. His mother states that he is so apprehensive about any medical treatment that his physician has prescribed phenobarbital to calm him. She states that she gave him a dose an hour ago and asks whether you think another dose is needed to calm him before the examination. What are the implications of this situation? What should you do? What should you tell the mother? Should you tell anyone else?

2. Jennifer Gilman has just received an IV injection of morphine sulfate because of extreme pain from injuries suffered in a car crash. As you take her x-ray images, what potential side effect should you be especially alert to identify? How would you recognize this effect? If you observed it, what would you do?

3. Mildred Danford, age 82, has just received an IV injection of 2 mg of diazepam. This is a low dose for an adult and does not usually produce untoward side effects, but Mrs. Danford's speech has become quite slurred and she is very drowsy. Could this be a side effect of the medication she received? What might account for her condition?

CRITICAL THINKING EXERCISES—cont'd

4. Ravi Sinha received his first dose of a new antibiotic medication before being transported to the imaging department. After he arrives, he begins scratching his forearms and complaining of itching on his back. Red blotches are apparent on his neck and his face. What type of reaction is Ravi experiencing? Give an example of a medication that may be needed to counteract this reaction.

14

Medication Administration

OBJECTIVES

At the conclusion of this chapter, the student will be able to:

- State the six rights of medication administration.
- Demonstrate the steps used in the administration of oral medication.
- List and describe five routes of medication administration.
- State the relative advantages and disadvantages of the three enteral routes of medication administration.
- Correctly chart the administration of a medication.
- Identify veins suitable for intravenous (IV) injections.
- State the flow rate, height of bag, and appearance of injection site that would indicate that an IV infusion is flowing correctly.

- Demonstrate the steps used to discontinue an IV infusion.
- List the steps to be taken when an IV infusion has infiltrated.
- State the average rate of flow for IV fluids expressed in drops per minute.
- Identify the sites used for intramuscular injections.
- List and demonstrate precautions for the safe administration of all parenteral medications.

OUTLINE

The Radiographer's Role
  Medication Orders
Dosage
Routes of Administration
  Enteral Route: Oral, Rectal, and Nasogastric Tube
  Medication Inhalation
  Topical Route

Sublingual and Buccal Routes
Parenteral Injections
Intravenous Route
Extravasation
Monitoring IV Fluids
Precautions for All Injections
Charting Medications

KEY TERMS

ampule	hydrostatic pressure	isotonic
angina pectoris	infiltration	normal saline
buccal	intermittent injection port	parenteral
cathartic	intra-arterial	standing order
diluent	intradermal	subcutaneous (SC)
enteral	intramuscular (IM)	sublingual
extravasation	intrathecal	topical
hematoma	intravenous (IV) infusion	transdermal

THE RADIOGRAPHER'S ROLE

Emphasis on acute care and shorter hospital stays has increased the percentage of patients who arrive at the imaging department with complex monitors and arterial lines in place. Some patients may have medication pumps to precisely govern the rate of intravenous (IV) infusions or to deliver measured amounts of drugs at regular intervals. If a pump is set up for patient-controlled administration of pain medication, the patient can release the agent as needed. IV infusions are very common. They deliver fluids and medications into a vein at a slow and constant rate by gravity flow. Radiographers may need to monitor these systems while patients are in their care, but the nursing service or IV therapy department is responsible for the initiation of most routine medication administration. Patients who must not miss a dose in their prescribed medical regimen will have their medications brought to them by a nurse.

Radiographers become more involved in medication administration when medications are given for radiographic procedures. These may include contrast agents injected or ingested to visualize soft-tissue structures on radiographic images; anesthetic agents injected before the insertion of needles into the spinal canal (epidural or intrathecal space) or into a joint capsule to cause insensibility to pain; and antianxiety or sedation agents given to calm the patient or relieve pain during invasive procedures and magnetic resonance imaging (MRI) examinations.

When there is a sudden change in a patient's status or when emergencies occur in the radiology suite, the radiographer must be able to quickly locate medications. One example might be a severe allergic reaction to a contrast medium. An acute angina attack, a sudden asthmatic episode, or an insulin reaction are other typical emergencies seen by radiographers where prompt administration of medication may be essential. The radiographer will be responsible for checking the allergic history of patients, preparing medication for administration, verifying patient identification, assisting the physician, and monitoring the patient after the medication has been given. If state regulations and hospital policies permit, radiographers might also be expected to administer and chart the medication or contrast medium.

> For your own protection, you must be familiar with the rules governing medication administration in your state and your institution.

Medication Orders

When medications are given in the imaging department, a physician selects the drug, determines the route of administration, and prescribes the exact dosage. Orders may be written or verbal and may sometimes be in the form of a standing order. Verbal orders are not acceptable in all states, and may not be permitted in some institutions, even if not prohibited by state law. Any verbal orders given in the radiology department should be written or countersigned by the physician before leaving the area. This aspect of patient care has a high potential for medicolegal problems.

A standing order consists of written directions for a specific medication or procedure, signed by a physician, and used only under the specific conditions stated in the order. Such orders are found in a Policy and Procedures Manual or Standing Orders book available for immediate reference in the radiology department. For example, many radiology departments have standing orders to administer a cathartic (strong laxative) preparation before certain radiographic examinations (see Chapter 17). In this case the standing order would state which examinations require the advance cathartic preparation, the name and amount of the drug, the time to be administered, and any patient conditions that would preclude implementation of the order. It would be signed by the radiologist and would be reviewed and countersigned on a regular basis. A sample of the patient instruction sheet might also be included.

The information in this section provides a basis for assisting the physician in medication administration, but it is not a substitute for directions from the physician. When preparing to administer medication, the first step is to verify patient identification. Two identifiers are needed; usually the patient's full name and birthdate are used. You may ask the patient to state name and birthdate, or check the patient's armband against the order. Next, check the order. If you have questions about the dosage or method of administration, check with the physician or your supervisor. Third, verify the medication and note the expiration date. Finally, check for allergies in the chart or obtain an allergy history from the patient. Remember to perform hand hygiene before preparing the medication. When preparing medications, the memory device in Box 14-1 will help you to avoid errors.

> No medication should ever be given without a physician's order.

BOX 14-1   The Six Rights of Medication Administration

1. The right dose
2. Of the right medication
3. To the right patient
4. At the right time
5. By the right route
6. With the right documentation

DOSAGE

The usual dose and safe dosage range for each medication is included in the information on the package insert, and is available online at http://www.clinicalpharmacology.com. Most hospital computer networks have a clinical pharmacology section where actions, indications, safe dosage, and compatibility are discussed. Physicians are not required to prescribe the usual dose and may specify a different dose for very good reasons, but when an order specifies a much higher dose than usual, be sure to verify the accuracy of the order before proceeding.

Some textbooks provide formulas for calculating pediatric drug dosage based on the child's age and the usual adult dose. No formula is provided here because of the risk of serious error. Some drugs are not approved for pediatric use. Others require a higher or lower dose than such formulas would indicate. When a medication or contrast medium is approved for pediatric use, the recommended pediatric dose according to the child's age and/or weight will be stated in the package insert and in medication references.

The metric system, with which you are already familiar, is usually used for measuring patient weight when calculating dosage and is also used for measuring medications. To convert a patient's weight from pounds (lb) to kilograms (kg), which are used in the metric system, divide the weight in pounds by 2.2, which is the number of pounds in a kilogram.

$$\text{Pounds (lb)} \div 2.2\ \text{lb/kg} = \text{kilograms (kg)}$$

Example

What is the metric weight of a child weighing 46 lb?

$$46\ \text{lb} \div 2.2\ \text{lb/kg} = 20.9\ \text{kg}$$

When medication is prescribed by weight, the formula for determining the total dose is:

$$\text{Dose/kg} \times \text{Weight (kg)} = \text{Total dose}$$

Example

If a dose of 4 mg/kg is prescribed, how many milligrams should be given to a child weighing 20 kg?

$$4\ \text{mg/kg} \times 20\ \text{kg} = 80\ \text{mg}$$

Liquid medications are measured in units from liters (L), slightly more than a quart, down to milliliters (mL), which are thousandths of a liter. One milliliter is equal to 1 cubic centimeter (cc), and 1 ounce equals 30 mL.

Because liquid agents are often diluted for use, the strength is expressed as a ratio of the amount of the drug to the total volume of solution. For example, 1:1000 indicates a dilution of 1 part drug to 1000 parts of water or other solvent.

If the active ingredient is a solid, it is measured by weight in grams (g), milligrams (mg), or micrograms (μg or mcg). The strength of solids dissolved in a liquid is designated in terms of weight per volume, often mg/mL. You may need to determine how much liquid will provide a given dose of a solid:

$$\text{Dose} \div \text{Strength} = \text{Volume}$$

Example

If the drug is supplied in a strength of 4 mg/mL, and you want to administer 10 mg, you will need 2.5 mL:

$$10\ \text{mg} \div 4\ \text{mg/mL} = 2.5\ \text{mL}$$

Conversely, you may need to know how much of a solid is delivered in a given volume of liquid:

$$\text{Strength} \times \text{Volume} = \text{Dose}$$

Example

If 2 mL of solution is given and the strength is 4 mg/mL, the dose would be 8 mg:

$$4\ \text{mg/mL} \times 2\ \text{mL} = 8\ \text{mg}$$

Practice these calculations so that you can do them quickly and flawlessly whenever you are required to prepare a parenteral medication.

ROUTES OF ADMINISTRATION

Enteral Route: Oral, Rectal, and Nasogastric Tube

The enteral route indicates administration of medication directly into the gastrointestinal tract via oral or rectal sites or via a nasogastric (NG) tube. When a patient is severely nauseated or unable to swallow, medications can be administered by rectum. Various forms of suppositories and enemas are available for this purpose. The rectal administration of suppositories and enemas is discussed in Chapter 17. Although medication can be absorbed directly through the rectal mucosa, portions may be expelled prematurely, making dosage unreliable. An effective alternative for these patients is to administer medications and liquid nutrition through an NG tube. The use of an NG tube is effective, and the dosage is easily controlled. NG tubes are discussed in Chapter 20.

The oral route of administering medication is common and familiar. Oral medications are supplied in a variety of forms, including tablets, capsules, granules, and liquids. Some tablets are chewable, but almost all medication should be swallowed with varying amounts of liquid, usually water. Liquid medications are usually taken with water as well. Granules are mixed with a specified amount of liquid. Follow the directions on the package insert.

Most medications that are taken orally dissolve in the stomach and then pass into the small intestine where the majority of the absorption takes place. The bloodstream then carries it to the liver via the portal venous system, which diminishes the therapeutic effect of the drug before it reaches the target tissue. This is called the *first pass effect*. Some oral medications are irritating to the stomach and are provided in an enteric or coated form that allows the tablet to pass through the stomach before dissolving. These medications should not be chewed or broken, because this would negate the benefit of the enteric coating.

> ! Oral medications with an enteric coating must be swallowed whole, not chewed, crushed, or broken.

One way to minimize errors when administering drugs is to establish a set routine and follow it unfailingly. The steps in Box 14-2 serve as a guide to establishing a procedure for the administration of oral medications.

Medication Inhalation

Some lung conditions are treated with inhalation therapy. Liquid medications are vaporized, administered by an inhaler or nebulizer, and inhaled by the patient. For example, albuterol is administered with a metered dose inhaler for asthma control. Respiratory therapists apply these treatments and instruct patients in proper techniques for self-administration of these medications at home. The inhalation route is also used for the administration of radioactive gases for nuclear medicine lung ventilation studies, and for general anesthetics during surgery.

Topical Route

The topical route of administration refers to the application of medication to the surface of the skin or mucous membranes. Some topical medications are applied for a local effect, such as when calamine lotion is used to relieve the itch caused by poison ivy.

Other topical medications are used for a systemic effect, and this type of administration is termed transdermal. These medications are applied to the skin in a paste form or on small adhesive disks that allow

---

BOX 14-2   Procedure for Oral Medication Administration

- Perform hand hygiene.
- Obtain the proper medication and read the label.
- Prepare the medication tray with a medicine cup and a glass of water (if appropriate).
- Read the label again.
- Show the physician the label, and pour the correct amount of medication directly into the medicine cup. When pouring liquids, hold the label against the palm of your hand so that it will stay clean and legible.
- If the physician requests that you administer the medication, check the patient's identification using two identifiers, stay with the patient, confirm that the medication is swallowed, and offer water, if permitted.
- Return the tray and discard the remaining water and medicine cup.
- Repeat hand hygiene.
- Chart the medication.

the medication to be absorbed through the skin into the bloodstream. One such topical drug, nifedipine, is used by patients with heart conditions to increase vascular dilation. Other examples include the transdermal nicotine patches used to treat symptoms of nicotine withdrawal when quitting smoking, fentanyl patches for pain control, and adhesive scopolamine disks to treat vertigo and to prevent motion sickness. In a hospital, these patches should be annotated with the time and date. It is important to notify the nursing service if a patch becomes detached while the patient is in your care.

Sublingual and Buccal Routes

These variations in the topical route involve placing the medication in contact with the mucosal membranes of the oral cavity. Although these medications are placed in the mouth, these are not considered oral or enteral routes. Drugs placed under the tongue (sublingual) or inside the cheek (buccal) can be absorbed into the blood through the oral mucosa and are immediately available without having to be digested and absorbed through the stomach or bowel.

When coronary arteries are unable to supply the heart muscle with sufficient nutrients and oxygen, this results in a crushing pain called angina pectoris. When the vasodilator nitroglycerin is administered sublingually, it is absorbed directly into the bloodstream, dilating the coronary arteries. This helps relieve the pain by improving circulation to the heart muscle. Patients with angina should have their medication with them at all times, including during imaging procedures. An emergency supply of nitroglycerin is usually stocked in the imaging department.

An example of buccal administration is the application of glucose paste inside the cheek of an unconscious patient suffering from an insulin reaction.

Parenteral Injections

Although patients may prefer to take medications orally, some drugs cause irritation of the gastrointestinal tract, cannot be absorbed by this route, or must be given by a route that will produce a very rapid response. By using a parenteral route, medications are injected directly into the body and bypass the gastrointestinal tract. Parenteral injections may be given in several ways and are classified as intradermal, subcutaneous (SC), or intramuscular (IM), according to the injection method used (Figure 14-1). Intravascular and intrathecal injections are also parenteral methods. Intravascular administration is classified according to the type of vessel into which the injection is made. IV injections are the most common type of intravascular administration, but intra-arterial injections are also included in this classification. The term intrathecal refers to injections into the spinal canal. This method is discussed in more detail in Chapter 19.

Parenteral medications are those that are introduced to the body by means of injection.

Parenteral Equipment

The equipment needed for each type of parenteral injection is summarized in Table 14-1. Hypodermic needles are supplied in various diameters and lengths. The gauge of a needle indicates the diameter of the bore, and the gauge increases as the diameter of the bore decreases. An

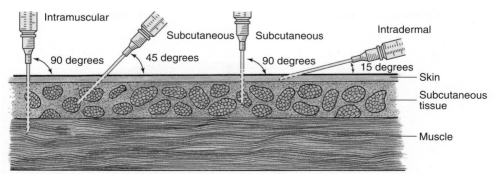

FIG 14-1 Methods of parenteral injection. (From Perry AG, Potter PA, Ostendorf WR. *Clinical nursing skills and techniques,* ed 8, St Louis, 2014, Mosby.)

18-gauge needle has a larger bore than a 22-gauge needle, and delivers a given volume of fluid more rapidly. A 22-gauge needle can be used for much smaller veins because it makes a smaller hole, and excessive bleeding or hematoma (collection of blood in tissues) are less likely to occur when it is removed. The length of hypodermic needles is measured in inches and may vary from 1/2 inch, used for accessing IV line ports and for intradermal injections, to 4 1/2 inches, needed for intrathecal injections. A 2 1/2-inch length is typical for IV needles, and the usual gauges range from 18 to 22 for adults.

As stated in Chapter 9, the widespread incidence of bloodborne infection has placed an emphasis on the prevention of accidental needlesticks. Occupational Safety and Health Administration (OSHA) regulations require the use of engineering controls to decrease the risk to health care workers from contaminated needlesticks and have led to the development of special devices to accomplish this purpose. These engineering controls include two types of devices: needleless systems for accessing established IV lines and sharps with a built-in safety feature or mechanism that effectively reduces the risk of an exposure incident. These sharps are called Sharps with Engineered Sharps Injury Protection (SESIPs for short). Examples of SESIPs are illustrated in Figure 14-2.

Injectors have been designed that can deliver a measured amount of medication through the skin by the use of a high-pressure jet. These injectors are said to be less painful, protect against accidental needlesticks, and have the advantage of being reusable for up to a week without resterilization. Jet injectors are considerably larger

TABLE 14-1	**Equipment for Parenteral Injections**			
	Intradermal	**Subcutaneous**	**Intramuscular**	**Intravenous**
Dose volume	< 1 mL	< 2 mL	< 5 mL	< 1 L
Needle type	SESIP hypodermic	SESIP hypodermic	SESIP hypodermic	SESIP butterfly needle or IV catheter
Needle length	5/8 inch	5/8 inch	1 inch	1 1/2 inches
Needle gauge	26 ga	23–25 ga	22 ga	18–20 ga

ga, Gauge; IV, intravenous; SESIP, Sharps with Engineered Sharps Injury Protection.

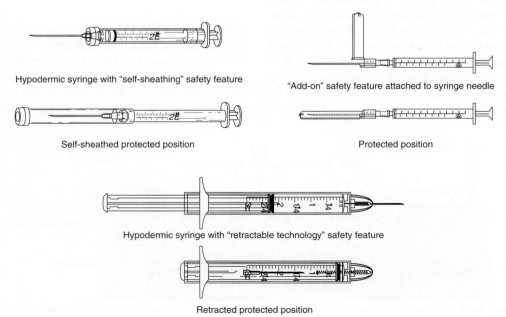

Hypodermic syringe with "self-sheathing" safety feature

Self-sheathed protected position

"Add-on" safety feature attached to syringe needle

Protected position

Hypodermic syringe with "retractable technology" safety feature

Retracted protected position

FIG 14-2 Examples of Sharps with Engineered Sharps Injury Protection (SESIPs).

than disposable syringes and are currently much more expensive to use. They are most practical for diabetics who require frequent administration of insulin and for use in mass immunization programs.

Disposable plastic syringes are supplied in individual sterile paper or plastic wraps, sometimes with a needle attached. Syringes consist of a barrel with a measurement scale on the outside and a plunger to force the contents through the needle. The plunger tip is usually made of latex.

Many frequently used medications are supplied in a small tube with attached needle. This unit holds a premeasured amount of medication and serves as the syringe barrel. It fits into a reusable holder with attached plunger. The tube is sealed with a latex plug that is advanced by pushing the external plunger, forcing the medication through the needle. These medication units may be supplied in large quantities and, although they are clearly labeled, may not be accompanied by the usual package insert. The medication unit is easily removed from the holder and discarded in one piece into a sharps container.

In recent years, an increasing number of individuals have become sensitized to latex. This has caused a return to the use of glass syringes for such patients. Glass syringes are not disposable and are sterilized before each use. Because the plunger is ground to fit the barrel precisely, both barrel and plunger may be marked with code numbers that must match for the syringe to work properly. When you open the wrap, you will need to assemble the two parts. To avoid contaminating the syringe, pick up the plunger by the handle only and insert it into the barrel. Needles are supplied separately. After selecting a suitable needle, twist the hub of the needle firmly onto the syringe and fill the syringe in the same manner as the disposable syringe. After use, discard the needle into the sharps container. The barrel and plunger must be separated and placed in a container with disinfectant until they can be sterilized.

Parenteral Routes

As stated previously, parenteral administration involves the direct injection of the medication into the body by one of several routes. IV administration is the parenteral route that offers the most immediate effect. As the medication is dispersed through the bloodstream, the latent time until it reaches the site of action is very short. This extremely important parenteral route is covered in detail later in this chapter.

Intradermal Injections

Intradermal injections are parenteral injections administered between the layers of the skin. This method was once used to test patient sensitivity to contrast media. Experience has proved that a complete history is a more accurate predictor of allergic reactions than the intradermal *skin test,* and most radiographers are not likely to perform this procedure. The anterior surface of the forearm is a typical site for intradermal injections. Only very small quantities may be injected intradermally, so a tuberculin syringe is used; it is finely calibrated and comes with a very small (26-gauge) needle. The tuberculin skin test introduced in Chapter 9 involves an intradermal injection to the anterior forearm.

Subcutaneous Injections

Subcutaneous (SC; under the skin) injections deliver medications into the fatty tissue layer beneath the skin. Usually a 5/8-inch needle with a gauge of 23 to 25 is inserted at a 45-degree angle. Syringes used for SC injections are usually 2 mL or smaller in size, because it is painful to inject a large quantity of liquid beneath the skin. The most convenient areas for SC injections are on the upper arm and on the outer aspect of the thigh.

Intramuscular Injections

Intramuscular (IM; into the muscle) injections are sometimes given in larger amounts than SC injections, up to 5 mL, and the needle size is also larger, usually 22 gauge. The injection is given into the deltoid muscle of the upper arm (Figure 14-3), the gluteal muscles in the hip area (Figure 14-4), or the vastus lateralis muscle of the lateral thigh (Figure 14-5). For children younger than 5 years of age, the vastus lateralis site is preferred to the gluteus site. Because the gluteus maximus muscle only develops fully through walking and running, a danger of damage to the sciatic nerve exists when injections are given into this area before the muscle is sufficiently developed. IM injections are not usually given into the anterior thigh because this site is extremely painful, and the discomfort may persist for several days.

> **!**   Do not give any IM injections into the anterior thigh. Children younger than 5 years of age should not receive IM injections into the gluteus maximus muscle.

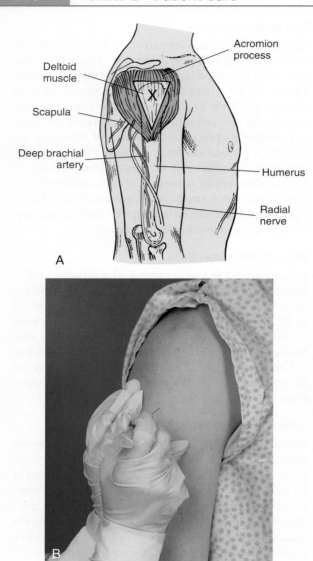

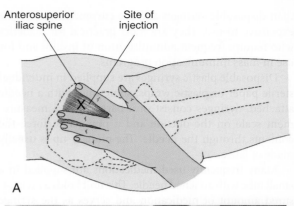

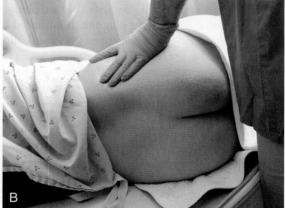

FIG 14-3 A, Anatomic view of deltoid muscle injection site. B, Site of intramuscular injection into deltoid muscle. (From Perry AG, Potter PA, Ostendorf WR. *Nursing interventions and clinical skills,* ed 6, St Louis, 2016, Elsevier.)

Intra-arterial Administration

Intra-arterial administration involves percutaneous access to the artery by a needle, frequently followed by catheter placement to permit injection at a specific anatomic site. Intra-arterial injections are performed by physicians, and radiographers are most likely to encounter this route of administration in the angiography suite.

FIG 14-4 A, Anatomic view of ventrogluteal muscle injection site. B, Injection into the ventrogluteal muscle avoids major nerves and blood vessels. (From Perry AG, Potter PA, Ostendorf WR. *Nursing interventions and clinical skills,* ed 6, St Louis, 2016, Elsevier.)

This procedure is performed under conditions of surgical asepsis and is described more fully in Chapter 22.

Intrathecal Administration

Intrathecal administration is the intraspinal method used when a contrast medium is to be injected through a spinal needle directly into the subarachnoid space. Myelography is the most common imaging procedure that requires the intrathecal method. The procedure is called a lumbar puncture and is performed by a physician using surgical asepsis. This procedure is described more fully in Chapter 19.

Preparation for Parenteral Administration

To prepare for parenteral injections, specifically intradermal, SC, and IM injections, the radiographer

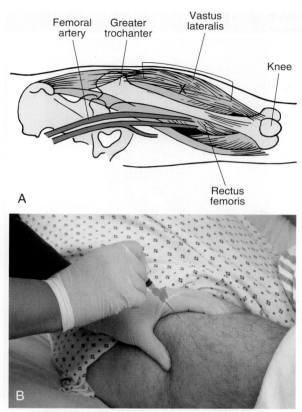

FIG 14-5 A, Anatomic view of vastus lateralis muscle injection site. B, Injection site into vastus lateralis muscle. (From Perry AG, Potter PA, Ostendorf WR. *Nursing interventions and clinical skills,* ed 6, St Louis, 2016, Elsevier.)

assembles the proper syringe, needle, and an alcohol wipe for cleansing the skin. Next, the medication is obtained and the label is read carefully. The medication label states the name of the medication and its strength, and gives an expiration date past which the drug should not be used. Be sure to keep the container until the medication is charted. When medications are not used frequently (such as in an emergency kit or on a crash cart), they should be checked often. Out-of-date supplies should be discarded and replaced. When supplies are used for an emergency, they should be replaced as soon as possible.

> **!** Never borrow medication or equipment from the emergency cart for routine use!

BOX 14-3 Parenteral Injection Procedure

- Greet the patient. Check patient identification and explain the procedure.
- Select the appropriate injection site.
- Perform hand hygiene and don clean gloves.
- Cleanse the selected area with an alcohol wipe.
- Hold the skin taut with your nondominant hand.
- Insert the needle at the correct angle, and pull back slightly on the plunger.
- If no blood is present, inject the medication.
- Withdraw the needle quickly, and wipe the injection site.
- Place the syringe with attached needle in a sharps container.
- See to the patient's comfort.
- Remove your gloves and perform hand hygiene.
- Chart the medication.
- Discard the container and any remaining medication.

A common rule of thumb is to read the label three times before administration: (1) when selecting the container, (2) while preparing the dose, and (3) just before injection. *This is essential to be absolutely certain that you have the correct drug and the proper strength, and that the expiration date has not been exceeded.* Also confirm that the vial is not damaged, that the medication has not changed color, and that there is no floating material. Draw the medication up into the syringe from the ampule or vial, or select the appropriate prefilled syringe unit. Follow the procedure outlined in Box 14-3.

> **!** For accuracy, read medication labels three times to be certain that you have the correct drug at the proper strength and that the expiration date has not been exceeded.

If the medication is supplied in a vial, use the method illustrated in Procedure 14-1. After checking the label, pull off the vial's protective cap, exposing the rubber stopper and taking care not to contaminate it. *Do not remove the outer retaining ring.* This ring is essential to prevent the rubber stopper from being forcibly ejected when drawing up the medication. Because this is a closed system, you must inject a volume of air equal to the amount of fluid you will remove. Remove the needle cover and pull down the plunger of the syringe to the desired reading. Insert the needle or needleless cannula through the stopper and inject air into the bottle. Invert the bottle, and make sure

PROCEDURE 14-1   LOADING SYRINGE FROM VIAL

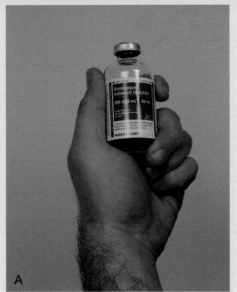

A, Check label for drug name, correct strength, and expiration date. Remove the vial's protective cap, but not the retaining ring. Do not touch the rubber stopper.

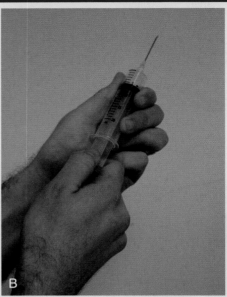

B, Pull back on plunger to desired dose reading.

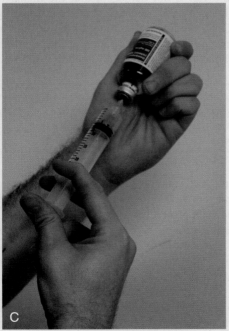

C, Inject air into air space in vial.

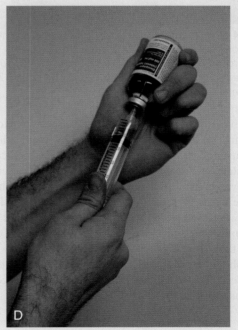

D, Tip vial downward to withdraw solution.

PROCEDURE 14-1   LOADING SYRINGE FROM VIAL—cont'd

E, Tap syringe to dislodge bubbles.

F, Eject remaining air and check that the dosage is accurate.

G, Recap needle using one hand only. Label the syringe. *Note:* Only sterile needles may be recapped.

the needle tip or cannula is below the fluid level. Then, pull down the plunger to the desired reading and check for bubbles. If there are any, dislodge them, eject the air from the syringe, and check to be certain that the dosage is correct. After removing the needle or disconnecting the syringe from the cannula, replace the needle cover using only one hand to decrease the likelihood of sticking yourself and contaminating the needle. If the medication will not be administered immediately, label the syringe so that there will be no question about what it contains.

The vial was originally designed as a multiple-dose container, but the frequency of contamination is so great that multiple uses are now restricted to use for the same patient on the same day. Vials of local anesthetic are sometimes used repeatedly for the same patient during a radiographic procedure. When using a vial after the first time, clean the stopper with an alcohol wipe. (Alcohol is not needed for the first injection because the stopper is sterile when the vial is opened.) When the procedure is completed, discard the vial and any remaining medication. Some vials are not meant for multiple uses and are marked accordingly. For medications dispensed in relatively small quantities (10 mL or less), vials have largely been replaced by preloaded syringes that are discarded after use.

Ampules are glass containers with narrow necks that are opened by breaking the glass. Although ampules are now used infrequently, you may encounter them in the radiology department as part of a sterile tray. When a drug is supplied in ampule form, a filtration needle is used to fill the syringe from the ampule to prevent the possibility of drawing up minute particles of glass. A small file is used to nick the neck of the ampule. The top then snaps off easily. Use a small gauze sponge to protect your fingers when opening the ampule because the glass may break unevenly and cut your hand (Figure 14-6). Next, securely attach the filtration needle to the syringe and remove the needle cover, taking care not to contaminate the needle. Place the needle tip in the ampule below the solution level and withdraw the required amount of the medication into the syringe. Hold the syringe to the light to check for air bubbles. If bubbles appear, hold the syringe with the needle pointing up and tap the side of the syringe. As the bubbles rise, they can be ejected with gentle pressure on the plunger. The removal of air is essential to accurate dosage measurement and may affect patient safety. Now read the label again. The ampule is retained until after the drug has been administered and charted. If the medication is not being administered immediately, label the syringe with the name and strength of the medication. Before the drug is administered, replace the filtration needle with an injection needle and show the physician the ampule and the syringe while stating aloud what has been done. After administration, the medication is charted and the ampule, together with any remaining medication, is discarded. Perform hand hygiene.

Injectable medications are supplied with adhesive labels for identifying the syringe after it has been filled. These labels usually include barcodes that can be scanned into electronic medication records. Some labels are supplied in a sterile wrap for use during sterile procedures. Apply the appropriate label to the syringe as soon as the medication has been drawn up. This is especially important if the medication is not going to be administered immediately.

Intravenous Route

IV fluids and medications are administered to meet specific needs. Patients respond rapidly to medication administration via this route. IV injection is used for delivering most emergency medications when an immediate response is critical.

Dehydrated patients may need fluid and electrolyte replacement. The most common replacement fluids are normal saline (NS; an isotonic solution of 0.9% sodium chloride in water) or a 5% solution of dextrose in water (D5W). These solutions are usually stocked in radiology departments. If you are starting or replacing IV fluids, be certain that the solution is correct. Less common solutions, or those containing medication, may need to be replaced by the nursing service. The IV route may be used to administer medications, parenteral nutrition, or chemotherapy. This is also the route used to

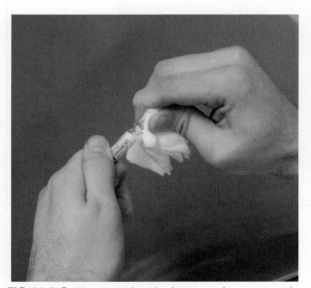

FIG 14-6 Protect your hand when opening an ampule. Break the ampule away from your face.

inject contrast media for radiographic examinations of the urinary tract and for some computed tomography (CT) studies, and to provide sedation during invasive procedures and MRI examinations. (See Chapter 19 for a discussion of contrast radiography, Chapter 20 for a discussion of central venous catheters and arterial lines, and Chapter 22 for CT and MRI procedures that may involve injections.)

Venipuncture may be accomplished with a hypodermic needle, a butterfly set, or an IV catheter (for example, Angiocath). The IV use of hypodermic needles is generally restricted to phlebotomy for obtaining laboratory samples and for single, small injections. A butterfly set is preferable to a conventional hypodermic needle for most IV injections and is often used to facilitate injections with a syringe. This apparatus consists of a needle with plastic projections that may be taped to the patient's skin after the needle is in place (Figure 14-7). This prevents

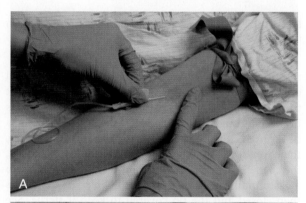

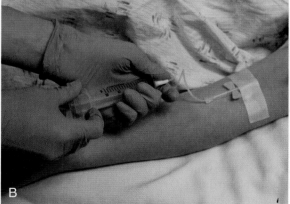

FIG 14-7 A butterfly set facilitates direct IV injection. **A,** Needle projections provide grip for venipuncture. **B,** Tubing provides needle stability during injection.

movement of the needle in the vein. Attached to the needle is a short length of tubing with a hub that attaches to a syringe. The syringe is filled from a vial or ampule and is then attached to the tubing. Before the butterfly needle is inserted into the vein, the tubing is filled with liquid from the syringe to avoid injecting air into the vein. This method has a distinct advantage because movement of the syringe will not cause movement of the needle, decreasing the likelihood that the needle's position in the vein will be compromised.

IV catheters are frequently used instead of butterfly sets when repeated IV injections or continuous infusions will be administered. The IV catheter is a two-part system consisting of a needle that fits inside a flexible plastic catheter. The catheter hub may have wing-shaped plastic projections similar to the butterfly set to aid in holding the needle during venipuncture. The needle portion is solid rather than hollow and serves both to stiffen the catheter for insertion and as a stylet to prevent blood backflow through the catheter. This combination unit is inserted into the vein, and the catheter is advanced by slipping it forward over the needle. The catheter is then secured with tape, the needle is withdrawn, and the catheter is connected to the supply system. IV fluid, medication, or a contrast medium can then be administered by syringe through an injection port on IV tubing from a hanging bottle or bag. Alternatively, if a continuous infusion is not needed, an **intermittent injection port** (sometimes called a *saline lock*) may be used. This is a small adapter with a diaphragm that is attached directly to an IV catheter.

One of the engineering controls mentioned previously to minimize hazards posed by needlesticks is the use of *needleless* systems (Figure 14-8). These systems facilitate blood draws and IV medication administration without the use of needles after an injection port or IV line has been established. An important feature of the system is a self-healing rubber substance used for medication vial caps, intermittent injection ports, and access ports on IV tubing. These caps and ports can be repeatedly penetrated by blunt plastic cannulas without damaging their integrity. The blunt cannulas are used to draw up medications and to access established IV lines for blood draws and medication administration. The use of a needleless system greatly reduces needle use and its attendant hazards in the health care setting.

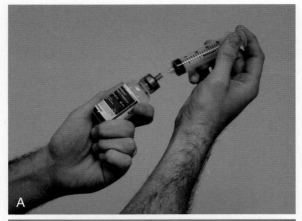

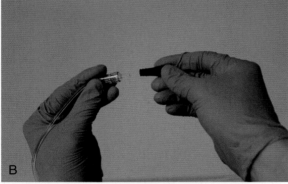

FIG 14-8 Needleless IV access system. A, Needle-free safety is facilitated with a vial adapter, as shown here fitted to top of multiple-dose vial. B, Threaded IV tubing connects to the needleless injection site.

When a procedure requires the IV infusion of a large volume of fluid, an IV pole and infusion set are needed. Setting up fluid administration equipment is not complicated but is another skill that improves with practice. IV solutions are provided in bottles and plastic bags (Figure 14-9). The bags have a cap over the sterile port through which the drip chamber of the IV tubing is inserted. The drip chamber is removed from its wrappings and inserted into the sterile port.

> **!** When connecting the tubing, take care not to contaminate either component.

Solutions supplied in bottles have a removable cap and sometimes a rubber diaphragm covering a rubber

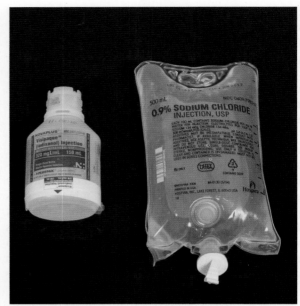

FIG 14-9 IV contrast media and fluids are packaged in bottles and in plastic bags.

stopper. The cap is removed, and the diaphragm is pulled off without touching the stopper. After ensuring that the clamp on the tubing is closed, the drip chamber is inserted through the stopper. Now the bottle or bag may be inverted and hung on the IV pole. When it is in place, the cover at the other end of the IV tubing is removed, the clamp is opened, and the fluid is allowed to run into a basin until the tubing is free of bubbles. The clamp is then closed and the tip covered to keep it sterile. See Procedure 14-2.

Starting an IV Line

The veins most often used for initiating IV lines are found in the anterior forearm, the posterior hand, the radial aspect of the wrist, and the antecubital space (Figure 14-10). Usually the antecubital veins on each arm are large enough and near enough to the surface to be easily seen. Although they may be the easiest to locate and to puncture, there are drawbacks to their use. Easy access to these veins is important in emergencies and for routine blood draws. Overuse, however, may cause these veins to become scarred or sclerotic, creating serious problems for patients receiving long-term care. When antecubital IV lines remain in place for some time, they become uncomfortable and inhibit the patient's ability

PROCEDURE 14-2   IV INFUSION SETUP

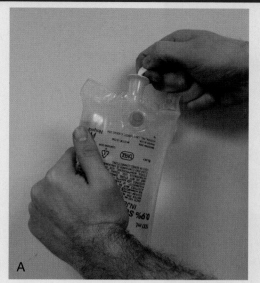

A, Remove protective cover from access port. Avoid contamination.

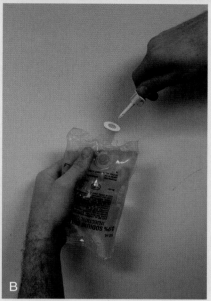

B, With tubing clamped off, insert drip chamber firmly into access port.

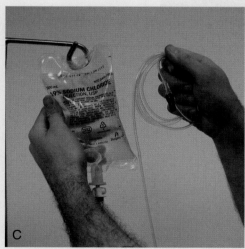

C, Invert bag or bottle, and suspend from pole.

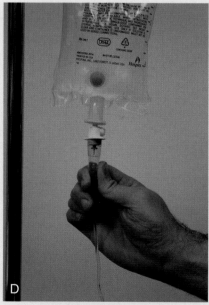

D, Pinch drip chamber to draw fluid into chamber. Fill chamber about half full.

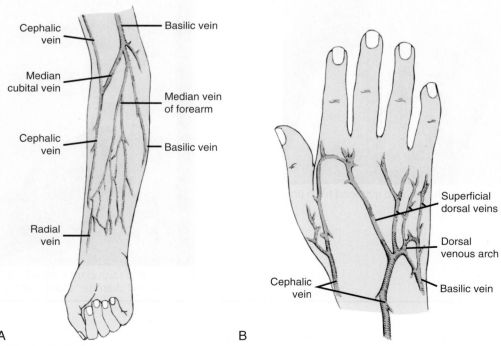

E, Unclamp to fill tubing and reclamp once air has been removed from the line. Setup is ready for attachment to IV catheter.

Cephalic vein

Basilic vein

Median cubital vein

Median vein of forearm

Cephalic vein

Basilic vein

Radial vein

Superficial dorsal veins

Dorsal venous arch

Cephalic vein

Basilic vein

A

B

FIG 14-10 Veins used for venipuncture. A, Veins of the anterior aspect of forearm. B, Superficial veins of the dorsal aspect of the hand.

to flex the elbow. Flexion at the elbow may crimp the catheter, preventing IV flow. For these reasons, the nursing service tends to use antecubital veins as a last resort. In imaging departments, the IV line is usually placed only for the duration of the procedure, and the use of antecubital veins is acceptable when necessary. A vein of adequate size is essential when a bolus of contrast will be delivered at a rapid rate (see Chapter 19). For children, this usually requires an antecubital site. When placing an IV line in an antecubital vein, a flexible IV catheter must be used and the elbow should be restrained in extension by attaching it to an arm board. Flexion of the elbow with a needle or catheter in an antecubital vein can rupture the vein, causing **infiltration** (leakage into surrounding tissue), hematoma, and scarring.

To select a vein, first secure the tourniquet proximal to the intended site. Instruct the patient to open and close the hand a few times and then hold a firm fist. These measures restrict circulation and enlarge the veins, making them easier to identify and to penetrate accurately. The ideal vein can be readily seen and palpated. It is at least twice the diameter of the needle or catheter you plan to use and does not appear to bend or curve for a distance at least equal to the length of the needle or catheter. If a suitable vein is not immediately apparent, let the arm hang down for a few seconds with the tourniquet in place, then gently slap the skin over the area where the vein should appear. This may increase the likelihood that the vein will stand out well. If a suitable vein is still not apparent, remove the tourniquet and repeat the process with the other arm. Procedure 14-3 shows the step-by-step process of starting an IV line using an IV catheter. Initiation of an IV line must be documented in the medical record.

PROCEDURE 14-3 VENIPUNCTURE USING IV CATHETER

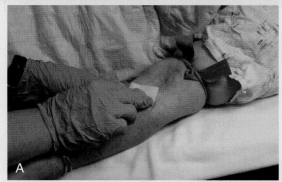

A, Perform hand hygiene and don protective gloves. After securing tourniquet and selecting vein, cleanse skin according to the protocol for your institution.

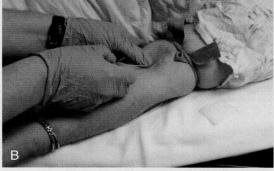

B, Hold catheter at an acute angle to skin and insert into vein.

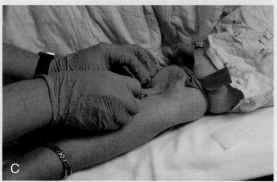

C, Blood return into catheter and hub indicates successful placement.

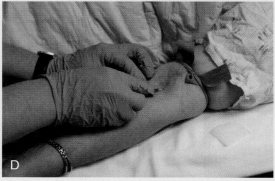

D, Advance catheter over stylet until hub is against skin.

PROCEDURE 14-3   VENIPUNCTURE USING IV CATHETER—cont'd

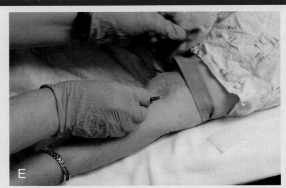

E, Release tourniquet.

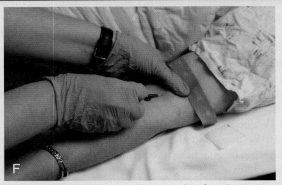

F, Holding pressure on vein near tip of catheter, remove stylet.

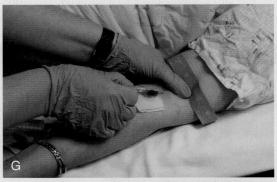

G, Connect delivery system to catheter.

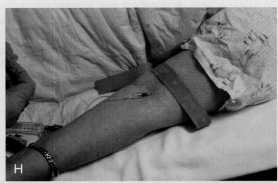

H, If system includes an injection port, attach port and syringe for flushing port. Injection port and flush syringe are provided as a unit.

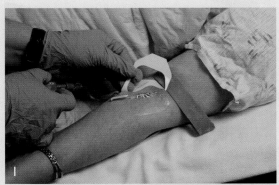

I, Tape catheter in place. Although it is usual for IV lines placed in imaging departments to be discontinued when the procedure is complete, if IV line will remain in place after procedure, treat site with antiseptic ointment and cover with protective film. Add a label with date, time, catheter gauge, and your initials.

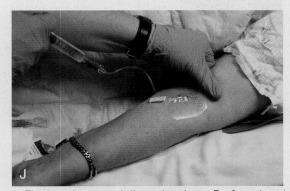

J, Flush catheter and discard syringe. Perform hand hygiene and chart initiation of IV line.

In addition to the steps illustrated, evidence-based practice suggests numbing the area before injecting. Several methods can be used to accomplish this before starting an IV: a topical anesthetic applied to the skin at the injection site, or an intradermal injection of bacteriostatic saline or local anesthetic at the injection site. Be aware that sometimes an intradermal injection at the IV site obstructs the vein.

As you practice with classmates, suitable veins may appear readily. In the clinical setting, however, it is often more difficult. Obese patients may have veins that are too deep to be seen or palpated, and elderly patients may have veins that are easily seen but roll under the skin or are too crooked to be suitable. For patients who have undergone a mastectomy, you should select a vein on the extremity opposite the side of the mastectomy site because these patients often suffer from lymphedema, which causes boggy tissue and may obstruct the vein. Patients with scarred and sclerotic veins from extensive IV therapy, especially chemotherapy, may require a non-routine approach.

Infants and children can present challenges when an IV line is needed. Their small veins are more difficult to see and feel, and the situation is often complicated by the child's refusal or inability to cooperate. Passive distraction, such as a movie, helps allay the fear that is often responsible for a child's distress. The use of an anesthetic at the injection site as described previously is optional, but topical anesthetics work well with IV ports and peripheral IV lines on infants and children. Infants or toddlers who are active and uncooperative may be immobilized using the same methods that are used to immobilize children for imaging (see Chapter 10). When the line is established, the arm or leg should be immobilized with an arm board. Use a padded plastic board in the appropriate size. Wrap with gauze and secure with tape (Figure 14-11).

Your competence and confidence will increase considerably with experience. You should attempt venipuncture only when you have a reasonable expectation of success, and seek more experienced help whenever you are in doubt. Most hospitals have an IV therapy department with specially trained and highly experienced nurses who will assist you with difficult situations. Some hospital policies state that all IV lines for chemotherapy patients and children younger than a certain age must be started by IV therapy personnel.

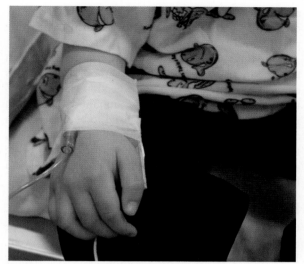

FIG 14-11 An arm board stabilizes the IV site on a toddler's arm.

> **!** If a particular patient's situation is beyond your skill level, or if you have attempted venipuncture on a patient twice unsuccessfully, call on the IV therapy department or consult another team member.

IV Medication Administration

When the IV line has been established, many IV medications can be administered through an intermittent injection port or through access ports on IV infusion tubing. Do not administer medications via specialty IV catheters such as peripherally inserted central catheters (PICC) (see Chapter 20). Specialty catheters may be accessed only by qualified nursing personnel. Before injecting through IV lines, check to be sure that the medications involved are compatible. Chapter 19 addresses the subject of compatibility between contrast media and common medications. After checking the patient identification and the medication label, draw the correct dosage into a syringe. Cleanse the port with alcohol, and inject the medication through the port. When an intermittent injection port is used, a small amount of flush solution is injected through the port to prevent blood from coagulating inside the catheter and to remove any residual medication that may not mix compatibly with the current injection. The system is flushed with sterile saline solution immediately after it is established and again before and after each use. Physicians may order the use of heparin solution as a flush for some patients.

Sometimes medications will be administered through the IV line using the *piggyback* method. This involves connecting a bag or bottle of medication via its own IV tubing to an existing IV line. The amount of medication may be considerable, or it may need to be dispersed in a large quantity of **diluent** (diluting liquid). In this case, the piggyback line is filled and clamped before being attached to the IV line; the IV line is then clamped, and the piggyback line is opened.

Extravasation

Occasionally IV fluids or medications may leak or be accidentally injected into the tissues surrounding a vein. Leakage may be caused by the rupture of the vein or by passage of fluid through intact vessel walls as a result of high injection pressure in a small vessel. Extravasation is also referred to as infiltration. The term *extravasation* refers to the fact that the fluid is outside the vessel, whereas infiltration indicates that it has diffused into the surrounding tissue. This condition may be both painful and dangerous. Some medications administered may be *vesicants*, agents that cause blistering if infiltrated into subcutaneous tissue. When extravasation occurs, the patient is likely to complain of discomfort, and you may observe swelling at the site. The following precautions help minimize the possibility of infiltration:

- Check for backflow of blood to be certain that the catheter is properly situated before injecting.
- Immobilize the catheter at the injection site.
- Stop the injection immediately if the patient complains of discomfort at the injection site, if you note swelling around the injection site, or if any resistance to injection is felt.

When infiltration does occur, you must remove the needle and attend to this problem before proceeding with an injection at another site. Assure the patient that the pain is only temporary. Maintain pressure on the vein until bleeding has stopped completely to avoid the additional complication of a hematoma at the site of the extravasation. After the bleeding has stopped, apply a cold pack to the affected area to help alleviate the pain. This will also cause constriction of the blood vessels in the area and help to keep the infiltrate localized. If cold packs are not readily available, a terry towel can be wrapped around ice cubes, or ice in a plastic bag can be applied. A dry towel should be wrapped around the bag to protect the skin and hold the bag in place. Replace the cold pack with another as soon as it melts. Ice packs are applied to the extravasation site for 20 to 60 minutes, repeated three times a day, until swelling is diminished. An incident report must be completed for any extravasation involving a potentially irritating medication or contrast medium. Advise outpatients to consult their physicians or to report to the emergency department if inflammation or discomfort persists.

At one time, hot packs were recommended for the treatment of all IV infiltrations because the increased circulation that results with heat helps the body to absorb the extravasated fluid more rapidly. Research now confirms that the safest and most effective treatment for infiltration of contrast media and other irritating substances is the application of cold packs, which tends to limit the area of involvement.

Discontinuing an IV Line

When you must discontinue an IV line, you will need a sterile adhesive bandage, bandage scissors, and cotton balls or gauze sponges. Follow the illustrations in Procedure 14-4. Perform hand hygiene, and explain the procedure to the patient. Wearing protective gloves, close the drip control and gently remove the adhesive tape holding the catheter. If it is necessary to cut the tape, take care not to cut the catheter, which may be doubled back under the tape. With the site exposed where the catheter enters the vein, remove the catheter with a long, smooth pull, and check that the catheter tip is intact when removed. Apply pressure to the site with a dry cotton ball or sponge. A dry contact is preferred to an alcohol wipe so that the adhesive bandage will stick to the skin. Maintain the pressure for one minute or until the bleeding stops, and then cover the site with a sterile adhesive bandage or secure the cotton ball to the site with tape. Discontinuation of the IV must be documented in the medical record. With the patient in a safe, comfortable position, dispose of the equipment in the proper container, remove your gloves, and repeat hand hygiene.

Monitoring IV Fluids

Patients who are receiving IV fluid administration may come to the radiology department with a standard IV set, or possibly a medication pump, in place. Patients with certain kidney diseases or cardiac problems will need to have their fluid intake closely monitored. For these

PROCEDURE 14-4 DISCONTINUING AN IV LINE

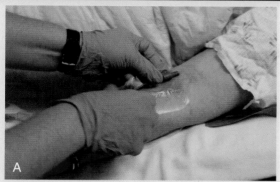

A, Wearing protective gloves, close the drip control and gently remove any tape. If you need to cut tape, take care not to cut the catheter.

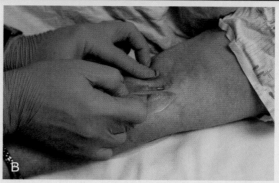

B, Expose the site where the catheter enters the vein.

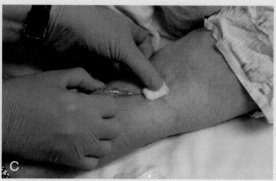

C, Holding a cotton ball gently over the puncture site, remove the catheter with a smooth pull.

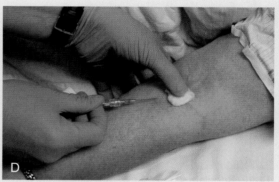

D, Check that the catheter tip is intact. Apply pressure to the site with a cotton ball for several seconds.

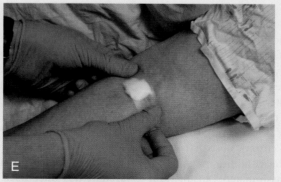

E, Firmly secure the cotton ball over the site with tape, or apply a sterile adhesive bandage. Repeat hand hygiene and chart that the IV has been discontinued.

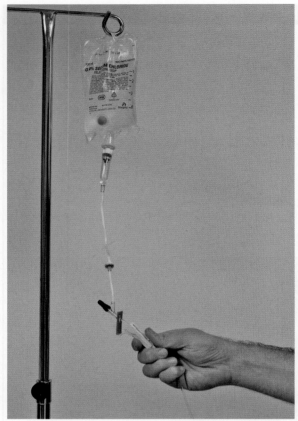

FIG 14-12 Regulate the IV flow rate using the clamp below the drip chamber. Practice improves precise regulation of drip rate.

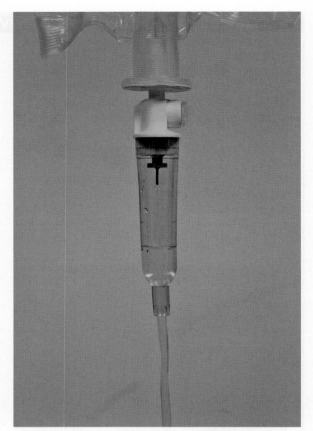

FIG 14-13 A microdrip chamber is used as part of an IV system for keeping a vein accessible without delivering an excessive amount of fluid.

patients especially, you must know how fast the IV set is supposed to run, not just how fast it was running when the patient entered the radiology department. Check the orders. If in doubt, call the nurse in charge of the patient.

Most patients easily tolerate 15 to 20 drops/min from a standard IV set. At this rate, the patient receives approximately 60 mL/h. If an IV infusion runs too fast, a patient with a condition such as chronic obstructive pulmonary disease or congestive heart failure may receive more fluid than can be readily assimilated, causing fluid to accumulate in the lungs (pulmonary edema). Because an IV set may also contain medication, the patient could suffer a toxic effect or an overdose. On the other hand, slow IV administration might result in inadequate medication dosage. The drip rate is controlled by a clamp below the drip meter (Figure 14-12) that can be opened

or closed to control the rate of flow. Practice using this control in the laboratory before confronting it in the clinical area. If you have changed the flow rate for any reason and are concerned about regulating it correctly, be sure to notify the nursing service when the patient is returned to their care.

You may encounter an IV dripping slowly with a microdrip set (Figure 14-13). The small size of the drops allows continuous flow at a reduced volume. This system was once used extensively to keep an IV line open for medication administration and is still used on occasion, especially for pediatric patients, but intermittent injection ports have largely replaced *keep open* IV lines.

When checking an IV set, remember to check the height of the bottle or bag. It should always be 18 to 20

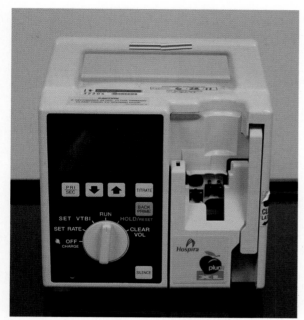

FIG 14-14 Medication pump. Models vary; you must be knowledgeable about those used in your clinical setting.

inches above the level of the vein. If the bag is inadvertently placed lower than the vein, blood will flow back into the catheter or tubing and may clot, causing the fluid to stop flowing. This frequently necessitates restarting the IV line at a new site. On the other hand, an IV solution that is too high may cause fluid to infiltrate into the surrounding tissues because of the increased **hydrostatic pressure** (the pressure exerted by fluid due to the force of gravity).

Always remember to check the area around the injection site. If it is cool, swollen, and boggy, the IV solution may have infiltrated. In the case of infiltration, turn off the IV set and treat the area for extravasation as previously described.

Medication pumps (Figure 14-14) are used for various reasons, including patient-controlled pain medication, parenteral nutrition, and continuous medication administration. If your clinical area deals frequently with patients on medication pumps, and especially if your work involves IV injections through lines governed by pumps, you must understand the operation of the specific pumps used in your facility. Medication

pumps can be plugged into an electrical outlet, but most pumps also have batteries that allow operation during transport. An alarm system is part of the pump and will emit a warning sound when the solution supply is low, when flow is interrupted, or when the battery power is weak. The ability to handle pumps competently is most easily acquired by hands-on practice under the direction of experienced personnel.

When a hanging supply of IV fluid is running low, or when the pump alarm signals an interruption in flow, you may be strongly tempted to work rapidly, complete the procedure, and return the patient promptly to the nursing service rather than cope with changes in the IV system. All too often this results in a nonfunctioning or "blown" IV line. For some patients, starting a new IV line presents no particular problem. Unfortunately, patients who are hospitalized and receiving IV fluid or medication frequently have the fewest suitable veins. This is particularly true of pediatric patients, whose tiny veins are fragile and difficult to access. Patients receiving chemotherapy or parenteral nutrition are also likely to present difficulties when a new site is needed. You can avoid some of these problems by following these suggestions:

- Call in advance, and inform the medication nurse if the procedure will be lengthy.
- Whenever possible, plug in the pump rather than relying on battery power.
- Watch IV fluid levels, and allow time for replacement before the IV fluid is exhausted.
- If an IV set does run out, or if the alarm sounds despite precautions, call the nursing service immediately rather than waiting until the patient is returned to the nursing unit.

Precautions for All Injections

Most needles and syringes are provided in sterile wraps, used once, and then discarded. One common on-the-job injury is an accidental skin puncture by a contaminated needle. As discussed in Chapter 9, Standard Precautions are essential for your safety as well as that of the patient. For this reason we strongly urge you to use caution and apply the following rules when dealing with parenteral equipment:

- Wear gloves when dealing with any object contaminated by blood or when inserting or removing an IV line.
- Dispose of all syringes and needles directly into a puncture-proof container without recapping.

- Use safety-designed needles and needleless devices whenever possible.
- Always follow established rules of aseptic technique.
- Read the label three times: (1) before drawing up the medication, (2) after drawing it up, and (3) with the physician before administration.
- Label the syringe with the medication name and strength (concentration) if the medication will not be administered immediately.
- Confirm patient identification using two identifiers before administration.
- Check for allergies.
- Monitor the patient carefully for side effects.

CHARTING MEDICATIONS

When a medication is given by a physician, or by a radiographer under the physician's supervision, it is always recorded in the patient's chart. The notation is made in the appropriate section of the chart and includes the date, time of day, drug name, dosage, and route of administration. A typical entry in the medication record might read: 10:50 am, Benadryl, 50 mg, PO. Each entry must include the identification of the person who charted it. Initials alone are not considered adequate identification. If the medication record calls for initials, there is another place in the chart, often on the same page, where each set of initials is identified with the signer's full name. For legal reasons, the radiographer who charts medication must use the exact procedure established by the institution.

If an emergency prevents the charting of medications at the time they are given, the radiographer should make a written notation of the time, drug, and dosage so that accurate information will be available when the charting is completed. If this is not done, the pressure of the situation may lead to confusion of the facts. The time, sequence, and dosage of several medications may be forgotten or charted incorrectly. Any medication prescribed or administered by a physician should be charted by the physician; if charted by the radiographer, the physician should countersign it. The legal significance of complete accountability in such situations cannot be overemphasized.

The administration of contrast media is charted as a medication. Following every examination that involves contrast media, the radiographer must

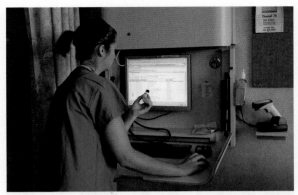

FIG 14-15 Medications may be charted in the computer by scanning the medication container, the patient's armband, and the caregiver's barcode identification.

enter into the patient's medical record the following information:
- Contrast agent's name and strength
- Volume administered
- Route of administration
- Date and time of administration
- Signature or approved identification

Contrast administration may also be confirmed by a specific statement in the radiologist's report.

When paper charts are used, physicians enter an account of the procedure and any medications given in the progress notes. The radiographer is responsible for checking that the drug, time, dose, and route of administration are clearly expressed. This avoids the possibility of duplication and provides guidelines for the nursing staff if follow-up care is needed. Some hospitals have a medication administration sheet on which all medications must be charted.

In medical centers with computerized charting, wireless barcode scanners are used to record patient identification, caregiver identification, and medication identification (Figure 14-15). The medication, date, and time are thus entered automatically into the electronic record. Depending on the situation, a nurse may add a notation of the dose and the route of administration. Radiographers may not have direct access to this system. In this case, written records may be scanned into the electronic record or the written record may be sent back to the nursing unit with an inpatient.

Charting routines vary. Familiarize yourself with the routine of your specific clinical area.

Based on the 2015 National Patient Safety Goals of The Joint Commission (TJC), health care workers are required to communicate a complete list of the patient's medications to the next provider of service. Therefore, a radiographer is required to inform the nurses of any medications administered to the patient, inclusive of contrast media. Similarly, a complete list of the patient's medications must be communicated to the imaging department prior to administration of any contrast media. Other patient safety goals that relate to medication include proper patient identification using two identifiers, and labeling all medications in surgical and procedural settings as stated in this chapter. The entire TJC Patient Safety Goals statement for 2015 is available at http://www.joint commission.org/hap_2015_npsgs/.

■ SUMMARY

- Before medication administration, you must check the order, check patient identification, check for allergies to the medication, verify that the medication is correct, and check that the expiration date has not passed.
- Dosages may be ordered in weight units, whereas the medication must be measured in liquid units. Some medications are prescribed according to the patient's weight in kilograms. If you administer medications, you must be able to calculate dosage accurately.
- The enteral route of drug administration involves direct placement of the medication into the digestive tract, orally, rectally, or via an NG tube.
- Medications placed under the tongue (sublingual) or inside the cheek (buccal) are absorbed into the bloodstream directly through the mucous membrane.
- Inhaled medication may be administered via inhaler or nebulizer to treat lung conditions and for certain nuclear medicine imaging studies and general anesthesia.
- The topical route refers to the application of medication to the skin. Topical medications may treat a skin condition or may have a transdermal effect, entering the circulation via the skin. Transdermal medications are usually administered via an adhesive patch.
- Parenteral injections are classified as intradermal (between skin layers), SC (under the skin, in the fat layer), or IM (within a muscle; usually the deltoid, the gluteus, or one of the thigh muscles). The volume of the injection often determines the type of parenteral injection, and the type of injection determines the length and gauge of the needle used.
- Medication administered via the IV route produces a very rapid response, which is why this route is commonly used to administer emergency medications. This route is also used to administer infusions for fluid and/or electrolyte replacement. Contrast agents are administered via this route for some x-ray, CT, and MRI examinations.
- An IV line is established using a butterfly needle or an IV catheter. If the line will be used over a period of time, it may be attached to an IV infusion set or an intermittent injection port. To use an injection port, cleanse the port with an alcohol wipe, flush with saline, inject the medication or contrast agent, and flush again with saline. Do not administer medications via specialty IV lines, such as a PICC. Document establishment of an IV line in the medical record.
- When IV fluids leak from a vein or are accidentally injected outside a vein, this is called infiltration. Precautions are needed to prevent infiltration because it is painful and may be dangerous. In case of infiltration, stop the injection or infusion immediately, maintain pressure on the vein until the bleeding stops, and treat the area with cold packs.
- To discontinue an IV line, wear gloves, close the drip control, remove any tape, pull the catheter from the vein, and apply pressure to the site with a cotton ball or gauze sponge. Cover the site with a sterile adhesive bandage. Document discontinuation in the medical record and note that the catheter was intact at the tip when discontinued.
- When monitoring IV fluids, note the flow rate, maintain the bag or bottle at a height of 18 to 20 inches above the vein, and notify the nursing service if the flow stops, the bag or bottle is nearly empty, or an alarm sounds on the medication pump.

- Charting of medications is a critical part of medication administration. The chart record must state the date, time, medication, dose, route of administration, and identity of the person administering the drug. This may be recorded in a paper chart record or entered electronically into the computer record. Be certain that any medication orders you receive are signed by the physician before leaving the area.

REVIEW QUESTIONS

1. Medications given in imaging departments are most often administered via the route that provides the most rapid response. This is the:
   A. SC route
   B. intradermal route
   C. IV route
   D. intrathecal route
2. A parenteral administration of 5 mL of Benadryl may be given IV or:
   A. intradermally
   B. SC
   C. IM
   D. any of the above
3. The average flow rate for infusion of IV fluids is:
   A. 5 to 10 drops/min
   B. 15 to 20 drops/min
   C. 40 to 50 drops/min
   D. 60 drops/min
4. The administration of a medication by means of a rectal suppository is an example of using which of the following routes of administration?
   A. Buccal
   B. Enteral
   C. Intradermal
   D. IM
5. A medication is prescribed according to the patient's weight in the metric system. The patient weighs 140 lbs. His weight in the metric system is approximately ___ kg.
   A. 308
   B. 110
   C. 64
   D. 28
6. The route of administration for any medication order is determined by referring to:
   A. the drug package insert
   B. the physician's order
   C. the patient's nurse
   D. the patient
7. When medication is injected into the spinal canal, the method of administration is called:
   A. IM
   B. SC
   C. intradermal
   D. intrathecal
8. A butterfly set is a specialty needle used for which of the following types of injections?
   A. Intradermal
   B. IV
   C. Intra-arterial
   D. IM
9. Leakage of IV fluid into the surrounding tissues is termed:
   A. infiltration
   B. angina pectoris
   C. hematoma
   D. hydrostatic pressure
10. Needleless medication systems and SESIPS are devices that provide:
    A. safety to patients by preventing overdose
    B. safety to hospitals by recording dosages correctly
    C. safety to health care personnel by preventing infections from needlesticks
    D. economy by minimizing medication waste

Answers can be found in the Answer Key on pages 429-431.

CRITICAL THINKING EXERCISES

1. Mrs. Short is a patient with moderately controlled epilepsy who complains of upper abdominal pain. She has remained NPO (*nil per os* meaning *nothing by mouth*) in preparation for this examination and did not take her medicine last night or this morning. As she enters the dressing room, she falls heavily to the floor in a major motor (grand mal) seizure. "Here, give her this medicine," her husband orders. "She takes it by mouth." Which routes of administration are most appropriate for such patients? Should you administer medicine from her purse? Why or why not? What risks are involved in giving oral medication to unconscious patients?

2. Mrs. Erbele, a 50-year-old woman who lives alone, fell from a step stool in her basement. She was unable to stand and remained on the floor until found by her daughter 48 hours later. She has been admitted to the emergency department with dehydration and a possible hip fracture. An IV of D5W is running at 60 mL/h when she is brought to the radiology department. In an attempt to assist as you and another radiographer transfer her to the x-ray table, she rolls onto one side. As you position her, you note that her IV has stopped dripping. What could have caused this? What should be checked first? What actions should you take? Should you discontinue the IV?

3. Janet Johnson, age 8, is scheduled for a head CT with contrast. She is reluctant to offer her arm for venipuncture. Although she is not crying, she is obviously very apprehensive. Her mother appears anxious as well, and states that there have been problems in the past when others have tried to access Janet's veins. What can you do to help Janet cope with anxiety? What factors would influence your decision as to whether you should proceed with venipuncture or call for help?

4. Dr. Kirkpatrick has ordered 50 mg of Benadryl IM for a patient experiencing a mild allergic reaction. The available supply of this medication is a liquid containing 20 mg/mL. How much of this liquid should you draw into the syringe? What length and gauge of needle would you use? Suggest a suitable injection site.

15

Emergency Response

EMERGENCIES

An *emergency* can be defined as a serious, unexpected event that demands immediate attention. Sudden deterioration in the status of any patient under your care is an acute situation requiring an appropriate response. Whether such a situation leads to a more serious problem may depend on your ability to act quickly and efficiently. Seen from this perspective, no patient problem can be considered trivial. You will experience many acute situations over the years, and you must be prepared to minimize the possibility of any further injury or complication.

EMERGENCY DEPARTMENT

The emergency departments (EDs) of most hospitals serve a variety of clients. Individuals with health insurance may use urgent care or surgical centers for minor emergencies. For the poor and uninsured, however, the ED often serves the additional function of family physician. Many such admissions to the ED present valid problems, even if they are not emergencies. This can rapidly overload both staff and facilities, especially in an urban setting. Establishing priorities and functioning effectively under such circumstances can demand intense application of your patient care and assessment skills. In addition to the material on trauma units in the following paragraphs, you will find information about the use of radiography in trauma units in Chapter 20.

TRAUMA UNITS

Many hospitals have specialized facilities called *trauma units*, which are part of the ED. There are three designated levels of trauma facility:

- Level I trauma centers care for all levels of injuries and are staffed around the clock with physicians, surgeons, and support personnel who are highly trained in the care and treatment of traumatic injuries. Level I hospitals have access to transfer facilities, such as helicopter rescue units, permitting the most seriously injured patients to reach the center in a relatively short time. A Level I hospital must be able to provide emergency radiography, fluoroscopy, computed tomography (CT), and magnetic resonance imaging (MRI) procedures around the clock. There must also be access to nuclear medicine studies, angiography, and sonography. Facilities for neurologic care must also be available.
- Level II trauma centers are the next level of trauma care. ED physicians are on 24-hour duty, as are emergency trained nurses and radiology staff. Surgical radiographic and fluoroscopic procedures must be available, as well as the ability to perform angiography, CT, and MRI procedures. Patients will be transferred to Level I facilities only if necessary.
- Level III trauma centers are smaller community hospitals that usually have an ED physician and radiographer on call at night. Trauma patients with life-threatening conditions will be transported to a Level I or Level II hospital as necessary.

Trauma units are designed to cope with life-threatening injuries. Many units have the resources to accept patients who have been airlifted directly to the unit from a considerable distance. Trauma units are usually staffed with one or more trauma physicians who receive highly specialized training in the diagnosis and treatment of traumatic injuries; trauma nurses, an anesthetist or respiratory therapist, radiographer(s), a phlebotomist, and one individual (usually a nurse) to act as a record keeper.

Research has proved that victims of massive trauma who survive their initial injury have a greater chance of recovery if their condition can be stabilized within the first hour after the accident (called the *golden hour*). For this reason, every minute is precious, and trauma teams work under great pressure. The care of highly trained personnel and the immediate availability of equipment for diagnosis and treatment have greatly improved the potential for saving lives.

The transport team, usually made up of qualified emergency medical technicians (EMTs), delivers the patient to the trauma unit as soon as an airway has been established, bleeding has been controlled, and the patient has been immobilized. The first assessments made by the physician at the trauma center involve evaluation of cardiac status, respiratory status, and the possibility of vertebral fracture. The danger of paralysis is so great that checking for spinal fracture ranks directly after **respiratory arrest** (cessation of breathing) and **cardiac arrest** (cessation of heartbeat) in terms of priority.

> **!** Trauma patients are transported on a rigid backboard and are not removed from it until the possibility of a spinal fracture has been ruled out.

Today's trauma imaging is done primarily in CT. If a trauma patient needs radiographs, protocols usually state that chest, pelvis, and lateral cervical spine images should be obtained. Images of the extremities are often acquired after the CT has been performed and the patient has returned to the trauma bay. The image receptors and grid cap for these images should be available in each mobile unit to avoid delays. In addition to mobile x-ray units, and possibly C-arm fluoroscopic units, trauma areas also have a CT scanner nearby and may have a small surgical suite immediately adjacent to them. Many EDs also include an emergency x-ray room.

The role of the radiographer in trauma radiography may be to take radiographs in the ED x-ray room, to operate the CT scanner, or to take radiographs with mobile equipment in the trauma bay while the patient is also being tested and treated by other members of the trauma team. Tips for adapting routine procedures for effectiveness in the ED are listed in Box 15-1. Radiographic items that may be helpful within a trauma setting are summarized in Table 15-1.

When trauma patients must be taken to the imaging department, their conditions have usually been stabilized. They have been thoroughly examined by a physician, any blood loss has been controlled, an airway has been established, intravenous (IV) fluids have been started, and medication for pain or blood pressure control has been given. A nurse usually accompanies the severely ill or injured patient when radiographs are taken on the way to the operating room, cast room, or intensive care unit (ICU).

Emergency patients are subject to sudden changes in condition and may go into shock. Treatment for shock is discussed later in Chapter 16. After the acute phase of an accident is over, many patients who were very brave experience a delayed emotional reaction. This may consist of uncontrollable crying or a compulsive urge to tell everyone about the accident. They may even have a physical reaction, such as fainting, trembling, or violent nausea. Your most positive action is to be available, offer nonverbal support, and watch carefully for any signs of a deteriorating physical condition. Your ability to speak calmly and work competently under pressure is reassuring.

When accident victims are brought to the x-ray room dressed in street clothes, it is sometimes necessary to remove their garments before the radiographic

TABLE 15-1	Trauma Radiography Equipment
Equipment	**Purpose**
Mobile x-ray unit	Allows imaging while the patient is in direct care of the trauma team; best method for critically injured patients who need constant supervision and cannot be transported to the radiography department
Cassettes • CR: (2–3) 14 × 17, (3–4) 10 × 12 • DR: multi-use plate in 14 × 17 or 17 × 17 size	For obtaining various necessary images, often several views of multiple body parts
Grid cap for cassette	To accommodate different body part thicknesses with respect to patient habitus
Cassette covers	Impermeable plastic covers to protect the cassette from becoming soiled with blood or body fluids
Lead aprons	For anyone assisting with the patient during imaging
Gonad shielding	For the patient during imaging, provided it does not interfere with the diagnosis
Protective apparel	Standard precautions: gloves, gown, splash-guard masks, and shoe covers plus disinfectant to wipe down the imaging equipment when finished
Identifying markers	Legal markers (right and left) and any additional markers to provide further information (arrow markers, lead BBs, positional markers)
Positioning aids	Tape and sponges (protected by an impermeable cover) to aid in accurate positioning
Pre-printed order(s)	Requisitions for the protocol radiographs (for example, chest x-ray) or for known injuries (such as femur, ankle) that are ordered in advance will save critical time when processing images and/or sending them to PACS

examination. Avoid cutting or tearing clothing whenever possible. Keep all the patient's personal possessions in one place. One easy system is to place everything in a plastic bag clearly identified with the patient's name, which is then placed on the stretcher or wheelchair with the patient. Check the procedure in your clinical area and be consistent in using it.

Box 15-1 offers helpful suggestions for trauma radiography.

MULTIPLE EMERGENCIES

Radiographers usually encounter only one emergency at a time. Occasionally, however, a single accident will have multiple victims, or several acute situations may develop simultaneously. In these cases, you must assess priorities. If you see that it may be difficult for you to cope alone, do not hesitate to call for assistance before the situation places any lives in jeopardy.

Although patients are usually admitted to the radiology department on a scheduled or first-come, first-served basis, exceptions must be made for emergencies. An order designated as **STAT** (from the Latin *statim*)

BOX 15-1   Trauma Radiography Tips

- Obtain information about patients and their injuries and preorder any imaging exams.
- Prepare the required radiographic and protective equipment (cassettes, cassette covers, lead aprons, gloves, gowns, markers).
- Assist the trauma team as much as possible in assessing the patient by providing an extra pair of hands or retrieving a warm blanket.
- Introduce yourself to patients and briefly explain what you need to image. Inquire about their mobility and ask for their assistance in positioning them, *if possible*.
- Provide radiation protection to any personnel required to stay in the room during imaging. Use pertinent gonad shielding on the patient unless it will interfere with the diagnosis.
- Seek assistance from the nurses or physicians in moving and positioning patients so that you do no further harm to them.
- Try to obtain the best images feasible with regard to the patient's condition. Two radiographs at 90-degree angles are required for all extremities, with the inclusion of at least one joint space for all long-bones.

---

must be done at once and indicates that the patient's well-being may be compromised by any delay. When more than one patient from the ED requires examination at the same time, the radiographer may need to determine which patient's status is the most urgent. Generally speaking, the highest priority is assigned to patients whose vital signs are unstable and whose immediate care depends on the results of the examination, such as those in severe respiratory distress. With two cases of apparently equal urgency, start with the patient who can be examined in the shortest amount of time, because this decision will result in the shortest total waiting period.

DISASTER RESPONSE

A *disaster* is an emergency of huge magnitude that creates an unforeseen, serious, or immediate threat to public health. It may be a natural event, such as a tornado, earthquake, flood, hurricane, or pandemic; or it could be accidental, as in the case of a plane crash or train wreck. Events of terrorism may be classified as man-made disasters.

Every hospital is required to have a carefully designed and written disaster plan, and each member of the health care team must be familiar with the plan and his or her role in it. Table 15-2 provides a standardized version of disaster code definitions. Disaster drills are regularly scheduled exercises that prepare the hospital staff to function effectively if the disaster plan must be implemented. A major disaster may involve all emergency services in the community, so your hospital may coordinate its drills with those of other agencies. You must be familiar with the plan for your institution and actively participate in the practice drills.

The process of identifying the victims, performing initial examinations, and assigning priorities for further care is called *triage*. A triage station is set up in a large area, such as a lobby. The triage officer, usually an emergency care physician, directs triage activity. Simplified methods of patient identification and record keeping are used to minimize the time required for paperwork. Typically, patients are assigned numbers that are written on tags and attached to their wrists or ankles. These are used to identify the radiographs and any required records.

Although disaster plans differ from hospital to hospital, certain elements are similar. A single person is responsible for the overall implementation of the plan.

TABLE 15-2   Standardized Emergency Code Communication

Code Name	Meaning
Red	Fire
Blue	Cardiac arrest or cessation of respiration
Orange	Hazardous material spill or release
Grey	Combative person
Silver	Weapon or hostage situation
Amber	Infant/child abduction
Internal triage	Internal disaster
External triage	External disaster
Rapid Response Team	Team response for a deteriorating medical condition
Trauma team	Team response for trauma patients
Code clear	Situation has been resolved

This person is immediately notified of the nature and scope of the disaster and evaluates the need for additional personnel, coordinating activities with other institutions and governmental agencies as required. A special communications network, established in advance, is used to notify all the necessary personnel who are not on duty. This system can be referred to as a *phone tree* and consists of a series of telephone calls, with each person called contacting three or four others before leaving home for the hospital. Text messaging may be substituted for phone calls. These methods provide rapid notification to many people without jamming the hospital telephone lines. As the health care team assembles, a group leader in each department will assign personnel to specific activities. In such a situation, you may be expected to perform services other than radiography, such as caring for less severely injured victims, answering the phone, or keeping records.

After the disaster is under control and normal procedures are reestablished, it is important to conduct a situational debriefing. Although this may appear bureaucratic, it provides an opportunity to summarize events and evaluate activities that could have been handled more efficiently. The intense pressure accompanying a disaster allows individuals to function far above their usual level of proficiency. Often this is followed by postsituational stress that can last for some time. Debriefing provides an opportunity to express fear, doubts, and grief, and can help avoid a prolonged reaction to such events.

Although victims of natural disasters, motor vehicle accidents, or other catastrophic events can arrive at the trauma unit at any moment, emergencies can also occur inside a health care facility. A staff member can suffer a serious fall, a visitor can suffer a cardiac event in the waiting room, or the condition of a patient on the x-ray table can suddenly deteriorate. Before we discuss any specific conditions, you should learn how to obtain assistance in an acute situation. The process of obtaining help will vary depending on your circumstances. When other team members are nearby, use a loud, firm voice to call for a specific person by name, for example, "Dr. Logan, please come to Room 3 immediately." Your control over the situation is reassuring to the patient and will be more effective than a distressed cry such as "Help!"

EMERGENCY CODE RESPONSE

Emergency Call Systems

When working alone, or when qualified assistance is not immediately available, you can obtain help by using the emergency call system. Each hospital has a procedure for summoning emergency help, and several different codes may be used to identify specific situations. The fire code mentioned in Chapter 7 is one example. Other codes may be used to announce the arrival of trauma patients in the ED or to cope with a situation that demands security personnel. If you need to summon help for a patient suffering from cardiopulmonary arrest, there is also a special code for this emergency (see Table 15-2).

Assisting the Emergency Response Team

Hospitals have a designated group of health care workers who respond to this type of code. The emergency response team, or code team, usually consists of one or more physicians, several nurses, a respiratory therapist, and an electrocardiographer.

When a code is called in the diagnostic imaging department, you must know your role and be completely familiar with what is expected of you with respect to your training. Once the emergency response team arrives and takes over, tell them the history of the situation and then stand by to follow their directions. There will be important tasks that you can perform. Record keeping is essential. Write down the time the emergency started and when the code team responded. You may be asked to record times and amounts of medications. It may be necessary to obtain equipment, call for other personnel, or monitor a telephone. It is important to keep unnecessary bystanders out of the way and to keep family members calm in an appropriate location, such as a waiting room.

You should practice going through each code procedure until you feel comfortable and can function professionally, even under very stressful circumstances. Recent research shows that **Rapid Response Teams** save lives. These teams are trained to intervene and assist caregivers before a patient's condition deteriorates to the point of a full-blown code condition.

> **!** You should call for help whenever you question the deterioration of a patient's condition.

Emergency Carts

Emergency carts, or *crash carts,* are rolling, multidrawered cabinets kept in strategic locations throughout the hospital (Figure 15-1). The code team usually brings the cart from the location closest to the patient. These carts vary somewhat, but each has certain essential items, such as airways, artificial ventilation equipment, emergency medications and the equipment for administering them, a board to slip under the patient when giving external cardiac massage, a blood pressure cuff, a stethoscope, and a defibrillator that can also serve as a cardiac monitor. Box 15-2 lists the equipment commonly found on an emergency cart. The cart should have a list of contents and should be inspected daily to ensure that emergency supplies are available for instant use and that their dates are within the expiry limits. Some hospitals seal the cart after supplies are replenished. *Never borrow equipment or supplies from the emergency set for routine use!* This practice results in the absence of life-saving items when they are most needed.

Table 15-3 lists the medications typically found on an emergency cart and can help to familiarize you with common emergency drugs and their actions. It is extremely important to learn both the proprietary (trade) and generic names. If a drug should be requested by its trade name, and the emergency stock is the generic equivalent by a different manufacturer, you must be able to quickly identify the correct medication by its generic name. This table is not meant to be a substitute for thorough knowledge of the contents of the emergency cart in your clinical setting.

Some emergency carts contain bags of IV solutions to which potent medications, such as lidocaine, have already been added. These medicated IV solutions should be stored in a different part of the cart so that they can be more easily differentiated from routine IV fluids. Because items may be stored incorrectly in the emergency cart, you must never select a medication or IV solution solely on the basis of its location. Always double-check the labels on any medications or solutions as you remove them from the cart.

> **!** Do not allow the urgency of the moment to interfere with the use of correct procedures.

After an emergency cart has been used, it must be restocked and prepared again for an emergency.

PATIENT ASSESSMENT

Patients come to the imaging department in widely varying states of health. As you use the skills you learned in Chapters 10 and 11, you will be able to assess patients and observe changes in their clinical signs and conditions. Individuals suffering from prolonged illness or trauma, or those weakened by extensive preparation for examination, may suffer a sudden, life-threatening change in status. Patients with a history of chronic cardiac or pulmonary disease are at greater risk when an invasive procedure is performed. Before any patient is injected with a contrast medium or subjected to an invasive procedure, a thorough history of previous cardiac events, allergies, chronic diseases, and medications should be taken. Baseline vital signs must also be taken and recorded.

Patients in the ED are classified as *nonurgent, urgent,* or *life-threatening.* Obviously, the most acute cases are seen first. Despite the specialized care available in the United States today, trauma is the most common cause of death for individuals younger than age 40. Deciding the order in which patients should receive treatment is ultimately the ED physician's responsibility.

> Trauma is the most common cause of death for individuals under 40 years old.

Families of trauma victims can be distraught and demanding when they perceive that others are being cared for first. On these occasions, your role is to reassure and explain to concerned individuals how priorities are set in such emergency situations.

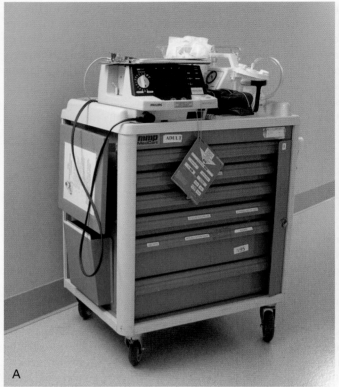
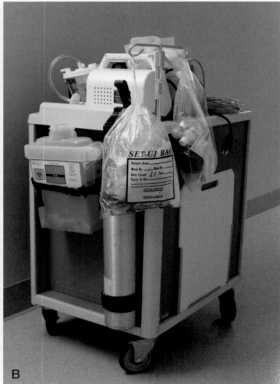
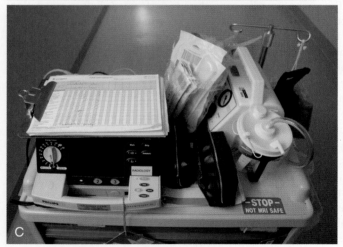

FIG 15-1 Emergency Cart. A, Front view. Drawers hold medications and small equipment. **B,** Additional equipment attached to back and sides: CPR backboard, intravenous pole, and oxygen tank. **C,** The top of the crash cart holds a defibrillator *(left),* a stethoscope and sphygmomanometer (in the case), and a portable suction unit *(right).* Note the cart contents checklist on top of the defibrillator.

BOX 15-2   Equipment Commonly Found on the Code Cart

Backboard	Needles, syringes
Bag valve mask	Pen, paper, checklist for
Blood collection tubes	cart contents
Blood pressure cuff	Protective gowns, eye-
Carbon dioxide detector	wear, masks
for ET tube placement	Scissors
Cardiac monitor	Sterile and nonsterile
Cutdown tray	gloves
Defibrillator	Stethoscope
Drugs according to institu-	Suction bottle
tional protocol	Suction catheters
Endotracheal tubes	Tongue blades
Flashlight	Tracheostomy tubes
Hemostat	IV solutions and tubing
Laryngoscope	IV cannulas

TABLE 15-3   Emergency Cart Medications

Agent	Action
Adrenalin (epinephrine)	Vasoconstrictor, increases cardiac output, raises blood pressure, aids respiration by relaxing the bronchioles
Amiodarone	Cardiac antidysrhythmic medication
Atropine	Respiratory/circulatory stimulant; dries up secretions
Calcium chloride	Combats tetany
Decadron (dexamethasone)	Anti-inflammatory
Dextrose 50%	Treats hyperkalemia
Dilantin (phenytoin)	Anticonvulsant
Glucagon	Reverses hypoglycemia
Heparin	Inhibits blood coagulation
Isuprel (isoproterenol)	Relieves bronchospasm
Levophed (norepinephrine)	Increases blood pressure, treats shock
Narcan (naloxone)	Opioid antagonist
Nitrostat (nitroglycerin)	Vasodilator, relaxes walls of blood vessels, increases circulation
Sodium bicarbonate	Combats acidosis
Solu-Medrol (methylprednisolone)	Anti-inflammatory
Sterile water	Diluent
Valium (diazepam)	Tranquilizer, antiseizure agent
Vasopressin	Vasoconstrictor
Verapamil	Cardiac antidysrhythmic medication, specific to paroxysmal supraventricular tachycardia (PSVT)
Xylocaine (lidocaine)	Anesthetic, cardiac antidysrhythmic medication

OXYGEN AND SUCTION

As a radiographer, you will encounter many patients who need supplemental oxygen. Because the need for oxygen and/or suction can be sudden and dramatic, you should be familiar with the mechanics of both wall-mounted and mobile systems. The administration of oxygen is noninvasive. Until a physician can evaluate the patient, it is appropriate to provide a low flow rate of oxygen to any patient who experiences acute anxiety accompanied by a rapid heart rate and shortness of breath. Oxygen is prescribed for patients with a wide range of illnesses and in any case of trauma that impairs oxygen uptake.

Oxygen Administration

Oxygen can be administered by various means. Tubing with nasal prongs (sometimes called a *nasal cannula*) is the simplest and most frequently used device for longer-term oxygen administration (Procedure 15-1). Always ensure that the oxygen is flowing through the tubing before placing it on the patient. The oxygen should be delivered at a rate of 1 to 6 L/min providing a 24% to 45% oxygen concentration. The oxygen supply can sometimes be warmed and/or humidified.

An oxygen mask is used to provide both oxygen and humidity. It is shaped to conform to the patient's face and held in place by an elastic strap. A simple face mask (Figure 15-2) is used primarily for short-term therapy because it is somewhat uncomfortable and the patient is unable to eat or drink when it is in place. It delivers oxygen concentrations that vary from 40% to 60%, depending on the fit and the oxygen flow rate. All departments should be equipped with pocket face masks in obvious locations in each room. Masks must be transparent for detection of regurgitation, a tight fit to the face, and furnished with an oxygen inlet. They should be available in a range of sizes to fit adults, children, and infants.

PROCEDURE 15-1   A NASAL CANNULA FOR THE ADMINISTRATION OF OXYGEN

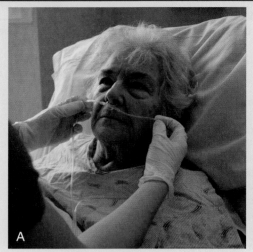

A, Position the prongs gently at nasal openings.

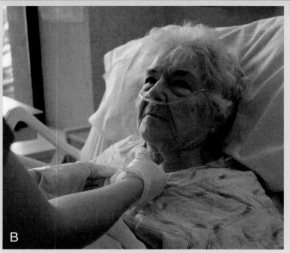

B, Wrap the tubes behind the ears and secure them together with fastener under the patient's chin.

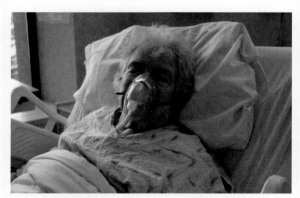

FIG 15-2 A simple oxygen face mask.

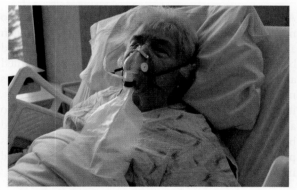

FIG 15-3 A nonrebreathing oxygen face mask.

To administer oxygen using a face mask, attach the mask to the oxygen supply and adjust the flow meter to deliver 1 to 10 L/min, as ordered. Place the mask over the nose and mouth, and slip the elastic band over the patient's head.

A nonrebreathing mask (Figure 15-3) has an attached reservoir bag that fills with 100% oxygen and a valve to prevent exhaled gas from being inhaled again. This mask can supply 100% oxygen to the patient when used properly. Partial rebreathing masks allow some exhaled air to enter the reservoir bag and can deliver oxygen at 40% to 70% concentrations.

High-flow masks are designed to administer the oxygen volume required by the patient and the concentration of oxygen is more accurately controlled. The Venturi mask (Figure 15-4) is an example of this type; it can deliver a controlled oxygen concentration of 24% to 60%. Because of the ability to precisely control the concentration of oxygen with this mask, it is recommended for patients with **chronic obstructive pulmonary disease (COPD)**. Physicians prescribe these specialized masks to meet specific patient needs.

An oxygen tent is used when a higher rate of humidity and oxygen is necessary than is available in the

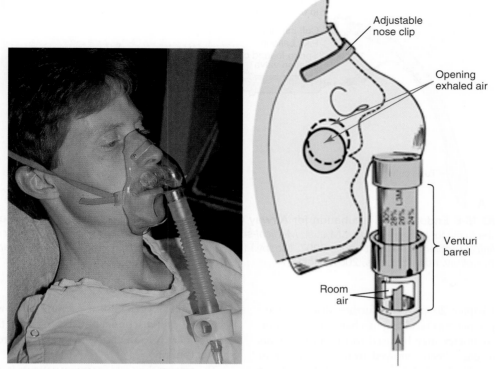

Adjustable
nose clip

Opening
exhaled air

Venturi
barrel

Room
air

FIG 15-4 A Venturi mask, an example of a high-flow oxygen mask. (From Potter PA, Perry AG, Stockert PA, Hall A: *Fundamentals of nursing,* ed 8, St Louis, 2013, Elsevier.)

ambient air. Tents are used most frequently in the pediatric department because children tolerate them better. If you are required to x-ray a patient in a tent, check with the nursing staff before turning off the oxygen, and complete the procedure as quickly as you can. Be sure to replace the tent and side rail. Ensure that the mist and oxygen are adjusted to the required levels before leaving the area.

Most patients receiving oxygen therapy function adequately with the aid of an oxygen supply and nasal prongs. Others, who require long-term respiratory support and airway management, may require endotracheal intubation or tracheostomy to maintain an open airway for oxygen administration.

Although the term **intubation** can refer to the placement of any tube, it is most commonly used to indicate the placement of an airway tube into the trachea. The usual placement is orotracheal intubation where, with the assistance of a laryngoscope, an endotracheal tube (ET tube or ETT) is passed through the oral cavity into

the trachea (Figure 15-5). However, placement through the nasopharyngeal cavity is sometimes used. The ETT is regarded as a very reliable method for protecting a patient's airway and ensuring that air can reach the lungs.

A **tracheostomy** is a surgical opening through the anterior neck into the trachea. An artificial airway that can be connected to the oxygen supply is inserted into the trachea through the tracheostomy. Both ETTs and tracheostomy tubes can be connected either directly to an oxygen supply or to a ventilator.

A **ventilator** is a mechanical respiratory device powered by compressed air that controls respiratory rate, volume of inspiration, and oxygen content. When positioning a patient with an artificial airway for a radiograph, take care not to disconnect or kink the tubing. An alarm on the ventilator alerts the staff to any sudden changes in respiration. If the alarm sounds while positioning the patient, do not turn it off. The nursing staff will monitor the procedure and help position the patient where

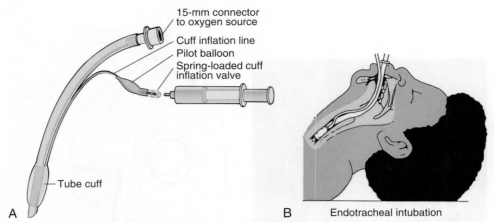

FIG 15-5 Endotracheal Intubation for Airway Control. A, Endotracheal tube. **B,** Endotracheal tube in place. (*A* From Lewis SM et al: *Medical-surgical nursing: assessment and management of clinical problems*, ed 7, St Louis, 2007, Mosby.) (*B* From Thibodeau GA, Patton KT: *Anatomy and physiology*, ed 6, St Louis, 2007, Mosby.)

necessary. Chapter 20 provides further discussion on radiography of patients receiving mechanical ventilation.

A pulse oximeter may be used to monitor patients who have recently been removed from a ventilator or whose oxygen level may be compromised. Knowledge of oxygen saturation values enables nurses to make changes in the oxygen flow rate as the patient's condition changes. Take care not to disturb the wires leading to the monitor when you move the patient.

In most imaging departments and acute care units, oxygen is available from a wall or ceiling outlet. An oxygen flow gauge for a wall unit is shown in Figure 15-6. The dial on the side, or within it, is used to adjust the flow rate, indicated by the level of the ball shown near the center of the gauge.

During transport, or in areas where oxygen is not otherwise available, portable oxygen units are used. You must be familiar with the operation of these units and the procedure for ensuring that they are immediately available when needed. The oxygen tank has an on/off valve including a dial indicating how much gas remains (Figure 15-7). A separate valve adjusts the flow rate, and an accompanying flow meter shows the delivery rate in units of liters per minute. *Both valves must be turned on to provide oxygen to the patient.* When transferring a patient, you may have to switch the oxygen supply from the wall outlet to the portable unit. First, note the flow rate. Open the main valve on

the portable oxygen tank and adjust the flow to the correct rate. Then disconnect the tubing from the wall unit and connect it to the portable tank. Be sure to turn off the wall supply.

The oxygen flow rate for many patients is 2 to 5 L/min. Severely compromised patients, such as trauma victims in shock, may receive oxygen at a much higher rate, up to 10 L/min. Patients with chronic lung disease should be provided with a Venturi mask, or if they are wearing nasal prongs, receive oxygen at a slower rate, less than 3 L/min. These patients must not receive a higher flow rate, because, unlike the case of normal patients whose blood carbon dioxide level controls their breathing reflex, it is the level of oxygen that controls the rate of respiration for these patients. High oxygen flow rates can depress their respiratory drive so that respiration becomes too slow for adequate ventilation. If you are caring for a patient who is already receiving oxygen, note the flow rate and check periodically that it is correctly maintained.

> **!** Patients with COPD should receive oxygen at rates *no higher* than 3L/min.

Suction

Mechanical suction is used when a patient is unable to clear the mouth and throat of secretions, blood, or

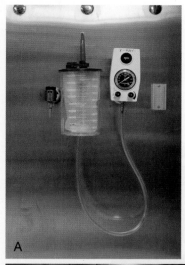

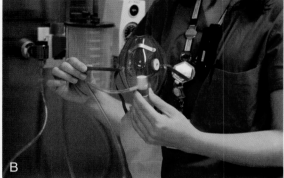

FIG 15-6 A, An oxygen flow meter, green unit, *left,* and suction system, *right,* at wall outlets. **B,** After turning on the oxygen and setting the flow rates, check to ensure oxygen is flowing through the tubing and then attach the mask or cannula.

- An adequate length of tubing connects the suction catheter to the receptacle.
- An assortment of disposable, flexible suction catheters is on hand for deep tracheobronchial suction by a qualified emergency response provider.
- A rigid pharyngeal catheter device (Yankeur) is available to clean foreign material from the mouth and pharynx.

Be alert to the need for suction whenever a patient feels nauseated, is bleeding from the mouth or nose, or is unable to swallow and cope with secretions because of a low level of consciousness. If a patient begins to aspirate mucus or vomitus, turn him/her immediately into the lateral recumbent position, don gloves and protective eyewear, and attempt to clear the airway manually. Remember to stand to one side when clearing an airway, because a sudden, violent expulsion of the obstructing material may spray your face. If a reflex cough does not clear the airway at this point, suction is needed.

It is unusual for a radiographer to work alone with an unconscious patient who is likely to aspirate. Such patients are usually accompanied by a nurse or physician, and your role is to assist in the procedure. Unwrap the appropriate suction tip, attach it to the suction apparatus, and turn on the suction. At this point, the nurse proceeds with suctioning while you hold the patient in position. When the emergency is over, clean or replace the receptacle and replace the disposable tip and tubing so that the suction unit will be ready for use when needed.

If you must suction the patient yourself, use your emergency call button or call for help while you unwrap the catheter and turn on the suction. After you have cleared the patient's mouth, pull the chin down and forward while inserting the suction catheter tip over the tongue in the midline. Do not insert the catheter forcibly, because you may injure the larynx. Use the suction tip called *a Yankeur* or *tonsil tip suction catheter* to clear the pharynx. Any suctioning beyond the pharynx should be done by a physician or someone trained in this procedure, such as those certified in advanced cardiac life support (ACLS).

vomitus. Most hospitals today have a wall-mounted suction apparatus (Figure 15-8), but some areas of the imaging department may still rely on moveable machines. You should know the location of the portable unit. If suction procedures were not part of your orientation, you must assume responsibility yourself for understanding and learning how to operate this equipment. When you are responsible for ensuring that the suction system is in working order, check that:
- The pump is working.
- The receptacle is connected to the pump.

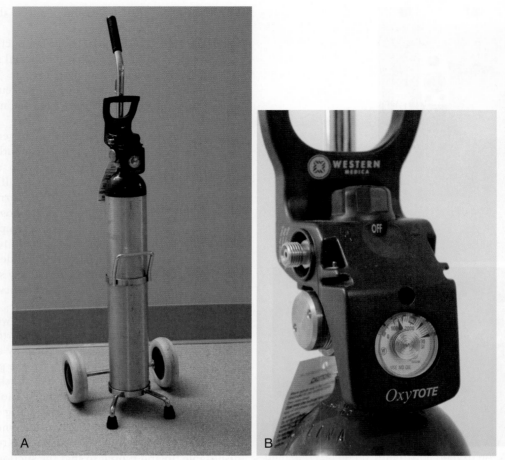

FIG 15-7 A portable oxygen system supports the oxygen needs of a patient during transport and in areas where oxygen is not otherwise available. A, Portable oxygen tank. B, Oxygen tank controls and gauge.

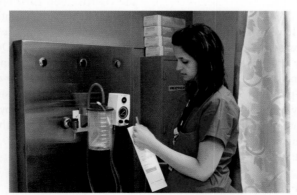

FIG 15-8 A wall-mounted suction apparatus ready for use.

SUMMARY

- An emergency is a condition that requires immediate attention. EDs in hospitals are staffed and equipped to handle emergencies. Certain hospitals are designated trauma centers. A Level I trauma center is prepared to handle all emergencies, including the most severe and life threatening.
- The basic rules of trauma radiography include arriving prepared in the trauma suite, obtaining diagnostic images by the least harmful method possible, and reducing radiation exposure to the patient and personnel. Take two 90-degree images of the site of interest and include as much of the injured area as possible.
- In the past, x-ray protocols dictated that chest, pelvis, and cross-table lateral cervical spine images be taken. However, most trauma patients now undergo only minimal radiographs, such as a chest x-ray, before going directly to the CT scanner. Films of the extremities will typically be acquired after the CT scan, either in the radiographic room or with a mobile unit in the trauma bay.
- All hospitals are required to have a disaster plan for handling a large number of emergencies at one time.

Radiographers must be familiar with the disaster plan for their facility and with their role in the plan.
- A standardized emergency code communication system is in place at every hospital. These codes are designed to be an efficient means of mass communication with the entire hospital staff.
- An emergency cart, or crash cart, should be readily available for use in an emergency. Typically, they are strategically placed throughout the hospital and contain essential items like airway access, medications, a cardiopulmonary resuscitation (CPR) board, a blood pressure cuff, other monitoring devices, and a defibrillator.
- Supplemental oxygen administration is a treatment for many conditions in which the oxygen supply to body tissues would otherwise be inadequate. Oxygen is usually administered through nasal prongs at a rate of 1 to 6 L/min.
- Suction equipment is used to clear the airway of liquid or semiliquid obstruction such as mucus or vomitus.

REVIEW QUESTIONS

1. Patients who are experiencing difficulty breathing and who do not have emphysema may safely receive supplemental oxygen though a nasal cannula at a flow rate of:
   A. 100%
   B. 1 to 6 L/min
   C. 5 to 10 L/min
   D. 10 to 20 L/min
2. Your patient collapses on the floor in front of you. After shaking him/her and calling his/her name without any response, you decide to activate the code system. Which standardized code would be the most appropriate code for you to call?
   A. Red
   B. Blue
   C. Orange
   D. Amber
3. Code Grey means:
   A. a combative patient
   B. the patient has an obstructed airway

   C. a hostage situation
   D. a hazardous material spill/release
4. The most appropriate type of oxygen administration device to provide a patient with 100% oxygen is:
   A. nasal prongs
   B. a partial rebreathing face mask
   C. a nonrebreathing face mask
   D. an oxygen tent
5. A procedure that is ordered as STAT should be performed:
   A. only when a physician is present
   B. before the day's end
   C. as soon as is practical
   D. immediately
6. During trauma radiography, care must be taken to:
   A. cause no further harm to the patient
   B. proceed with imaging as slowly as possible
   C. obtain textbook quality images by moving the patient into standard positions
   D. manipulate the patient into position as quickly as possible

7. Equipment that may be necessary for trauma radiography includes:
   A. positioning aids such as tape and/or sponges
   B. cassette covers
   C. lead aprons and shielding
   D. all of the above

8. The primary purpose of an impermeable cassette cover is to:
   A. cushion the patient from the hard cassette
   B. keep the cassette free from blood and body fluids
   C. allow the cassette to slide better under the patient
   D. avoid the need to disinfect the equipment after the examination

9. Trauma patients should only be removed from a backboard if/when:
   A. their spines have been cleared by a physician
   B. they ask to be removed
   C. they need to vomit
   D. they need to use the restroom

10. The purpose of the Rapid Response Team is to:
    A. transfer patients rapidly from one location to the next
    B. treat patients before their condition deteriorates
    C. investigate and monitor patient complaints
    D. prevent patients from exiting the building

Answers can be found in the Answer Key on pages 429-431.

CRITICAL THINKING EXERCISES

1. Suppose it was necessary to "call a code" and the patient has been successfully resuscitated. What tasks remain to be completed before and after the patient leaves the department?

2. Three requisitions come across on the printer for three different patients in the Emergency Room; each one is ordered STAT. The first patient has an abdominal series ordered for possible bowel obstruction. The second patient needs a foot x-ray to rule out the presence of a foreign body, and the third patient has a chest x-ray ordered for syncope. Describe the order in which you would image these patients and list the reasons why.

3. You have gone to get a patient from the ED who is receiving oxygen. While disconnecting various monitoring devices, you notice the pulse oximeter is measuring an 80% saturation rate and the monitor's alarm is sounding. What does this mean? Is it safe to take the patient to the x-ray room for the examination? What steps can you take to ensure the patient is receiving the required amount of oxygen?

4. The intensive care unit has ordered an abdominal x-ray series on Mrs. Klipp to rule out the presence of a bowel obstruction. She was admitted to the unit for a ground level fall in which she hit her head and is now in a cervical collar. Additionally, she seems somewhat disoriented, and suffers from extreme nausea. She cannot sit up because her spine has not been cleared. While performing the x-rays, Mrs. Klipp says she thinks she may throw up. Describe how you would assist her if she does vomit. In which position should you place her to prevent aspiration? What equipment may be necessary to help clear her airway?

16

Dealing with Acute Situations

OBJECTIVES

At the conclusion of this chapter, the student will be able to:

- Discuss the procedures for assisting patients during attacks of respiratory distress, myocardial infarction, stroke, asthma, epistaxis, angina, nausea, and syncope.
- List the four levels of consciousness and explain how the Glasgow Coma Scale can contribute to defining these levels.
- List the precautions to be taken in handling patients with possible fractures of the spine, ribs, or extremities.
- Recognize the signs of shock and respond appropriately.

- Explain the differences between syncope and vertigo.
- Contrast diabetic coma or hyperglycemia and insulin shock or hypoglycemia.
- Contrast diabetic ketoacidosis with hyperosmolar hyperglycemic nonketotic syndrome.
- Discuss seizure disorders, including the safety precautions and observations to be recorded.
- Identify the need for CPR; recognize the indications for using an AED and list the steps involved.

OUTLINE

KEY TERMS

anaphylaxis
angina pectoris
anoxia
asthma
cardiac arrest
cardiac tamponade
cerebrovascular accident (CVA)
concussion
defibrillator
dehiscence
embolus

epistaxis
erythema
evisceration
hemorrhage
hemothorax
hyperglycemia
hypoglycemia
myocardial ischemia
myocardial infarction (MI)
pleural effusion
pneumonia

pneumothorax
pulmonary edema
respiratory arrest
stridor
syncope
thoracentesis
thoracotomy
thrombus
tremor
urticaria
vasovagal

The clinical situations discussed in this chapter are circumstances encountered by radiographers in an acute care setting. Each has the potential to result in serious harm to the patient if not recognized and treated correctly, or when appropriate precautions are not observed. These conditions will often require you to request help, but first you must recognize the problem and the need for intervention.

RESPIRATORY EMERGENCIES

Airway Obstruction

Blockage of a patient's airway is a life-threatening situation. The obstruction may be caused by a solid object, but in a hospital setting is more likely to involve liquid or semiliquid material. This may be mucus, blood, or vomitus that cannot be expelled by a patient who is unconscious or semiconscious and this situation requires an immediate response. Call the code for a respiratory emergency and prepare suction for use. The emergency response and the use of suction are discussed in Chapter 15.

Respiratory arrest caused by choking can occur, for example, when an older person has difficulty chewing food, such as a piece of meat. To avoid embarrassment, the person may swallow the meat whole, causing it to lodge in the larynx. The combination of talking while eating and poorly fitting dentures may predispose individuals to choking incidents.

When any foreign body lodges in the opening of the trachea, victims becomes quite agitated, their faces become congested, and they may tear at their collars or clutch at their throats. Because the lungs hold more air than is normally used during respiration, the reserve supply can be used to help dislodge the foreign body by using a technique called the abdominal thrust (Heimlich Maneuver). Ask, "Are you choking?" If the person cannot speak but nods the head to indicate "yes," you need to perform the Heimlich Maneuver. Tell the person what you are about to do. Place your arms around the victim's waist from behind. With your thumb on the outside of your fist, place the fist on the abdomen just below the sternum, and with the other hand grasp your wrist. Quickly and forcefully apply pressure upward against the diaphragm just below the ribs (Procedure 16-1). This will compress the lungs and will frequently expel the aspirated object. Never insert your fingers into the mouth of a conscious patient in an effort to retrieve an obstructing object. A severe bite injury can occur or the obstructing material may be forced farther into the throat during the struggle. If any foreign material is visible in the mouth of an unconscious patient, use gloved fingers to grasp the tongue and lower jaw. Insert the index finger of the other hand at the base of the tongue and sweep it forward to clear the obstruction. This should never be done for children if the obstruction is not clearly visible and easily accessible.

> **!** *Never* perform a blind finger-sweep as it may force the object further into the throat.

Children more frequently aspirate foreign objects such as large wads of chewing gum, buttons, small toys, or coins that have been held in the mouth. Many of the

PROCEDURE 16-1   ABDOMINAL THRUST (HEIMLICH MANEUVER)

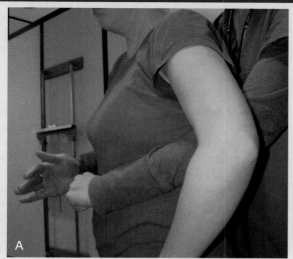

A, Encircling the victim from behind, place the knuckles of your left fist over solar plexus.

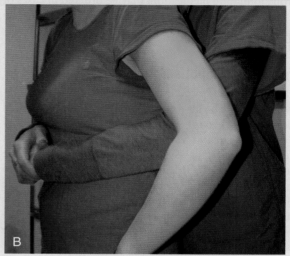

B, Grasp the left wrist with the right hand. Squeeze forcefully and quickly against diaphragm.

deaths from foreign body aspiration occur in children less than 1 year of age. Consumer product safety standards regulating the minimum sizes for toys and toy parts for young children have markedly decreased the incidence of fatal aspiration incidents.

Foreign body obstruction should always be suspected in children when there is a sudden onset of coughing or **stridor** (a harsh sound on inspiration). In infants, if respiration and coughing stop:

1. Turn the infant prone with the head lower than the trunk.
2. Support the head by firmly holding the jaw.
3. Deliver up to five forceful back blows between the shoulder blades using the heel of the hand.
4. While supporting the head and neck, turn the infant over, head lower than torso.
5. Place the two middle fingers on the sternum just below the nipple line.
6. Administer five thrusts over the sternum, taking care not to press over the liver.
7. Repeat steps as necessary until help arrives.

For children ages 1 to 8 years old, you may use the same Heimlich Maneuver as in the case of adults, with a series of quick subdiaphragmatic thrusts. Use your good judgment in determining the amount of force, however, because young children have a relatively large and

unprotected liver. The smaller the child, the greater the chance that damage to the liver may occur.

Reactive Airway Disease

The term *reactive airway disease* is not a specific diagnosis; it is a general term used to describe the conditions characterized by coughing, wheezing, or shortness of breath with an undetermined cause. When these symptoms are present, asthma is one of the possible causes. Some doctors use the terms "reactive airway disease" and "asthma" interchangeably, but they are not necessarily the same thing.

Asthma is difficulty in breathing caused by bronchospasm. Asthmatic attacks are sometimes related to allergies and are frequently precipitated by stress. If the radiologic procedure is new or frightening, dyspnea may result. Most individuals with chronic asthma carry a metered dose inhaler with a bronchodilating medication. Patients with asthma should take their medication with them into the examining room.

In the event of an acute episode of reactive airway disease, call for assistance. The usual treatment is to administer oxygen to keep the O_2 saturation level above 92%. The administration of albuterol by inhaler or nebulizer and parenteral administration of corticosteroids may be ordered by the responding physician. Subcutaneous injections of epinephrine or terbutaline (Brethine), a bronchodilating medication, may be ordered in cases of a severe attack. Although it is frightening for both the patient and the radiographer, a single such attack is seldom fatal.

Pulmonary Embolism

Another respiratory emergency that the prudent radiographer should be aware of is the lung condition called *pulmonary embolism* (PE). A pulmonary embolus is a substance such as a blood clot, fat, or air that travels through the vascular system and lodges in one of the pulmonary vessels. This interrupts the flow of blood to the lungs, increasing the pressure on the right ventricle of the heart. Part of the lung can die as a result of this obstruction, and if the blockage is massive enough, the patient can go into shock. A PE occurs most frequently as a complication of a thrombus formation in one or both lower extremities. The clot forms on the vessel wall and then breaks loose, causing one or many emboli. The signs and symptoms of PE are nonspecific, meaning they are similar to other respiratory or cardiac emergencies, so this respiratory emergency can often be overlooked or its discovery may be delayed.

There is a high index of suspicion of a PE when risk factors are present. Some risk factors include recent surgery or trauma of the lower extremity, smoking, heart failure, chronic obstructive pulmonary disease, cancer, prolonged immobilization, and pregnancy. Patients with unexplained dyspnea, tachypnea, or chest pain may be referred for a chest radiograph, although the purpose may actually be to rule out any other underlying causes, since most initial chest radiographs are negative for the presence of a PE unless the embolus has been present long enough to cause tissue necrosis. Computed tomography angiography (CTA) (see Chapter 22) of the chest is the primary method for detecting a PE. The treatment includes anticoagulation therapy, such as the administration of heparin and/or warfarin, and supportive measures such as oxygen and pain relief. In severe cases, the surgical removal of the embolus may be required.

CARDIAC EMERGENCIES
Acute Coronary Syndrome

Acute coronary syndrome (ACS) is an umbrella term used to cover a group of clinical symptoms that may indicate acute myocardial ischemia. Myocardial ischemia is a condition where an insufficient blood supply to the heart muscle results from coronary artery disease. ACS thus includes a spectrum of clinical conditions ranging from chest pain to a life-threatening heart attack. Electrocardiography is used to assess the nature and severity of ACS (see Chapter 11).

Myocardial Infarction

Myocardial infarction (MI) is the medical term for what is also called a heart attack. When a coronary artery becomes occluded, a portion of the heart wall becomes ischemic, and the heart muscle supplied by the artery will die if the blood flow is not quickly restored.

When a patient complains of sudden, intense chest pain, often described as a crushing pain, you should assume that he/she is having a heart attack until it is proved otherwise. Patients may underestimate the importance of this type of pain and assume instead that the sudden onset of pain is terrible heartburn or indigestion. Pain may be referred to the left arm, jaw, or neck. These patients often become diaphoretic, have an irregular heartbeat, become pale, and may feel nauseated and short of breath. In occasional cases of MI, these symptoms are present with little or no pain. You must prevent further damage by minimizing patient exertion. Call a physician, stay with the patient, and assist him/her to a comfortable position. If the patient has shortness of breath, raise the head of the bed or stretcher and administer oxygen at 2 to 4 L/min. The treatment for MI varies and may include the administration of pain medication, aspirin, oxygen, and often vasodilating and/or clot-dissolving drugs.

> **!** If a patient experiences an MI while in the imaging department, avert any further damage by preventing the patient from exerting him/herself and call for help.

Angina Pectoris

Angina pectoris, often shortened to "angina," occurs when the coronary arteries are unable to supply the heart with sufficient oxygen. These episodes of chest pain are precipitated by exertion or stress and are usually relieved by rest or the sublingual administration of nitroglycerin (see Chapter 14). The discomfort caused by angina varies from a vague ache to an intense crushing sensation. It is frequently mistaken for indigestion, because it often presents as pain under the sternum. If the substernal pain is not immediately relieved with rest, inform the radiologist and prepare a dose of a vasodilating medication such as nitroglycerin. A second dose may be ordered 5 minutes later. Although you may not be permitted to administer the medication, you should have the dosage on hand to assist a qualified person, such as a physician or nurse. An emergency supply of nitroglycerin is usually stocked in the imaging department.

Cardiac Arrest

For health care workers, one of the most anxiety-producing situations is to discover an unconscious patient or observe a patient suddenly lose consciousness. When this occurs, it is important to initiate the "shake and shout" maneuver. Patients who have simply fainted will respond if you call out their name and give them a gentle but firm shake. If there is no response, feel for the carotid pulse and observe for respiration. If the patient has stopped breathing, or if no pulse is detected, an emergency code must be initiated to summon an emergency response team immediately.

> **!** If a patient is unresponsive and no pulse or respiration can be detected, initiate an emergency code immediately and begin CPR.

Under most circumstances, the emergency response team will arrive less than a minute after being called. Time is vital, because the lack of effective circulation to the central nervous system can cause irreparable brain damage in 3 to 5 minutes. While awaiting the code team, you should proceed with cardiopulmonary resuscitation (CPR). As stated in Chapter 15, you must allow the emergency response personnel to take over immediately when they arrive. They will initiate or continue CPR. Stand by to keep record of any medication administration and/or defibrillation. Your help may be needed to connect the patient to the cardiac monitor. The monitor is connected by means of electrode wires that snap onto adhesive disks, which are attached to the patient's upper and left lateral torso (see Chapter 11). The wire electrodes and adhesive pads are stored with the monitor. Learn to check the monitor and its related supplies in your area. You should know how to connect a patient to the monitor, print a tape of the monitor reading, and change the tape when necessary. Because cardiac monitors vary, use

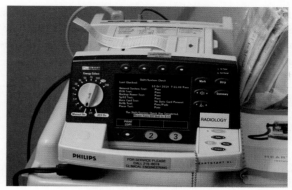

FIG 16-1 Defibrillator.

of this equipment should be part of your departmental orientation and in-service instruction.

Defibrillation

With the help of the cardiac monitor, the code team may determine that the **defibrillator** (Figure 16-1) is needed. This machine administers an electric shock to correct an ineffectual cardiac rhythm. The defibrillator does not need to be plugged in because it has an auxiliary battery system for use beyond the reach of electrical outlets. It must be turned on and set at the proper voltage. Two paddles attached to the machine make contact with the patient's chest. The paddle surfaces must be covered with disposable pads to protect the skin and facilitate the electrical contact. Some facilities use posterior and anterior gel pads for chest contacts; others place a paddle on each side of the chest. Once the defibrillator pads are in place, they can be used to assess cardiac rhythm by means of a special "quick look" mode option. When the equipment and the team are ready, CPR is interrupted, and the defibrillator operator announces that he or she is about to deliver a shock. The operator will give a warning "chant," such as, "I'm clear. You're clear. All clear." The operator then makes a visual check to ensure that no one is in contact with the patient or the patient's bed or stretcher. A distance of two feet is adequate. If the first shock is not successful, defibrillation may be repeated.

The initial rhythm in sudden **cardiac arrest** is usually ventricular tachycardia, followed by ventricular fibrillation. Ventricular fibrillation will convert to asystole (the heart will stop beating) within just a few minutes. Rapid defibrillation greatly increases the probability of a successful outcome. More than 50% of the victims of ventricular fibrillation can survive following early CPR if defibrillation takes place within three to five minutes. Even with early CPR, fewer than 10% of victims will survive if defibrillation cannot be initiated within 10 minutes after they collapse.

> More than 50% of ventricular fibrillation victims will survive CPR if defibrillation occurs within 3 to 5 minutes of collapse.

One device for treating cardiac arrest is the *automatic external defibrillator (AED)*. This device is very effective when used by personnel who only have a limited amount of training and is easier to learn to use than a conventional defibrillator. AEDs are becoming more commonly available in public places such as airports and restaurants. Some of these defibrillators are completely automatic and have the ability to analyze cardiac rhythm, identify ventricular tachycardia and fibrillation, and automatically deliver a shock. There is also a semiautomatic version in which the operator presses a button to start the rhythm analysis. If the AED identifies ventricular fibrillation, the need for shock is indicated, and the operator will press the shock control. The use of AEDs has been reduced to six simple steps:

1. Turn on the power.
2. Attach the adhesive pads to the victim's chest.
3. Attach pads to machine cables.
4. Clear the area.
5. Turn on the rhythm analysis. AEDs require 5 to 15 seconds to analyze the rhythm. The patient must not move during this time. Activating the analysis will also charge the AED if the rhythm is ventricular fibrillation.
6. Press the shock control to deliver the shock, if indicated.

While different brands and models of defibrillators have a variety of features, including different monitors, paper strip readouts, and operating instructions, the application of the device is simple. If your institution uses AEDs, periodic instruction will be provided. Your participation in both CPR and AED classes can help you to be prepared and effective in cardiac emergencies.

Cardiopulmonary Resuscitation

CPR is the basic life support system used to ventilate the lungs and circulate the blood in the event of a respiratory or cardiac arrest. Correct instruction in CPR is a vital part of your professional education. Your class should be given by a certified instructor, and you should take responsibility for updating your CPR card regularly. We have chosen not to provide CPR instruction here, because recommendations are updated frequently and printed materials are easily obtained from the American Heart Association or the American Red Cross. We do believe that practice on a resuscitation mannequin is essential. Your local college, fire department, and hospital in-service department may also offer courses taught by certified instructors that include lectures, videos, and practice time, plus review and testing sessions.

Even if you are certified in adult CPR, do not attempt CPR on infants or children unless you are also currently certified in pediatrics specifically. The American Heart Association's Basic Life Support (BLS) course for health care providers includes the techniques for adults, children, and infants. Most health care facilities require all imaging personnel to be BLS certified upon employment.

Occasionally, a patient who has had a *laryngectomy* is seen in the radiology department. These individuals have a permanent opening in the trachea (tracheostomy) and have had their larynx removed. They are unable to talk normally. They may have learned esophageal speech (the ability to swallow air and form words while belching it back), or they may use an artificial larynx (see Chapter 6). Care must be taken not to obstruct the airway. If a patient with a tracheostomy undergoes cardiopulmonary arrest, you must ventilate through the tracheostomy using a bag valve mask when doing CPR.

TRAUMA

Head Injuries

Trauma physicians will often start an assessment of a patient working from the head down to the feet. The doctor will verbally dictate a HEENT (head, eyes, ears, nose, and throat) examination before moving down the rest of the body. Patients who have received a blow to the head may have sustained a serious injury, even when there are no external signs of trauma. Damage may occur with or without a skull fracture. The brain is soft, has a rich blood supply, and is suspended in cerebrospinal fluid within the skull. A severe blow to the head causes the brain to bounce from side to side, resulting in injury on the side opposite the blow. This is called a *contrecoup* injury. A mild to moderate amount of damage, characterized by "seeing stars" or a very brief loss of consciousness, is called a **concussion**. If bleeding or swelling occurs inside the skull, a rise in intracranial pressure (ICP) may cause seizures, loss of consciousness, or respiratory arrest. Incidentally, similar symptoms may also occur in patients with increased ICP related to brain tumors.

As mentioned in Chapter 11, four levels of consciousness (LOC) are generally recognized and are described as follows:

1. Alert and conscious
2. Drowsy, but responsive
3. Unconscious, but reactive to painful stimuli
4. Comatose

> **!** LOC changes can reflect a variety of causes: alcohol consumption, drug overdose, pain medication, and insulin coma, among other things. Always bring an LOC change to the attention of a physician.

The Glasgow Coma Scale is a numerical scale that can be used to objectively assess changes in a patient's level of consciousness over time (Table 16-1). A patient who is alert and oriented when admitted, but then becomes increasingly incoherent, drowsy, and stuporous, may be showing signs of increased ICP. The earliest signs of increasing pressure may be irritability and lethargy, frequently associated with a slowing pulse and slow respiration. Notify the attending physician immediately if you suspect a change in LOC. Remember that an unconscious patient must have side rails in place, should not be left alone, and must be constantly monitored to maintain an airway.

Some trauma patients are under the influence of alcohol. Their condition may vary from inappropriate jocularity to an alcoholic stupor, or they may be argumentative or verbally abusive. It is easy to assume that an unconscious intoxicated patient has only "passed out" because of a high level of blood alcohol, but these patients are just as subject to sudden changes in their conditions as nonintoxicated persons. Be especially alert to LOC changes in these patients, because the effects of alcohol may obscure important signs. Patients taking pain medication, or those who are insulin dependent and have gone too long without insulin, may exhibit similar signs and symptoms.

TABLE 16-1	Glasgow Coma Scale	
Action	**Response**	**Score**
Eyes open	Spontaneously	4
	To speech	3
	To pain	2
	None	1
Verbal response	Oriented	5
	Confused	4
	Inappropriate words	3
	Incomprehensible sounds	2
	None	1
Motor response	Obeys commands	6
	Localized pain	5
	Flexion withdrawal	4
	Abnormal flexion	3
	Abnormal extension	2
	Flaccid	1
Highest possible score		15

Spinal Injuries

Every trauma patient is considered to have a potential spinal injury and must be evaluated by the emergency department (ED) physician before being moved. As stated in Chapter 15, trauma patients are transported to the hospital on a rigid backboard to prevent potentially hazardous movement of the spine. Even slight movement of a patient with a spinal fracture may cause pressure on the spinal cord, resulting in paralysis or death.

A cross-table lateral radiograph of the cervical spine is taken and evaluated by a physician before moving the patient from the backboard. When there is question of a cervical spine injury, a rigid cervical collar may be applied before the patient is moved. Additional x-ray exposures should be made without moving the patient whenever possible, especially if there is a question of a spinal fracture at any level. When a change of position is required, the three-person log roll is a good method of obtaining a lateral position while maintaining the alignment of the entire spine in the same plane without twisting or bending (Procedure 16-2). *If a patient is in a cervical collar, one person should remain at the head and stabilize the neck during the log roll.*

> **!** Patients with possible cervical spine fractures are immobilized with cervical collars and other radiolucent devices. These must remain in place during the initial radiographic examinations and until a physician has determined that it is safe for them to be removed.

PROCEDURE 16-2 "LOG-ROLL" TURNING METHOD FOR PATIENTS WITH SPINAL INJURIES

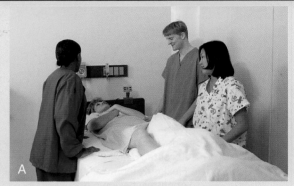

A, Position three lifters as shown. Lift the edge of the table pad or sheet.

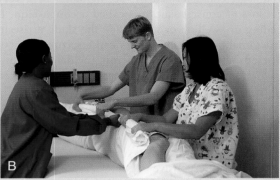

B, Maintaining the head and spinal column in one plane, turn the patient into a lateral position and place your hands on the shoulder and hip to stabilize. If a patient is in a cervical collar, one person should remain at the head and stabilize the neck during the log roll.

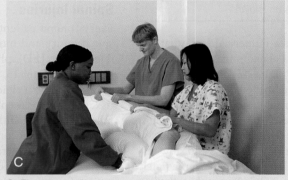

C, Flex the patient's knees to help maintain the position. Pillows may be placed along the patient's back for support.

Chest Injuries

Motor vehicle accidents and falls are two of the most common causes of chest injuries seen in the imaging department. Deaths caused by crushing or penetrating wounds of the thorax make up a significant number of trauma deaths each year. Fractured ribs are intensely painful and may be life threatening if a lung or blood vessel is punctured by the fracture fragments. If a **hemothorax** (blood in the pleural space) or **pneumothorax** (air in the pleural space) results, the lung may collapse, greatly reducing the available surface for oxygen exchange.

The treatment for either pneumothorax or hemothorax involves a **thoracotomy**, a procedure in which a surgical opening is made through the chest wall and a tube is inserted between the visceral pleura and the parietal pleura. The tubing may be connected to a water seal chest drainage system that assists the lung to expand by removing fluid or air from the pleural space (Figure 16-2). The term for this process is **thoracentesis.** The chest drainage unit is set or hung below the level of the bed or stretcher. Although the tubing is long enough to allow the patient a certain amount of movement, the unit is below the staff's usual level of vision.

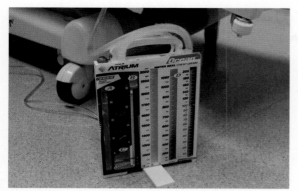

FIG 16-2 Disposable commercial chest drainage system. Take care not to disturb this unit or its attachments. It may sometimes be out of sight under the edge of the bed.

> **!** It is essential to be aware of a chest drainage unit, not to put tension on the tube or allow it to become kinked, and to always keep the unit below the level of the patient's chest.

When taking a radiograph, assess the situation carefully before moving the patient. If the patient becomes short of breath, cyanotic, or complains of chest pressure, notify the nursing staff immediately. Further discussion of treatment situations involving chest tubes and drainage units is found in Chapter 20.

Multiple rib fractures may result in a *flail chest*, a condition in which the structural integrity of the chest wall is lost and the lung collapses. When working with patients injured this severely, observe closely for signs of shock or **hemorrhage** (excessive bleeding). After their condition has been stabilized, these patients may be positioned supine or recumbent on the injured side. This allows the uninjured lung maximum expansion and facilitates adequate respiration. These patients must not be positioned for radiographic examination without the assistance of the trauma team or ICU staff.

A blunt blow to the chest may cause bruising of the heart and hemorrhage into the pericardium. This serious condition is called **cardiac tamponade.** As the pericardial sac fills with fluid, it prevents the heart from expanding and soon results in a critical situation. Because little exterior trauma may be apparent, this cause for serious concern should be considered whenever the driver in a motor vehicle accident has hit the steering wheel.

Extremity Fractures

Trauma involving the long bones of the body can be classified into two categories: (1) compound fractures, in which the splintered ends of bone are forced through the skin, and (2) closed fractures. Compound fractures are usually partially reduced and a dressing applied before radiographic examination. Fractures may also be classified according to the nature of the injury. Some common fracture types are illustrated in Figure 16-3.

There are many ways of temporarily immobilizing fractures of the long bones of the extremities. The two legs may be fastened together for stability during transportation (self-splinting), or a stiff object, such as a board or rolled-up magazine, may serve as a splint. Ambulances often carry pneumatic splints, which are air-filled sleeves that protect and immobilize the extremity.

> **!** Splints should not be removed except under the physician's direct supervision.

When you have to position a fractured extremity that is not supported by a splint, maintain gentle traction while supporting and moving the arm or leg. Two people may be required to support and position patients with a potential long bone fracture, because the extremity must be supported at sites both proximal and distal to the injury. It is important to minimize movement of the fracture fragments. This helps limit pain, prevent damage to the soft tissues around the fracture site, and avoid the initiation of a muscle spasm that could interfere with the physician's attempt to reduce and immobilize the fracture more permanently. Movement of the fracture fragments can tear the surrounding soft tissues, nerves, and blood vessels, seriously complicating the patient's condition.

Special care is required when positioning extremities following the application of a plaster cast. Undue pressure on a fresh (wet) cast may cause it to change shape. Lift the cast by placing your open hands underneath it; never grasp it from above. Observe the patient's fingers or toes for evidence of impaired circulation. They should be warm, pink, and sensitive to touch and pressure. Coldness, numbness, or lack of normal coloration should be reported to the physician immediately. Swelling inside the cast and subsequent pressure may compromise circulation and cause permanent nerve and tissue damage if it is not relieved promptly.

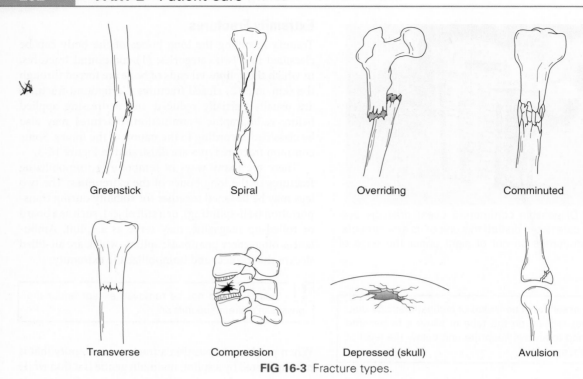

Greenstick   Spiral   Overriding   Comminuted

Transverse   Compression   Depressed (skull)   Avulsion

FIG 16-3 Fracture types.

Wounds

Patients with open wounds have usually been treated before you see them in the radiology suite. Bleeding has been controlled, and dressings applied. Your primary responsibility in the case of open wounds is to maintain the dressings and report promptly any significant amount of fresh bleeding. This is usually considered to be the amount of bright red blood sufficient to soak through a fresh dressing. If a laceration or incision opens, causing severe hemorrhaging, apply direct pressure to the site of bleeding while summoning immediate assistance.

Postsurgical Wound Dehiscence

Patients who have had major surgery may require radiographic examination. Wound dehiscence occurs when a suture line separates. It may be partial or superficial when it involves only the outer layers of the wound, or it may be complete, involving all layers of the wound. Complete dehiscence of a wound may lead to the protrusion of the underlying tissues through the wound, or to evisceration (loss of organs from a body cavity). While evisceration is rare, it may result when extensive suture

lines spread apart or split, particularly when infection has weakened the tissues or when an obese patient who has had extensive abdominal surgery experiences a sudden strain such as a fall or a severe attack of coughing or vomiting. When dehiscence occurs, the patient may tell you that something has given way and may complain of pain, or a rush of liquid may saturate the dressings. If this occurs, ease the patient to a semirecumbent position to take the strain off the abdominal area and summon a physician immediately.

If postsurgical patients are ambulatory or able to assist themselves onto the table, stand nearby to steady them and prevent a fall. An abdominal binder consisting of a wide elastic belt with a Velcro closure can be applied to help support the abdominal tissues postoperatively. Unless there are specific orders to the contrary, leave abdominal binders in place during radiographic examinations, because these supports help prevent wound dehiscence. If you must remove the binder, wait until the patient is comfortably situated on the radiographic table. Replace the binder before the patient is transferred back to the stretcher or wheelchair.

TABLE 16-2   Main Types of Shock and Their Causes

Type of Shock	Cause
Hypovolemic	Loss of blood from injury or internal hemorrhage, loss of plasma from burns, or other cause of severe dehydration
Neurogenic	Injury to the nervous system caused by head or spinal trauma
Cardiogenic	Cardiac failure caused by interference with the heart function; may be caused by embolism, cardiac tamponade, or complications from anesthesia
Septic	Massive infection, usually by gram-negative bacteria
Anaphylactic	Contact with foreign substances, usually proteins, to which the individual has become sensitized (including bee stings and some medications); iodine contrast agents for radiographic imaging may precipitate a similar response

Burns

Although burns themselves do not require radiographic evaluation, burn patients may also have traumatic injuries such as fractures. Burns are frequently associated with respiratory complications. The inhalation of hot gases may result in **pulmonary edema** (swelling of the respiratory tract caused by trapped excess fluid), **pleural effusion** (fluid in the pleural space), or the development of **pneumonia** (inflammation of the lungs), which must be monitored radiographically.

Burns can be categorized by the cause of injury, the percentage of body surface involved, and the depth of tissue destruction. The depth of burns is classified as first, second, third, or fourth degree. A first-degree burn involves the epidermis only. The skin is red, warm, tender, and painful. There may be swelling, but there is no blistering. A second-degree burn involves the dermal layer, but there is not enough damage to prevent the growth of new epidermis during healing. Pain, swelling, and blisters may be extensive and require medical attention. Full-thickness or third-degree burns extend deep into the subcutaneous tissues and destroy nerve endings. The skin appears charred, or white and lifeless. Such burns can be caused by scalds or exposure to steam. The subcutaneous tissue, dermis, and epidermis are involved, and skin transplants may be required. Full-thickness, or fourth-degree burns involve the skin, fat, muscle, and sometimes bone. The charred skin may be completely burned away. Extensive surgical debridement and grafting are commonly necessary, and sometimes amputation is required.

When a burn patient needs a radiograph, coordinate your examination with the nursing staff to ensure that the patient has received pain medication about 30 minutes before the procedure. If the burns are extensive, the patient may be under protective precautions to avoid infection. You may wish to review this technique in Chapter 9.

Burn patients may have grafts or healing skin that is extremely tender. Such tissue is easily damaged during transfers or positioning, so you should allow these patients to move themselves as much as possible. Use a transfer sheet (see Chapter 12) to avoid abrasion and ask for help if necessary.

SHOCK

Shock is a general term used to describe a failure of circulation in which the blood pressure is inadequate to support the perfusion of oxygen to the vital tissues, and the removal of the by-products of metabolism.

Shock is a dangerous, potentially fatal condition. Early signs of shock are pallor, low blood pressure, increased heart rate and respiration, and restlessness or confusion. There are five main types of shock, categorized according to the cause, which may be medical or traumatic: hypovolemic, septic, neurogenic, cardiogenic, and allergic (anaphylactic). These types of shock are described in the following sections and are summarized in Table 16-2.

Hypovolemic Shock

Hypovolemic shock, or low-volume shock, occurs when such a large amount of blood or plasma has been lost that an insufficient amount of fluid is available to fill the circulatory system. This may result from an external hemorrhage, lacerations, plasma loss from burns, or severe dehydration from any cause. Internal blood loss, such as bleeding into the peritoneum from trauma or a perforated gastric ulcer, can also cause hypovolemic shock. Severe dehydration from vomiting, diarrhea, or extreme diuresis can also contribute to hypovolemic shock. Low-volume shock is treated with fluid replacement, oxygen administration, and medication to promote vasoconstriction.

Septic Shock

Septic shock occurs when a massive infection, such as one caused by gram-negative bacteria, produces toxins that increase capillary permeability and vasodilation, causing the blood pressure to drop sharply. Although radiographers seldom encounter this type of shock, you may see cases in the intensive care unit or ED. In addition to antibiotic therapy, emergency treatment for the shock itself must be initiated immediately (see section on recognizing and treating shock).

Neurogenic Shock

Neurogenic shock, the failure of arterial resistance, causes blood to pool in the peripheral vessels. It occurs in reaction to an injury to the nervous system and is an acute situation that demands immediate, drastic intervention. Patients with head or spinal trauma must be monitored closely for a decrease in blood pressure, which is often the first indication of this type of shock.

Cardiogenic Shock

Cardiogenic shock results from cardiac failure or interference with heart function. A pulmonary embolus or a reaction to anesthesia may initiate such an event. In trauma patients, cardiac tamponade may be the precipitating factor. As stated earlier in this chapter, this occurs when a blow to the chest causes hemorrhage into the pericardium. The resulting pressure interferes with the heart's pumping ability.

Allergic Shock or Anaphylaxis

Allergic shock, also called **anaphylaxis** or anaphylactic shock, occurs when individuals are exposed to foreign substances to which they have become sensitized. An allergic reaction develops, directly affecting the blood vessels and other tissues. The blood pressure falls rapidly, severe dyspnea caused by respiratory obstruction from edema may develop, and death can result if this is not recognized and treated rapidly. Bee stings and injections of certain medications, including iodinated

contrast media, are the most common causes of anaphylactic reaction. In the imaging department, this is most likely to occur during or immediately after the injection of a contrast medium containing iodine (see Chapter 19).

Recognizing and Treating Shock

The following symptoms indicate some degree of shock in any or all combinations:
- Restlessness and a sense of apprehension
- Increased pulse rate
- Pallor accompanied by weakness or a change in thinking ability
- Cool, clammy skin (except in patients with septic or neurogenic shock)
- A fall in blood pressure of 30 mm Hg below the baseline systolic pressure
- Decreased urination
- Increased and shallow respiration

You are responsible for recognizing the symptoms of impending shock, knowing the location of emergency medical supplies, and being thoroughly familiar with the code routine of your institution. The physician may call on your knowledge of medications and your skill in medication administration during treatment. The radiographer's role in suspected shock is as follows:

1. Stop the procedure.
2. Assist the patient to a dorsal recumbent position to avoid a fall; elevate the feet to increase the blood flow to the brain. If dyspnea is present, elevate the head also.
3. Obtain help; notify the radiologist, physician, or nurse; when in doubt, call a code. It is much better to be mistaken than to have a patient die because of inadequate treatment.
4. Check the blood pressure.
5. Assist a dyspneic patient with oxygen.
6. Be ready to perform CPR.
7. Assist the code team or physician where necessary.
8. Chart the occurrence, the treatment administered, and the patient's response on an incident report form and/or in the chart.

> You are responsible for recognizing the symptoms of impending shock, knowing the location of emergency medical supplies, and being thoroughly familiar with the code routine of your institution.

TABLE 16-3   Treatment for Allergic Reactions Depends Upon the Severity of the Reaction

Severity of Reaction	Symptoms	Treatment
Mild	Warmth, flushing, metallic taste, coughing, nausea	No treatment is needed, because symptoms will resolve quickly without treatment.
Moderate or intermediate	Erythema, urticaria, bronchospasm	Antihistamine administered orally, intravenously, or intramuscularly. When bronchospasm is present, the inhalation of a bronchodilating medication may be indicated.
Vasovagal	Diaphoresis, hypotension, bradycardia	Place patient in dorsal recumbent position with the feet elevated 20 degrees and the head elevated slightly if breathing is a problem. Intravenous fluids and atropine may be administered if bradycardia is present.
Severe (anaphylaxis)	Warmth, tingling, itching of palms and soles, dysphagia, and throat constriction; progresses rapidly to laryngeal and bronchial edema, leading to respiratory arrest, cardiac arrest, or seizures; may be fatal if not treated promptly	Maintain the airway and call a code. Epinephrine is the drug of choice and is administered intravenously. Other medications and intravenous fluids may be prescribed as well.

Syncope

Fainting, or **syncope,** is a very mild form of shock that sometimes occurs when fright, pain, or unpleasant events are beyond the coping ability of the patient's nervous system. The blood pressure falls as the diameter of the blood vessels increases and the heart rate slows. When the blood pressure is too low to supply the brain with oxygen, the patient faints. Placing the patient in a dorsal recumbent position with the feet elevated usually relieves this type of shock. Patients who have been under NPO orders for 12 hours and are feeling anxious and stressed may undergo syncope.

Patients who feel faint should be assisted into a sitting or recumbent position. If a chair is not within reach, ease the patient to the floor. If the patient does not respond immediately, spirits of ammonia held under the nose usually bring a rapid return to consciousness. Small, crushable vials of ammonia are usually kept in imaging departments for this purpose and a physician's order is not required for their use. A physician should assess anyone who has more than a momentary loss of consciousness before the examination is resumed.

Psychological Shock

Psychological shock is the term for mental trauma caused by psychological events, as in "shell shock," now known as *posttraumatic stress disorder.* Although it is called "shock," psychological shock is far different from other types of shock with respect to its signs, symptoms, and treatment. Psychological shock can cause sudden changes in mood and behavior long after the traumatic event, but is very unlikely to create an emergency situation for radiographers.

MEDICAL EMERGENCIES

Reactions to Contrast Media

This section addresses patient reactions to contrast agents, particularly intravenous (IV) injections of contrast media containing iodine. Most reactions to contrast media are considered to be allergic responses. The symptoms and treatments for allergic reactions are summarized in Table 16-3. These reactions can range from mild to severe. It is not possible to accurately predict which patients may have an allergic response to a contrast medium. For this reason, once the intravascular line has been established, the initial injection of a very small amount of contrast medium is followed by a pause to allow any symptoms of an impending allergic reaction to appear. The length of time before the remainder of the injection will vary with radiologists and with the patient's allergy history.

> ❗ An appropriate history is helpful, but a patient who has had no adverse reaction to an iodine contrast agent at one time could experience a reaction on a subsequent occasion.

The cause of reactions to iodinated contrast agents has been studied at length but is still unknown. These reactions have been shown not to result from the formation of antibodies, which is the usual cause of allergic responses. Reactions occur most frequently following the intravascular administration of the large doses of ionic iodinated contrast medium used during such examinations as excretory urography, angiography, and enhanced CT studies. A greater risk of reaction is associated with IV administration than with arterial injections. Patients who are allergic to food and airborne particles are twice as likely to be affected, and those suffering from asthma are three times as likely to suffer an adverse reaction. Severe reactions are not common, occurring in approximately 1 out of 14,000 cases. Fatal reactions to contrast media are quite rare, with an incidence of approximately 1 in 40,000 cases. This represents a significant reduction in incidence since the introduction of nonionic and low-osmolar contrast agents (see Chapter 19).

Intravascular agents require special precautions, because adverse reactions can occur with devastating speed. Radiographers must be alert for the onset of these reactions and be prepared if they occur. Patients suspected of being sensitive are often premedicated with an antihistamine such as diphenhydramine (Benadryl), which is sometimes supplemented with a specific type of antihistamine called an H-2 blocker, such as cimetidine (Tagamet). A corticosteroid such as cortisone (Solu-Medrol), an anti-inflammatory, may be included in the premedication regimen. Although most reactions occur almost immediately, delayed responses may be seen and should be anticipated for at least 30 minutes after the injection. In rare instances, reactions have occurred as long as several hours after the injection. Interestingly, patients do not experience allergic reactions under general anesthesia. One investigator, A.F. Lalli, demonstrated a connection between anxiety and adverse reactions. He speculates that the deterrent effect of antihistamine drugs may be caused as much by the soporific (sleep-causing) effect of the antihistamine as by its specific action. To alleviate anxiety as a factor in potential adverse reactions, you must tell the patient what to expect without causing alarm.

Most patients experience a feeling of warmth during the injection of an ionic iodinated contrast medium and may feel flushed for 1 to 3 minutes afterward. A metallic taste in the mouth is another short-term sensation that can occur. If other minor symptoms such as nausea, vomiting, or coughing occur, provide an emesis basin, alert the radiologist, and continue to observe the patient carefully. These mild reactions pass quickly and may not produce vomiting if the patient is relaxed. No treatment is usually necessary.

An intermediate reaction is characterized by **erythema** (reddening of the skin), **urticaria** (hives), and/or bronchospasm. The physician should be notified while you remain with the patient. The usual treatment is to administer an antihistamine medication such as diphenhydramine orally, intramuscularly (IM), or IV, depending on the severity of the reaction. If hives are severe, cimetidine may also be given. Bronchospasm, especially when seen as an isolated sign, can be treated with two or three deep inhalations of a bronchodilator, such as albuterol. Some physicians prefer to give epinephrine at this point, especially if hypotension is present.

A **vasovagal** reaction to a contrast medium may be triggered when the injected agent stimulates the vagus nerve, causing cardiovascular changes resulting in increased vasodilation of arterioles. This can cause diaphoresis, hypotension, and sinus bradycardia. A steady drop in blood pressure can cause unconsciousness and may be life threatening. Place the patient in the supine position with the feet elevated about 20 degrees and the head elevated about 10 degrees; notify the physician. IV fluids and atropine can be administered if bradycardia is present. Atropine is an anticholinergic medication that acts as a vasoconstrictor, increasing the heart rate and elevating blood pressure. Anticholinergic medication blocks the action of acetylcholine, a neurotransmitter with many effects, including slowing of the heart rate and lowering the blood pressure. Atropine reverses these effects. Its action is similar in some respects to that of epinephrine, but it is more effective in response to a vasovagal reaction. Anticholinergic drugs increase the blood pressure and heart rate.

A severe allergic reaction is called **anaphylaxis** or anaphylactic shock. This life-threatening condition may result in respiratory or cardiac arrest and, less often, in seizures. The early symptoms of anaphylaxis include a sense of warmth, tingling, itching of palms and soles, dysphagia (difficulty swallowing), constriction in the throat, a feeling of doom, an expiratory wheeze, and then progression into laryngeal and bronchial edema.

The drug of choice for the treatment of anaphylaxis is epinephrine. Corticosteroid injections (Solu-Cortef or Solu-Medrol), the antihistamine diphenhydramine (Benadryl), and the H-2 inhibitor cimetidine (Tagamet) are drugs that may also be ordered, in addition to the infusion of IV fluids. Treatments for shock, respiratory and cardiac arrest may also be appropriate and are outlined elsewhere in this chapter. At the onset of anaphylaxis, the radiographer should alert the radiologist and call a code.

Chapter 19 provides more information about contrast media and reactions to various types of contrast agents.

Drug Reactions

A drug reaction can range in severity from a sudden bout of dizziness to cardiac arrest. The seriousness of the reaction can be found at any point along this continuum. The nature of the symptoms will determine the appropriate treatment. Treatments for the various conditions seen in response to drug administration are found throughout this chapter.

Not all drug reactions result from parenteral administration or even from prescribed medications. Individuals who have been sensitized to an over-the-counter medication may be just as prone to an allergic reaction as those receiving an IV medication, although the effects of the IV will appear faster.

Diabetic Emergencies

Patients who have diabetes are seen for the same variety of problems that bring other patients to the imaging department. Because diabetes is sometimes associated with circulatory problems, these patients may be candidates for arteriograms as well as for more routine procedures. The diabetic patient can often be identified by means of a medical information bracelet, such as Medic-Alert. These bracelets are also worn by individuals with other medical conditions that may require emergency treatment. The bracelet states the nature of the problem and can also indicate the appropriate emergency response. Some of these bracelets include a phone number or Internet address where medical personnel can obtain additional information about the patient's medical history in an emergency.

Diabetes Insipidus

There are two distinct kinds of diabetes: diabetes insipidus (DI) and diabetes mellitus (DM). DI is a disease induced by problems with the kidneys or pituitary gland causing glucose to be excreted in the urine while blood glucose levels remain normal. DI is characterized by polyuria and thirst. If untreated, the subsequent dehydration (water depletion) may result in fever, vomiting, and convulsions. Emergency responses to both vomiting and convulsions are discussed in other sections of this chapter. Fluid replacement is essential.

Diabetes Mellitus

DM is characterized by an inability to metabolize blood glucose. Insulin is a hormone normally produced in the pancreas in response to food intake. Insufficient insulin prevents the use of glucose by the muscles, causing the glucose level in the blood to rise, a condition called hyperglycemia. When the muscles cannot use glucose, the body breaks down fat for muscular contraction, and the by-products of fatty acid metabolism form ketone bodies. When excess ketone bodies appear in the blood, ketoacidosis develops. The body attempts to compensate for the acidosis by hyperventilation (air hunger) and the loss of minerals and water in the urine. When the blood glucose level is very high, sugar also "spills over" into the urine. The individual who is terribly thirsty, urinates copious amounts frequently, and has fruity-smelling breath may be approaching diabetic coma. It is characterized by a relatively slow onset. This condition is diagnosed by blood and urine tests and treated with diet, exercise, and medication, such as insulin or oral hypoglycemic agents.

There are two major classifications of DM: type I and type II. Type I, or insulin-dependent diabetes, may be characterized by a lean individual under age 25 who produces little or no insulin and may develop circulatory impairment of vision, the kidneys, or the extremities. Family history appears to be of minor importance. Autoimmune, genetic, and environmental factors are involved in this type of diabetes. Blood glucose levels must be closely monitored, and insulin is administered parenterally. Diabetic coma is more likely to occur with type I DM.

Type II DM, on the other hand, occurs most commonly in the obese individual over the age of 40 with a marked family tendency. This type of diabetes usually responds to oral hypoglycemic medications and to changes in diet and lifestyle.

TABLE 16-4 Diabetic Crises

Crisis	Cause	Symptoms	Treatment
Diabetic coma	Food consumption in excess of the dietary allowance Fever, infection, stress Insufficient insulin	Increased thirst Increased urinary output Decreased appetite Nausea, vomiting, weakness, confusion, coma	Inform physician Administer sugar-free liquids if conscious Insulin may be administered
Insulin reaction	Insufficient food following insulin administration Excessive exercise	Headache Hunger Cold, clammy skin Diaphoresis Tremors Tachycardia Impaired vision Personality change Loss of consciousness	Administer food or liquid with a high sugar content Glucagon may be administered Inform the physician immediately

Hyperosmolar hyperglycemic nonketotic (HHNK) syndrome is a severe condition that can occur when patients with neglected type II DM become dehydrated and hyperglycemic. This may be induced by sepsis, fluid loss from either dehydration or diuresis, by an MI, by oral or parenteral hyperalimentation solutions, or by IV glucose overload. The level of consciousness can vary from initial confusion to coma or seizures. Treatment includes fluid administration to rapidly expand the intravascular volume, thus increasing the circulation and urine output.

Hypoglycemia

A diabetic patient who has taken insulin but eaten no food may develop hypoglycemia, or low blood sugar. Unlike the slow onset of a diabetic coma, hypoglycemia is characterized by a sudden onset of weakness, sweating, tremor (quivering), hunger, and, finally, loss of consciousness. While the patient is still alert and cooperative, hypoglycemia can be quickly treated by giving the patient a small amount of candy or sweet fruit juice. Squeeze tubes containing a measured amount of glucose may be stored with the emergency medications. These prepackaged doses of glucose are useful because the gel-like material can be placed inside the patient's cheek. This decreases the risk that a semiconscious or confused patient will aspirate it, as may be the case with candy or juice. A parenteral injection of 0.5 to 1.0 mg of glucagon may be ordered if hypoglycemia is severe,

especially when the patient is unconscious. An IV infusion of dextrose solution may be ordered if the patient does not respond to the glucagon.

Report the occurrence of hypoglycemia to the physician. You must help the hypoglycemic patient to sit or lie down until the sugar takes effect. Occasionally, individuals with the same symptoms may be adamant that they do not have diabetes. They may have hypoglycemia without diabetes. The treatment is the same. Table 16-4 summarizes the physical findings associated with high blood sugar, indicative of approaching diabetic coma, and low blood sugar, which may signify an impending insulin reaction.

Cerebrovascular Accident

A cerebrovascular accident (CVA), also called a *stroke*, is the term for interruption of the blood supply to the brain. It occurs most frequently in the elderly, but may occur at any age. A rupture of a cerebral artery can cause hemorrhage into the brain tissue, or an artery may become occluded, impeding circulation to the area beyond the occlusion. The symptoms may occur very suddenly or may develop over a period of hours. Warning signs, easily remembered with the acronym FAST, include:

- Facial Droop
- Arm weakness on one or both sides
- Speech difficulty
- Time to call 9-1-1

Other symptoms may include:

- Extreme dizziness
- Severe headache
- Difficulty in vision or deviation in one eye
- Temporary loss of consciousness

These symptoms may be only temporary, but they should be reported immediately to a physician. The most promising outcome for a stroke patient is to be treated within 1 hour of the onset of the stroke. The patient should be helped into a recumbent position with the head elevated. Do not leave the patient, but summon assistance and have the emergency cart and oxygen at hand. Monitor the vital signs every 5 minutes or as ordered by the physician.

Transient ischemic attacks (TIAs), sometimes called "ministrokes," present similar symptoms, but usually last only minutes or a few hours at most. These temporary attacks should not be ignored, because they are frequently the precursors to more permanent damage.

Seizures

Seizures occur as a result of a focal or generalized disturbance of brain function and are accompanied by a change in the LOC. Patients with seizure disorders may come to the imaging department for any reason but are often seen for examinations such as a cerebral arteriogram or CT scan. A major motor (tonic-clonic or *grand mal*) seizure may be preceded by an aura or premonitory sign. The patient may say, "I'm going to have a spell," and should be assisted to a supine position as rapidly as possible. Frequently the seizure is signaled by a hoarse cry when air is forced past the vocal cords by a sudden contraction of all the abdominal and chest muscles.

When a tonic-clonic seizure occurs, your first duty is to keep the patient as safe as possible. Notify a physician immediately, request assistance, and do not leave the patient. If the patient is on an imaging table, your first concern is to prevent a fall. Remove any objects that may be hazardous, and place padding under the patient's head. Do not attempt to restrain the patient, and do not try to force objects into the patient's mouth.

! During a seizure, your first duty is to keep the patient as safe as possible and provide protection from harm by placing padding under the head and preventing a fall. *Do not attempt to restrain the patient or force objects into his/her mouth.*

A loss of consciousness and a rigid arching of the back are followed by alternate relaxation and rigidity of the muscles until the seizure passes and the patient slowly regains consciousness. While the patient is unconscious, involuntary voiding and defecation may occur. As the seizure passes, turn the patient to a lateral recumbent position to prevent aspiration of secretions, and remain with him/her to provide reassurance and assistance. In the immediate period following the seizure (postictal period), the patient may be somewhat irritable or confused and may wish only to sleep.

Less intense partial (focal) seizures may cause severe, uncontrollable tremors. This condition often causes extreme anxiety and hyperventilation in a conscious patient. These seizures are exhausting to the patient and may persist for over an hour without treatment. Instruct the patient to breathe slowly, and place a paper bag over the patient's nose and mouth if the hyperventilation is otherwise uncontrollable.

Another type of seizure, called *petit mal* or absence seizure, is characterized by a brief loss of consciousness during which the patient stares or may lose balance and fall. Many patients are unaware that they undergo this loss of consciousness.

Patients taking anticonvulsant medication may not have seizures for long periods. Most of these medications have a relatively slow excretion rate, which allows the patient to miss a dose or two without precipitating an attack. On the other hand, fatigue, apprehension, and the demands of a rigorous preparation for examination may initiate a seizure in a previously stable patient.

Realize that the seizure will run its course. It is most important for you to protect the patient from harm and to be an accurate observer. Note when the seizure began and how long it lasted. Did it involve both sides of the body equally, and did the contractions start in one area and progress from one extremity to another? These observations can help the physician reach an accurate diagnosis.

Remember that not all seizure-prone individuals have the same diagnosis. Seizures may be a reaction to drug sensitivity, infection, epilepsy, tumor, or fever. Myths and superstitions about seizure disorders have only recently begun to be dispelled. There is no direct, consistent correlation between seizures and mental acuity, emotional instability, or heredity.

Alcoholics hospitalized for medical treatment do not always reveal the extent of their alcohol addiction to their physicians. After 48 hours, they may suffer withdrawal symptoms, including visual and auditory hallucinations and tremors. Some may also experience major motor seizures. Barbiturate or benzodiazepine withdrawal can contribute to seizure activity as well.

Vertigo and Orthostatic Hypotension

A "light-headed" or dizzy sensation is common after prolonged bed rest; orthostatic hypotension is the usual cause. This results from the same basic mechanism that causes syncope, or fainting, discussed earlier in this chapter. Blood pools in the extremities when the torso is elevated and causes a transient cerebral anoxia (lack of oxygen). This condition can usually be avoided by having the patient sit up gradually. This sensation frequently affects elderly patients, so remain close to them and provide support when a change in position is necessary.

Vertigo has a different cause. The patient does not feel light-headed but describes the room as moving or whirling. These patients frequently cling to the table and will fall if not assisted to lie down. They may also experience violent nausea. This sensation is usually attributed to either an inner ear disturbance or to a lesion in the brain or spinal cord. A sudden onset in a patient who does not have a history of vertigo should be reported immediately to the physician, because this may be associated with a TIA or CVA. Alcohol or certain drugs may affect individuals in a similar manner and should also be called to the physician's attention.

Epistaxis

A nosebleed, or epistaxis, can be rather frightening to the patient but is usually not serious. Remove eyeglasses when necessary, and provide an ample supply of tissues. Instruct the patient to keep the head level, breathe through the mouth, and squeeze firmly against the nasal septum for 10 minutes. An ice pack applied to the bridge of the nose can help slow the flow of blood. The patient should not lie down, tip the head back, blow the nose, or talk. Provide an emesis basin, instructing the patient to spit out blood that runs down the nasopharynx rather than swallow it. If bleeding lasts for more than a few minutes, inform the

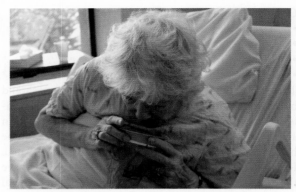

FIG 16-4 A patient with nausea is assisted to a sitting or lateral recumbent position and given a receptacle for emesis.

physician, who may want to apply more direct treatment.

Nausea and Vomiting

Nausea and vomiting are frequently encountered, and a well-prepared radiographer learns to cope easily with this situation. Occasionally patients may feel nauseated for a specific reason, such as after swallowing a barium preparation. Vomiting can sometimes be prevented by the radiographer's reassuring presence and by breathing suggestions. "Breathe through your mouth, taking short, rapid, panting breaths," or "Take some long, slow, deep breaths through your nose," are both effective instructions. These suggestions are helpful because they encourage a focus on breathing that distracts the patient from the nausea until it passes. Antiemetics can be requested to alleviate excessive nausea or control vomiting to facilitate the completion of a radiographic examination.

If a patient expresses the need to vomit, provide an emesis basin or disposable receptacle immediately. Bring the patient a clean receptacle before removing the soiled one. Provide tissues and water to rinse the mouth. It is especially important to support the patient in a sitting or lateral recumbent position to avoid the aspiration of vomitus (Figure 16-4). A lateral recumbent position is safest for the patient with nausea who is unable to sit up. If the patient loses consciousness, be sure to turn the head to the side and clear the airway. Wear gloves when handling soiled emesis basins or cleaning up after a patient has vomited.

■ SUMMARY

- Respiratory emergencies include choking events and asthma attacks. Asthma attacks require the administration of oxygen and/or a bronchodilating medication.

- Cardiac events can include angina pectoris (chest pain caused by constriction of the arteries of the heart), heart attack caused by occlusion of the arteries of the heart (MI), or cardiac arrest (complete cessation of the heartbeat). Angina is treated by the sublingual administration of nitroglycerin. The treatment for heart attacks varies and can include the administration of pain medication, aspirin, oxygen, and often vasodilating drugs. In the case of cardiac arrest, a code is called, and CPR and/or defibrillation are administered.

- Victims of trauma are usually cared for by emergency personnel and stabilized before being transported to the imaging department. Radiographers should be cautious to avoid further injury when handling patients who suffer from burns, wounds, or fractures. They should also be alert for changes in patient status that may indicate shock or increased intracranial pressure. Cervical spine precautions must be observed until the possibility of a cervical spine fracture has been ruled out.

- Shock is a serious condition of low blood pressure that can be caused by blood loss, infection, allergy, cardiac distress, or central nervous system trauma. Shock may begin with restlessness and a sense of apprehension, followed by an increased pulse rate, pallor, weakness, a change in thinking ability, and a drop in blood pressure. The radiographer who identifies signs of shock should stop the examination, place the patient in a recumbent position with the feet elevated, and summon qualified help.

- Syncope is a mild form of shock in which a patient feels faint and loses consciousness. Assist the patient to a safe position. If the patient does not respond quickly, administer spirits of ammonia to bring about a return to consciousness.

- Medication and contrast agents containing iodine may cause allergic reactions. Their treatment requires prompt recognition and measures appropriate to the severity of the reaction.

- Diabetes insipidus is a disease induced by problems with the kidneys or pituitary gland causing excess glucose to be excreted in the urine while blood glucose levels remain normal.

- Diabetes mellitus, both type I and type II, is a condition in which the body does not produce enough insulin or cannot use its own insulin, causing sugars to build up in the blood. Hyperglycemia has a slow onset and may eventually cause coma when untreated. It is treated by administering insulin or oral hypoglycemic agents. Hypoglycemia, also called insulin shock, occurs when the insulin treatment is not accompanied by adequate food intake. It is treated with the administration of glucose.

- A CVA (stroke) may be signaled by severe headache, dizziness, paralysis, weakness, difficulty in speaking, changes in vision, or a loss of consciousness. The prompt recognition of symptoms and treatment with clot-dissolving medication is indicated for strokes caused by the occlusion of cerebral vessels. Surgical intervention is used to treat hemorrhagic stroke caused by a rupture or leakage of a vessel in the brain.

- Types of seizures include petit mal (absence), focal, and grand mal (tonic-clonic). The principal treatment for all types is to keep the patient safe from injury until the seizure passes. Medication such as diazepam or lorazepam can be administered in cases of prolonged or repeated seizures.

- Vertigo is a sensation that the room is spinning. Patients with this condition should be assisted to sit or lie down; some may experience nausea.

- Orthostatic hypotension is a transient dizziness that sometimes occurs with a sudden change in position. Patients subject to this condition should rise slowly and be supported when first standing.

- In the case of epistaxis, or nosebleed, instruct the patient to squeeze firmly against the nasal septum for 10 minutes. The patient should not lie down, blow the nose, or talk, and should spit out rather than swallow any blood that runs down the nasopharynx.

- Focusing on breathing will sometimes help to prevent vomiting in a patient with nausea. Provide an emesis basin and assist the patient to a sitting or lateral recumbent position.

REVIEW QUESTIONS

1. While you are positioning Margaret Dunne for an upright chest radiograph, she collapses against you and slowly slips to the floor. The first thing you should do is:
   A. call a code.
   B. "shake and shout."
   C. get the emergency drug box.
   D. start CPR.

2. John Gaffney is sitting in the waiting room waiting for his wife to get dressed following a radiographic examination. Mr. Gaffney looked well when he arrived at the department, but when you go to tell him that his wife will be out in a moment, you notice that he is pale, diaphoretic, and seems distracted. When you ask if he is all right, he says, "Gee, I don't know. I can't seem to get my breath." Which of the following actions is not appropriate?
   A. Help him to lie down
   B. Call for help
   C. "Shake and shout"
   D. Check for a diabetic identification bracelet

3. A patient who reports that he feels as if the room is spinning is experiencing:
   A. a heart attack.
   B. hypoglycemia.
   C. postural hypotension.
   D. vertigo.

4. Epistaxis is another name for:
   A. a seizure.
   B. a nosebleed.
   C. syncope.
   D. angina

5. While taking radiographs on a trauma patient, you should be especially alert for signs of:
   A. absence.
   B. syncope.
   C. hypoglycemia.
   D. shock.

6. Shock resulting from blood loss is called:
   A. hypovolemic shock.
   B. septic shock.
   C. cardiogenic shock.
   D. neurogenic shock.

7. Which of the following treatments is appropriate when a patient is experiencing syncope?
   A. The administration of sweet fruit juice
   B. Assist the patient to lie down and elevate the feet
   C. Use of an AED
   D. Call a code and begin CPR

8. When a diabetic patient has taken the usual dose of insulin, but has not eaten, he/she may feel faint and weak and may show signs of sweating and tremors. The term for this condition is:
   A. diabetic coma.
   B. hyperglycemia.
   C. hypoglycemia.
   D. epistaxis.

9. CVA is the abbreviation for a term that refers to:
   A. an interruption of the blood supply to the brain.
   B. a heart attack.
   C. a type of seizure.
   D. a type of fracture.

10. When a patient experiences a seizure, your first priority is to:
    A. keep him/her safe.
    B. call for help.
    C. finish the examination.
    D. restrain the patient.

Answers can be found in the Answer Key on pages 429-431.

CRITICAL THINKING EXERCISES

1. A motor vehicle accident brings three victims to the ED, and all three need radiographs.
   - Dave Black has abrasions and pain in his right leg.
   - Paul White has displacement of his left shoulder and has become increasingly cross and drowsy.
   - The driver of the car, Mary Green, has no visible injuries but complains of a painful sternum.
   Which patients would cause you the most concern? What would you do?

2. What signs alert you that a patient is experiencing airway obstruction? Would you give CPR?
3. What a week in the imaging department! Three patients exhibited symptoms of shock:
   - Mrs. Doble was having an excretory urogram.
   - John Dix was having a radiographic examination for minor injuries suffered in a motor vehicle accident in which his daughter was killed.
   - Jacob Marsan nearly amputated his own leg when he dropped a circular saw.

   What type of shock was most likely in each case? How would the treatment differ for these three patients?
4. List 4 types of fracture. What kinds of problems may occur when fracture fragments move? What precautions will help prevent these problems?

17

Preparation and Examination of the Gastrointestinal Tract

OBJECTIVES

At the conclusion of this chapter, the student will be able to:

- Explain the purpose of contrast media use in gastrointestinal (GI) studies.
- List three types of patients whose GI studies should be scheduled as early in the day as possible.
- Discuss the purpose of bowel preparation for various studies and select a method appropriate for the patient's age and condition.
- List two steps you could take to make barium more palatable for oral administration.
- List the temperature, amount of fluid, and height at which the bag should be hung when preparing for administration of cleansing enemas and barium enemas.
- Position a patient correctly for enema administration.

- List three indications and two contraindications for radiographic examinations of the upper gastrointestinal tract.
- List three indications and two contraindications for radiographic examinations of the lower gastrointestinal tract.
- Compare and contrast procedures for routine upper GI series, double-contrast upper GI series, and hypotonic duodenography.
- Give two reasons for discontinuing the examination or preparation of a patient having lower GI studies.
- Discuss complications that could arise during an examination for Hirschsprung disease.

OUTLINE

304

KEY TERMS

abscess	fistula	mucosa
cathartic	gastritis	peristalsis
commode	gastroesophageal reflux disease	peritonitis
congenital megacolon	(GERD)	polyp
Crohn disease	hemorrhoids	pylorospasm
diverticulitis	hiatal hernia	spasm
diverticulosis	Hirschsprung disease	stricture
diverticulum (*pl.* diverticula)	hygroscopic	suppository
duodenitis	hypervolemia	ulcer
dysphagia	inflammatory bowel disease	ulcerative colitis
enema	(IBD)	Valsalva maneuver
esophagitis	irritable bowel syndrome (IBS)	varices (*sing.* varix)
esophagram	irrigation	viscosity

This chapter focuses on the use of barium sulfate ($BaSO_4$, often simply called barium) as a contrast medium in examination of the gastrointestinal (GI) tract. It also discusses the preparation and follow-up care for contrast studies of the GI tract and for the other abdominal soft-tissue examinations discussed in Chapter 19.

Radiographic examination of the GI tract requires visualization and differentiation of soft tissue structures. Because soft tissues are more difficult to demonstrate than bony structures, substances are introduced into the body that absorb radiation to a different degree than the tissues themselves. These substances are called contrast media (contrast medium *sing.*) and may generally be classified into three groups:
1. Barium sulfate products
2. Water-soluble iodine compounds
3. Gases

Many soft-tissue examinations using contrast media require some type of advance preparation. The purpose may be to ensure that the procedure will not cause untoward side effects, such as nausea, but the principal reason for preparation is to cleanse the GI tract so that gas, food, or fecal material will not obscure the structures to be demonstrated radiographically.

Some preparations require several steps to ensure optimum visualization.

SCHEDULING AND SEQUENCING

One of the more challenging problems shared by nursing services and imaging departments involves the scheduling of multiple diagnostic procedures that may all be ordered at one time by the referring physician. With outpatients, communication involves the imaging department and the nurse or receptionist in the physician's office. Consultation may be needed to decide how many procedures can be done in one day and how to sequence them in such a way that they will not interfere with each other. For example, an upper GI series usually results in barium scattered throughout the intestinal tract for several days. Even tiny amounts of residual barium cause complications in radiographic examinations of the urinary tract, where tiny opacifications are diagnostically significant. Residual barium in the digestive tract also causes unacceptable artifacts on abdominal computed tomography (CT) scans. For these reasons, barium studies are scheduled last in any series of imaging procedures.

Some departments may schedule a series of several examinations in one day for patients who are able to tolerate this approach. In some ways, this may be less stressful, resulting in a single bowel preparation, a single period of fasting, and perhaps a shortened hospital stay. However, a debilitated patient can tolerate only a limited schedule with recovery time between procedures. In addition, radiologists prefer various scheduling practices. For some, it may be common procedure to schedule gallbladder sonography and both upper and lower GI studies on the same day. Others may insist on 2 or 3 days for completion of the same examinations. Whatever the practice in your institution, it should be stated in the procedure manual and the standing orders and be easily available to those involved in scheduling, ordering, and planning preparation.

When fiberoptic studies, such as gastroscopy or sigmoidoscopy, are ordered in conjunction with radiographic examinations requiring barium, fiberoptic studies are usually done first. This avoids the possibility of the barium interfering with visual assessment during the fiberoptic examination. Patients undergoing gastroscopy should have nothing by mouth (NPO) for 12 hours preceding the examination. They usually receive sedation and a muscle relaxant before the physician inserts the gastroscope. When an upper GI series is to follow, allow sufficient time for the patient to become responsive and alert before administering the barium, because oral administration of barium to a sedated patient increases the risk that the patient may aspirate the barium.

When sequencing diagnostic procedures, any thyroid assessment tests must be performed before administration of any iodinated contrast medium, because iodine can cause inaccurate results in thyroid tests for at least 3 weeks. Box 17-1 provides a guide to sequencing multiple diagnostic studies for patients undergoing a comprehensive workup.

An additional consideration in patient scheduling involves deciding which patients to schedule first in the morning and which to schedule later in the day. Imaging departments always begin the daily routine with patients who must fast in preparation for examination so that they will not have to go without food for too long. When several fasting patients are scheduled, you may have to decide which study to perform first. Emergency patients have priority, followed by pediatric and geriatric patients, because they have the most difficulty being NPO for long periods of time, and extended fasting may interfere with their recovery.

BOX 17-1   Guide to Sequencing Order for Diagnostic Studies

1. All radiographic examinations not requiring contrast media and any laboratory studies for iodine uptake
2. Radiographic examinations of the urinary tract
3. Radiographic examinations of the biliary system
4. Lower gastrointestinal series (barium enema)
5. Upper gastrointestinal series

Note: CT studies requiring IV contrast may be done any time after blood has been drawn for iodine uptake studies. CT studies of the abdomen or pelvis should precede examinations involving barium.

When scheduling multiple studies involving administration of iodine contrast, care must be taken that the total maximum dosages of iodine compounds are not exceeded (see Chapter 19).

Give priority to diabetic patients who must postpone their insulin until their morning meal. Remind them to postpone their morning insulin until the examination is complete, even if they have an early appointment. If an emergency should cause a delay, the patient who has had insulin may suffer a reaction (see Chapter 16).

ENSURING COMPLIANCE WITH PREPARATION ORDERS

For inpatients, the nursing service is primarily responsible for performing patient preparation. You have a duty to ensure that standing orders for preparations are current and to check with both the patient and the chart to ensure that the orders have been carried out before the examination.

Preliminary radiographs without contrast agents, sometimes called scout images, are often taken to evaluate patient preparation. These images may also reveal abnormalities before the administration of contrast media. Caution at this point may avoid the needless repetition of an examination because of inadequate preparation. Unnecessary repeat studies waste time, money, and energy in the radiology department and result in additional radiation exposure and inconvenience to the patient. Take care to avoid such repetitions so that patients will have confidence in the care they receive.

Although radiologists establish the procedures, the imaging department supervisor is usually the person who ensures that orders are distributed and properly followed. A representative of the imaging department should meet regularly with the nursing staff to provide rationale and clarify any questions regarding preparations. Radiographers tend to assume that "nurses know all about these things," yet preparation for radiography is not a significant part of their education. Nurses usually learn about the rationale for the examinations and the particulars of preparation on the job. Person-to-person follow-up is especially important whenever a standard procedure has been changed or when the two departments have recurring problems concerning preparations.

When instructing an outpatient regarding preparation for an examination, it is helpful to have printed instructions prepared in advance. If more than one alternative is printed on any given paper, be certain to indicate, both orally and in writing, which instructions are to be followed. Review the sheet with the patient slowly, explaining any words or procedures that may not be familiar. Have the patient restate the instructions to ensure there is a clear understanding of what is to be done. If the patient is too young, too ill, confused, or incapable of understanding and following the instructions, give the instructions (oral and written) to the person who will be responsible for assisting the patient. Instructions for preparation may be given online, which is convenient for many patients, but may not be ideal for all. If this method is used, written instructions must be available for patients who do not have computer access, and all instructions must include the telephone number of the imaging department so that the patient or the patient's caregiver may call if any questions arise.

When scheduling and giving instructions over the telephone, it is especially important to have patients repeat the instructions in their own words. This ensures that they have understood the instructions. Patients may sometimes say, "Yes, yes," in an effort to sound cooperative, even if they do not understand what you have said.

PREPARATION FOR EXAMINATION

Specific preparations vary among institutions and radiologists, so refer to the procedures at your institution. The most common radiographic preparations are for cleansing purposes. Certain examinations almost invariably require cleansing preparation, the primary one being the barium enema or lower GI study. For this examination, the inner lining of the large intestine must be clean and free of all fecal matter. It is a complex undertaking to cleanse all of the irregular surfaces of the bowel, and this task usually requires several steps. These may include diet, cathartics, suppositories, or enemas, and the process often consists of several or all of these methods. Once mastered, these techniques may be applied to preparations for other examinations. For example, cleansing preparation is also required for studies of the urinary tract (see Chapter 19).

Diet

An examination scheduled well in advance offers the opportunity to employ diet as an effective preparation. Patients may be placed on a low-residue diet for several days preceding the examination. At the same time, liquid intake, particularly water, is encouraged or forced, resulting in rapid transit of waste through the digestive tract and less residue in the bowel. For the 24 hours immediately before the examination, the patient's diet may be restricted to clear liquids. These are foods that are entirely absorbed through the intestinal wall, leaving no residue. A clear liquid diet may consist of consommé or bouillon, apple juice, gelatin, and tea. Some soft drinks may also be taken. A good rule to follow is to avoid any food or drink that is not transparent. Milk products are definitely to be avoided, because they curdle during digestion, producing high-residue solids.

Fasting is another dietary regimen that may be used in patient preparation for radiographic examinations. The NPO order is usually instituted for a limited period, approximately 8 to 12 hours before the procedure, but the fasting period may vary depending on the patient's age and the policies in place in the imaging department. Fasting ensures that the stomach will be empty at the time of examination, which is important for two reasons:

1. If the stomach is to be examined, it must be empty and "clean" so that it will produce an accurate radiographic image of its inner surfaces.
2. If the examination might cause nausea, as intravenous (IV) contrast agents occasionally do, the patient is less likely to vomit. Fasting decreases the possibility that vomitus may be aspirated.

Cathartics

Cathartics are strong laxative preparations often prescribed to aid in cleansing the bowel. There are five principal types: bulk, lubricant, emollient, saline, and stimulant. Bulk cathartics are made from various types of fiber, such as psyllium seed husks, and lubricants include oily substances, such as mineral oil. Emollient cathartics are actually stool softeners that lower the surface tension of feces, allowing water and fat to penetrate for ease in evacuation. These types are not commonly used in bowel preparation for imaging studies. Saline and stimulant cathartics are used extensively. Saline types, particularly magnesium salts, change the osmotic forces of the colon, increasing the fluidity of the intestinal contents by enhancing water retention and indirectly increasing the motor activity of the bowel. Stimulant cathartics act directly to increase the motor activity of the intestinal tract. Stimulant cathartics tend to be stronger and somewhat more irritating than saline cathartics.

Common cathartics for bowel preparation include bisacodyl (Dulcolax), a strong stimulant cathartic in tablet form, and citrate of magnesia, a saline cathartic in the form of a carbonated beverage. Polyethylene glycol (for example, Miralax) is an osmotic preparation in powdered form that is mixed by the patient with a large amount of liquid. The standing orders may specify one or more of these drugs. Commercial bowel preparation kits are available and may be used in your institution. They may contain one or more types of cathartics, a suppository, a low-volume enema, and illustrated instructions in several languages.

Research has demonstrated that increased fluid intake enhances the effectiveness of cathartics and aids in minimizing patient discomfort. For this reason, standing orders for cathartics are accompanied by a fluid intake schedule that usually recommends at least 8 ounces of water or clear liquid every 2 hours between noon and midnight on the day preceding the examination.

Strong cathartics may cause patients to experience painful **spasms** (involuntary muscle contractions) of the bowel and irritation of the intestinal lining. Persistent diarrhea may last through the night, preventing sleep. Although patients may find this preparation uncomfortable and inconvenient, its effectiveness in cleansing the bowel usually outweighs these considerations.

The procedural manual and the standing orders will state a usual dosage of a specific cathartic, but a degree of flexibility in this regard is essential. Exercise caution in implementing an aggressive preparation for elderly or frail patients who are likely to experience an adverse effect. In addition to providing a gentler alternative for the debilitated patient, those with chronic or acute diarrhea may require a lower dosage or less active preparation than is usually given. When decreasing the routine strength or amount of cathartics, the use of a low-residue diet and increased fluid intake become critically important to the success of the preparation. Conversely, those patients who have chronic constipation or are habituated to the use of laxatives may require a more active drug or a higher dose of the prescribed cathartic. A brief history of the patient's bowel habits helps in assessing whether the usual preparation is appropriate.

Always advise patients of the nature of the action expected from the cathartic when it is given.

Suppositories

A rectal **suppository** is a semisolid nugget of medication that is inserted into the rectum to stimulate peristaltic action in the colon and promote evacuation of the distal portion of the lower bowel. To insert a suppository, wear disposable gloves and insert the suppository gently into the anus with one hand while holding the buttocks apart with the other hand. Using one finger, gently push the suppository past the internal sphincter and approximately 2 to 3 inches into the rectum in a superior-anterior direction. Be certain that the suppository rests in contact with the rectal **mucosa** (lining membrane), since it will not be effective if lodged in a fecal mass. Almost immediately, the patient will have an urge to defecate. If the patient acts upon this urge too quickly, the result will be evacuation of the suppository only. Encourage the patient to retain the suppository for at least 30 minutes before evacuation.

Cleansing Enemas

Enemas are another method of bowel cleansing that is sometimes prescribed in preparation for radiographic examination, although they are not used as frequently today as in the past. This procedure consists of filling the colon with liquid to aid in dislodging and flushing out any fecal contents remaining in the lower intestinal tract. In the case of an inpatient, the nursing service carries out orders for enemas in the patient's room. Outpatients usually implement the orders at home. Occasionally, however, this duty is assigned to a radiographer. You should be familiar with this procedure in case you are assigned this duty and so that you can instruct patients who need advice on taking enemas at home. An understanding of this procedure provides a basis for learning the technique of administering the barium enema, which is routine for every radiographer.

The liquid used for a cleansing enema may be tap water or soapsuds in water. Normal saline solution, glycerin in water, and olive oil are also used occasionally. The equipment needed consists of an enema bag with attached tubing, a disposable rectal catheter, and apparatus from which to suspend the enema bag. An IV pole is especially useful for suspending the bag because of its mobility and its height adjustability. For a tap water enema, fill the container with 1000 mL of tepid (105° F) water from the tap. If soapsuds are ordered, add 30 mL of liquid castile soap and mix well. Castile soap is a very pure product and is ideal for this purpose; other soap products are likely to contain additives that may be irritating or toxic to the bowel and should not be used. Attach the rectal catheter to the tubing and, holding the catheter over the sink, open the clamp. When the tubing and catheter have filled completely with the liquid, close the clamp. Filling the tubing and catheter before administration prevents instillation of air into the colon. You will also need a water-soluble gel to lubricate the catheter tip. If the patient is unable to walk to the bathroom, obtain a bedpan, toilet tissue, and cleansing towelette and keep them at hand.

When you are ready, explain the procedure to the patient and give instructions for assuming the Sims' position (left anterior oblique) (Figure 17-1). Cover the patient with a bath blanket for warmth and modesty. Avoid exposing the patient more than is necessary. Hang the enema container approximately 18 inches above the level of the table. The proper height is important because the position of the enema bag regulates the liquid flow pressure. When the bag is too high, the increased hydrostatic pressure may produce a flow that is too rapid, causing abdominal cramping. Excessive pressures could also cause serious harm to patients with conditions that weaken or inflame the bowel, such as **diverticulitis** or **ulcerative colitis.**

To insert the rectal catheter, wear disposable gloves, spread the buttocks with your fingers, and gently push the lubricated tip through the anus, directing it superiorly and anteriorly into the rectum 2 to 4 inches. When inserting a rectal catheter in a female patient, take care to ensure that the catheter enters the anus and not the vagina. At first, point the tip in the general direction of the umbilicus. If you encounter any resistance to

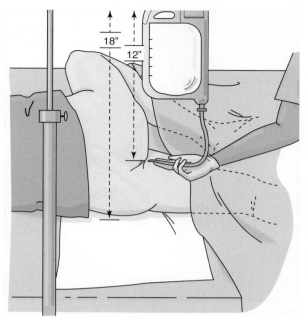

FIG 17-1 Patient and equipment placement for enema administration. (From Sorrentino SA. *Mosby's textbook for nursing assistants*, ed 8, St Louis, 2012, Mosby.)

the insertion of the catheter, do not exert more force. It may be helpful to gently direct the tip posteriorly to accommodate the posterior flexure of the rectum (Figure 17-2) or to permit a bit of the liquid to flow before attempting to advance the catheter. Sometimes feces in the rectum prevent proper insertion. In this case, ask the patient to defecate before continuing with the enema. If extensive **hemorrhoids** (enlarged rectal veins) or other pathologic conditions interfere with catheter insertion, seek the assistance of a nurse or physician.

When the catheter is properly situated, open the clamp, allowing the liquid to flow. If the patient complains of abdominal cramping, lower the enema container or stop the flow temporarily and encourage the patient to relax by breathing through the mouth and panting lightly. Spasms of the bowel may occur during enema administration and often produce discomfort as well as an urge to defecate. The patient may feel "full" and believe that no further liquid can be tolerated. A spasm often occurs after the administration of about 200 mL of liquid, which is the approximate amount required to fill the sigmoid colon. When viewing the

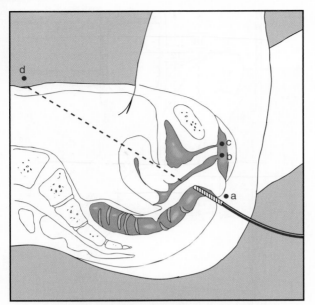

FIG 17-2 Rectal anatomy in relation to other anatomic structures (female patient). **A,** Anus. **B,** Vaginal orifice. **C,** Urethral orifice. **D,** Umbilicus.

fluoroscopic image during a barium enema examination, you will have an opportunity to observe this occurrence. If the patient has received less than 400 mL of the enema, you can be certain this feeling is caused by spasm rather than actual filling of the colon. A brief pause, perhaps with a change of position, should relieve the spasm and allow the procedure to continue. When the bag is empty, or if the patient complains of fullness after the administration of at least 750 mL, stop the flow and remove the catheter. Encourage the patient to hold the enema for 10 minutes, if possible, before going to the bathroom.

Assist the patient to the bathroom or onto the bedpan and allow as much privacy as is consistent with patient safety. When patients require help onto the **commode** (toilet), use the same face-to-face assist learned in Chapter 12 for helping patients into wheelchairs. Make certain that the back of the gown is clear of the seat. Ensure the patient's safety and then leave the patient alone, calling attention to the emergency call button if one is available. Check with the patient at frequent intervals. If the patient or gown has become soiled, provide a clean gown, a warm, wet washcloth, a towel, and assistance with cleansing, as needed. A pleasant, helpful attitude reassures patients

who may feel very embarrassed about having soiled themselves.

Permit ample time for the patient to expel the enema. This is very important because spasm of the colon may deceive the patient into thinking that evacuation is complete. If the patient has expelled only a part of the enema and is unable to expel the remainder, encourage some physical activity. Standing up and walking around the room for a few minutes usually results in relaxation of the spasm, allowing the patient to complete the evacuation.

One large enema that fills the entire colon is much more effective than several small ones that fill only the sigmoid colon and are discontinued at the first sign of discomfort. If the order calls for "enemas until clear," repeat the procedure up to a total of three times or until no solid material can be detected in the stool. If you are checking for this result, instruct the patient not to flush the commode.

When inspecting the stool, you may see evidence of bleeding. A black, tarry substance is indicative of blood from the upper GI tract. Fresh, red blood may result from hemorrhoids or pathologic conditions in the colon. When there is more than a trace of blood in the stool, report this finding immediately, and continue with additional enemas only on the direct order of a physician. Because visualization of the causative lesion may be the reason for the examination, the physician may want the preparation to be continued or perhaps modified to fit the patient's condition.

The sodium phosphate (Fleet) enema is a complete, disposable enema unit containing a salt solution that is highly efficient as an evacuant. It is very effective for the distal portion of the large bowel, but does not contain enough fluid to cleanse the entire colon. This enema is sometimes used as a final step in a more comprehensive regimen and is often the method of choice for impromptu use in the radiology department when the patient's previous preparation has not been adequate. Complete instructions come with the product and are easily understood by radiographers and most outpatients.

When excessive amounts of gas and feces are present, cleansing preparation may be desirable for examinations of the sacrum and coccyx. Standing orders seldom specify this application. With emphasis on limiting radiation exposure, especially to the pelvic area, bowel cleansing before sacrum and coccyx radiography may deserve reconsideration. A Fleet enema for this purpose is inexpensive, easy to give, and relatively tolerable for the patient. It may decrease the number of repeat exposures while increasing diagnostic accuracy.

CONTRAST MEDIA AND OTHER DIAGNOSTIC AIDS FOR GASTROINTESTINAL EXAMINATIONS

Barium Sulfate

Barium sulfate is an inert inorganic salt of the chemical element barium. It is used exclusively for radiography of the GI tract and is administered either orally or rectally. Barium is packaged in many forms, ranging from 100 lb drums of plain barium sulfate to premeasured packets containing a finely pulverized form of the medium combined with artificial flavoring and coloring. Barium sulfate must not be administered in powder form. The dry powder is mixed with water just before use, forming a suspension that may be thick or thin, depending on the proportions of barium and water. Barium is also supplied in concentrated liquid suspensions, and this is the type of product that is most commonly used. These suspensions may be ready to use or may require dilution. Instructions for specific applications are provided with the products. Barium is also supplied in tubes in the form of an oral paste for studies of the pharynx and the esophagus.

The barium itself has no flavor, but many patients find it difficult to swallow because of its chalky consistency. For oral administration, it is most palatable when cold and offered with a drinking straw, which helps prevent it from coating the mouth.

For rectal administration (barium enema), disposable enema kits are available that include a plastic bag, enema tubing, and a rectal catheter. A liquid barium suspension may be poured into a disposable enema bag and diluted, if required, with tepid water. Some kits contain powdered barium, to which the radiographer must simply add water and shake vigorously. The bags are usually printed with graduated markings to aid in measuring the water as it is added. A bead at the junction of the bag and the tubing may prevent premature emptying of the bag. After mixing the barium in the bag, squeeze at the junction to dislodge the bead and allow the tube to fill. If the unit has a clamp rather than

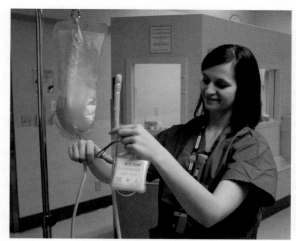

FIG 17-3 Close the clamp while filling the bag, then open it briefly to allow the tube to fill.

a bead to prevent flow through the tubing, close the clamp while filling the bag and open it briefly to allow the tube to fill (Figure 17-3).

The proper viscosity (thickness) of the barium suspension is important in GI examinations. Studies of the esophagus require a thick mixture, whereas single-contrast barium enemas demand a thin one. Radiologists' preferences vary regarding the proportions to be used in regulating viscosity. This can usually be controlled with sufficient accuracy by following established standard measurements for the amounts of barium and water to be combined for each study. Suggested proportions for various applications (indicated by the weight of barium sulfate per volume of water [w/v]) are provided in Table 17-1.

Because barium sulfate is an inert compound, it does not react chemically with the body to any appreciable extent. Allergies to barium itself are almost never a problem, and few side effects occur. If oral barium preparations contain coloring or flavoring additives, it may be standard practice to check with patients about possible allergies to these substances. The principal problem complicating the use of barium is its hygroscopic nature (that is, its tendency to absorb water). When mixed with water, it slowly absorbs the liquid and tends to solidify in the same manner as plaster of Paris, although to a lesser degree. The normal function of the colon, which is to absorb water from the bowel contents, tends to increase this problem. Care must be taken so that patients with restricted bowel action do not develop a bowel obstruction as a result of barium impaction. Inactive geriatric patients are most prone to this problem. To decrease the risk of these complications, patients should increase intake of fluids and bulk in their diet. A laxative or cathartic preparation may also be prescribed following barium studies of either the upper or lower GI tract.

Instances of allergic reactions to latex (rubber) products, including a few severe anaphylactic responses to latex enema tips, have been reported. Products have now been introduced that do not contain latex, and these have largely replaced latex enema tips. If your facility uses latex tips, you may need to take a patient's allergy history before barium enema studies (see Chapter 19).

Iodinated Media

Special water-soluble iodine compounds, such as Gastrografin and Hypaque Sodium Oral, are available for contrast examinations of the GI tract. The radiologist will determine when these media are needed. These media are used only in special cases when the administration of barium sulfate may be contraindicated. They are especially useful when a rupture of the GI tract is suspected, such as perforated ulcer or ruptured appendix, because these compounds can be absorbed into the bloodstream from within the peritoneal cavity. For this reason, they are also advantageous when the risk of

TABLE 17-1	Barium Sulfate Oral Suspension Dosage Recommendations		
	Examination	**Usual Dose**	**Barium Concentration (w/v)**
Adult and adolescent (usually applicable to geriatric patients, but may be modified by physician)	Esophagus, single contrast	5-150 mL	60%-155%
	Esophagus, double contrast	15-140 mL	60-250%
	Stomach and duodenum, single contrast	240-360 mL	40-120%
	Stomach, double contrast	Initially, 75-120 mL for gastric coating	200-250%
		After gastric coating is observed and radiographs are taken, an additional 150–300 mL may be administered	40-80%
	Entire small intestine, oral administration with follow-through imaging	480-700 mL	40-80%
	Enteroclysis	500-2400 mL	24-50%
Pediatric	Upper GI, single contrast	Dosage must be individualized by physician	50-100%
	Upper GI, double contrast	Dosage must be individualized by physician	200-250%
	Entire small intestine, oral administration with follow-through imaging	Dosage must be individualized by physician	50-100%
	Enteroclysis	Dosage must be individualized by physician	20-30%

Note: Suspension should be mixed vigorously just before administration.
Data from www.drugs.com/mmx/barium-sulfate.html

perforation during the procedure is a concern, and they are indicated when abdominal surgery is likely in the immediate future. Barium sulfate extravasation (leakage) into the peritoneal cavity cannot be absorbed and therefore presents a much more serious complication than water-soluble contrast agents. The iodinated media may be used when there is a high risk of barium impaction, and they are also occasionally used for neonatal studies. In cases of suspected perforation, some radiologists will begin the procedure with a water-soluble contrast agent. When no perforation is identified, they may repeat the examination with barium, which provides greater radiographic contrast.

Compared with barium, iodinated contrast media are more expensive and generally produce less radiographic contrast. Hyperosmolar ionic iodinated media are not without risk either (see Chapter 19). Serious dehydration and complications from aspiration can result. These media are therefore contraindicated for examinations of the esophagus or when a fistula (abnormal passageway) connecting the esophagus and the trachea is suspected. A nonionic, low osmolar contrast medium can be used in place of barium when esophageal perforation or esophageal-tracheal fistulas are being ruled out.

Air Contrast

Barium and iodine compounds provide positive contrast; that is, they absorb more radiation than surrounding tissues and make a white or light shadow on the image. Air and gases, on the other hand, absorb less radiation and produce negative contrast, or dark shadows. When used in combination for double-contrast GI examinations, the barium coats the mucosal lining of the alimentary canal, while the air fills the lumen. The result is a high degree of contrast, which tends to enhance visualization of the GI mucosa.

Glucagon

Glucagon is one of the drugs used to treat hypoglycemia. In addition to increasing the level of blood glucose, it causes relaxation of the smooth muscle of the GI tract. This effect is useful as a diagnostic aid in examinations of the GI tract because it slows peristalsis (contractions that propel food through the digestive tract) and prevents cramping. Anticholinergic drugs, such as atropine, have a similar effect, but glucagon is most commonly used for this purpose because of a lower incidence of side effects.

Commercially prepared glucagon is a polypeptide hormone identical to naturally occurring human glucagon. It is supplied in lyophilized (freeze-dried) form as part of a kit that includes a diluent and specific instructions. The drug is mixed with the diluting solution immediately before use. When using glucagon, follow the general instructions in Box 17-2.

Table 17-2 lists recommended dosages, routes of administration, and anticipated timing of effects. Because the stomach is less sensitive to the effect of glucagon, 0.5 mg (0.5 units) IV or 2 mg (2 units) intramuscular (IM) are recommended for examinations of

---

BOX 17-2 Guidelines for Administration of Glucagon

- The diluent is provided for use only in the preparation of glucagon for parenteral injection and for no other use.
- Glucagon should not be used at concentrations greater than 1 mg/mL (1 unit/mL).
- Reconstituted glucagon should be used immediately. *Discard any unused portion.*
- Reconstituted glucagon solutions should be used only if they are clear and of a water-like consistency.
- Parenteral drug products should be inspected visually before administration to check for particulate matter and discoloration.

From *Clinical Pharmacology* at http://www.clinicalpharmacology.com

---

TABLE 17-2 Effects of Dose and Route of Administration on Response to Glucagon

Dose	Route of Administration	Time of Onset of Action	Approximate Duration of Effect
0.25-0.5 mg (0.25-0.5 units)	IV	1 min	9-17 min
1 mg (1 unit)	IM	8-10 min	12-27 min
2 mg* (2 units)	IV	1 min	22-25 min
2 mg* (2 units)	IM	4-7 min	21-32 min

*Administration of 2 mg (2 units) produces a higher incidence of nausea and vomiting than does lower doses.
From *Clinical Pharmacology* at http://www.clinicalpharmacology.com
IM, Intramuscular; *IV*, intravenous.

the stomach, duodenum, and/or small bowel. For colon examinations, the recommended dose is 2 mg (2 units) IM approximately 10 minutes before the procedure. The most common side effects of glucagon administration are nausea and vomiting, which are most likely to occur with doses of 2 mg (2 units).

UPPER GASTROINTESTINAL STUDIES

Studies of the upper gastrointestinal tract may be ordered for a number of reasons (Table 17-3). The study may include only the esophagus (esophagram) or the entire portion of the digestive tract between the pharynx and the the duodenum.

Perhaps the purpose that first comes to mind is detecting the possibility of ulcer formation. Ulcers are lesions or sores affecting the mucous lining of the GI tract and may occur in any portion of it. Ulcers may cause pain, but become even more serious when they bleed, causing anemia and sometimes hemorrhagic shock. Another cause of bleeding in the upper GI tract

is a condition known as esophageal varices. These are enlarged veins in the lower part of the esophagus that occur most often in patients with serious liver disease. They are usually asymptomatic unless they bleed. Bleeding in the upper GI tract results in dark or black blood with a tarry consistency in the bowel movement. Emesis during an upper GI bleed typically has the appearance of coffee grounds.

The terms esophagitis, gastritis, and duodenitis refer to infection or inflammation of the esophagus, stomach, or duodenum, respectively. Gastroesophageal reflux disease (GERD) is a type of esophagitis that occurs when stomach contents breech the esophageal sphincter, bringing stomach acid into contact with the more delicate mucosa of the esophagus. GERD can cause substernal pain that is sometimes mistaken for heart pain, and often causes an intense sensation of heat in the throat, commonly called heartburn. A hiatal hernia, which is the protrusion of a portion of the stomach into the thoracic cavity (Figure 17-4), can also cause heartburn. This occurs when the upper

TABLE 17-3 Conditions, Indications, and Contraindications Pertinent to Gastrointestinal Examinations

Examination	Conditions	Indications/Symptoms	Contraindications
Esophagrams - Adult and Adolescent	Varices, neoplasm, GERD, hiatal hernia, obstruction, foreign body, stricture, or perforation	Atypical chest pain (substernal), dysphagia, heartburn, black tarry stool	Perforations of any portion of the gastrointestinal tract, acute bowel obstruction, severe constipation, pregnancy, severe dysphagia
Upper GI Studies	Ulcers, gastritis, hiatal hernia, GERD, neoplasm	Nausea, vomiting, gastric bleeding, weight loss, anemia, abdominal pain	
All Small Bowel Studies	Obstruction, tumor, fistula, IBD/IBS	Abnormal bleeding, malabsorption, abdominal pain, unexplained weight loss, diarrhea, abdominal masses	
Lower GI Studies	IBD/IBS, neoplasm, diverticulitis	Chronic diarrhea, constipation, cramping, gas, bloating, lower abdominal pain, passing of red blood, mucus, or pus	Suspected bowel perforation, severe ulcerative colitis, pregnancy, toxic megacolon, acute abdominal pain
Pediatric GI Studies (in addition to conditions and indications listed above for adults)	Congenital syndromes, suspected motility disorders, great vessel anomalies, post-surgical evaluation, malrotation, intussusception	Recurrent pneumonia, failure to thrive	

portion of the stomach pushes up through the hiatus, the opening in the diaphragm through which the esophagus passes before reaching the stomach. Gastritis can occur as a result of overproduction of stomach acid, sometimes due to bacterial infection, and may be the precursor of ulcers.

Structural problems such as **diverticula** (pocket formations in mucous membranes), **strictures** (narrowing of the lumen of the GI tract), and **polyps** (growths that occur on mucous membranes) can cause upper GI symptoms, as can neoplasms, which may be either benign or malignant. These conditions may cause difficulty moving foods through the pharynx or esophagus, which is classified as a *motility disorder*. Motility disorders are characterized by symptoms that include **dysphagia** (difficulty swallowing), chest and/or abdominal pain, and unexplained vomiting and/or indigestion.

Contraindications for an upper GI series include, but are not limited to, perforations of any portion of the gastrointestinal tract, acute bowel obstruction (see page 319), severe constipation, pregnancy, and severe dysphagia that would be likely to cause aspiration of barium into the lungs.

Routine Upper Gastrointestinal Series

An upper GI series is a fluoroscopic and radiographic examination of the esophagus, stomach, and duodenum. Barium is typically used as the contrast medium for this study and is administered orally. Patient preparation is usually quite simple, consisting of an NPO order for approximately 8 hours before the examination. Some radiologists prefer that patients not smoke on the day of the examination, because smoking may increase gastric

secretions, resulting in liquid dilution of the contrast medium in the stomach. For the same reason, patients should avoid chewing gum. Figure 17-5 demonstrates the importance of adequate preparation for an upper GI study.

The examination usually begins with the fluoroscopic table in the upright position and the patient standing on the footboard. While the patient drinks the barium, the radiologist observes the fluoroscopic image of the esophagus. The table is then placed in the horizontal position, and the recumbent patient is turned into various positions to coat the lining of the stomach and to demonstrate all aspects of the mucosal lining of the stomach and proximal duodenum. The table may also be placed in the Trendelenburg position, and the patient asked to stop breathing and bear down as if having a bowel movement. This is called the **Valsalva maneuver** and is sometimes useful in the diagnosis of hiatal hernia.

The patient care role of the radiographer in this examination consists of preliminary explanations and instructions, handing the patient the cup of barium, receiving the cup when the patient has finished it, and assisting the patient to assume various positions as directed by the radiologist during fluoroscopy. The examination is occasionally delayed when the barium in the stomach does not empty into the duodenum because of **pylorospasm** (constriction of the sphincter muscle between the stomach and the duodenum). In this event, place the patient in the right anterior oblique position, which allows gravity to assist the normal flow of gastric contents. Following the fluoroscopic examination with spot images, the radiographer may take images with the overhead tube.

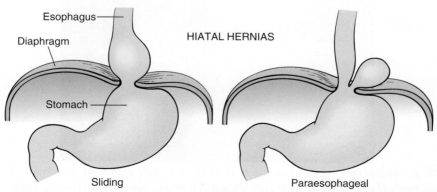

FIG 17-4 Hiatal hernia. (From Damjanov I. *Pathology for the health professions*, ed 3, St Louis, 2006, Elsevier Saunders.)

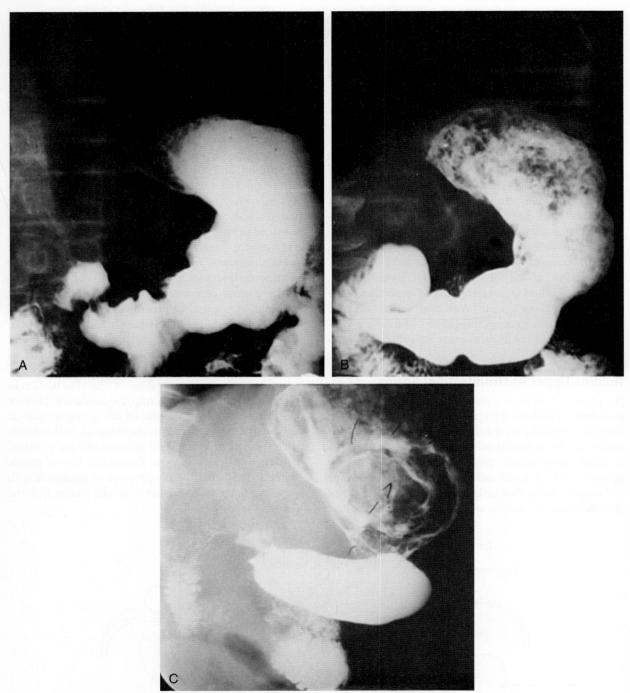

FIG 17-5 A, Normal radiograph of stomach. **B,** Upper GI study with food in stomach. **C,** Cancer of the stomach. Note the similarity in appearance of B and C. (Courtesy of Harvey Tracy, Swedish Hospital, Seattle, WA.)

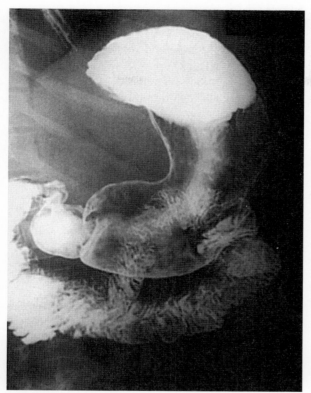

FIG 17-6 Double-contrast upper gastrointestinal study. (From Long BW, Rollins JH, Smith BJ. *Merrill's atlas of radiographic positioning & procedures*, ed 13, St Louis, 2016, Mosby.)

Double-Contrast Upper Gastrointestinal Study

Double-contrast examination is another method used to evaluate the upper GI tract. The examination is "double-contrast" because it uses both barium or an iodinated medium to provide positive contrast, and gas which is a negative contrast agent. This combination enhances visualization of the mucosal surface (Figure 17-6) and involves some variation in procedure compared to the routine upper GI series. At the beginning of the examination, the patient is given a gas-producing substance in the form of a tablet, powder, or carbonated beverage. This is followed by a small amount of a high-density barium mixture. The patient may feel the need to belch but should be instructed to try not to do so, because the gas must be retained in the stomach to provide radiographic contrast.

Glucagon may be injected IM or IV before examination to induce relaxation of the stomach and duodenum for improved visualization. The technical aspects of this procedure are essentially the same as for the routine upper GI series.

Hypotonic Duodenography

This examination is useful for the detection of lesions in the duodenum distal to the duodenal bulb and for the diagnosis of pancreatic disease. It involves passing a tube through the mouth or nose and into the duodenum after the administration of glucagon to relax the GI tract and halt peristalsis. Barium and air are injected through the tube via syringe to provide radiographic contrast. The procedure is similar to the enteroclysis examination of the small bowel discussed in the following section, the differences being the placement of the tube and the extent of bowel to be evaluated. The use of this study is declining. Double-contrast upper GI examinations are more likely to be used for evaluation of the duodenal loop, and ultrasound, CT, needle biopsy, or endoscopic retrograde cholangiopancreatography are used for pancreatic evaluation. These imaging methods are discussed in Chapters 19 and 22.

SMALL BOWEL STUDIES

There are two basic methods of introducing contrast into the small bowel for radiographic evaluation: oral and enteroclysis, or small intestine enema, in which an intestinal tube is used to instill the contrast.

Oral Method

The most common method of studying the small bowel is the oral method. For this study, the patient drinks the barium suspension, and a series of timed radiographs follows its progress through the small bowel. The first radiograph is usually taken 15 minutes after the ingestion of the barium, and subsequent radiographs are taken at 15- to 30-minute intervals until the entire small bowel is visualized (Figure 17-7). A small bowel follow through is complete when the cecum is visualized in the right lower quadrant. Fluoroscopy with spot films may be used at any time during the procedure to study portions of the intestine as they become opacified with the contrast medium. Ice water, coffee, tea, or a food stimulant may be used to increase intestinal motility and speed the filling of the small bowel. Often this procedure follows an upper GI series, utilizing a single dose of barium for both studies. A limited study of the small bowel may be a routine part of the upper GI series, consisting

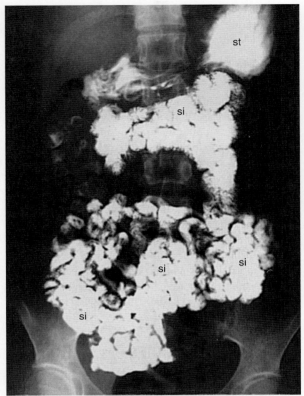

FIG 17-7 Small intestine 30 minutes after oral ingestion of barium. (From Long BW, Rollins JH, Smith BJ. *Merrill's atlas of radiographic positioning & procedures*, ed 13, St Louis, 2016, Mosby.)

of a single radiograph of the abdomen taken 30 to 60 minutes after barium ingestion.

Enteroclysis

Enteroclysis is the injection of nutrient or medicinal liquid into the small bowel. For the radiographic procedure, a special catheter with a stiff wire guide (Bilbao or Sellink tube) is inserted through the mouth or nose and advanced to the distal portion of the duodenum. Barium is injected through the tube under fluoroscopic control at a flow rate of approximately 100 mL per minute. Fluoroscopy and spot film radiography are followed by routine radiographs (Figure 17-8). Once the contrast has reached the cecum, air or methylcellulose may be injected through the tube to provide double contrast.

Thorough cleansing of both the large and small bowel is essential to the success of the enteroclysis

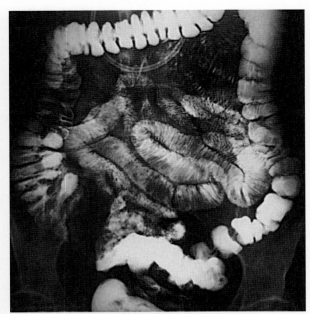

FIG 17-8 Enteroclysis procedure demonstrates contrast filling of both small bowel and colon. (From Long BW, Rollins JH, Smith BJ. *Merrill's atlas of radiographic positioning & procedures*, ed 13, St Louis, 2016, Mosby.)

study and must be accomplished without the use of enemas, because enema fluid may be retained in the small bowel and degrade the quality of the visualization. The routine preparation is usually a combination of diet and cathartics.

EXAMINATIONS OF THE LOWER GASTROINTESTINAL TRACT

Fluoroscopic/radiographic examination often plays a significant role in the diagnosis of conditions that affect the colon and rectum. Some indications for lower GI studies are similar to those for the upper GI tract (Table 7-3). For example, inflammation and ulcerations of the mucosa can also affect the colon and can be quite serious. These manifestations are termed **inflammatory bowel diseases (IBDs).** When chronic irritation and inflammation cause bouts of diarrhea, cramping, and gas, but do not cause physical changes in the bowel tissue, the condition is termed **irritable bowel syndrome (IBS).** When chronic inflammation results in small open sores on the mucosal surface of the colon or rectum, the condition is known as ulcerative colitis. Another form of IBD, **Crohn disease,** is

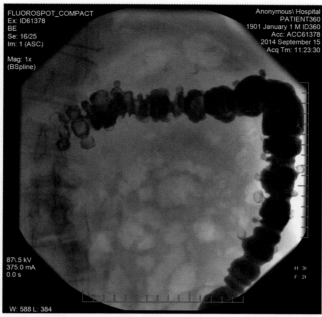

FIG 17-9 Fluoroscopic spot film showing diverticula in the transverse and descending colon.

an autoimmune disease that causes damaging inflammation and may affect the entire gastrointestinal system. All of these conditions typically produce symptoms of chronic diarrhea, constipation, cramping, bloating, pain, and/or the passing of blood, mucus, or pus. Blood originating in the colon or rectum is red in color, as opposed to the black appearance of blood from the upper GI tract.

> Red blood in the stool indicates bleeding from the colon or rectum, whereas black tarry stools are typical of bleeding from the upper GI tract.

As stated previously, diverticula are pouches or pockets that form in the walls of the digestive tract. The presence of diverticula in the colon is termed **diverticulosis** (Figure 17-9) and is a common condition in the aging population. Although diverticulosis is often asymptomatic, it is not unusual for fecal matter to become lodged in the diverticula, causing the inflammation known as diverticulitis. Approximately 25% of patients suffering from acute diverticulitis develop complications. These may include bowel obstruction due to scarring, a fistula between portions of the bowel or between the bowel and the bladder, or an **abscess**. An abscess is a painful,

localized collection of pus that can occur in the colon when swelling causes obstruction of a diverticulum, preventing drainage and allowing the proliferation of bacteria.

Polyps or tumors, malignant or benign, can impede the passage of intestinal contents through the bowel. Such problems are characterized by symptoms of bloating, lower abdominal pain, changes in bowel habits, and the passage of blood in the stool. In the case of a tumor, particularly colon cancer, signs often include unexplained weight loss, and the condition may have a profound effect on general health.

Bowel obstruction is a condition of partial or complete blockage of the digestive tract that may be caused by scar tissue. Although adhesive scars often result from surgery, they can also occur with no history of surgery as a result of inflammatory disease As surgical or inflammatory lesions heal, tissues may stick together, forming adhesions, which are attachments that change the configuration of the intestine and cause motility disorders. Bowel obstruction may affect the small intestine as well as the colon.

When motility disorders affect newborns or small children, barium enema studies may be performed to detect congenital anomalies, malrotation of the bowel,

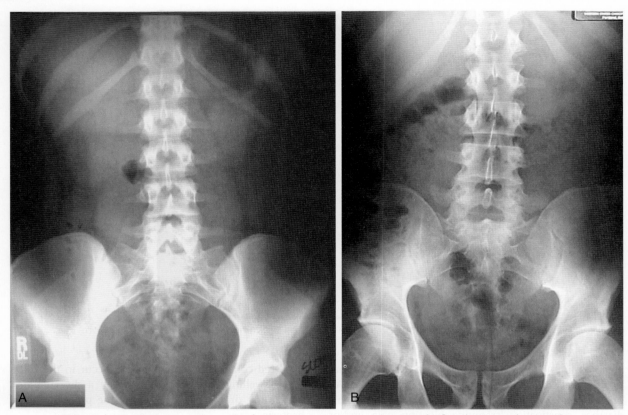

FIG 17-10 Preliminary radiographs for barium enema examination. **A,** Good preparation results in very little gas or fecal matter within the abdomen. **B,** Extensive gas and fecal material shows a lack of adequate preparation.

or intussusception (a serious disorder in which the intestine "telescopes" upon itself, allowing part of the intestine to slide into an adjacent portion). These conditions may also affect the small bowel.

Contraindications for a barium enema include, but are not limited to suspected bowel perforation, severe ulcerative colitis, pregnancy, toxic megacolon, and acute abdominal pain.

Routine Barium Enema

A barium enema (BE) is a routine fluoroscopic and radiographic examination of the colon. Barium sulfate is instilled under fluoroscopic control, followed by the taking of radiographic images, evacuation of the barium, and the taking of post-evacuation radiographs.

A preliminary radiograph of the abdomen may be taken before the instillation of barium (Figure 17-10). This "scout" image has diagnostic value from the

radiologist's viewpoint and may also provide technical assistance to the radiographer. In addition, it affords a further opportunity to assess the efficacy of the preparation. If fecal material is seen in the colon on this image, further preparation may be required for an optimum study. If glucagon is routinely used, it is usually administered intramuscularly following evaluation of the preliminary radiograph. Glucagon induces colon relaxation and reduces patient discomfort, which may allow the radiologist to perform a more satisfactory examination.

The administration of the BE is very similar to the procedure for the cleansing enema, with several significant exceptions:

- A larger amount of liquid is prepared for a BE than for a cleansing enema, usually 1200 to 1500 mL.
- The enema bag is suspended a greater distance above the table, usually 24 to 30 inches. This is necessary

because the greater viscosity of the barium suspension requires greater hydrostatic pressure to maintain an adequate flow rate.

- A larger rectal catheter is used. This may be a disposable plastic enema tip or a disposable retention catheter with an inflatable cuff (Figure 17-11).

The retention catheter helps the patient retain the barium for the duration of the study. Some radiology departments use retention catheters for all patients. In other facilities, the radiographer must decide when a retention catheter is required. Patients who are alert, competent, and cooperative may be more comfortable with a plain enema tip. Others may feel more secure with a retention cuff in place. The patient's expectation regarding enema retention may help you decide which tip to use. The cuff of the retention catheter is inflated with an air pump. Most disposable retention catheter kits include a disposable pump in the form of a plastic bag that is squeezed to inflate the cuff. Follow the directions provided with the unit. Over-inflation of the catheter cuff may injure or rupture the rectum, which could be very hazardous to the patient. To minimize this risk, the radiologist can inflate the cuff under fluoroscopic control at the beginning of the procedure.

Place the patient in the lateral recumbent or left Sims' position for insertion of the enema tip. Don protective gloves, and insert the lubricated tip as instructed for the cleansing enema. If a retention catheter is used, inflate the cuff unless it is the radiologist's practice to do so. After the tip is situated, place the patient in the supine position in readiness for the fluoroscopic study. The radiologist will indicate when to start and stop the barium flow. After fluoroscopy, routine radiographs are taken (Figure 17-12).

When the study is complete, remove the tube and escort the patient to the bathroom. If a retention catheter is used, be certain to deflate the cuff before attempting to remove the catheter. It may be beneficial to place the bag below the level of the table and allow part of the barium to drain back into the bag before removing the catheter. Alternatively, the catheter may be clamped and disconnected from the bag and removed from the rectum after the patient is seated on the commode.

Most BE examinations include one or more post-evacuation radiographs (Figure 17-13). The best result

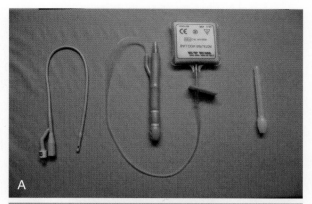

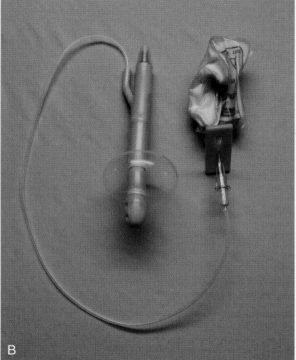

FIG 17-11 An assortment of enema catheters. **A,** Left to right: Foley (urinary) catheter (which may be used for pediatric enemas and for enemas through colostomies), retention catheter with inflatable tip, and disposable enema tip. **B,** Retention catheter with tip inflated. Disposable inflation device **(on right)** is included with product.

is obtained when the patient has evacuated the barium as completely as possible. As with the cleansing enema, allow ample time (at least 5 minutes) for evacuation and encourage physical activity if appropriate.

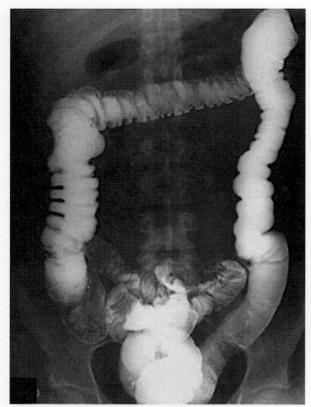

FIG 17-12 Barium enema study demonstrates lumen of colon (anteroposterior projection).

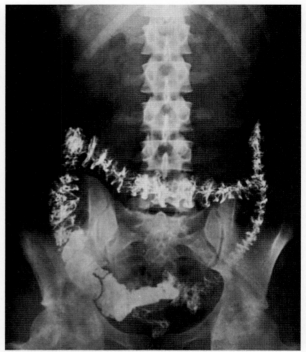

FIG 17-13 Post-evacuation radiograph shows the mucosal pattern of the colon (posteroanterior projection). (From Long BW, Rollins JH, Smith BJ. *Merrill's atlas of radiographic positioning & procedures*, ed 13, St Louis, 2016, Mosby.)

Barium Enema Considerations and Precautions

Patients with Colon Enlargement

Radiographers may need to provide special care to patients with unusual conditions who are undergoing BE examinations. Lower GI studies are important in diagnosis and evaluation of these conditions, but they may also prove hazardous.

One example is the patient with an enlarged colon, often caused by chronic constipation. An extreme example of colon enlargement is the infant or child who has **congenital megacolon** (colon enlargement present at birth), also called **Hirschsprung disease.** This condition involves a segment of distal colon in which no peristalsis occurs because of a neurologic deficiency. This causes chronic constipation and resulting enlargement of the colon to an extreme degree (Figure 17-14).

Whenever the colon is enlarged, the increased area of the mucosal lining provides greater opportunity for rapid, excessive absorption of water from the barium suspension. This predisposes these patients to barium impactions. The radiologist may decide to use an aqueous iodine contrast in place of barium. If barium is used, follow-up care to avoid impaction is essential. This may involve diet, forced fluids, cathartics, and/or cleansing enemas, similar to the preparation for the examination.

When colon enlargement causes excessive fluid absorption during a BE, a massive change in the fluid concentration in the blood, known as fluid overload or **hypervolemia,** may result. While this is not common, you should be alert to the onset of physical distress and shortness of breath with patients who have congestive heart failure. In such cases, extreme fluid overload could lead to total physical collapse.

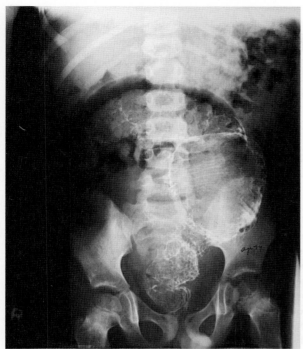

FIG 17-14 Barium enema study (post-evacuation): child with Hirschsprung disease. (From Ballinger PW, Frank ED. *Merrill's atlas of radiographic positions and radiologic procedures*, ed 10, St Louis, 2003, Mosby.)

The hazards of excessive water absorption can be reduced by mixing the barium with normal saline solution instead of tap water. Normal saline is a solution of 0.9% sodium chloride (table salt) in water; prepare it by dissolving 2 level teaspoons of salt in 1 liter of tepid water.

Potential Colon Perforation

As previously mentioned, any condition that causes weakening, inflammation, or degradation of the intestinal walls increases the possibility that perforation of the colon could occur during enema administration. In the case of a barium enema, extravasation of barium into the peritoneal cavity causes a very serious complication known as barium **peritonitis** (inflammation of the peritoneum, the lining of the abdominal cavity). Patients who are particularly at risk include the elderly, patients receiving long-term steroid medication, and those with diverticulitis or ulcerative colitis.

Precautions involve lowering the enema bag to maintain a relatively low flow pressure and/or using aqueous iodinated media instead of barium, when indicated. A rigorous bowel preparation may not be appropriate for patients at risk of bowel perforation. Instead, several days of a clear liquid diet may be substituted for the usual preparation.

Ostomies

Another situation requiring special knowledge and skill in the performance of a BE involves patients with ostomies, that is, colostomies or ileostomies. These patients have undergone surgical resections of the colon for the treatment of disease, trauma, obstruction, or birth defect. As explained in Chapter 10, the distal end of the remaining functioning bowel (proximal colon or, if the entire colon has been removed, the distal ileum) terminates in an artificial opening in the abdominal wall called a stoma. The stoma appears as a small hole surrounded by a rosette of mucosal tissue similar in appearance to the lining of the mouth. Because the patient has no voluntary control over the stoma, fecal matter is automatically expelled through this opening. In the case of a "double barrel" colostomy, there are two stomas: the distal end of the proximal segment and the proximal end of the distal segment. Fecal matter is expelled from the proximal segment and mucus from the distal portion.

The location of the stoma is determined by the nature of the surgery and the size of the bowel portion that has been removed. Figure 17-15 illustrates the common types of colostomy and ileostomy and lists the characteristics of each that may be of concern to radiographers. To determine a patient's ostomy type, check the history section of the chart. For the sake of simplicity in the material that follows, we will refer to all of these artificial openings into the GI tract as colostomies.

Colostomies may be temporary or permanent. Sometimes a temporary colostomy is performed to allow the distal portion of the bowel to rest and heal. The remaining bowel portions may later be surgically reconnected (anastomosis). If the distal portion of the bowel must be removed, the colostomy is permanent.

Patients with colostomies must wear a colostomy bag, which is a receptacle that fits over the stoma and is sealed to the skin surrounding it. Appliances for this purpose are designed to receive fecal matter, minimize

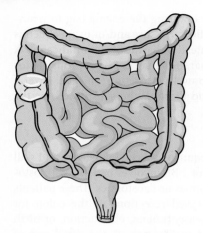

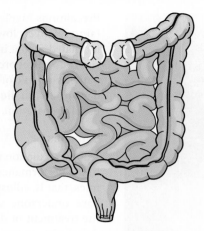

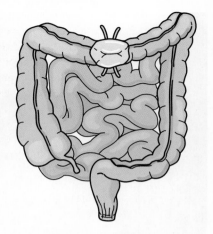

The **ascending colostomy** is done for right-sided tumors.

The **transverse (double-barreled) colostomy is** often used in such emergencies as intestinal obstruction or perforation because it can be created quickly. There are two stomas. The proximal one, closest to the small intestine, drains feces. The distal stoma drains mucus. Usually temporary.

The **transverse loop colostomy** has two openings in the transverse colon, but one stoma. Usually temporary.

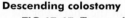

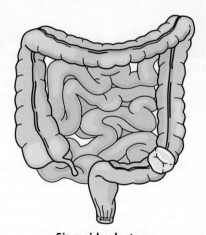

Descending colostomy

Sigmoid colostomy

FIG 17-15 Types of ostomies. (From Monahan FD, et al. *Phipps' medical-surgical nursing: Health and illness perspective*, ed 8, St Louis, 2007, Mosby.)

odor, and protect the skin surrounding the stoma. Fecal matter expelled from a colostomy may be highly odorous and irritating to the skin. The more proximal the colostomy, the more severe these problems tend to be. Patients with colostomies may be quite sensitive about this condition, and it is important to avoid any display of disgust or revulsion while caring for them. Until you are confident with the procedure, you should work with an experienced radiographer.

Patients who have had a colostomy for any length of time are accustomed to performing their own colostomy care and are often most comfortable when they are allowed to empty their colostomy bag and cleanse the area themselves. Many colostomy patients irrigate their stoma daily to initiate a bowel movement at a convenient time. This allows them to wear a smaller bag or simply a protective cover. If a cleansing enema is necessary, the competent colostomy patient may do a much more effective job than the radiographer. If you must perform an irrigation (cleansing enema) on a colostomy patient, the procedure is essentially the same as that for the colostomy BE (described in the following paragraphs), except that water is used instead of barium.

A special catheter is needed for the colostomy BE. A urinary retention (Foley) catheter may be used, since it is smaller than a rectal catheter and has a small inflatable cuff to hold it securely in place. Don disposable gloves, remove the colostomy bag, and cleanse the area. Place the patient in the supine position, and lubricate the catheter tip. Insert the catheter tip approximately 4 to 6 inches into the stoma. It is held in position by inflating the cuff with a syringe. The radiologist usually inserts the catheter and inflates the cuff. If it is your duty, insert the catheter gently and do not force it if you encounter any resistance. When the catheter is properly situated, use a syringe to inflate the catheter cuff to hold it snugly in place. Take care not to overinflate the cuff; 5 to 10 mL of air is usually sufficient. Special enema kits for colostomies are commercially available and may be used instead of the Foley catheter. One manufacturer's directions for such a kit, including illustrations, are shown in Figure 17-16.

A colostomy enema may require 500 to 700 mL of barium. The barium is instilled under fluoroscopic control as the radiologist directs. When the examination is complete, drain as much barium as possible back into the enema bag, deflate the catheter cuff, and remove the catheter. Provide the patient with an emesis basin or disposable colostomy bag in which to empty the barium. A suitable bag is a part of most disposable BE colostomy kits. If you are using this type of product, the bag will be in place during the examination, and the barium can be easily drained into it following the study.

The patient then requires the necessary supplies to cleanse the area and apply a fresh colostomy bag. Give instructions to outpatients in advance so that they can bring the necessary supplies from home to replace the colostomy bag after the examination. Chapter 10 provides instructions for assisting a patient to apply a fresh colostomy bag.

Occasionally, the distal portion of the remaining colon may be studied. For this part of the examination, the procedure is the same as for any routine BE except that much less barium is needed. Following this study, it may be necessary to irrigate the distal colon to remove the barium, because this part of the colon is no longer active in the elimination process.

Double-Contrast Barium Enema

Some radiologists prefer the enhanced visualization of the mucosal lining provided by double-contrast studies for some or all of the colon examinations they perform (Figure 17-17). A special barium mixture may be purchased for this purpose, or a preparation is thoroughly mixed to provide a suspension that is very smooth and somewhat thicker than for single-contrast studies. After the colon is filled, examined, and partially evacuated, air is instilled via the enema tip using a special insufflation device or an air pump, such as the bulb used with a sphygmomanometer. Air must be instilled slowly to avoid cramping and patient discomfort. After the study, the patient returns to the bathroom to evacuate the air and any residual barium.

Disposable double-contrast enema kits are available commercially. After routine instillation of barium, these kits allow barium to be siphoned back into the bag by lowering the bag below the height of the table. Thus, evacuation is accomplished without removing the patient from the fluoroscopic table. Air retained in the bag may then be instilled into the colon by turning the bag upside down and squeezing it gently. Some kits are supplied with a special enema tip that has a double lumen, allowing separate passages for air and barium and providing better control of air instillation.

Defecography

Defecography is a procedure for the evaluation of patients with defecational dysfunction. It is also known as evacuation proctography or dynamic rectal examination. Kits for this procedure include a high-density barium sulfate paste with a special injector to instill the barium. No patient preparation is needed. After the barium is instilled into the rectum, the patient is seated on a special radiolucent commode in front of the fluoroscopic unit. Video recording or serial spot films of the defecation process produce images in the lateral projection.

FOLLOW-UP CARE

As mentioned earlier, bowel care is very important after all barium studies because of the tendency

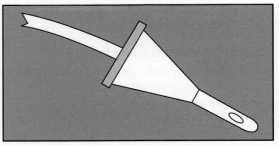

STEP 1: Lubricate the catheter tip with the water-soluble jelly (provided) and slide the catheter through the cone shield. Be sure the small end of the cone shield taper is pointing toward the blunt end of the catheter.

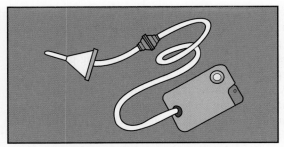

STEP 2: Attach the catheter to a standard barium solution bag by using the 5-1 connector that is attached to the catheter.

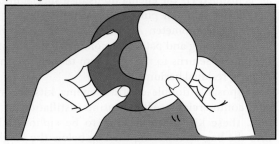

STEP 3: Remove the release paper from the adhesive ring on the irrigation sleeve.

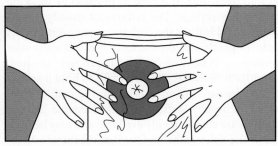

STEP 4: Attach the irrigation sleeve to the skin around the stoma.

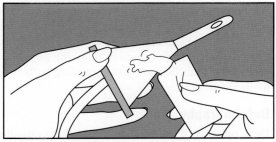

STEP 5: Lubricate the soft cone shield with the water-soluble jelly included in the kit.

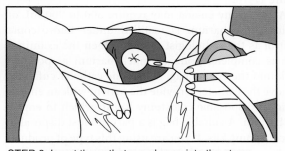

STEP 6: Insert the catheter and cone into the stoma through the top opening of the irrigation sleeve.

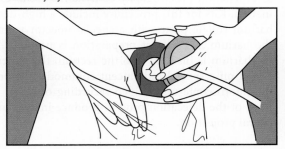

STEP 7: Cone may be held in place to retain the barium.

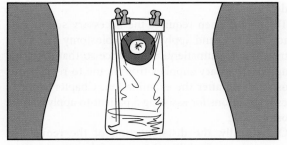

STEP 8: At the end of the procedure, fold the bottom of the sleeve to its top and clip in place with the two (2) clips enclosed.

FIG 17-16 Instructions for use of commercial barium enema colostomy kit. (Courtesy of Mentor Urology, Santa Barbara, CA.)

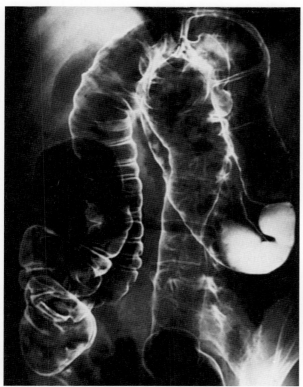

FIG 17-17 Double-contrast barium enema enhances visualization of mucosal pattern (oblique projection). (From Long BW, Rollins JH, Smith BJ. *Merrill's atlas of radiographic positioning & procedures*, ed 13, St Louis, 2016, Mosby.)

of barium to clump and harden in the bowel. This may cause constipation and, in severe cases, barium impaction with resulting bowel obstruction. To prevent these complications, instruct patients to increase their intake of fluids and high-bulk foods following barium examinations. It is also a common practice to administer a cathartic preparation following the examination. This may be a liquid, such as milk of magnesia or citrate of magnesia, or a tablet, such as bisacodyl. For inpatients, the nursing service may administer the medication when the patient returns to the unit. For outpatients, the radiographer may administer the cathartic when the examination is completed, or the patient may simply be instructed to take a laxative on returning home.

If the departmental policy is merely to prescribe a laxative and leave its procurement and administration to the patient, you must be very specific when explaining the rationale for this instruction. Otherwise, the patient who has just undergone a major catharsis in preparation for the examination may not feel inclined to heed the advice and may not follow through as directed. Some hospitals have found that the most effective method of ensuring compliance is for the radiographer to administer the cathartic to every outpatient on completion of the examination. If this is your duty, use the method for oral administration of medication described in Chapter 14.

SUMMARY

 Advance preparation is essential for most examinations of the GI tract. Diet, cathartics, enemas, and suppositories are used, alone or in combination, in preparation protocols.

- Contrast media are used to aid in visualization of the mucosal surfaces of the GI tract. Barium sulfate, sometimes in combination with air, is most commonly used, but ionic and nonionic iodinated media may be indicated for certain conditions.
- Glucagon is a drug used to relax smooth muscles and reduce peristalsis; it is administered IV or IM for various imaging studies of the GI tract.
- Conditions that may be diagnosed using upper gastrointestinal examinations include irritation or infection

of a portion of the upper digestive system: esophagitis, gastritis, or duodenitis. When severe, these conditions may result in the formation of ulcers. Causes may include GERD in the esophagus or excess production of acid in the stomach. Motility disorders may be caused by hiatal hernia, polyps, diverticula, or tumors. Symptoms that typically provide indications for upper GI studies include unexplained vomiting, indigestion/ heartburn, dysphagia, chest pain, upper abdominal pain, and black, tarry stools.

- A routine upper GI series is a study of the esophagus, stomach, and duodenum. A fasting patient drinks a barium sulfate mixture during fluoroscopic examination and spot imaging. The radiographer may obtain images with the overhead tube following the fluoroscopic examination.

- A double-contrast upper GI study is similar to the routine study except that, in addition to the barium, the patient also swallows a tablet, powder, or carbonated beverage to produce gas in the stomach.
- Hypotonic duodenography is a study that involves passing a tube into the duodenum after the administration of glucagon. Both barium and air are injected through the tube via a syringe to examine both the duodenum and the pancreas.
- The methods for radiographic examination of the small bowel involve oral ingestion of barium or instillation of barium via catheter into the duodenum. The latter method is termed enteroclysis.
- Conditions that may be diagnosed using lower gastrointestinal examinations include IBDs such as IBS, ulcerative colitis, and Crohn disease. Diverticulitis and its complications are also common sources of problems diagnosed with these

examinations, as are polyps and tumors. Symptoms of these conditions that typically serve as indications to order lower GI studies include lower abdominal pain, chronic diarrhea, constipation, gas, cramping, bloating, and/or the passing of red blood, mucus, or pus.

- The lower GI series, or BE, is a routine procedure for studying the colon. Barium or an iodinated medium, and sometimes also air, is introduced rectally during fluoroscopy. Radiographs are made before and after evacuation of the contrast medium.
- BEs on patients with colon enlargement, ostomies, and conditions that may predispose them to colon perforation require special precautions.
- Along with instructing the patient to drink plenty of fluids, cathartics may be administered following barium studies to prevent constipation or barium impaction resulting from hardening of the barium within the colon.

▌ REVIEW QUESTIONS

1. Preparation for an upper GI series usually involves:
   - A. cathartics
   - B. suppositories
   - C. enemas
   - D. nothing by mouth for 8 hours
2. A medication used to reduce peristalsis and prevent cramping for GI studies is:
   - A. glucagon
   - B. Glucophage
   - C. Gastrografin
   - D. barium sulfate
3. A position that assists the gravity flow of barium from the stomach is:
   - A. supine
   - B. prone
   - C. right anterior oblique
   - D. left posterior oblique
4. Oral administration and enteroclysis are methods of administering the contrast medium for examination of the:
   - A. esophagus
   - B. stomach

   - C. small bowel
   - D. colon
5. Follow-up care after an upper GI series or other barium study usually involves:
   - A. a clear liquid diet
   - B. cleansing enemas
   - C. a cathartic such as citrate of magnesia
   - D. glucagon
6. When performing a barium enema on a patient with Hirschsprung disease, safety concerns may require mixing the barium with:
   - A. glucagon
   - B. normal saline
   - C. iodine contrast
   - D. a gas-producing powder
7. A suppository is most likely used in preparation for which of the following examinations?
   - A. Barium enema
   - B. Hypotonic duodenography
   - C. Oral small bowel series
   - D. Upper GI series

8. A Foley catheter would be useful in performing which of the following examinations?
   A. Double-contrast barium enema performed through the rectum
   B. Barium enema performed through a colostomy
   C. Enteroclysis
   D. Double-contrast upper GI series
9. Which of the following examinations requires barium and air to be injected into the GI tract via a catheter?
   A. Double-contrast upper GI series
   B. Routine BE
   C. Hypotonic duodenography
   D. Defecography
10. Which of the following contrast media preparations would be appropriate for a GI examination when there is likelihood of colon perforation, or when GI surgery is immediately anticipated?
   A. Barium sulfate mixed with normal saline
   B. Barium sulfate mixed with a carbonated beverage
   C. An iodinated contrast medium
   D. Normal saline with glucagon

Answers can be found in the Answer Key on pages 429-431.

CRITICAL THINKING EXERCISES

1. Leah McKelvey calls from Dr. Rahaman's office to schedule a series of examinations for Martha Logan. Ms. Logan needs to have a chest radiograph, an excretory urogram study of the urinary tract involving IV administration of an iodine-containing contrast medium, and an upper GI series. She also needs to stop by the clinical laboratory to have fasting blood samples drawn for multiple blood chemistry tests. Leah wants to know whether this can all be done on the same day. Is this possible? Explain to Leah the advantages and disadvantages of scheduling these examinations on one day, compared to two or more separate appointments. In what order should these examinations be done?
2. Eleanor Buss, age 70, is an outpatient and has just arrived for her barium enema appointment with her daughter, who will be waiting to drive her home after the procedure. Mrs. Buss seems to be very anxious and nervous and is uncertain whether she wants to have the examination. List possible causes of Mrs. Buss's anxiety. What would you say to her?
3. Richard Meyerson, age 42, stops by the radiology department to arrange an appointment for a barium enema examination. The history on his requisition form states that Mr. Meyerson had colon surgery 6 months ago and has a sigmoid colostomy. Explain to Mr. Meyerson what will be involved, how he should prepare, and what he should bring with him to the examination.
4. Nathan Purdy, age 55, is scheduled for a barium enema. Upon reviewing the preliminary radiograph, the radiologist notes that there is excessive fecal material in the colon and instructs you to reschedule the examination. Tell Mr. Purdy why the examination must be rescheduled, and explain what he must do to ensure a good result.

18

Surgical Asepsis

OBJECTIVES

At the conclusion of this chapter, the student will be able to:

- Compare and contrast medical asepsis, disinfection, and sterilization.
- List four types of sterilization used in clinical settings, describe each, and state their principal applications.
- Correctly identify sterility indicators on sterile packs.
- Demonstrate correct procedure for establishing a sterile field.
- Demonstrate correct procedure for adding items to a sterile field without contaminating the field.
- Demonstrate correct procedure for preparing the skin for a sterile injection procedure such as an arteriogram or a myelogram.
- Demonstrate correct procedure for open sterile gloving.
- Demonstrate correct procedure for performing a surgical hand scrub/handrub.
- Demonstrate correct procedure for sterile gowning with closed gloving.
- Demonstrate correct procedure for removing a dressing and for applying a sterile dressing.

OUTLINE

Sterilization
    Chemical Sterilization
    Autoclaving
    Conventional Gas Sterilization
    Gas Plasma Technology
    Sterility Indicators
Sterile Fields

Skin Preparation
Donning Surgical Attire
Surgical Hand Scrub
    Traditional Method
    Alcohol-based Handrub Method
Sterile Gowning and Gloving
Removing and Applying Dressings

KEY TERMS

autoclave
free radical
sterile conscience

sterile field
sterilization
surgical asepsis

surgical hand scrub
surgical handrub

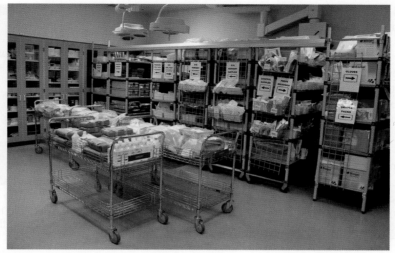

FIG 18-1 Storage area for sterile items in the central sterile supply department.

In Chapter 9 we defined medical asepsis as a method of reducing the number of pathogenic microorganisms in the environment and intervening in the process by which they are spread. **Surgical asepsis,** on the other hand, is the process of creating and maintaining an area that is completely free of pathogens. **Sterilization** is the complete destruction of all organisms and spores from equipment used for patient care or procedures. The sterile linens, gloves, and instruments used in surgery may be the first examples that come to mind, but many other procedures require sterile equipment, including lumbar punctures, catheterizations, and injections, as well as the care of some immunocompromised patients.

It should be clarified that, although the surgical suite contains sterile areas, radiographers who are called to this area to obtain radiographs or operate the C-arm fluoroscope do not wear sterile attire. Before entering, they dress in clean scrub clothes and wear a cap and surgical mask. Sterile gowns and gloves are not required because the radiographer avoids contact with the sterile field. Radiography in surgery is discussed in detail in Chapter 21.

Sterile items used in imaging departments are usually obtained from central sterile supply (Figure 18-1). Most disposable items, such as small syringes, intravenous sets, and catheterization sets, are sterile when purchased and are protected by a paper or plastic wrap. Reusable items, such as instruments and glass syringes, are wrapped, sterilized, and reissued by central sterile supply. Trays for surgical procedures may also be prepared in this way.

STERILIZATION

Although the radiographer is seldom directly involved in the process of sterilization, it is helpful to understand the methods that may be used. Four methods of sterilization are used, some of which are more reliable than others: chemical, autoclaving (steam), gas, and gas plasma.

Chemical Sterilization

Chemical sterilization involves the immersion and soaking of clean objects in a bath of germicidal solution followed by a sterile water rinse. The effectiveness of this process depends on solution strength, temperature, and immersion time, all of which are difficult to control accurately. Contamination of the solution or the object being sterilized may occur and is not easily detectable. For these reasons, chemical sterilization is one of the less satisfactory methods for providing surgical asepsis and is not recommended. If chemical sterilization must be used, follow the chemical manufacturer's instructions completely. Chemical sterilants are often used to achieve high-level disinfection of devices that come in contact with the mucous membranes, such as flexible, fiberoptic endoscopes. High-level disinfection can be accomplished in less than an hour and is effective at destroying microorganisms, but will not kill spores.

Autoclaving

An autoclave is a device that provides steam sterilization under pressure, the most commonly used sterilization method. It is also the quickest and most convenient means of sterilization for items that can withstand heat and moisture. High temperatures (250° F to 275° F [121° C to 135° C]) can be achieved under pressure, making this an extremely effective method.

> Steam sterilization by means of an autoclave is the most common and most effective method for most surgical instruments and trays.

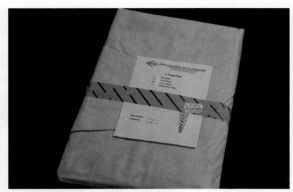

FIG 18-2 Sterility indicators. The tape that seals this pack was originally a plain, light color. The stripes appeared on the tape when conditions for sterility were achieved.

Conventional Gas Sterilization

Items that would be damaged by high temperatures are usually sterilized with a mixture of gases (Freon and ethylene oxide) heated to 135° F (57° C). Gas sterilization is used primarily for electrical, plastic, and rubber items, and for optical ware. Telephones, stethoscopes, blood pressure cuffs, and other equipment used in isolation rooms may be sterilized in this manner. This treatment is very effective but has one significant drawback: The gases used are poisonous, so they must be dissipated by means of aeration in a controlled environment. Because aeration is a slow process, it is important to send items for gas sterilization to central sterile supply well in advance of the time they will be used. A note indicating the date and hour the item is needed will help the staff plan their workload effectively.

Gas Plasma Technology

Because of the toxic fumes and residues of ethylene oxide sterilization, a safer method of sterilizing heat- and moisture-sensitive items is used where the need to sterilize a large volume of such equipment makes this method cost effective. Items are cleaned, wrapped, and placed in a compact mobile unit where low-temperature hydrogen peroxide gas plasma diffuses through the wrapped instruments and effectively kills both microorganisms and spores.

Gas plasma is formed within the sterilizing unit when vaporized hydrogen peroxide is subjected to radio-frequency energy, changing the vapor into a low-temperature plasma. The plasma then breaks down into free radicals (atoms with unpaired electrons in their outer shells). These free radicals destroy the microorganisms by stripping their atoms of electrons. Upon completion of the sterilization cycle, the remaining free radicals are converted into nontoxic by-products, primarily water and oxygen.

Because the gas plasma system uses very low heat and moisture, it can effectively sterilize endoscopes, fiberoptic devices, microsurgical instruments, and powered instruments. Another advantage is greater safety for central sterile supply department workers because there are no toxic fumes, by-products, or residues, and no handling of chemicals. For these reasons, gas plasma technology has significantly reduced the use of ethylene oxide, but it cannot completely replace this method. Gas plasma cannot sterilize instruments that have long, narrow lumina, and it cannot be used for powders, liquids, or any cellulose materials, such as paper, cotton, or linen.

Sterility Indicators

Most forms of hospital sterilization use chemical indicators to identify that a pack has been sterilized (Figure 18-2). Indicators are placed inside and outside the pack to show that the gas, steam, or gas plasma has penetrated to all surfaces. Indicators change color when the required conditions have been met.

> Radiographers are responsible for correctly recognizing the sterility indicators used in their clinical facility.

In addition to chemical indicators, hospitals use biological indicators (BIs) to ensure that all forms of microbial life are destroyed during the sterilization process. BIs are closed containers that contain different species of nonpathogenic spore-forming bacilli, each resistant to a specific sterilization process. The appropriate container is placed inside the unit with the instruments during sterilization. Inability to culture the spores following sterilization confirms that the instruments are free of all microbial life. BIs are used in each load that includes implantable devices and for quality control on a routine daily or weekly basis, depending on hospital policy.

Suppliers of commercial sterile packs use gamma radiation from cobalt-60 or an electron beam to destroy microorganisms and spores. Commercial packs also contain indicators and expiration dates to confirm their sterility.

STERILE FIELDS

A **sterile field** is a microorganism-free area prepared for the use of sterile supplies and equipment. It should be prepared on a clean, dry, flat work surface in an area that poses minimal risk for contamination and is within easy reach of the physician. Preparations must be made before starting a procedure that requires sterile technique, and the radiographer may be responsible for assembling the needed equipment. Sterile procedure in the imaging department usually involves the use of a sterile pack that includes most of the items needed for a specific procedure. Additional items, if needed, may be added to the sterile field after it has been established. The first step in preparing a sterile field is to confirm the sterility of packaged supplies and equipment (Figure 18-3).

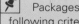 Packages are considered sterile if they meet the following criteria:
- They are clean, dry, and have not been opened or punctured.
- Their expiration date has not been exceeded.
- Their sterility indicators have changed to a predetermined color, confirming sterilization.

Most procedures today use disposable equipment wrapped in paper or plastic. Directions on the packages are usually clear and precise, and taking time to read them in advance will increase your self-confidence

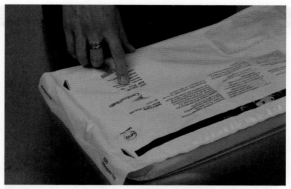

FIG 18-3 Always check expiration dates before opening sterile packs.

when assisting the physician. Nondisposable equipment that has been processed by central sterile supply is double-wrapped in cloth or heavy paper and sealed with indicator tape. All packs are wrapped in a standardized manner and are always opened using the following method (Procedure 18-1):
- Place the pack on a clean surface within reach of the physician. Check the expiration date and sterilization indicator.
- Inspect the sterile item for the integrity of its cover; look for punctures, tears, discoloration, or any sign that the package may be contaminated.
- Just before the procedure begins, break the seal and open the pack.
- Unfold the first corner away from you; then unfold the two sides.
- Pull the front fold down toward you and drop it. Do not touch the inner surface.
- The inner wrap, if there is one, is opened in the same manner.
- You have now established a sterile field.

Nondisposable sterile items wrapped separately may now be added to the sterile field. Standing back from the table, grasp the object through the wrapping with one hand. With the other hand, open the wrapping, allowing it to fall down over your wrist. Unwrap in the same order as when opening the pack. Hold the edges of the wrapper with your free hand, and drop the object onto the sterile field without releasing the wrapper (Procedure 18-2).

Disposable sponges, gloves, and other small items are supplied in "peel-down" paper or plastic wraps and may be added to the sterile field. Following the

PROCEDURE 18-1 ESTABLISHING A STERILE FIELD

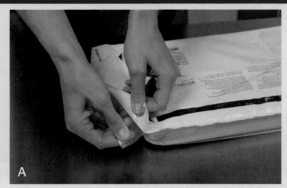

A

A, When opening a commercial pack with a sealed cover, remove the cover first. When opening a double-wrapped pack, begin with the following step (B).

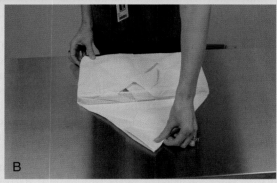

B

B, Open the wrap by opening the first corner away from you. Note that handling of the corners in this way contaminates the edge of the wrap. For this reason the outer 1″ border of the inside of the wrap is no longer considered sterile.

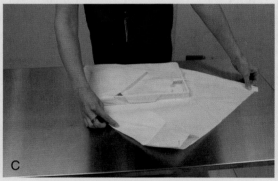

C

C, Open one side by grasping the corner tip.

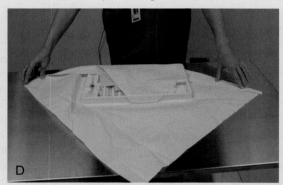

D

D, Open second side in same manner.

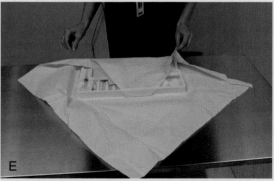

E

E, Grasp fourth corner carefully to avoid contaminating the field.

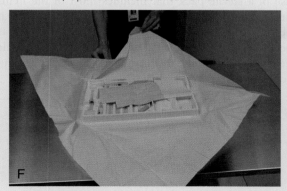

F

F, Pull the remaining corner toward you. If there is an inner wrap, open it in the same manner. A sterile field is now established.

PROCEDURE 18-2 ADDING A DOUBLE-WRAPPED ITEM TO A STERILE FIELD

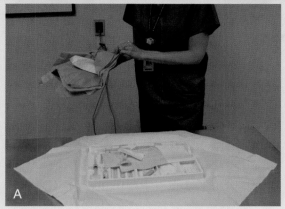

A, Holding item in nondominant hand, open outer wrap; open first fold away from your body.

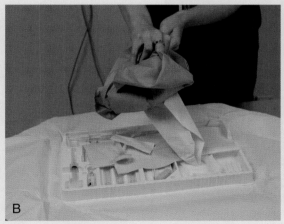

B, Avoid contamination of the field by holding corners of outer wrap while dropping item onto tray. Take care to avoid placement near the outer edge of the field.

PROCEDURE 18-3 ADDING A DISPOSABLE ITEM TO A STERILE FIELD FROM A "PEEL DOWN" WRAP

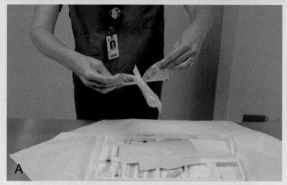

A, Separate wrap according to package instructions.

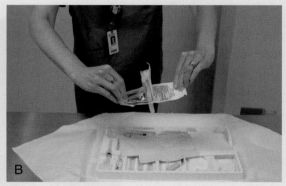

B, Invert package, allowing item to drop onto field. Take care to avoid placement near the outer edge of the field.

instructions, separate the package layers, invert the package, and allow the object to fall onto the sterile field without contaminating the object or the sterile field (Procedure 18-3).

It may be necessary to add a liquid medium, such as Betadine, to a sterile tray. After double-checking the label, position the label toward your hand to prevent it from becoming stained by the liquid, open the spout, and squirt the first few drops into the waste-basket or sink. By discarding the first small amount poured, you "wash" the container's lip and avoid the

possibility of contaminating the tray (Procedure 18-4). Then, pour the required amount into the sterile receptacle on the tray, show the physician the label, and close the spout.

When a radiographer must manipulate items in a sterile field, a sterile transfer forceps may be used. Unwrap the forceps, grasping the handles firmly without touching the remainder of the instrument. Keep the forceps above your waist and in your sight at all times. After use, place the tips in a sterile field with the handles protruding so you can use them again. Do not reach across the sterile field.

If a procedure must be postponed, do not open the tray. If it is already open, cover it immediately with a sterile drape or discard it, because airborne contamination

PROCEDURE 18-4   ADDING LIQUID TO A STERILE FIELD

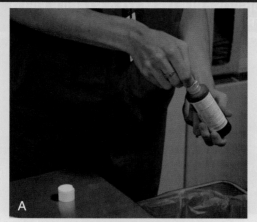

A, Check label and open bottle.

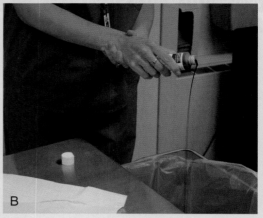

B, Cleanse lip of container by pouring or squirting small amount into waste container.

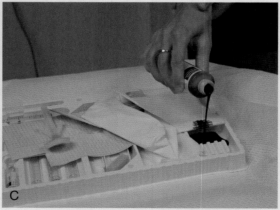

C, Pour required amount into receptacle on tray, taking care not to contaminate the sterile field.

is just as serious as a break in sterile technique. Box 18-1 summarizes the principles of surgical asepsis.

Standard principles of asepsis are listed in Box 18-1. We cannot overemphasize the importance of developing a "sterile conscience," which refers to an awareness of sterile technique and the responsibility for telling the person in charge whenever you contaminate a field or observe its contamination by someone else. The inconvenience of reestablishing a sterile field often makes beginning students reluctant to speak out about apparent breaks in technique. Physicians and coworkers may not seem to appreciate your challenge at the moment, but your professionalism and concern for the patient's

welfare will be reflected in the confidence that team members place in your aseptic technique.

> When you work in or near sterile fields, you have an ethical responsibility to be aware of sterile technique and to tell the person in charge when you contaminate the field or observe its contamination by someone else.

Upon completion of the procedure, don gloves and thoroughly clean all reusable items before returning them to central sterile supply. Items must be free of all residues so that the sterilizing agent can penetrate to all surfaces.

Thorough cleaning is very important and is most easily accomplished when done promptly. Discard disposable items, placing needles in the sharps container and the rest of the items in a biohazard bag.

SKIN PREPARATION

Procedures that involve puncture or incision of the skin require special skin preparation. Skin preparation must sometimes be performed in medical imaging departments and is required for invasive radiologic procedures such as lumbar puncture for myelography and arterial catheterization for angiography. These imaging procedures are described in more detail in Chapter 19.

The purpose of skin preparation is to minimize the introduction of pathogens to the body via the puncture or incision, thus reducing the likelihood of infection. Although it is not possible to sterilize the skin, a high degree of microbial dilution is accomplished by means of proper skin preparation. Preparation includes cleansing thoroughly and removing hair if necessary, followed by applying an antiseptic solution such as Betadine or Zephiran and surrounding the prepared area with sterile drapes. The prepared area is usually a circle approximately 12 inches in diameter with the puncture or incision site at its center. The physician will specify the exact site. The procedure is outlined in Box 18-2. Hair removal is not always required for skin preparation, and *shaving is only done on the specific order of the physician in charge.*

BOX 18-2   **Preparing the Skin for Sterile Procedures**

1. Obtain a "skin prep set" and a bottle of antiseptic for painting the skin. The preparation set includes a basin, liquid soap such as pHisoderm, gauze sponges, razor, towel, forceps, and medicine cup.
2. Perform hand hygiene.
3. Place the patient in a comfortable position and ensure privacy.
4. Explain what is to be done.
5. Expose an area slightly larger than the preparation site, keeping the patient as completely covered as possible to provide comfort and modesty.
   Note: If hair removal is not ordered, omit steps 6 and 7.
6. If hair removal is ordered, use a dry razor to shave a small area at a time. Hold the skin taut with one hand and shave with short, firm strokes in the direction of hair growth. The same concept applies if using an electric razor.
7. Wipe the area with a sterile gauze sponge wetted with alcohol, removing all the hair.
8. Perform hand hygiene and don sterile gloves.
9. Pour a little of the antiseptic into a waste container to cleanse the lip of the bottle.
10. Fill the medicine cup with antiseptic.
11. Grasp several gauze sponges with the forceps and dip them into the antiseptic.
12. Paint the skin with the antiseptic, starting in the center of the area and working outward in a circular pattern. Do not scrub harshly, but remember that friction is more effective than soap in cleansing the skin. Discard the sponge.
13. Allow the skin to dry.
14. Repeat steps 12 and 13.
15. Open the pack containing the sterile drape or sterile towels. The physician, wearing sterile gloves, will drape the area surrounding the prepared site.

> The purpose of skin preparation is to minimize the introduction of pathogens to the body via the puncture or incision, thus reducing the likelihood of infection.

DONNING SURGICAL ATTIRE

Surgical attire must be donned before entering the areas where surgical scrubbing, gowning, and gloving take place. This attire usually consists of a pair of scrub pants, scrub shirt, cap or hood, and a mask, but may vary with the institution to include shoe covers* and protective eyewear. Put on the hood or hair cover first and cover all hair. Then, don scrub clothes and put on shoe covers. Next, put on the mask. Position it at the bridge of the nose; tie the upper ties, then the lower ties, making sure that its lower edge is under the chin. With the mask in place, don glasses, goggles, or eye shield, if needed. Make sure that eyewear fits snugly against the forehead and face and that vision is clear.

SURGICAL HAND SCRUB

The ability to perform a **surgical hand scrub** is necessary when the radiographer is asked to assist with a sterile procedure by working within a sterile field. Before donning a sterile gown and gloves, the radiographer performs this special type of hand hygiene to remove as many microorganisms as possible from the skin of the hands and forearms through both mechanical and chemical means.

You should not scrub or assist with any sterile procedure if you do not feel well or if you have an upper respiratory infection. Do not scrub if there are skin problems involving your hands or arms. Wounds and hangnails tend to ooze serum, which encourages rapid bacterial growth and increases the danger of infection to the patient. Before you begin, examine your hands to be certain that the nails are short and free of polish,* the cuticles are in good condition, and there are no cuts or skin problems. Remove all jewelry* from your hands and forearms.

Traditional Method

Your institutional policies will govern the selection of materials provided for surgical scrubbing and the method to be used. The soap may be in a wall-mounted container controlled by a foot or knee lever. An antimicrobial soap or detergent that is effective against both gram-positive and gram-negative microorganisms is used. These agents act rapidly and continue to inhibit microbial growth in the hours following the scrub.

---

*There is some controversy as to whether it is necessary to wear shoe covers and also whether it should be required to remove nail enamel or simple rings from fingers. Use the procedure established by your institution. When in doubt, the conservative approach ensures safety: Wear shoe covers and remove nail polish and all jewelry.

The extent of the scrub may be determined by timing the steps or counting brush strokes.

Before you begin, open a sterile gown pack and a pack of sterile towels, unless there is a scrub assistant to do this for you. Obtain two brushes and a disposable fingernail cleaner. A properly executed surgical hand scrub using the timed steps method is illustrated in Procedure 18-5. The steps are listed in Box 18-3. Keep in mind that the basic principle of a surgical scrub is to wash the hands thoroughly, and then to wash from a clean area (the hands) to a less clean area (the arms).

Alcohol-Based Handrub Method

In the 2002 Centers for Disease Control and Prevention (CDC) guidelines regarding hand hygiene, the CDC recognized the alcohol-based handrub technique as an appropriate alternative to the traditional surgical scrub described above. This method is as effective in reducing the bacterial counts on hands as the traditional method. Box 18-4 lists the steps in the handrub procedure.

The handrub method is performed in two stages. Begin by turning on the water and adjusting it to a comfortable, warm temperature. Perform a prewash by wetting the hands and forearms and lathering with a nonantimicrobial agent from the fingertips to 2 inches above the elbow. Clean fingernails under running water and discard nail cleaner. Rinse hands and arms under running water and thoroughly dry them with a paper towel. The second stage is the application of an alcohol-based **surgical handrub** product that provides a very high level of disinfection that persists for a prolonged period of time. Follow the manufacturer's instructions. Aseptic principles for the alcohol-based surgical handrub are the same as those listed for the surgical hand scrub in the previous paragraph.

STERILE GOWNING AND GLOVING

Sterile gowning takes place before sterile gloving and after donning surgical attire and performing a surgical hand scrub. To don the sterile gown, the radiographer follows the procedure shown in Procedure 18-6. The surgical assistant is usually responsible for assisting other members of the team with donning gowns and gloves.

There are two methods of gloving for sterile procedures: the open method and the closed method. The closed method is illustrated as a part of the sterile gowning

PROCEDURE 18-5 TRADITIONAL SURGICAL HAND SCRUB PROCEDURE (COUNTED STROKE METHOD)

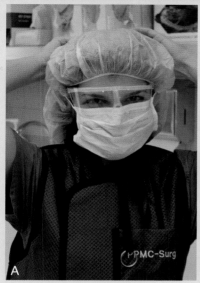

A, Wearing surgical attire, cap or hood, shoe covers, and mask, don protective eyewear and/or lead apron, if needed.

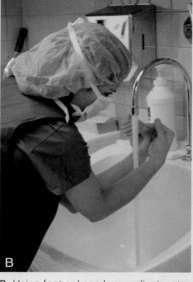

B, Using foot or knee lever, adjust water flow and temperature. With hands above elbows, wet hands and forearms. Avoid splashing your clothing.

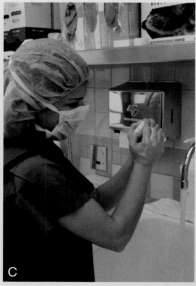

C, Add antimicrobial soap and more water as needed to make a lather. Thoroughly wash hands and arms. Use brush to scrub nails and hands (about 1 minute for each hand). Discard brush.

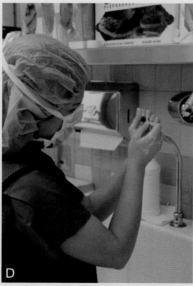

D, Clean under fingernails with fingernail cleaner. Discard cleaner.

Continued

PROCEDURE 18-5   TRADITIONAL SURGICAL HAND SCRUB PROCEDURE (TIMED STEPS METHOD)—CONT'D

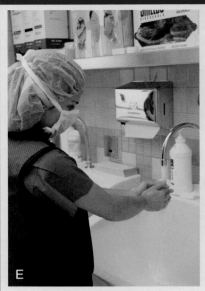

E, Rinse hands and forearms.

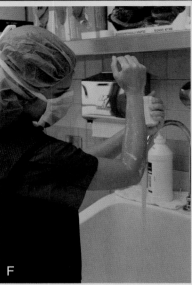

F, With the second brush and antimicrobial soap, time a 3-5 minute scrub on one hand and arm following instructions of the soap manufacturer. Visualize each finger, hand, and arm as having four sides. Wash all four sides of each thoroughly, keeping hand elevated and elbow down.

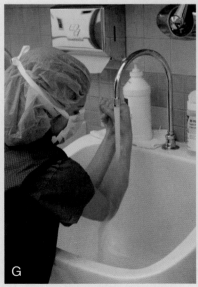

G, Rinse, keeping hands above elbows. Repeat scrub for the other hand, fingers, and arm. Rinse again.

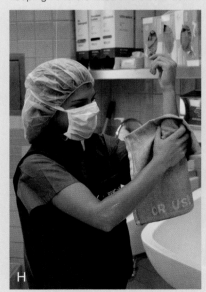

H, Dry thoroughly with a sterile towel, starting with the fingers. Avoid contaminating the towel.

BOX 18-3 Surgical Hand Scrub: Traditional Method

1. Wear surgical attire and appropriate personal protective equipment.
2. Using foot or knee lever, adjust water flow and temperature.
3. Wet your hands. Add a few drops of antimicrobial soap and more water as needed to make a lather.
4. Wash your hands and forearms thoroughly. Use one brush and soap to clean your hands and nails, and clean under your nails with the nail cleaner under running water.
5. Rinse your hands and arms thoroughly, keeping your hands higher than your elbows. Take care to avoid splashing your scrub clothes, because the dampness may later moisten your sterile gown, causing contamination.
6. Using the second brush and more soap, the actual scrub begins. Following instructions of the soap manufacturer, scrub the first hand and arm for 3 to 5 minutes. Rinse. Add more soap and repeat for the other hand, fingers, and arm. The prescribed number of brush strokes is usually 15 strokes to the nails of each hand and 10 strokes to each area of the skin, which usually takes about 5 minutes.
7. The fingers, hands, and arms should be visualized as having four sides, and each side must be effectively scrubbed. Starting with the fingernails, scrub them vigorously, holding the brush perpendicular to the nails. Then scrub all sides of each finger, the palms, and the backs of the hands. Divide each forearm into thirds and use a circular motion to scrub each side of the forearms and elbows, up to 2 inches above the elbows.
8. Keep your hands above your elbows while scrubbing and add small amounts of water as needed to maintain a good lather. When scrubbing is complete, discard the brush.
9. Rinse your hands and arms thoroughly from fingertips to elbows in one motion, allowing the water to drain off at the elbows. Turn off the water with the foot or knee control.
10. Keeping your hands above the elbows and away from your body, enter the surgical suite by backing through the door.
11. To dry, grasp the corner of a sterile towel and step back from the field, allowing the towel to fall open. Bend forward at the waist and hold your arms away from your body and above your waist. Dry your hands, then your arms, thoroughly, rotating the towel as required.
12. Take care not to contaminate the sterile field, the towel, or your hands.
13. You are now ready to don a sterile gown and gloves.

BOX 18-4 Surgical Scrub: Alcohol-based Handrub Method

1. Wear surgical attire and appropriate personal protective equipment.
2. Using foot or knee lever, adjust water flow and temperature.
3. Wet hands and arms, and lather with approved non-antimicrobial agent.
4. Clean fingernails under running water using disposable nail cleaner; discard nail cleaner.
5. Rinse hands and arms under running water.
6. Dry hands and arms using a paper towel.
7. Dispense the manufacturer's recommended amount of alcohol-based handrub into the palm of one hand. *Do not use water with the handrub.*
8. Dip the fingertips of the opposite hand into the handrub and work it under the nails.
9. Spread the remaining handrub evenly over the hand and forearm to just above the elbow, covering all surfaces.
10. Using additional handrub, repeat steps 7-9 with the other arm.
11. Repeat steps 7-10, if recommended.
12. To facilitate drying, continue rubbing antiseptic handrub into hands until dry.
13. Keep scrubbed hands and arms in view and avoid contamination; allow to air dry completely before donning a sterile gown and gloves.

technique illustrated in Procedure 18-6. The open method is used by radiographers when sterile gowning is not required, and is depicted in Procedure 18-7.

When removing the gloves, invert them as you pull them off and perform hand hygiene.

REMOVING AND APPLYING DRESSINGS

In many health care institutions today, radiographers are called upon to perform tasks that were once performed solely by nurses. You may be directed by a physician to

PROCEDURE 18-6   STERILE GOWNING WITH CLOSED GLOVING TECHNIQUE

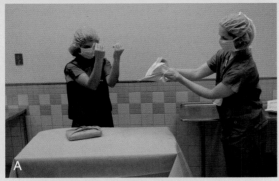

A, Assistant opens gloves and sterile gown pack.

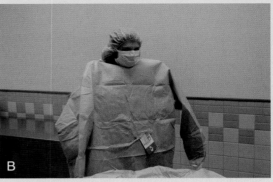

B, Lift folded sterile gown and step back from table. Allow gown to unfold with the inside of the gown toward you.

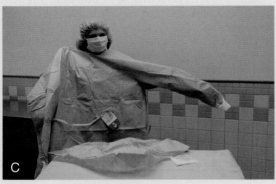

C, Insert arms into sleeves.

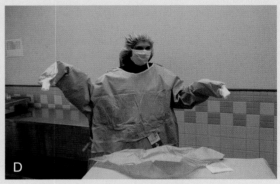

D, Do not allow hands to protrude through cuffs.

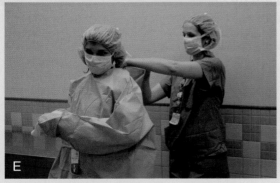

E, Assistant fastens gown at neckline and fastens non-sterile ties inside back of gown at waist level.

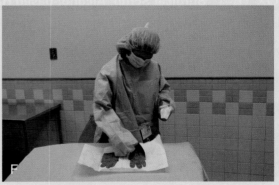

F, With dominant hand remaining inside sleeve, pick up glove for nondominant hand.

PROCEDURE 18-6 STERILE GOWNING WITH CLOSED GLOVING TECHNIQUE—CONT'D

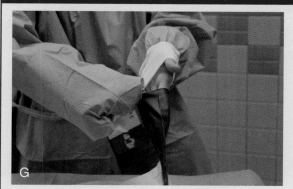

G, Insert nondominant hand into glove. Keep fingers within sleeve until glove is in place.

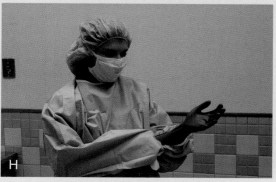

H, Stretch cuff of glove over cuff of gown.

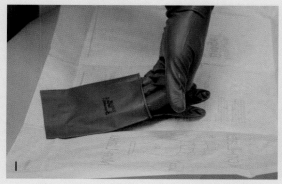

I, With nondominant hand, pick up second glove.

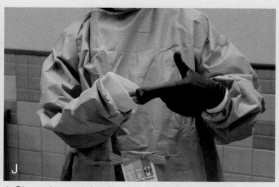

J, Place glove on dominant hand while keeping fingers within sleeve.

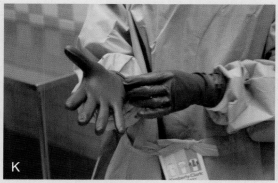

K, Stretch cuff of glove over cuff of gown. Adjust sleeves under gloves for fit and comfort.

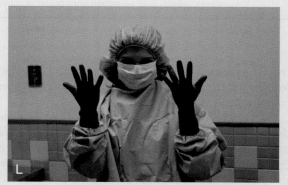

L, Closed gloving is complete. Remember to keep hands above waist level.

Continued

PROCEDURE 18-6   STERILE GOWNING WITH CLOSED GLOVING TECHNIQUE—CONT'D

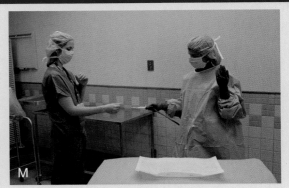

M, Separate outer sterile waist tie from gown and pass tie with tab to assistant.

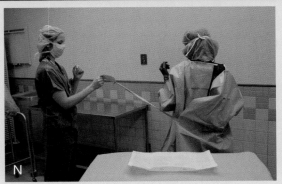

N, Turn in a circle to wrap tie around your waist.

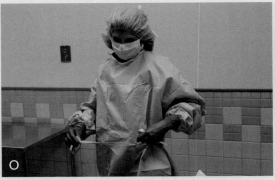

O, A sharp tug on the tie will separate it from the contaminated tab, allowing you to fasten the tie without contaminating your gown or gloves.

remove a patient's dressing, and it may also be your duty to apply a fresh dressing when the examination has been completed.

To remove a dressing, first perform hand hygiene, don gloves, and inform the patient of what you are about to do. Use care in removing the dressing to prevent cross-contaminating the wound and yourself. Remove the dressing gently to avoid hurting the patient. Place the soiled dressing in a plastic bag and seal it before adding it to the biohazard container. Remove your gloves following the same procedure used with isolation techniques (see Chapter 9), and perform hand hygiene.

The application of a new dressing requires sterile technique. Begin by preparing your supplies: sterile gloves, sterile drape, sterile gauze, and tape. You may also need some normal saline to clean the area around the wound. When you have assembled everything you will need, proceed by following the steps outlined in Box 18-5.

PROCEDURE 18-7 OPEN GLOVING TECHNIQUE

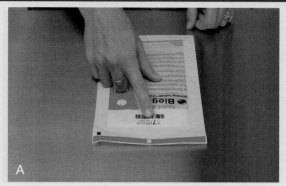

A, Perform hand hygiene. Obtain gloves and check for correct size.

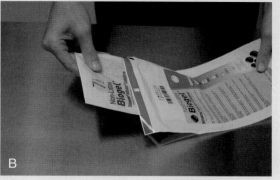

B, Open outer wrap to remove folded inner wrap.

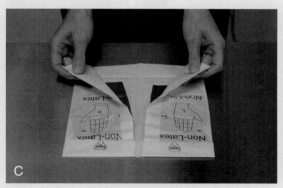

C, Expose gloves with open ends facing you.

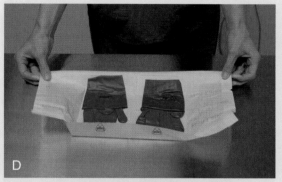

D, Open inner wrap completely, taking care not to contaminate the gloves or the wrap immediately surrounding the gloves.

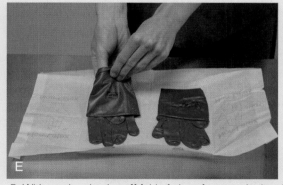

E, With one hand, grip cuff fold of glove for opposite hand.

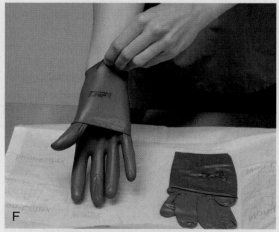

F, Put on first glove, touching only inner surface of folded cuff.

Continued

PROCEDURE 18-7   OPEN GLOVING TECHNIQUE—CONT'D

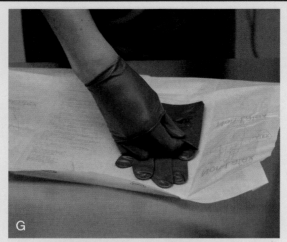

G, Using gloved hand, grasp second glove under cuff.

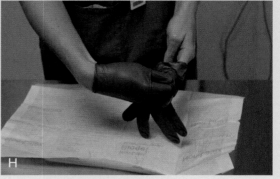

H, Insert hand into second glove.

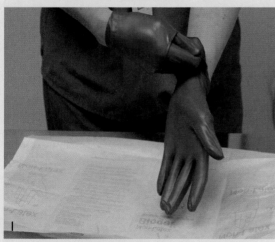

I, Put on second glove, and unfold cuff.

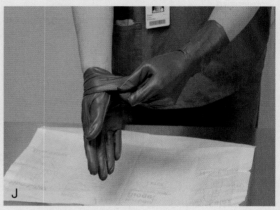

J, Insert fingers under cuff of first glove, and unfold cuff.

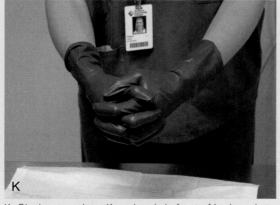

K, Gloving complete. Keep hands in front of body and at safe distance from uniform to avoid contamination.

BOX 18-5 Applying a Sterile Dressing

- Tell the patient what you plan to do.
- Perform hand hygiene.
- Tear several strips of tape to a convenient length.
- Open the sterile drape pack, placing the drape near the patient.
- Partially open the drape by pulling from the corners. This creates a small sterile field for your other sterile items.
- Open the dressing package and add the sterile dressing to your sterile field.
- If you will need to cleanse around the wound, drop sterile gauze sponges into your field for this purpose.
- To moisten the gauze sponges, open a small vial of sterile normal saline solution. Recheck the label and pour a small amount of the saline over the sponges. Do not allow liquid to soak through to the sterile towel. Check the label for the third time before discarding the vial.
- Don sterile gloves using the open method described for sterile gloving.
- Use the moist sponges to clean gently around the wound.
- Allow the area to dry completely.
- Apply the dressing over the wound and secure it with tape.
- Cover the patient.
- Dispose of any waste.
- Remove your gloves and perform hand hygiene.

SUMMARY

- Surgical asepsis is the process of creating and maintaining an area that is completely free of pathogens. Sterilization is the complete destruction of all organisms and spores from equipment used for patient care or procedures.
- Surgical asepsis is often associated with the surgical suite, but it is also used whenever any invasive procedure, such as a lumbar puncture or urinary catheterization, is performed. Surgical asepsis can also be employed when caring for immunocompromised patients.
- Establishing a sterile field, performing a surgical scrub, and donning sterile attire to assist with an invasive procedure, such as an angiogram, are all examples of practicing surgical asepsis. It is part of each radiographer's education to learn the practice of surgical aseptic technique.
- Four different methods may be used to sterilize supplies and equipment: chemical, autoclaving, ethylene oxide gas, and gas plasma. Each method has advantages and disadvantages as well as recommended applications. Sterility and biological indicators are used to ensure that all packs are properly sterilized and all forms of microbial life are destroyed during the sterilization procedure.
- A sterile field is a microorganism-free area prepared for the use of sterile supplies and equipment. The sterility of packages and supplies must be confirmed before establishing a sterile field, and they must be opened properly to prevent contamination. Once a sterile field is established, other sterile items and liquids can be added, following proper procedure. To maintain the integrity of the sterile field, the health care worker must follow the standard principles of surgical asepsis.
- A surgical hand scrub is a specific method of reducing the number of organisms on the hands and forearms and minimizing microbial growth in the following hours. It is practiced without fail before donning sterile gown and gloves to work in a sterile field. There are two basic methods: the traditional scrub using a brush and antimicrobial soap and the alcohol handrub method that involves washing with a nonantimicrobial soap, drying the skin, and applying a surgical alcohol-based skin rub.
- Sterile gowning and gloving are necessary in certain circumstances for work within a sterile field. Following the surgical hand scrub/handrub, a sterile gown is put on with the help of an assistant. As part of the gowning procedure, sterile gloves are donned using the closed gloving method.
- Open gloving is the method used when complete sterile attire is not required. After performing hand hygiene, the glove package is opened, and the gloves are donned without contaminating their outer surfaces.

- Radiographers may be asked to remove dressings before procedures and to apply sterile dressings following procedures. While wearing protective gloves, remove the dressing with care so as not to hurt the patient, then place the dressing in a sealed plastic bag before discarding it in a biohazard container.

- To apply a new dressing, the radiographer assembles and prepares the needed items, establishes a small sterile field in which to place the sterile items, and dons sterile gloves using the open gloving method. Aseptic technique is used to clean around the wound if needed, apply a sterile dressing, and secure it to the patient's skin.

REVIEW QUESTIONS

1. The standard principles of surgical asepsis include:
   A. not passing between the surgeon and the sterile field.
   B. never reaching across a sterile field.
   C. discarding items that become contaminated.
   D. all of the above.

2. Which of the following methods of sterilization is the quickest and most convenient method for items that can withstand heat and moisture?
   A. Conventional gas sterilization
   B. Autoclaving
   C. Chemical sterilization
   D. Gas plasma technology

3. The fastest and safest method for sterilizing items that cannot withstand heat is:
   A. chemical sterilization.
   B. gas sterilization using Freon and ethylene oxide
   C. gas plasma technology.
   D. autoclaving.

4. Which of the following sterilization methods requires the dissipation of poisonous gas?
   A. Gas plasma technology
   B. Chemical sterilization
   C. Gas sterilization using Freon and ethylene oxide
   D. Dry heat

5. A microorganism-free area prepared for the use of sterile supplies and equipment is called a(n):
   A. aseptic area.
   B. surgical pack.
   C. central sterile supply.
   D. sterile field.

6. When a sterile procedure is delayed, which of the following is NOT an appropriate method of dealing with the sterile tray?
   A. If the tray is not open, do not open it
   B. If the tray is open, set it aside and avoid touching it
   C. If the tray is open, cover it with a sterile drape
   D. If the tray is open, discard it

7. When you contaminate a field or observe its contamination by someone else, the ethical awareness that requires you to tell the person in charge is referred to as a:
   A. sterile conscience.
   B. aseptic consciousness.
   C. surgical validation.
   D. sepsis response.

8. The surgical handrub is an alternative to:
   A. sterile gloving.
   B. the surgical hand scrub.
   C. protective gloving.
   D. the open gloving technique.

9. When preparing for a surgical procedure that requires complete sterile attire, which of the following steps takes place after the surgical hand scrub?
   A. Put on surgical mask
   B. Put on surgical gown
   C. Open a pack of sterile towels
   D. Cover hair with cap or hood

10. Which of the following is NOT worn by a radiographer when performing imaging procedures in surgery?
    A. Surgical mask
    B. Cap or hood
    C. Scrub clothes
    D. Sterile gown

Answers can be found in the Answer Key on pages 429-431.

CRITICAL THINKING EXERCISES

1. Two special needles need to be sterilized for a procedure that is scheduled for tomorrow morning. The autoclave is apparently broken and will not function. What options might be available that would enable you to have the necessary equipment sterile and ready when needed?

2. Describe the process of preparing a patient's skin for a sterile injection. If the physician has ordered hair removal as part of the prep, how and when should this be done?

3. After cleansing the patient's skin, you have established a sterile field with a lumbar puncture tray in preparation for a myelogram procedure. While the radiologist is discussing the procedure with the patient, he accidentally backs into the tray table and his elbow contaminates the sterile field. What should you say? What should you do? How might this have been prevented?

4. A patient is waiting on the x-ray table, and a sterile field has been established. The physician has not arrived and you are planning to leave the room to call her. What measures can you take to ensure that the sterile field is not contaminated in your absence?

Contrast Media and Special Radiographic Techniques

OBJECTIVES

At the conclusion of this chapter, the student will be able to:

- Name four types of contrast media and give two examples and two applications for each.
- List four types of adverse responses to contrast media injections.
- Demonstrate how to take an appropriate history before the injection of an iodinated contrast medium.
- Describe the radiographer's role in performing an IV urogram.

- Name the blood chemistry tests that may be significant in patients scheduled for urography.
- Describe three methods used to introduce contrast media into the biliary system.
- Describe the procedure for the injection of contrast media for myelography.

OUTLINE

KEY TERMS

aqueous
arthrography
bolus
cholecystectomy
cholecystitis

cystogram
diuretic
ionic
manometer
myelography

nephrogram
nonionic
osmolality
stent
viscosity

As Chapter 17 has shown, special agents may be used to enhance the radiographic contrast of soft tissues. Among these are barium sulfate, air, gases, and various iodine compounds. While Chapter 17 discusses primarily barium sulfate products and their use in the gastrointestinal tract, this chapter focuses on procedures using contrast media other than barium outside the gastrointestinal system. Special knowledge and skill in patient preparation, contrast media administration, and patient monitoring are required to perform these procedures. Some of these examinations are very sophisticated and it is not within the scope of this book to deal with the specifics of each. The exact techniques vary greatly among departments and radiologists, and procedures are subject to change. Some of these studies, however, are so integral to the radiographer's work that they are performed routinely. A more thorough understanding of them will help you form the judgments required for professional performance in these situations.

CONTRAST MEDIA

Air and Gases

The mass density or atomic weight of a substance determines the degree to which it will attenuate radiation. Air and gases are very light and therefore absorb x-rays to a significantly lesser degree than do soft tissues; as a result, structures containing gases appear black or very dark on a radiographic image. This appearance is referred to as a negative contrast, and air and gases are called negative contrast agents. Cavities filled with air show a clear outline of the surrounding soft tissues, which have a lighter gray appearance because of their greater degree of radiation absorption. In addition to double-contrast studies of the colon and stomach, air or gas is sometimes used as a contrast agent in **arthrography** (contrast studies of joints), as illustrated in Figure 19-1. Gas may be used as a contrast agent in **myelography** (visualization of the spinal canal) for those patients who are allergic to iodinated contrast media. Gas is also used to fill the peritoneal cavity for fiber optic studies of various organs, including the female reproductive system and the biliary system.

Gas for radiographic contrast must be nontoxic and readily absorbed by the body, but not so rapidly that it disappears before the study is complete. Carbon dioxide (CO_2) meets these criteria. CO_2 has clear advantages over room air as a diagnostic gas because the body absorbs it much faster than the nitrogen in air. It is commercially available in small cartridges for individual applications or in large, pressurized cylinders that are more practical for departments using large quantities for double-contrast enemas as well as other studies.

> Carbon dioxide is a common, effective, and safe gas that serves as a negative contrast agent, one that appears dark on the radiographic image.

In the past, gas was introduced into the spinal canal to delineate the ventricles of the brain (pneumoencephalography) or directly into the ventricles for the same purpose (ventriculography). These examinations have

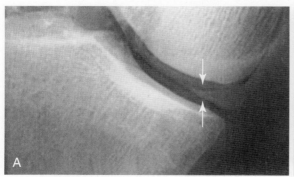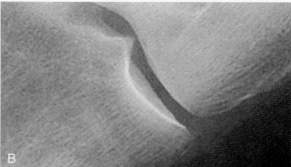

FIG 19-1 A, A pneumoarthrogram shows the use of injected air to provide a negative contrast *(arrows)* in a joint space, delineating the knee cartilage. **B,** Similar knee radiograph without contrast. Cartilage is not visible. (From Frank ED, Long BW, Smith BJ: *Merrill's atlas of radiographic positions and radiologic procedures,* ed 12, St Louis, 2011, Mosby.)

now been replaced by less invasive procedures, such as computed tomography (CT) and magnetic resonance imaging (MRI) examinations (see Chapter 22).

Iodinated Media

Most organs and blood vessels have x-ray absorption characteristics which are very similar to those of the surrounding soft tissues. This causes their radiographic images to be only faintly distinguishable, if visible at all. With an atomic number of 53 and a mass number of 127, iodine is a heavy element compared to the composition of the body. Iodine compounds, therefore, absorb radiation to a greater degree than blood or soft tissues, causing any organ or blood vessel containing the contrast agent to stand out by appearing white or much lighter than the surrounding tissues. This radiopaque appearance is referred to as positive contrast, the opposite of the radiolucent, dark, or negative contrast seen with air or gas. Iodine compounds delineate many different structures more clearly than noncontrast radiography. Figure 19-2 illustrates the use of an iodinated contrast medium to visualize the internal structures of a kidney. Look for other examples of enhanced visualization using positive contrast agents throughout this chapter.

> Positive contrast agents such as barium sulfate and iodine compounds absorb more radiation that the surrounding tissues and therefore appear white or light on the radiographic image.

Most iodinated contrast agents are **aqueous**; that is, water is the principal solvent for the iodine compound.

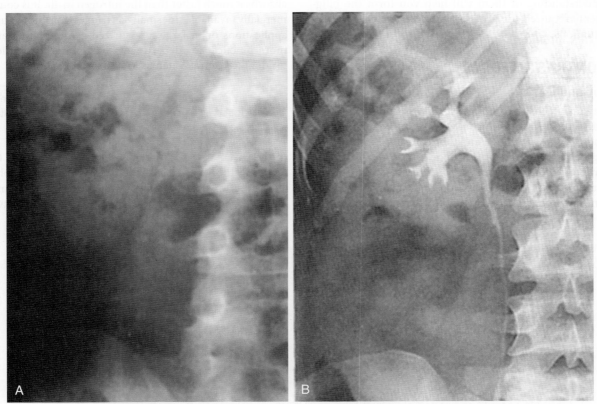

FIG 19-2 A, Right upper quadrant of the abdomen without contrast agent. Kidney outline is faintly visible. **B,** Right upper quadrant of the abdomen with positive contrast from iodinated medium filling the internal structures of kidney. The internal structures are clearly seen, as is the faint outline of the kidney. (From Frank ED, Long BW, Smith BJ: *Merrill's atlas of radiographic positions and radiologic procedures*, ed 12, St Louis, 2011, Mosby.)

These agents mix readily with blood and other body fluids. These are the only contrast media suitable for intravascular injection.

Aqueous iodine compounds are by far the most frequently used contrast agents other than barium. These media are stocked in the radiology department in a wide variety of types, volumes, and strengths (Figure 19-3). Although some of these products are approved for one specific purpose, many have broader applications. These multipurpose agents may be administered intravenously (IV) for urography, intraarterially for angiography (visualization of vessels), or injected directly into the structures to be visualized, such as the common bile duct for cholangiography or a joint capsule for arthrography.

Table 19-1 lists procedures that use contrast agents. Appendix J provides an extensive list of contrast agents used for diagnostic imaging. Specific information on content, strength, contraindications, and precautions for all of these products can be found in the drug package inserts and in common drug references.

Iodinated Contrast Media Administration

A contrast medium can be administered slowly by means of a diluted, high-volume IV infusion, or in the form of a **bolus** injection. A bolus refers to a substantial IV dose delivered rapidly. Timing is important. A bolus may be injected using a syringe attached to an IV catheter or butterfly set. The contrast enhancement for CT scans may involve a bolus, an infusion, or both. Pressure injectors can be programmed to supply a rapid bolus at first, followed by a slower infusion of the remaining contrast.

The procedures for venipuncture and access to intravenous lines are illustrated in Chapter 14. Information about the administration of contrast for specific procedures is found later in this chapter and in Chapter 22.

Characteristics of Iodinated Media

All water-soluble iodine contrast media are carbon-based organic chemicals composed of molecules containing iodine atoms and various combinations of other atoms. These molecules vary in size, and some contain more iodine atoms than others. Figure 19-4 illustrates the chemical structure of typical iodine contrast molecules. These products differ with respect to certain characteristics of their strength and chemical nature that affect their clinical performance. These characteristics include iodine concentration, osmolality, viscosity, and toxicity.

Iodine Concentration

Many different iodine concentrations of contrast agents are available, and the concentration required for any

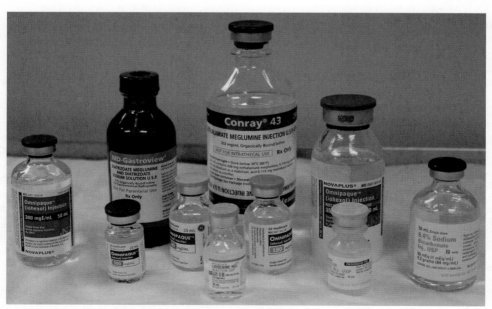

FIG 19-3 An assortment of iodinated contrast agents.

TABLE 19-1 **Imaging Studies Using Contrast Media**

Examination	Route of Administration	Structures Visualized	Examples of Contrast Media Used
Angiography			
Aortography	Arterial catheter	Abdominal or thoracic aorta	Omnipaque 350, Optiray 350
Angiocardiography	Arterial catheter	Heart and surrounding great vessels	Imagopaque 350, Iomeron 350, Visipaque 320
Digital subtraction angiography (DSA)	Arterial catheter	Cerebral vasculature, aorta, and branches	Iomeron 300, Imagopaque 350, Omnipaque 140
Digital subtraction angiography (DSA)	Intravenous	Cerebral vasculature, aorta, and branches	Iomeron 350, Conray-43
Peripheral arteriography	Arterial catheter	Arteries of the extremities	Visipaque, Hexabrix, Isovue-300, MD-76
Peripheral venography	Intravenous	Veins of the extremities	Conray-43, Imagopaque 200 or 250, Visipaque 270
Cerebral angiography	Arterial catheter	Cerebral vasculature	Optiray 240, Visipaque 270
Selective visceral arteriography	Arterial catheter	Renal, celiac, splenic, or coronary arteries, for example	Hexabrix, Imagopaque 300, MD-76, Optiray 320
Biliary System			
Cholangiography, operative and postoperative	Direct injection via laparoscope	Common bile duct	Conray, Reno-60, Hypaque Meglumine 60%, Hypaque 76
Cholangiogram, postperative	Direct injection via T-tube	Common bile duct	Conray, Reno-60, Hypaque Meglumine 60%, Hypaque 76
Endoscopic retrograde cholangio-pancreatography (ERCP)	Catheter via endoscope	Common bile duct and pancreatic duct	Conray, Reno-60, Hypaque Meglumine 60%, Hypaque 76
Percutaneous transhepatic cholangiography (PTC)	Direct injection	Common bile duct	Conray, Reno-60, Hypaque Meglumine 60%, Hypaque 76
Spinal Studies			
Myelography	Intrathecal injection via lumbar puncture	Spinal canal (subarachnoid space)	Omnipaque 180, Isovue 200, Isovue 300
Discography	Direct injection	Intervertebral disk	Conray, Reno-60, Hypaque Meglumine 60%, Hypaque 76
Urinary Tract Studies			
Excretory urography	Intravenous	Kidneys, ureters, and bladder	Iomeron 350, MD-76, Optiray 240, Reno-60, Omnipaque 300–350, Visipaque 320, Reno-Dip (infusion), Conray-43, Hypaque 60%
Retrograde urography	Ureteral catheters via cystoscope	Kidney pelves, calyces, and ureters	Hypaque-Cysto 30%, Iomeron 200, Cysto-Conray II, Cystografin, Reno-30
Cystourethrography	Direct injection via Foley catheter	Urinary bladder and urethra	Hypaque-Cysto 30%, Iomeron 200, Cysto-Conray II, Cystografin, Reno-30
Gastrointestinal Studies			
Esophagram	Oral administration	Esophagus	Barium sulfate products
Upper GI series	Oral administration	Esophagus, stomach, and duodenum	Barium sulfate products, Gastrografin, Hypaque Sodium Oral Powder, MD-Gastroview

TABLE 19-1   Imaging Studies Using Contrast Media—cont'd

Examination	Route of Administration	Structures Visualized	Examples of Contrast Media Used
Lower GI series	Rectal catheter	Colon	Barium sulfate products, Hypaque Sodium, Gastrografin, MD-Gastroview
Small bowel series	Oral administration or enteroclysis	Small intestine	Barium sulfate products, Gastrografin, Hypaque Sodium Oral Powder, MD-Gastroview
Miscellaneous Studies			
Arthrography	Direct injection	Joints (for example, knee, shoulder, ankle)	Conray, Visipaque 320, Hypaque Meglumine 60%, Hypaque 76
Computed tomography (CT)	Intravenous	Contrast enhancement of anatomy examined	Imagopaque 300, Conray-30
Computed tomography (CT)	Oral administration	Contrast enhancement of GI tract	Gastrografin, Hypaque Sodium Oral Powder, MD-Gastroview
Hysterosalpin gography	Direct injection via cervical cannula	Uterus and fallopian tubes	Iomeron 300, Sinografin
Lymphography	Direct injection into lymphatic vessels in feet	Lymph vessels and lymph nodes	Ethiodol
Magnetic resonance imaging (MRI)	Intravenous	Brain, spinal cord, and vascular structures	Magnevist, ProHance (these paramagnetic agents are not iodinated.)

GI, gastrointestinal.

given application depends largely upon the degree to which it will be diluted by body fluids. For example, a high concentration is needed to study the aorta, where dilution by a large volume of blood is a factor, whereas a lower concentration is adequate for the visualization of veins and smaller arteries. Greater concentrations have a greater viscosity and greater osmolality and tend to be more toxic.

> The iodine concentration determines the degree to which the medium will attenuate x-rays, with higher concentrations producing a greater degree of positive radiographic contrast.

Osmolality

Osmolality refers to the number of particles in solution per kilogram of water. The osmolality of human blood is about 300 milliosmoles per kilogram (mOsm/kg), whereas the osmolality of water-soluble contrast media ranges from 300 mOsm/kg to more than 1000 mOsm/kg.

Injecting an IV solution that exceeds the osmolality of human blood (termed a hyperosmolar solution) affects the body as a result of an alteration in osmotic pressure. These effects are discussed in a later section of this chapter.

Contrast media that are formed from a chemical structure that contains more iodine atoms per molecule can provide the desired contrast with fewer molecules and, therefore, have a lower osmolality. Because osmolality is largely responsible for the adverse effects of contrast media, the risk is reduced when the osmolality is lowered.

Some contrast media molecules dissociate into two charged particles when placed in a solution, resulting in a higher osmolality. This process is called ionization, and media whose molecules dissociate in this way are termed ionic. Media whose molecules remain whole in solution are termed nonionic.

To compare the relative osmolality of both ionic and nonionic contrast agents, it is helpful to use a ratio of the number of iodine atoms to the number of particles.

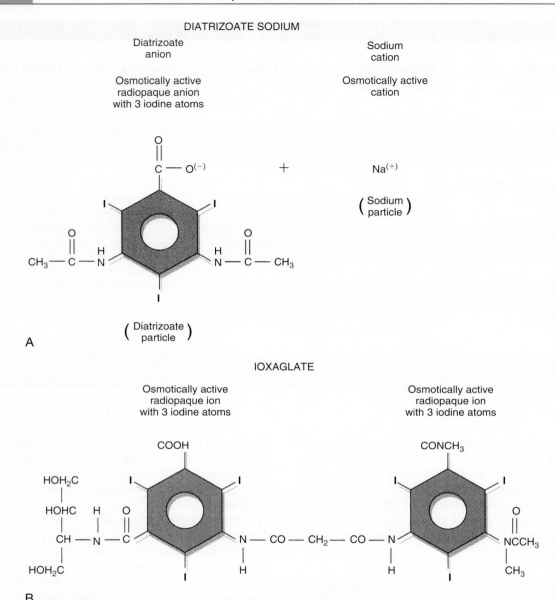

FIG 19-4 Molecular structure of some typical iodine contrast agents. **A,** Representation of high-osmolar ionic contrast agent. Diatrizoate sodium contains one osmotically active negative particle (anion) and one osmotically active positive particle (cation), for a total of two osmotically active particles when in solution. Diatrizoate sodium contains three iodine (I) atoms per two osmotically active particles, to constitute a ratio of 3:2, which equals 1.5. **B,** Representation of low-osmolar ionic contrast agent. Ioxaglate contains a total of six iodine atoms per two osmotically active particles, to constitute a ratio of 6:2, which equals 3.0.

IOPAMIDOL

FIG 19-4, cont'd C, Representation of nonionic contrast agent. Iopamidol does not dissociate into anions and cations in solution. It contains only one osmotically active particle to constitute a ratio of 3:1, which equals 3.0.

For instance, a compound such as diatrizoate meglumine with a ratio of 3:2 contains three iodine atoms and will dissociate into two particles in solution. When the ratio is divided, the numerical value is 1.5. Compare this with a nonionic medium such as iopamidol (tradename Isovue or Niopam) that also has three atoms of iodine in each molecule, but does not dissociate; it has a 3:1 ratio, or a numerical value of 3. The higher the numerical value of the ratio, the lower the osmolality for any given iodine concentration. When a compound has a lower osmolality, fewer particles are injected intravenously, resulting in fewer or less severe adverse effects for the patient. Some of the newer contrast media have an osmolality equal to that of human blood (deemed an isotonic or isosmolar solution) and rarely cause any adverse effects. Commercial names for various types of contrast media are provided later in this section.

> Contrast agents with a low osmolality tend to be less toxic than those with a high osmolality.

Viscosity

Viscosity is a measure of the resistance of fluid to flow. Liquids with a high viscosity are sometimes described as "thick" or "syrupy," while those with a low viscosity may be thought of as "thin" or "watery." Viscosity is determined by the number of particles in a solution, the size of the particles, and the attractions among the particles. Agents with high iodine concentrations tend to be more viscous. Viscosity is also affected by the specific nature of the molecule. This characteristic is an important consideration in determining the flow rate, injection time, and appropriate needle size. Solutions with a high viscosity require greater injection pressures for administration. Viscosity may be reduced somewhat by warming the medium to body temperature before injection.

Toxicity

As discussed in Chapter 14, the term *toxicity* refers to the potential of an agent to cause harm. The toxicity of a contrast medium on body tissues and organs is related to the chemical configuration of the molecules, the iodine concentration, the osmolality, ionization characteristics, the rate of injection, and the dosage administered. Contrast media that are nonionic, have a low osmolality with a low iodine concentration, and are injected slowly tend to be less toxic and less likely to result in adverse reactions or side effects. Intraarterial injections of contrast media tend to produce fewer toxic effects than IV injections.

Types of Iodinated Media

Two common, versatile, water-soluble iodine compounds are diatrizoate meglumine and diatrizoate sodium. Each chemical has advantageous properties. The sodium salts are made up of relatively small molecules and contain more iodine per molecule, so in equal concentrations they are more radiopaque than their meglumine counterparts. Meglumine (methylglucamine) salts are somewhat less toxic and more soluble in water. They are also more viscous. Some contrast agents, such as Renografin-60 and Hypaque 76, contain both chemicals. These agents, which have been in use for decades, are ionic compounds and are now referred to as *high-osmolar contrast agents (HOCAs),* because of their relatively high osmolality compared with the newer generation of water-soluble iodine contrast media.

In the 1980s, low-osmolar contrast agents (LOCAs) were introduced to the radiology market. Although these products were ionic, they delivered a relatively high concentration of iodine with fewer particles in solution than the conventional contrast media. The first of these agents was metrizamide (Amipaque), and its primary application was for intrathecal injection for myelography. Metrizamide was followed by LOCAs for multipurpose use, such as meglumine ioxaglate (Hexabrix). Many newer LOCAs are also nonionic. Examples include iopamidol (Isovue and Niopam) and iohexol (Omnipaque). Iodixanol (Visipaque) is a nonionic contrast medium defined as isosmolar because its osmolality is equal to that of blood. These agents are less toxic than conventional contrast media and are less likely to stimulate an anaphylactic response. They are also more comfortable for the patient, producing less heat and discomfort when injected. They are particularly desirable for angiographic cardiac catheterization studies (special procedures where a contrast medium is injected through a catheter to show the coronary arteries of the heart), because they are less likely to cause irregularities in cardiac function. Furthermore, iodixanol is often the contrast medium of choice when patients are experiencing mild to moderate renal insufficiency, because it is less nephrotoxic.

Risk factors that may influence the choice or dosage of media include any history of compromised renal, cardiac, or respiratory function or a history of allergies. The weight given to these risk factors varies with the institution and physicians involved. Nonionic contrast agents and other LOCA products were very expensive when they were first introduced. Today, however, these agents are comparable in cost with HOCA products. For this reason, most radiology departments use LOCAs for most procedures and for all patients whose allergy history or physical condition places them at greater risk. Isosmolar agents such as Visipaque are more expensive than the nonionic LOCAs, and because of the higher cost, they may be specified only for high-risk patients, such as those with poor kidney function or cardiac problems.

> Low osmolality contrast agents are used routinely for most procedures requiring iodinated contrast media. Isosmolar agents are used for high-risk patients.

Pharmacodynamics and Adverse Responses

When water-soluble media are injected intravascularly, they circulate in the blood and are excreted by the kidneys. When injected into other structures, they are absorbed gradually into the bloodstream before being excreted. The adverse reactions that may occur in response to contrast media injections can range from mild and transient to severe and life threatening. The pharmacodynamics of contrast media responses involve the effects of osmolality, ionization, and molecular toxicity.

Osmolality affects the body as a result of the tissue response to osmotic pressure. Because water passes through cell membranes in the direction of the highest particle concentration (osmosis), media with a higher osmolality tend to cause dehydration of blood cells and of the cells of the blood vessels and surrounding tissues. Subsequent circulation causes a reversal of this process, changing the hemodynamics (blood flow) of the red blood cells and in the capillary lining. These changes may produce adverse effects on pulmonary artery pressure, blood volume, and cardiac output.

Ionization also affects toxicity and is a factor to be considered when using ionic media. The central nervous system is sensitive to increased levels of ions in the blood, which may interfere with the normal electrical activity of the body. The resulting risk includes the possibility of seizures and cardiac dysfunction. Generalized effects frequently seen in response to ionic media include a sensation of warmth spreading throughout the body, light-headedness, nausea, and vomiting.

Histamine is an organic nitrogen compound that serves as a neurotransmitter. It triggers immune responses and allergic reactions. When histamine is released in response to a contrast injection, it causes allergic or anaphylactoid (anaphylactic-like) responses, but this is not usually the result of antigens in the blood, as is the case with most other allergic reactions. This is apparent because allergic responses to contrast agents do not occur in anesthetized patients. These findings suggest that anaphylactoid reactions to contrast agents are the result of a central nervous system response. Because ionic media have a much more powerful effect on the central nervous system than nonionic media, ionization may also account for the higher incidence of allergic responses to the ionic media.

Toxicity may occur as a result of an excessive dose or failure of the renal system to excrete the media. It may also result when a contrast medium is combined with an incompatible medication. When iodine media are mixed directly with incompatible medications, the contrast agent may undergo a chemical change, resulting in solid particles that precipitate with a potential for very serious consequences. Research has not established the results of all the possible combinations of contrast agents and medications, but precipitate formation has been noted with some combinations of contrast media and the following common medications: diphenhydramine, papaverine hydrochloride, cimetidine, and protamine (see Chapter 13). To avoid the possibility of this complication, flush the IV or arterial catheter with saline both before and after the injection of the contrast medium.

> **!** Always flush catheters with saline, both before and after injection of a contrast medium, to avoid toxicity due to incompatibility of medications.

Precautions

Because procedures involving IV, intraarterial, or intrathecal administration of iodine contrast clearly involve risk, an informed consent is usually required, and a careful history is essential. Patients may have allergic reactions to contrast agents because of a sensitivity to iodine or some other component of the contrast medium. Toxic responses, either mild or severe, may occur in patients with poor heart or kidney function or may result from an overdose of the contrast agent.

Renal failure or compromised renal function impairs the patient's ability to eliminate the contrast medium and may result in a toxic response. As stated in Chapter 11, urea and creatinine are products of cellular metabolism that are excreted by the kidneys, and high blood levels of these substances indicate impaired renal function. Therefore, radiographers must check the blood chemistry section of a patient's chart to ensure that the blood urea nitrogen (BUN) and creatinine levels are within normal limits. The usual normal ranges for adults are considered to be approximately 6 to 20 mg/dl for BUN and 0.6 to 1.5 mg/dl for creatinine. Creatinine levels of 2.0 mg/dl or greater may constitute a contraindication for the administration of iodine contrast agents. *Report abnormal test levels to the radiologist before the administration of iodinated contrast.* In outpatients, screen for a history of kidney failure, kidney disease, or diabetes, and report any positive responses. The policies of many institutions state that elderly patients and those with histories of kidney problems or diabetes must have BUN and/or creatinine tests performed before the administration of iodinated contrast media.

> **!** Laboratory tests of BUN and creatinine levels are checked before contrast injections to avoid the possibility of nephrotoxicity. Report any abnormal test levels to the radiologist before beginning the examination.

Patients with diabetes must be identified because this disease predisposes the patient to renal complications. It is especially important to be alert to the possibility that diabetic patients may be taking medications containing metformin hydrochloride, such as Glucophage, Glucovance, Metaglip, or Avandamet, which are agents prescribed to manage hyperglycemia. Metformin products must be withheld on the day the contrast medium is administered and for at least 48 hours afterward. At that point, metformin therapy is resumed only when the attending physician has determined through testing that the patient's renal function is normal. Diabetic patients may suffer acute renal failure as a result of the contrast medium. With inadequate kidney function, metformin could build to dangerous levels in the blood, causing lactic acidosis, a potentially fatal change in the blood pH.

! Diabetic patients who take medications containing metformin must have this medication withheld prior to a contrast injection, and for 48 hours afterward, to avoid the possibility of metformin toxicity if the contrast agent causes problems with their kidney function.

Contrast agents cause vasodilation, which may produce dangerous changes in blood pressure and cardiac output. Radiographers must identify patients with heart disease before contrast administration, because these patients are at greater risk of an adverse response.

Because excessive doses of contrast media may have a toxic effect, it is a radiographer's duty to ensure that the maximum dosages of contrast agents are not exceeded. While an overdose of a contrast agent is unlikely when routine procedures are followed for a single examination, an overdose may become an issue when injections must be repeated because of errors or problems in angiographic studies or when multiple examinations are ordered. Patients may be scheduled for more than one iodine contrast examination in a limited period in several different departments, such as radiography, cardiovascular laboratory, or CT. For instance, a patient brought to the emergency department with chest pain and dyspnea may be suspected of having a pulmonary embolus and sent to CT for a chest scan with contrast of the vessels. Depending on the findings of this study, the patient may be admitted and transferred to the care of another physician who orders a pulmonary angiogram. The total cumulative contrast dose for multiple procedures may exceed the 24- to 36-hour maximum dose, usually 250 mL. Ideally, records should be kept, transferred with the patient, and read by those who order additional tests, but it is essential for the radiographer to check the patient's chart and double-check by asking the patient whether any other tests have been done recently. Recent contrast examinations should be brought to the attention of the radiologist, who will determine if contrast is necessary for subsequent examinations and whether the proposed study would result in an overdose.

As discussed in Chapter 11, the history you take must document allergies. Of particular concern are previous allergic responses to medication, especially to contrast agents, and a history of asthma. Patients who have experienced asthmatic attacks in the past are three times more likely than others to respond to a contrast medium with an anaphylactoid reaction.

BOX 19-1 Checklist for a Precontrast History

1. History of kidney disease or kidney failure. Check patient chart for BUN and creatinine levels.
2. History of diabetes. If yes, check for a metformin medication.
3. History of heart disease or hypertension. Check current blood pressure.
4. Iodine contrast studies within the past 48 hours? If yes, check to determine when, which agent, concentration, and dose. Provide this information to radiologist.
5. Any history of allergy.
6. Any history of asthma.
7. Previous allergic reaction to contrast medium. If yes, what agent and what reaction?
8. Current medications. Note particularly any beta blockers, antihypertensive medications, or metformin products.

Another common history question involves any routine medications the patient may be taking. Radiologists sometimes want to know whether the patient is taking beta blockers or antihypertensive drugs. A statement of routine medications may provide clues to various conditions of interest for which the patient is being treated.

Although some radiologists prefer to take the history themselves, most institutions use a written form for this purpose. A summary of the essential elements for a precontrast history is provided in Box 19-1. If the patient's history suggests a high risk of adverse response, a nonionic contrast medium may be indicated and/or the procedure may be preceded by the administration of an antihistamine or corticosteroid drug to reduce the risk of reaction. If the patient has a history of allergy to iodine and has not been premedicated, the procedure may be cancelled and another imaging modality, such as ultrasound or non-contrast spiral CT, substituted.

Because most allergic responses occur within a very short time after injection, a minute amount of the contrast medium may be injected intravenously, followed by a pause during which the patient is carefully observed. If no symptoms are noted, the injection is then continued. You must be prepared to respond to a reaction from the test dose, because serious allergic responses have been reported in sensitive individuals with only 1 mL of the medium injected.

Severe reactions to contrast media are not common, but they do occur. Although the physician should be

BOX 19-2   Reactions to Iodinated Contrast Media

Reaction Type	Signs and Symptoms	Response
Common reaction	Feeling of warmth, flushing, metallic taste, nausea, vomiting, coughing	No treatment necessary; symptoms resolve rapidly. Prevent aspiration of emesis if patient vomits.
Intermediate reaction	Erythema, urticaria, bronchospasm	Notify physician; prepare antihistamine or epinephrine if ordered.
Vasovagal reaction (intermediate)	Vasodilation, diaphoresis, hypotension, bradycardia	Notify physician; place patient in dorsal recumbent position with feet elevated 20 degrees; elevate head slightly if breathing is a problem; prepare intravenous fluids or atropine if ordered.
Severe reaction, anaphylactic shock	Respiratory or cardiac arrest, seizures, hypotension. Onset characterized by warmth, tingling, itching palms, throat constriction, feeling of doom, followed by expiratory wheeze and laryngeal and bronchial edema. May be fatal if not treated promptly.	Maintain airway and call a code; treat as for shock, respiratory or cardiac arrest, as symptoms require.

within the immediate area, radiographers often note the first signs of a reaction. Your ability to cope with such emergencies depends on your recognition of the symptoms and your knowledge of the actions and treatment to follow. Box 19-2 sets out descriptions of symptoms and the appropriate responses to the varying degrees and types of reactions to contrast media.

! Emergency supplies and equipment must be readily available whenever iodinated media are injected.

State laws or regulations may govern whether radiographers are allowed to start IV lines and/or perform IV injections. Institutional requirements or prohibitions may exist as well. In most situations when radiographers are permitted to administer IV contrast, some sort of certification and/or skill verification is required. Be familiar with the standards of your hospital, and keep your qualifications current. See Chapter 14 for IV injection procedures.

CONTRAST EXAMINATIONS OF THE URINARY SYSTEM

Excretory Urography

Excretory urograms are sometimes called IV urograms (IVUs) or IV pyelograms (IVPs). The term *pyelogram* is derived from roots signifying visualization of the kidney pelvis and was once the common name for this study. Because the scope of the examination includes the entire urinary tract, *urogram* is a more accurate term and is now the most commonly used.

An excretory urogram is a functional study of the urinary system accomplished by the injection of a water-soluble nonionic iodine contrast medium, such Omnipaque 300 or 350, Isovue 300, or Visipaque 320. The contrast agent mixes and circulates with the blood until it reaches the kidneys, which excrete it as a component of the urine. The contrast medium first opacifies the outer portion of the kidney as it fills the tiny vessels and glomeruli in the cortex and collecting tubules in the medulla. This imparts a hazy opacification to the entire kidney structure, which quickly disappears with normal function. Images made within the first 3 minutes after injection to visualize this phase are referred to as **nephrograms** and are used in the evaluation of hypertensive patients.

As the kidneys excrete the contrast medium, it is channeled into the calyces and pelves of the kidneys, clearly outlining these structures. As the pelves fill, the opacified urine begins to flow through the ureters and into the bladder (Figure 19-5). This process occurs within 15 to 20 minutes with normal kidney function. Thus each portion of the urinary tract may be visualized in turn by the timing of the imaging sequence. A urinary tract obstruction or infection may require an extension

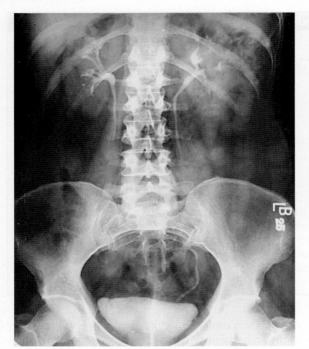

FIG 19-5 Excretory urogram. (From Long BW, Rollins JH, Smith BJ: *Merrill's atlas of radiographic positioning & procedures*, ed 13, St Louis, 2016, Elsevier.)

of the timing of the study in order to visualize the internal structures of a diseased kidney.

> An excretory urogram is a functional study of the urinary system consisting of radiographic images taken following the intravenous injection of a water-soluble nonionic iodine contrast medium.

The preparation for urography usually includes cleansing of the bowel to avoid gas and fecal shadows that could obscure structures of interest. Nothing by mouth (NPO) orders are given to avoid nausea and to create a moderate degree of dehydration, resulting in a greater concentration of the contrast medium in the kidneys. Be familiar with your departmental policy on the withholding of medications before the examination. For instance, drugs that have a diuretic effect (promoting increased urination) may be withheld, because they tend to dilute the contrast agent with body fluids during excretion. As mentioned earlier,

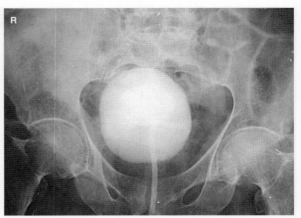

FIG 19-6 Cystogram. (From Long BW, Rollins JH, Smith BJ: *Merrill's atlas of radiographic positioning & procedures*, ed 13, St Louis, 2016, Elsevier.)

diabetic patients taking antihyperglycemic agents containing metformin must also have this medication withheld.

In preparation for the injection, check the emergency supplies and equipment and set up the IV medication tray (see Chapter 14), including the vial of contrast medium, a syringe, and an appropriately sized IV catheter or butterfly needle. The dosage varies depending on the medium used, the radiologist's preference, and the patient's weight and age.

After explaining the procedure and injecting the contrast medium, the radiographer proceeds with the technical aspects of the examination. If a radiologist is to inject the contrast medium, the radiographer performs the introductions and assists with the injection where necessary. The patient must be continually and closely monitored for any signs of an adverse reaction to the contrast agent.

Cystography

Several other studies of the urinary tract deserve mention. The cystogram provides contrast imaging of the internal contours of the bladder. The bladder is filled by retrograde injection of a water-soluble iodine medium through a urinary catheter (Figure 19-6) and examined using fluoroscopy and/or radiographs.

Voiding cystourethrograms (VCUGs) examine both the bladder and the urethra. The bladder is filled with contrast as when performing a cystogram, the catheter is removed, and fluoroscopy with spot films records the contours of the urethra and the action of the bladder as the patient voids. This procedure is useful to identify urethral obstruction in males and for the diagnosis of vesicoureteral reflux (urine backflow from the bladder into the ureters) in both males and females. This study is more commonly performed on children than on adults. Some institutions have specialized equipment for measuring the urinary force and flow rate, and these measurements may be taken in conjunction with the VCUG study.

When a cystogram is ordered, the patient is usually sent to the radiology department with a retention catheter in place. If an outpatient study is being carried out, or if the catheter must be replaced, the hospital will have a specific standing order indicating who will insert the catheter. A nurse or nursing assistant may be requested to come to the imaging department for this duty, or the radiologist or urologist may catheterize the patient. In some hospitals, this procedure is performed by radiographers who have been trained in catheterization technique (see Appendix K). Multimedia training aids, lab instruction, and practice with anatomic models will assist you in learning catheterization theory and technique.

The chief concern when performing a cystogram is the possibility of introducing bacteria into the urinary tract, thus causing an infection in a patient with an already compromised urinary system. A cystogram is a minor sterile procedure that does not require sterile gowning. When the catheter is in place, the contrast medium (Cystografin or Hypaque-Cysto) is poured into a 50- to 100-mL catheter-tip syringe and allowed to flow by gravity through the catheter and into the bladder. Depending on the specific protocol of your institution, this procedure may be repeated several times until the desired quantity has been instilled. Some radiologists use relatively small quantities of the contrast agent. Others prefer the bladder to be completely filled and distended.

> **!** Strict sterile procedure is required when performing cystograms to avoid the possibility of initiating a urinary tract infection.

The radiographer's role includes explaining the procedure to the patient, assembling the necessary equipment and supplies, assisting the physician with the injection, and completing the technical aspects of the procedure.

In some departments, cystography may be performed solely by radiographers. Box 19-3 provides suggested procedures for performing both routine cystography and VCUG studies.

Cystography may be performed in conjunction with a cystoscopic procedure (fiberoptic study of the bladder). Under these circumstances, the patient is sedated and a surgical nurse assists the physician. The radiographer's role is almost exclusively technical. These procedures are usually performed in a cystourology room that is part of the surgical suite.

Retrograde Urography

Another urographic examination, often performed in conjunction with cystoscopy, is the retrograde urogram (formerly called retrograde pyelogram). Under cystoscopic visualization, long, slender catheters are inserted into the ureters, and a water-soluble iodine compound such as Reno-30 is injected into the kidney pelves through the catheters. This study provides radiographic visualization of the anatomic form of the pelves, calyces, and ureters (Figure 19-7). Because this procedure carries a much lower risk of a reaction to the contrast medium than procedures involving IV injections, it is sometimes ordered instead of an excretory urogram for patients at risk of an allergic response or those with high BUN or creatinine levels. Most hospitals have a cystourology room in the surgical suite with special equipment for performing these studies. The surgical staff provides the patient care; the radiographer's role is similar to that of performing a surgical cystogram and is almost exclusively technical.

CONTRAST EXAMINATIONS OF THE BILIARY SYSTEM

Before the 1990s, biliary problems, such as stones in the gallbladder or common bile duct or acute **cholecystitis** (inflammation of the gallbladder), were treated with open surgery only. Today, there are safer and less invasive treatment methods for many biliary problems. Fiber optic devices such as the laparoscope and the endoscope are now used in both the diagnosis and treatment of biliary disease, so patients who are not good candidates for surgery can now be successfully treated. With better treatment options available, the diagnostic information required to make treatment decisions becomes more complex. Physicians may need to know the size, number, location, and composition of gallstones, whether the cystic duct is patent, and whether there are any anomalies in the structure of the biliary ducts. A number of possibilities exist for obtaining this information. Contrast radiography, ultrasound examination, cholescintigraphy (a nuclear medicine procedure), CT studies (especially spiral CT IV cholangiograms), and MRI examinations of the biliary system may all play a role in this complex process.

Traditionally, a diagnosis of right upper quadrant pain began with an oral cholecystogram. Today, the initial procedure is usually an ultrasound examination,

followed by further studies when necessary, as determined by the initial findings.

> Sonography is usually preferred as the first step in the diagnostic evaluation of the gallbladder.

Intravenous Cholangiography

At one time, the IV cholangiogram (IVC) was the preferred method of examining the common bile duct, but a relatively high degree of risk is associated with the

---

BOX 19-3   Procedures for Cystography and Voiding Cystourethrography

Cystography

1. Obtain all necessary equipment, and position it conveniently.
2. Place the patient on the table in the supine position, and cover him or her with a sheet, allowing access to the catheter.
3. Explain the procedure.
4. Fill the syringe with contrast medium.
5. Perform hand hygiene. Put on gloves.
6. Using antiseptic, cleanse the end of the drainage tube connecting the catheter to the urine collection bag. This is essential to prevent potential infection if the catheter is to be left in place and reattached to the collection bag after the procedure.
7. Separate the catheter from the drainage tubing, taking care not to contaminate either end. Protect the end of the tubing with dry, sterile gauze or a sterile plastic cover.
8. Place the tubing so it will not be contaminated. Hold the catheter in your nondominant hand.
9. Place the syringe tip into the end of the catheter. Hold catheter and syringe in the vertical position to prevent air from being injected into the bladder, and allow the contrast medium to flow into the bladder by gravity. It is not necessary to push the plunger of the syringe.
10. The contrast will be instilled under fluoroscopic control. When the bladder is full, clamp the catheter.
11. Remove gloves. Repeat hand hygiene.
12. Complete the fluoroscopic and radiographic imaging of the full bladder.
13. When the study is complete, perform hand hygiene, put on gloves, and unclamp the catheter. Allow the contrast/urine to drain into a disposable container.

14. Cleanse the end of the catheter with antiseptic. Reconnect to the drainage tubing, taking care not to contaminate the ends.
15. Remove equipment. Remove gloves, and perform hand hygiene.
16. Assist the patient from the radiographic table.
17. Charting should include the amount of urine discarded if the patient is under orders to have the intake and output (I&O) recorded.

Voiding Cystourethrography (VCUG)

Follow Steps 1 through 12 above.

13. When the full bladder imaging is complete, position the patient in preparation for imaging while voiding. Female patients will be positioned supine; male patients will be in the posterior oblique position. Take care that the penis does not superimpose the femur.
14. Repeat hand hygiene, and put on clean gloves.
15. If the retention catheter has a balloon, deflate the balloon. This may be accomplished by using scissors to snip off the balloon valve and allowing the water to drain into a basin or by using a 10-ml syringe and needle to withdraw the water through the valve. Do not unclamp the catheter itself.
16. Remove the catheter by pulling gently, sometimes before or during voiding, depending on the radiologist's preference. Discard the catheter and clamp.
17. Proceed with the established procedure for imaging the voiding process. Usually the urine is collected in a disposable pad, basin, urinal or towel that has been placed to absorb it without interfering with the image of the urethra.
18. When the study is complete, cleanse the genital area with a towel and see to the patient's comfort.
19. Remove gloves, and repeat hand hygiene.

contrast used. Today, IV cholangiograms using spiral CT with nonionic contrast media provide safer, quicker, and more comprehensive visualization. Percutaneous transhepatic cholangiography (PTC), T-tube cholangiography, endoscopic retrograde cholangiopancreatography (ERCP), magnetic resonance cholangiopancreatography (MRCP), and ultrasound studies also provide information about the common bile duct.

Percutaneous Transhepatic Cholangiography

Percutaneous transhepatic cholangiography (PTC), sometimes called thin-needle cholangiography, involves placing the tip of a long, thin needle through the patient's right side, through the liver, and directly into the common bile duct. An injection of 20 to 40 mL of a multipurpose contrast medium of 50% to 60% strength is introduced through the needle under fluoroscopic control for the visualization of the biliary system.

The radiographer's role is to assist the radiologist with the skin preparation and the sterile techniques required for the injection and to complete the procedure's technical aspects.

PTC presents a risk to the patient and is usually attempted only when immediate information is required and more conservative approaches are impractical or have been unsuccessful. The possible complications include leakage of bile into the peritoneal cavity, hemorrhage, pneumothorax, and sepsis (infection).

T-Tube and Surgical Cholangiography

After surgical cholecystectomy (removal of the gallbladder), a tube is sometimes left temporarily in the patient. This flexible rubber tube is about the size of a drinking straw in the shape of a T. The crossbars of the T extend into the hepatic and common bile ducts. The base of the T passes through the stump of the cystic duct or a tiny surgical opening in the common bile duct and exits through a small opening left in the original incision (Figure 19-8).

The T-tube serves primarily as a drain for bile until the postsurgical edema in the common bile duct subsides and bile can pass normally into the duodenum. It also serves as an avenue for the administration of a contrast agent if it is necessary to examine the biliary system postoperatively. This study may be performed to detect residual calculi in the hepatic or common bile duct, but it is most frequently used to determine the patency of the ducts before removing the drain.

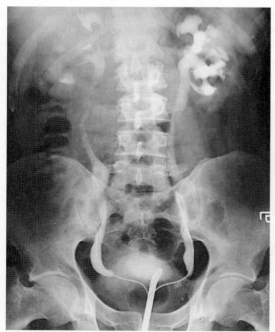

FIG 19-7 Retrograde urogram. (From Long BW, Rollins JH, Smith BJ: *Merrill's atlas of radiographic positioning & procedures*, ed 13, St Louis, 2016, Elsevier.)

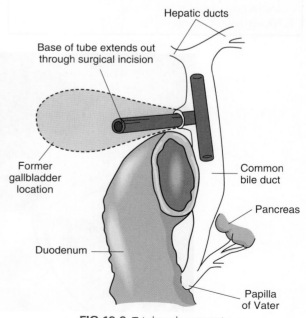

FIG 19-8 T-tube placement.

A postoperative study done in the radiology department requires the radiographer to assume a more prominent role. The procedure is summarized in Box 19-4. You should review the availability and contents of the emergency supply kit before any procedure involving a contrast agent, however, reactions to this study are extremely rare.

BOX 19-4 Postoperative T-Tube Cholangiography Procedure

1. Perform hand hygiene.
2. Fill a 30-mL syringe with the contrast medium, a multipurpose aqueous iodine preparation such as Renografin-60 or Hypaque Meglumine 60%, taking care that there is no air in the syringe. (Air bubbles injected into the biliary system are often indistinguishable from residual calculi.)
3. Attach a sterile graduated adapter (Christmas tree adapter) to the syringe.
4. Clamp off the distal portion of the T-tube with a hemostat.
5. Insert the adapter securely into the distal end of the T-tube, taking care to avoid contamination of the adapter and to prevent air in the tubing.
6. The radiologist will inject the contrast medium under fluoroscopical control and take spot films of the biliary system.
7. When the imaging is complete, reclamp the T-tube and remove the adapter.
8. Repeat hand hygiene.

A surgical cholangiogram may be performed in conjunction with a cholecystectomy to ensure that any calculi remaining in the ducts are detected and removed before closing the incision. During surgery the radiographer's duties are strictly technical. Patient care is carried out by the anesthesiologist, and the contrast injection is performed by the surgeon, with assistance from the surgical team (see Chapter 21).

Endoscopic Retrograde Cholangiopancreatography

ERCP is a fiber optic examination of the common bile duct performed with an endoscope. The patient is sedated and the back of the throat anesthetized. The tubular portion of the endoscope is then passed through the patient's mouth (Figure 19-9), down the throat, and through the stomach into the duodenum. A small catheter is passed through the endoscope into the distal end of the common bile duct through the papilla of Vater. Contrast is injected through the catheter, and spot films or digital images record the cholangiogram radiographically.

Attachments for the gastroscope include a "stone basket" for the removal of biliary calculi and a tiny rotary blade for excising any scar tissue or other obstructions. Sometimes the papilla of Vater will be widened (sphincterotomy) with the use of electrocautery (cut with electricity) or a small plastic tube called a stent is left in the papilla to facilitate the passage of stones and bile drainage.

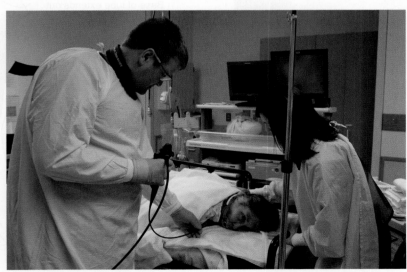

FIG 19-9 Radiographer assists radiologist or endoscopist with endoscopy for ERCP examination.

ERCPs may be performed in the radiology department or in a minor surgical setting using the C-arm fluoroscope, with the patient under deep sedation (if tolerated). Some departments have a dedicated suite with fluoroscopic and endoscopic equipment for performing this procedure.

OTHER CONTRAST EXAMINATIONS

Myelography

The myelogram is an examination using contrast media to visualize the internal surfaces of the spinal canal. This study helps in the diagnosis of conditions characterized by deformity or crowding of the spinal canal, such as spinal cord tumors and intervertebral disk herniations. Fluoroscopic spot films record the areas of interest. A CT study may be performed after the myelogram to obtain axial images of the spinal canal while the contrast is still present.

The injection portion of the procedure is called a spinal tap or **lumbar puncture** and involves the insertion of a needle into the subarachnoid space where a contrast medium is then injected for the myelogram. The usual medium is a water-soluble, nonionic contrast agent, such as Omnipaque or Isovue-M. The aqueous medium forms a homogeneous mixture in spinal fluid and outlines the nerve roots as the fluoroscopic table is tilted into various positions. The water-soluble contrast agent is readily absorbed from the spinal fluid and excreted via the urinary tract. This characteristic is a disadvantage in a prolonged procedure because the contrast medium may begin to disappear before the study is complete. For this reason, it is important to avoid delays between the time of injection and the examination.

The radiographer's role during a lumbar puncture and myelogram is to assist the physician. In preparation, the radiographer assembles the following items:

- A sterile myelogram tray or lumbar puncture tray
- An antiseptic for the skin preparation (for example, Betadine)
- An ample supply of the contrast medium
- Sterile gloves for the physician (two pairs)
- A sterile spinal manometer and specimen tubes (if necessary and not included on the tray)
- Additional spinal needles possibly added to the tray to meet the physician's preferences

When these items are ready, the patient is positioned according to the physician's preference, either prone (possibly with a bolster under the abdomen) or laterally recumbent with the hips flexed and knees drawn up toward the chin. In either position, the objective is to provide convenient access to the puncture site for the physician while providing maximum lumbar flexion to separate the spinous processes at the level of the injection (Figure 19-10). The site is selected under fluoroscopy by the physician and is frequently the L2-L3 or L3-L4 interspace. This portion of the spinal canal is below the level of the spinal cord and is readily accessible in most patients. The physician or the radiographer may prepare the skin (see Chapter 18). The physician then drapes the area and proceeds with the puncture. The radiographer may be asked to position the fluoroscope tower and table during the examination while the physician is in sterile gloves.

When the physician is ready to make the injection, the radiographer prepares the vial of contrast medium,

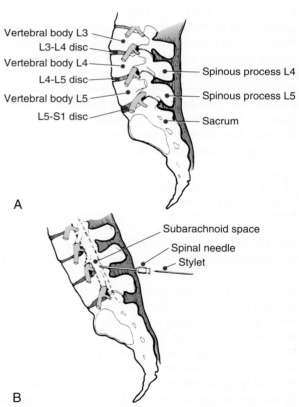

FIG 19-10 Lateral aspect of lumbar spine. **A,** Normal posture. **B,** Spinal flexion separates spinous processes, allowing needle access to the subarachnoid space.

shows the physician the label, and holds the container steady at a slight angle to facilitate withdrawal into the syringe. After the injection, the needle is withdrawn from the spine, and the fluoroscopic examination proceeds.

During the fluoroscopic portion of the study, the radiologist will tilt the table, causing the contrast agent, which is heavier than the spinal fluid, to move by gravity in the spinal canal and fill the areas of clinical interest. Do not forget to check the footboard and shoulder guard on the fluoroscopic table to ensure that they are secure before the table is tilted. These supports will provide safety for the patient as the table tilts. Lock the fluoroscope tower so that it will not accidentally collide with the patient. The patient's head must be kept above the level of the spine, and the head of the radiographic table should not be lowered more than 15 degrees. The patient is usually in a prone position during the examination. When the cervical region is to be studied, the patient's neck is extended with the chin supported on a radiolucent sponge. This position prevents the contrast agent from flowing into the cerebral region, causing an adverse effect, such as a headache. Observe the patient for any change in appearance that may indicate a change in status. Listen for any complaint, and provide reassurance. Occasionally, a patient may faint during the lumbar puncture or subsequent myelogram. Seizures and allergic reactions are rare, but may occur at any time from the moment of injection to as long as 8 hours afterward.

> **!** Check the footboard and shoulder guard to ensure that they are secure before tilting the table.

The lumbar puncture procedure may also include the measurement of spinal pressure using a spinal manometer. This device for measuring fluid pressure is a sterile, graduated glass tube. When attached to the spinal needle with the stopcock (flow valve) open, fluid rises in the tubing to a height that indicates the pressure of the spinal fluid within the spinal canal. When measuring spinal fluid "opening" pressure, the physician states the pressure reading aloud, and the radiographer records the value for later inclusion in the patient's medical record and the radiologist's report. The stopcock is then closed, and the manometer is detached from the needle. The closing pressure may also be obtained.

When a sample of the spinal fluid is removed, it is placed in sterile specimen tubes. The radiographer is responsible for ensuring that the specimens and requisition form are delivered promptly to the laboratory. The radiographer can delegate this duty to another member of the team while continuing to assist the radiologist. The person who delivers the specimens must be instructed to notify the medical technologist that a spinal fluid specimen has been delivered. This is very important, because a delay in processing the specimen may invalidate the results. Many facilities require signed documentation indicating that laboratory specimens have been delivered and received.

A loss of spinal fluid with the resulting lowered spinal fluid pressure tends to cause severe headaches following lumbar punctures. This discomfort can be minimized by controlling activity and encouraging fluid intake for 24 hours after the examination. A stretcher is required for transport out of the department as the patient is kept supine with his or her head elevated 20 to 30 degrees for the first 4 to 8 hours. Activity may be restricted for an additional 16 hours. Failure to keep the head elevated allows the contrast medium to flow upward to the hypothalamus, causing severe nausea with vomiting and potential dehydration.

> Increased fluid intake, slight head elevation, and limited activity are steps taken to minimize the headache and nausea following a lumbar puncture.

Contrast Arthrography

Arthrography, or contrast radiography of the joints, is a special procedure used to detect injury and disease of the joint cartilage as well as any abnormalities of the joint capsule (Figure 19-11). The contrast medium for these studies may be a gas, one of the water-soluble iodine compounds (50% to 60%), or a combination of both (double-contrast arthrography). The shoulder and hip are the most common sites for this study, but the knee, ankle, and other joints can be examined arthrographically as well.

Patient care for these examinations consists mainly of providing an explanation and support to the patient and assisting the radiologist with both the injection procedure and the manipulation of the fluoroscope tower. The necessary items are available commercially in a sterile disposable tray, to which you may need to add an

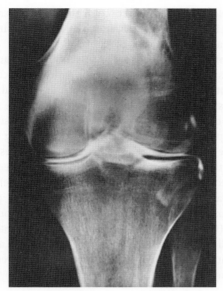

FIG 19-11 Contrast arthrogram of knee.

antiseptic for preparation of the skin, contrast media, a local anesthetic, and gloves for the radiologist.

After the injection, you may be asked to assist the patient to perform a range of joint movements to distribute the contrast agent. You may also be called upon to wrap the extremity with an elastic bandage to maintain an even pressure on the area for contrast localization and optimal visualization. The wrap must be firm but not too tight. Periodically check the distal portion of the wrapped extremity for any signs of decreased circulation, including numbness, discoloration, or swelling, that may indicate that the bandage is too tight. Bring any of these signs to the radiologist's attention. Fasten the wrap with adhesive tape rather than the usual metal clips, which are radiopaque and may obscure an anatomic area of interest.

The radiologist may stress the joint during the arthrographic procedure, using considerable pressure. Sometimes this is required for the contrast to reach the damaged areas or fill splits in the joint cartilage for adequate visualization. This procedure can be quite painful, so stay close to the patient and provide plenty of support and reassurance. After the examination, have a wheelchair present for transporting the patient out of the department and instruct him or her to avoid using the injected joint, as rest will allow the contrast to dissipate more quickly.

Contrast arthrography is not as common as it once was because of the increased use of CT and MRI arthrography studies to evaluate the soft tissue components of joints. For MRI studies, a paramagnetic contrast agent (gadolinium) may be introduced into the joint under fluoroscopic control before the patient is imaged in the MRI department.

Therapeutic and MRI joint injection procedures are similar to injections for contrast arthrography, however, they require only a small amount of the contrast medium to confirm the correct needle placement before administering medications or MRI contrast.

SUMMARY

- Gases such as air and CO_2 provide negative (dark or radiolucent) contrast for imaging studies that may include arthrography and myelography.

- Positive (radiopaque) contrast for studies of structures outside the gastrointestinal tract is accomplished using a variety of iodine compounds. Aqueous iodine media are miscible with body fluids.

- The osmolality (the number of particles in solution per kilogram of water) of aqueous iodine compounds determines whether they are classified as HOCAs, LOCAs, or as isosmolar contrast agents. They are designated ionic if their molecules dissociate into two or more charged particles and as nonionic if their molecules remain whole in solution. Ionization and osmolality affect the toxicity of contrast media.

- Compromised renal, cardiac, or respiratory function and a history of allergies are risk factors for iodine contrast agent injection.

- To avoid toxic or allergic reactions to contrast media, a specific history is taken, BUN and/or creatinine levels are checked, and care is taken to ensure that maximum dosages are not exceeded. Radiographers must be prepared to respond to adverse reactions.

- Excretory urography is a radiographic examination of the urinary tract by means of an aqueous contrast medium injected intravenously. Retrograde urography provides radiographic images of the internal structures of the kidneys and ureters by means of a contrast agent which is injected directly through catheters placed in the ureters.

- Cystography is radiographic imaging of the bladder following an injection of a contrast medium through a urinary catheter. A VCUG is similar to a cystogram with the added feature of imaging the urethra while the patient voids.
- Radiographic imaging of the gallbladder has been largely replaced by sonography. Several radiographic studies of the biliary system show the biliary ducts: IV cholangiography using spiral CT; percutaneous transhepatic cholangiography involving direct injection of a contrast medium through a long, thin needle; and T-tube cholangiography in which a contrast agent is administered through a T-shaped tube that has been surgically placed during a cholecystectomy. Imaging of the biliary system and pancreatic duct can also be accomplished by means of an ERCP with a contrast agent injected through an endoscope that enters the common bile duct through the gastrointestinal tract.

- Myelography is a fluoroscopic and/or CT examination in which a contrast medium is injected into the spinal canal by means of a lumbar puncture.
- Arthrography involves the injection of an aqueous contrast medium and/or gas or gadolinium contrast agent to provide visualization of the internal structures of joints using fluoroscopy and/or MRI.
- The duties of radiographers for these contrast imaging procedures vary considerably depending on the preferences of the radiologist and the policies of the health care institution. In addition to the technical aspects of the procedures, the radiographer must be familiar with the principles of effective patient communication (Chapter 6), medical history taking (Chapter 11), physical assessment (Chapter 11), sterile techniques (Chapter 18), medication administration (Chapter 14), and emergency response (Chapters 15 and 16).

▮ REVIEW QUESTIONS

1. When molecules of water-soluble iodine contrast do not dissociate but remain whole in solution, the medium is described as:
   A. ionic
   B. nonionic
   C. HOCA
   D. viscous

2. Blood chemistry values that provide information pertinent to the administration of iodine contrast agents include:
   A. blood glucose and total cholesterol
   B. high-density lipoprotein cholesterol and BUN
   C. BUN and creatinine
   D. blood glucose and bilirubin

3. Which of the following examinations provides images of the urethra?
   A. VCUG
   B. IVU
   C. BUN
   D. PTC

4. PTCs, ERCPs, and T-tube cholangiograms are examinations that may be performed to show the:
   A. gallbladder
   B. spleen
   C. common bile duct
   D. ureters

5. A sterile manometer and specimen tubes might be needed when preparing to perform a(n):
   A. cystogram
   B. myelogram
   C. excretory urogram
   D. arthrogram

6. Diabetic patients who are to receive an iodine contrast agent should have their medication withheld if it contains:
   A. glucose
   B. insulin
   C. metformin
   D. beta blockers

7. Iodine compounds injected into a blood vessel are excreted from the blood by the:
   A. colon
   B. liver
   C. pancreas
   D. kidneys

8. The risk of a severe allergic response to an iodine contrast injection is greatest with patients who have a history of:
   A. asthma
   B. heart disease
   C. diabetes
   D. kidney failure

9. The effect of a diuretic medication is to:
   A. reduce blood glucose levels
   B. promote urination
   C. reduce histamine levels
   D. prevent nausea

10. A cystogram is a radiographic study of the:
    A. gallbladder
    B. common bile duct
    C. soft tissues of a joint
    D. urinary bladder

Answers can be found in the Answer Key on pages 429-431.

CRITICAL THINKING EXERCISES

1. Meg Munsey's allergy history states that she has experienced several mild asthmatic attacks that were attributed to a pollen allergy. During an excretory urogram, she becomes agitated and short of breath. What should you do?

2. Your supervising technologist has asked you to prepare the supplies and tray for a urinary catheterization and cystography. What technique must you follow? Why is this technique important?

3. George LeForte is gowned and ready for his cervical myelogram. What should you do to prepare for the injection procedure? How should Mr. LeForte be positioned for the contrast injection? What should you watch for as you monitor his condition after the injection? What is your responsibility with regard to his spinal fluid specimens? What instruction should he receive for follow-up care?

4. The package insert information supplied with Mallinckrodt's Optiray, a multipurpose water-soluble iodine contrast agent, provides the following information on the pediatric dosage for excretory urography:

Children: *Optiray 320 at doses of 0.5 to 3 mL/kg of body weight has produced diagnostic opacification of the excretory tract. The usual dose for children is 1 to 1.5 mL/kg. Dosage for infants and children should be administered in proportion to their age and body weight. The total administered dose should not exceed 3 mL/kg.*

The radiologist has requested a dose of 1 mL/kg for an 8-year-old child weighing 60 pounds. What is the volume of contrast to be administered? Is this order consistent with the manufacturer's recommendations? What is the recommended *maximum* dosage for this child?

Note: You may find it helpful to review the information on dosage calculation in Chapter 14.

20

Bedside Radiography: Special Conditions and Environments

OBJECTIVES

At the conclusion of this chapter, the student will be able to:

- Demonstrate the appropriate procedure for gathering information before performing a bedside radiographic examination.
- List three situations in which bedside radiography may be preferable to examination in the imaging department.
- State the purposes of gastric, nasoenteric, tracheal, and thoracic suction.
- List the precautions to be taken when doing a bedside examination of a critical neonate in the intensive care unit (NICU).
- List four important factors to be noted during an initial survey before radiography in the intensive care or coronary care unit.

- List three types of special beds or mattresses that can be seen in special units, and state the precautions to be used when doing mobile radiography with each type.
- List three essential precautions to be taken with patients who have a tracheostomy.
- Demonstrate the procedure for discontinuing gastric suction.
- List and describe two types of central venous catheters.
- Identify the correct locations for the tips of Swan–Ganz, Groshong, and PICC catheters.
- State the consequences of dislodging a thoracic tube, and explain how to avoid this occurrence.

OUTLINE

Mobile Radiography
Special Care Units
    Postanesthesia Care Unit
    Emergency Trauma Unit
    Neonatal Intensive Care and Newborn Nursery
    Intensive Care and Coronary Care Units
Treatment Situations Involving Specialty
  Equipment

Special Beds and Mattresses
Orthopedic Traction
Tracheostomies
Mechanical Ventilation
Nasogastric and Nasoenteric Tubes
Closed Chest Drainage
Specialty Catheters
Pacemakers

KEY TERMS

atelectasis
central venous catheter (CVC)
coronary care unit (CCU)
decompression
enclosed incubator
intensive care unit (ICU)
nasoenteric (NE)

nasogastric (NG)
neonate
neonatal intensive care unit (NICU)
orthopedic traction
osseous

peripherally inserted central catheter (PICC)
postanesthesia care unit (PACU)
tracheostomy
tracheotomy

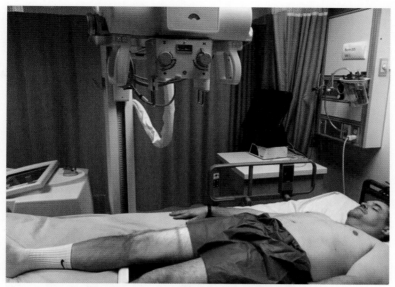

FIG 20-1 A mobile radiographic unit in use.

MOBILE RADIOGRAPHY

Thus far in the text, we have primarily discussed patient care in the radiology department. This chapter deals with bedside imaging and the conditions encountered when radiography or fluoroscopy is needed outside the imaging department. Emphasis is given to patient conditions usually seen in special care units but which may occasionally be encountered in the radiology department or other areas of the hospital.

Hospital radiology departments are equipped with mobile x-ray generators. These are used primarily for bedside radiography and may also be used in the surgical suite. Studies done with this equipment are frequently called *portable examinations,* but this is not a very accurate term. Portable means "capable of being carried," and few x-ray machines fit this description. When equipment is on wheels or capable of being moved around, *mobile* is the better word. Two types of units are generally used: the mobile radiographic unit (Figure 20-1) and the C-arm mobile image intensifier, a fluoroscopic unit (Figure 20-2). The C-arm unit produces dynamic images for real-time viewing and is also capable of producing radiographs of a relatively small anatomic area.

Bedside radiography is ordered when a patient's condition makes transfer to the radiology department difficult or hazardous. It is often more advantageous to perform bedside radiography for patients in special care units, **orthopedic traction** (treatment to correct bone deformity), and isolation (see Chapter 9 for isolation procedures). As mobile radiography equipment has significant technical limitations compared with the facilities in the diagnostic imaging department, it is seldom possible to do bedside examinations with the same ease and radiographic quality possible in the radiology suite. If the examination ordered can be done in the radiology department with a better outcome, the radiographer should consult the nurse in charge on the advisability of moving the patient. If the attending physician has ordered a mobile study, however, the examination must be done that way, or the physician's consent must be obtained to change the order.

With the exception of abdominal or single-view chest radiographs, bedside examinations are seldom routine. Standard positioning may not be possible, and situations often demand creative, innovative approaches. The skills gained by observing and assisting experienced radiographers will help you learn to handle these difficult situations competently.

The following list provides general guidelines for performing any bedside examination:

- Check with the nurse in charge to inquire about the patient's condition and any special considerations. Teamwork with the nursing staff is crucial in overall patient care.
- Confirm the order in the patient's chart, if applicable.

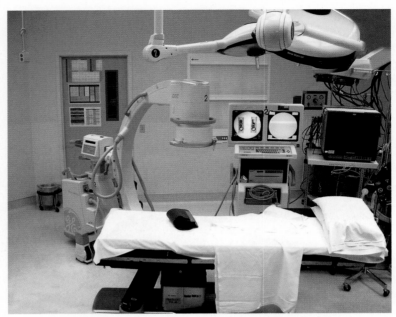

FIG 20-2 A typical setup of a C-arm fluoroscopic unit.

- Always greet the patient, check the name and birth date on the patient's wristband, and inspect and prepare the room before bringing in the x-ray equipment. This includes temporarily dismissing a patient's visitors for the duration of the examination.

These guidelines will be expanded as needed to meet special care unit requirements in the sections that follow.

SPECIAL CARE UNITS

Intensive care, coronary care, neonatal intensive care, postanesthesia care, and trauma units in the emergency department (ED) are considered special care units. Patients in these settings are in critical condition and need continuous monitoring and care by specialized nurses and physicians.

Postanesthesia Care Unit

The postanesthesia care unit (PACU) is sometimes referred to as *postanesthesia recovery* (PAR) or simply the "recovery room." It is located just outside the surgical suite, allowing for the unimpeded transfer of patients and immediate access to surgeons, anesthesiologists, and operating room nurses. Special dress is generally not required for personnel entry. PACUs may also be located near critical care units for the expeditious transfer of patients requiring continuous monitoring when they leave the PACU.

The PACU is designed and staffed for close observation and care of patients following operative procedures that require an anesthetic agent. Each patient admitted is retained until the effects or possible complications of anesthesia have been eliminated. Because of the effects of the anesthesia and pain medication, patients in this unit are generally not fully responsive. They may be receiving oxygen, with or without a ventilator. They may also have central venous catheters (CVCs) and various drainage tubes. These treatment situations are frequently seen in the intensive care unit and are described in detail in a later section of this chapter. A nurse will be nearby to assess the patient's condition and provide intravenous (IV) fluids, medication, and simple comfort measures.

> Following general anesthesia, surgical patients are monitored in the PACU until the effects of the anesthesia have resolved.

These patients are often monitored radiographically. Erect or semierect chest radiographs are frequently requested to show line placement or diagnose a possible pneumothorax or atelectasis. Anteroposterior and cross-table lateral images of osseous (bony) structures are sometimes ordered to check artificial joints, the alignment of fractures, and the placement of fixation hardware. The mobile x-ray unit is used to demonstrate these anatomical areas. The nurse will inform you of any patient precautions and will assist you during the examination if necessary.

Patients in the PACU often complain of being cold. This is because of the effects of anesthesia, premedication, and the cool atmosphere of the operating suite and PACU. Keep patients covered with warming blankets during examination whenever possible. While obtaining images, follow the same precautions described later in this chapter for patients in the intensive care unit (ICU) or coronary care unit (CCU).

Emergency Trauma Unit

Patients with severe trauma are often x-rayed in the trauma room as part of the total assessment of their injuries. The patient is immobilized on a backboard and placed on top of the trauma bed until radiographic images rule out fractures or spinal injury. Mobile x-ray examinations of the cervical spine, chest, and pelvis are commonly ordered. The radiographer must wear a lead apron and must also don protective attire over the lead apron to prevent contact with the patient's blood or body secretions. Assessment and stabilization of the patient create a flurry of activity as nurses, physicians, and laboratory, respiratory therapy, and electrocardiography (ECG) technicians perform their specialized tasks. The radiographer must carefully maneuver the x-ray equipment around these other professionals, position the image receptor, center the x-ray tube, and obtain the images as efficiently as possible. Only minimal movement of the patient can be tolerated. Disturbance of the equipment, tubes, and lines used to monitor and treat the patient must be avoided. Lead aprons must be provided for staff members who cannot leave the patient.

> The trauma physician establishes the priorities in the trauma unit. Although imaging may be critically important, it must sometimes be delayed while the team works to stabilize the patient. Be alert to the needs of other team members for access to the patient.

Trauma patients arrive at the ED in a variety of emotional and physical conditions. They may be agitated, intoxicated and belligerent, or in an altered state of consciousness (confused, drowsy, or comatose). They may have bone piercing their skin, large and gaping wounds, fractured and distorted extremities, partially severed body parts, or severe burns.

As a beginner student, you will always work beside an experienced radiographer until you develop the knowledge, skill, perseverance, and patience required for this unique setting.

Neonatal Intensive Care and Newborn Nursery

Although most newborns arrive in perfect health, some have serious problems and are placed in the neonatal intensive care unit (NICU). Premature and low–birth-weight infants, or those with health problems, may require frequent imaging. For example, pediatric respiratory distress syndrome (PRDS) or newborn atelectasis (failure of the lungs to expand completely) may require chest radiographs for evaluation. Newborns with cardiac, urinary tract, gastrointestinal, congenital, or skeletal anomalies may need chest, abdomen, or osseous studies. Skull radiographs may be requested for infants with neurologic problems. Even infants in the newborn nursery who are not in critical condition sometimes require a radiograph, for example, when a clavicle fracture is suspected at birth or a chest radiograph is required to confirm aspiration pneumonia.

The neonate (newborn) at risk may be placed in an open incubator under a radiant warmer (Figure 20-3) or in an enclosed incubator. The enclosed incubator (Figure 20-4) may be used because this closed environment provides extra warmth, moisture, and oxygen while reducing exposure to airborne infection.

> **!** Do not open a closed incubator or handle a newborn unless a nurse or physician is present.

Procedure

Even when protective precautions are not in place, attention to the general principles of medical asepsis is essential for the infant's safety. Infants needing radiography may require protective precautions to avoid nosocomial infections. These include disinfecting the x-ray equipment before coming into the unit, hand hygiene, and possibly covering your uniform with a gown. A mask is generally not necessary, and gloves are worn only if you handle the baby. Refer to the infection control guidelines established by your institution. There are generally fewer restrictions on handling and positioning babies who are not in critical condition.

The neonate at risk must be radiographed within the enclosed incubator. A nursing staff member will usually assist. Some enclosed incubators are designed with

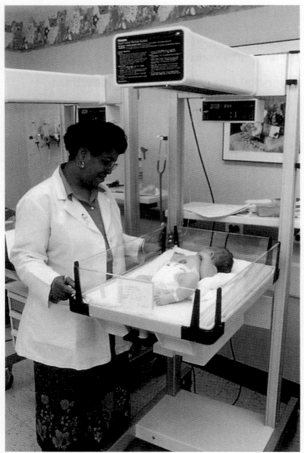

FIG 20-3 Open incubator with a radiant warmer for infants at risk. (From Wong DL, Hockenberry-Eaton M, Wilson D, Winkelstein ML, Schwartz P: *Wong's essentials of pediatric nursing,* ed 6, St Louis, 2001, Mosby.)

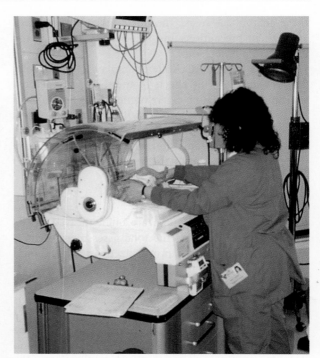

FIG 20-4 The enclosed incubator provides warmth, moisture, and oxygen while premature infants and those at risk gain maturity and strength. (From Wong DL, Hockenberry-Eaton M, Wilson D, Winkelstein ML, Schwartz P: *Wong's essentials of pediatric nursing,* ed 6, St Louis, 2001, Mosby.)

a sliding tray below the unit for cassette placement. If you must open the unit to place the image receptor (IR), it is imperative that you work quickly to preserve the warmth of the infant. The IR is covered and placed under the patient by the nurse, who positions him/her according to the radiographer's instructions. If the infant is in an open incubator with a radiant warmer, remember to move these lamps out of the way before centering the x-ray tube. Before making the exposure, provide a gonad shield for the infant, a lead apron for yourself, and one for the nurse, if necessary. Remember to don gloves if you must hold or handle the neonate. If the infant is on a ventilator, do not turn it off to eliminate respiratory motion and do not apply tension to the ventilator tubing; you may accidentally disconnect it from the ventilator. (See the section on mechanical ventilation later in this chapter.) Shared radiographic items (such as R/L markers, gonadal shields, and the IR) should be disinfected and/or placed inside a protective covering before coming into contact with the patient.

Intensive Care and Coronary Care Units

The ICU and CCU are special care units designed for patients in critical condition whose treatment and status require frequent monitoring. Depending on the size of your institution, the ICU may be subdivided into medical, surgical, trauma, neonatal, and pediatric units. The CCU may also be subdivided, with patients recovering from cardiac surgery in one area and those receiving medical and nonsurgical treatment (e.g., balloon angioplasty) in another.

Today's ICUs and CCUs are equipped to monitor the heart's electrical activity, cardiac output, cardiovascular function (through the placement of special catheters), blood pressure (through placement of an arterial line), internal body temperature, oxygenation, intracranial pressure, and ventilation. Continuous support equipment, such as cardiac assist devices (for example, aortic balloon pump) and dialysis machines may also be connected to patients in ICUs and CCUs.

The ICU and CCU are familiar places to radiographers. Many patients in these units require frequent radiographic monitoring with mobile units. Chest radiographs are most often called for, but other examinations and/or imaging procedures may also be requested. For example, you may be asked to bring the C-arm mobile image intensifier to the ICU for bronchoscopy or to the CCU for placement of a central venous catheter or a pacemaker.

The inexperienced radiographer entering these units need not expect great difficulty in coping with the acutely ill patient. Because there is always adequate staff to provide constant patient care, the radiographer's duties are limited almost exclusively to technical considerations. The special problems faced in this environment may be twofold: dealing with your own anxiety about confronting near-death situations and manipulating an assortment of life-sustaining equipment connected to the patient and to other equipment by a network of cords, cables, pumps, tubes, and lines (Figure 20-5).

Procedure

Before bringing your equipment into the ICU or CCU, confer with the nurse in charge. You will be more successful in obtaining a diagnostic radiograph and minimizing any harm to the patient if you coordinate your efforts with those of the nursing staff. Explain what you need to do to accomplish the procedure and inquire about any necessary precautions. As a case in point, patients with head injuries in the trauma ICU are often kept in a semierect position to minimize intracranial pressure. Lowering the head end of the bed and proceeding with your imaging without checking with the nurse can be life-threatening to these patients.

Assessing how well the patient can cooperate with the procedure is the next step. Speak to patients, even when they are not responsive, and provide a brief explanation and calm reassurance as you work. Assume that patients can hear you, and avoid making any qualitative remarks about their condition or continuing a personal discussion during the examination. All communication should be kept professional.

As space is sometimes limited, you may need to move some equipment to make room for the x-ray unit. Check the bed rails and the area under the bed to locate cords, tubes, and drainage receptacles so that you will be aware of their location and not damage them accidentally as you move equipment. Some ICUs and CCUs have an overhead system that provides support for monitors, oxygen, suction, and compressed air for the ventilator. A freely movable unit containing bottles for chest tube drainage and nasogastric suction may be located at the head of the bed. These innovations allow more room and mobility when it is necessary to move the bed or to care for the patient from the head of the bed. If the bed must be moved, obtain help from the nursing service. Usually, two people are needed to move the bed safely without placing undue stress on the cables and tubes connected to the patient. When a mobile C-arm and monitor are used, locate the most convenient electrical outlet and decide where to place the equipment. The beds in the ICU and CCU are usually "fluoro capable" (radiolucent), permitting operation of the C-arm through the bed.

When the plan is clear and the area is ready, bring in the x-ray equipment and complete the study as efficiently as possible. Because drainage tubes, IV lines, and dressings all have a tendency to leak, cover the IR with a plastic or cloth cover and don gloves before lifting or turning the patient. Check that all lines and tubes are clear as you place the IR under the patient. Using a plastic cassette cover and sliding the IR under the draw sheet, or between the mattress and the sheet, may facilitate placement. Always employ radiation protection measures for yourself and others. Correct procedure requires all nonessential staff to leave the immediate area. Provide lead aprons for the remaining staff, place a gonad shield on the patient if applicable, and announce "X-ray!" before making the exposure. When the examination is complete, carefully return everything to its original location and allow visitors to return to the room.

> **!** Accidentally dislodging lines or tubes is a common and dangerous error. Check that all lines and tubes are clear as you position the patient and the equipment.

The monitoring units have auditory and visual signals that are activated by a change in the patient's condition or position or when there are equipment problems. An alarm may indicate that a patient is breathing too

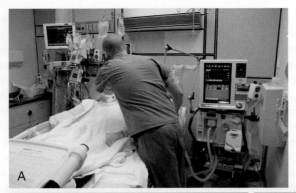

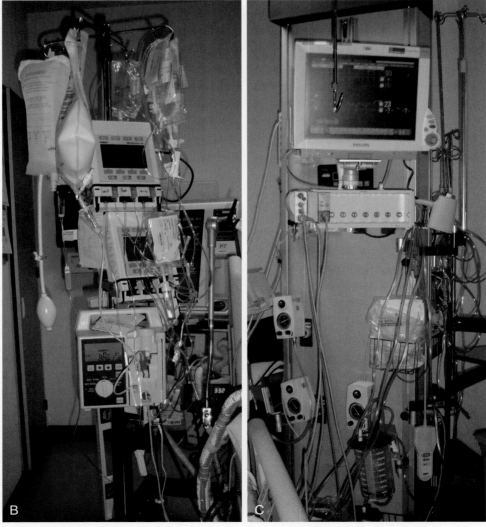

FIG 20-5 Critical patients within the ICU may require a variety of life-sustaining equipment. A, A patient in ICU is surrounded by an array of technical equipment. B, Typical IV stand in the ICU supports multiple medication pumps and bags of IV fluids. C, This ICU tower supports a vital signs monitor, access valves for oxygen and pressurized air, oxygen administration equipment, and suction equipment.

fast, the blood pressure or pulse rate is too low, or a tube or line has become dislodged or disconnected from the patient or the equipment. When an alarm is activated while positioning the patient, check the patient's condition before summoning the nurse. Do not manually turn off the alarm. If the alarm does not terminate within 15 seconds, a nurse will come to check the patient.

Patients with ventilators, heart monitors, and other specialized equipment may be found in different parts of the hospital but are most frequently encountered in the ICU or CCU. Whatever their location, patients being monitored need the same precautions and attention to detail as those in a specialized unit.

TREATMENT SITUATIONS INVOLVING SPECIALTY EQUIPMENT

Special Beds and Mattresses

Many patients in ICU, CCU, and long-term care units are relatively immobile and have circulation problems. Several innovative devices are used to improve circulation in immobilized patients. Alternating pressure mattresses, air mattresses, rocking beds, and various types of wave, flotation, and bead mattresses are among the equipment that can enhance the well-being of patients who are unable to tolerate being moved in the usual manner. The continual changes in position and pressure promote healing and decrease requirements for frequent turning of patients from side to side.

When bedside radiography is needed for patients on special beds, consult the nursing staff to see exactly what equipment is being used. Beds that have a rocking motion or waves of alternating pressure need to be turned off during x-ray exposures to avoid motion blur on the radiograph. Air mattresses must be fully inflated to firm up and level the bed before placing the IR under the patient.

Some patients need to lie on an alcohol- or water-filled pad to raise or lower body temperature. It is important to place the IR on top of the pad to avoid artifacts that interfere with the image. Be especially careful not to snag the pad while positioning the IR.

The surfaces of Mylar warming blankets or pads (also known as aluminized, solar, or space blankets) are very effective in reflecting body heat back toward the patient's body. Again, you must use care in placing the IR between the patient and the reflecting surface without damaging the Mylar. The "Bair Hugger" is another version of a warming blanket. It has two layers. The layer in contact with the patient is a flat, non-woven fabric; above this lies a series of connected plastic tubes that are filled with warm air. An attached electrical unit, controlled by a thermostat, supplies the air. Because the blanket does not contain any metal parts, radiographs can be taken without removing it. Use care to avoid damaging the plastic.

> Specialty mattresses and blankets are quite expensive and can easily be damaged. It is your duty to recognize them and to use appropriate precautions.

Orthopedic Traction

Orthopedic traction is a mechanical method using weights to provide a constant pull on part of the body for therapeutic reasons. In the past, fractured long bones, such as the femur, were placed in traction to maintain the alignment of bone fragments as they healed. Today, however, traction is used only until the muscle spasm subsides and the bone is surgically immobilized with a pin or plate. This permits a cast to be applied and allows the patient to convalesce at home.

When doing an x-ray examination, you should never attempt to alter a patent's traction. A sudden release of traction may result in serious harm to the patient. Even an accidental bump against the bed or the traction weights may cause severe pain. Since patients are usually aware of which movements are tolerable, let them assist as much as possible with any moving or lifting. Often the traction apparatus includes a trapeze bar that the patient grips to assist in elevating the torso. If you have any doubt about any particular movements, ask the nursing service.

Tracheostomies

A **tracheotomy** is a surgical procedure that creates an opening into the trachea to provide a temporary or permanent artificial airway. This opening, through which a tube may be placed, is called a **tracheostomy** (Figure 20-6). A tracheotomy may be necessary because of an obstruction in the upper respiratory tract caused by laryngospasm, cancer of the larynx, or burns in the mouth and throat. Another reason may be to provide controlled respiration with a ventilator in patients with respiratory collapse caused by paralysis, pulmonary edema, trauma, or adult respiratory distress syndrome (ARDS).

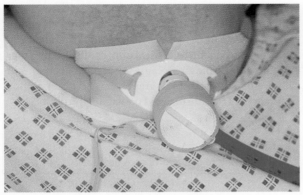

FIG 20-6 Tracheostomy. (From Scully C: *Medical problems in dentistry*, ed 6, Oxford, 2010, Churchill Livingstone.)

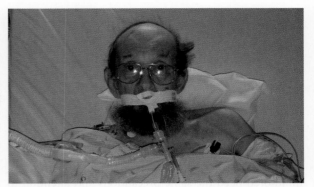

FIG 20-7 A patient with an endotracheal tube in place for mechanical ventilation.

Patients with new tracheostomies are monitored in the ICU. Because these patients require frequent suctioning to keep the tube free of secretions, close monitoring and immediate access to suction equipment are required. For these reasons, a nurse will accompany these patients when they are brought to the diagnostic imaging department.

The tapes holding the tracheostomy tube are never untied because a sudden cough can expel the tube, and the edges of the tracheostomy may close sufficiently to obstruct respiration.

> **! TRACHEOSTOMY PRECAUTIONS**
>
> - Monitor tracheostomy patients closely.
> - Never untie the tapes holding a tracheostomy tube in place.
> - Have suction equipment and supplies immediately available.

Mechanical Ventilation

Patients who need mechanical assistance with respiration are intubated; that is, an endotracheal tube is passed through the mouth and into the trachea (Figure 20-7). The tube is then connected to a ventilator (mechanical respirator), as illustrated in Figure 20-8, which assists breathing either by supplementing the patient's breath or by forcing respiration under pressure. Ventilators may also be connected directly to tracheostomies.

When performing a radiographic examination of the chest or abdomen, do not turn off the ventilator to eliminate the respiratory motion. If the ventilator is controlling both the rate and the volume of breathing, you may be able to determine when a brief pause in respiration will

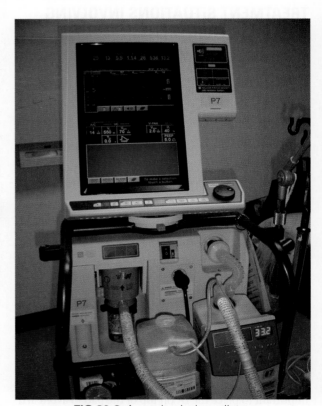

FIG 20-8 A mechanical ventilator.

occur by paying attention to the breathing rhythm. If the exposure time is short and your sense of rhythm is good, you will be able to take a motion-free exposure.

> Never disconnect or turn off a ventilator.

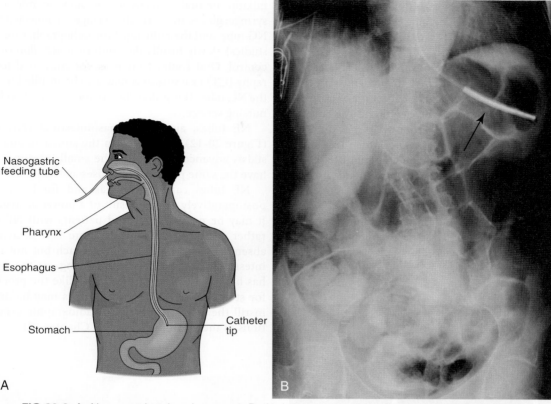

FIG 20-9 A, Nasogastric tube placement. **B,** Abdomen radiograph shows a nasogastric feeding tube in the stomach *(arrow)*. (A From Perry AG, Potter PA, Ostendorf WR: *Nursing interventions and clinical skills*, ed 6, St. Louis, 2016, Elsevier.)

Position the patient carefully without applying tension to the ventilator tubing so you do not disconnect it from the endotracheal or tracheostomy tube or ventilator. If the ventilator alarm is activated during the positioning and the patient appears distressed, notify the nurse immediately. Protect yourself when positioning patients on ventilators. Wear gloves and avoid placing your face too close to the patient's head and neck area. These precautions will help prevent contamination by mucus if the tubing disconnects.

Patients may also be ventilated manually by a nurse or respiratory therapist with an Ambu bag, a device that is squeezed regularly by hand to force respiration. This method can be used briefly during the time between intubation and setting up the ventilator. Manual ventilation, often referred to as *bagging,* may also be used while the patient is being transferred for diagnostic studies. Ambu bags are also used by nuclear medicine

technologists to instill radionuclides for ventilation studies.

Nasogastric and Nasoenteric Tubes

Another treatment situation that may be encountered in the ICU and elsewhere involves the insertion of **nasogastric (NG)** or **nasoenteric (NE)** tubes. These tubes are passed through the nose and down into the stomach or small intestine.

Nasogastric tubes are passed into the stomach (Figure 20-9) and have several purposes:
- Feeding
- Decompression
- Radiographic examination

It may be necessary to feed a patient with an NG tube when trauma, disease, an altered state of consciousness, or a surgical procedure (for example, tracheostomy) prevents normal swallowing. A commonly used feeding tube is the Dobbhoff nasogastric feeding tube (Figure 20-10) which has a smaller lumen and is more flexible than the NG tubes used for decompression.

Decompression, the removal of gas and secretions by suction, is prescribed to prevent vomiting in patients who have recently had surgery or have an intestinal obstruction. The Levin and the Salem–Sump tubes are the most common NG tubes used for this purpose. The Levin is a single-lumen tube with several holes near its tip. The Salem–Sump tube is a radiopaque double-lumen tube. One lumen is used to remove the gastric contents; the other functions as an air vent (Figure 20-11).

The NG tube may also be used to administer medication and for the radiographic examination of the stomach. The radiographer draws up a thin barium mixture or oral aqueous iodine solution into a large syringe; gloves are worn, the syringe is connected to the NG tube, and the radiologist (or radiographer for some studies) slowly instills the contrast under fluoroscopic control. Oral contrast mixtures for computed tomography (CT) examinations may also be instilled through the NG tube. This is done before the examination by the nursing service.

NE tubes, also called nasointestinal (NI) tubes (Figure 20-12), are placed in the stomach, and peristalsis advances them into the small intestine. They have the same potential purposes as NG tubes.

NE tubes can remove gas and fluid occurring postoperatively or as a result of a bowel obstruction. It may be necessary to feed patients with NE tubes rather than NG tubes when there is a decrease or absence of peristalsis in the stomach but not in the intestines, delayed gastric emptying, or the patient has had a gastric resection. Much like the procedure for studying the stomach, NE tubes may be used to instill the contrast media for radiographic examinations of the small intestine (see Chapter 17).

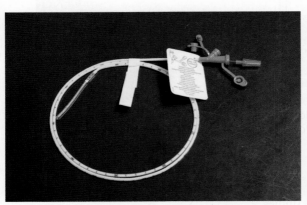

FIG 20-10 Dobbhoff nasogastric feeding tube.

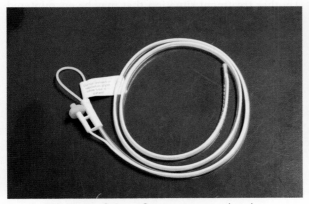

FIG 20-11 Salem–Sump nasogastric tube.

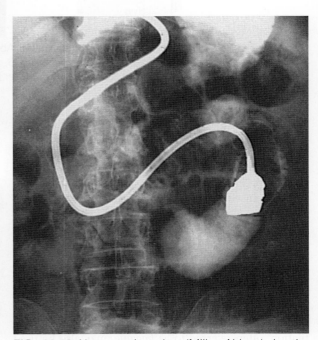

FIG 20-12 Nasoenteric tube (Miller–Abbott) in the small bowel. Note the aqueous iodine contrast medium injected through the tube to outline the intestine just distal to the opaque weight at the tube tip.

Some typical nasoenteric tubes include the Miller–Abbott, Harris, and Cantor tubes. The Cantor and Harris tubes have a single lumen with one opening for drainage. The Miller–Abbott has a double lumen, one for drainage and the other for a balloon. The balloon is weighted to simulate a bolus of food and promotes peristalsis to advance the tube into the small intestine. NE tubes are frequently localized radiographically; they may be placed fluoroscopically if advancement beyond the stomach is difficult.

When performing bedside radiography of a patient with an NG or NE tube, there is little cause for concern except to avoid disturbing the tube. It is uncomfortable when tugged on and very messy if the drainage end is dislodged from the bottle or the suction machine.

When the tube is connected to suction for decompression, it can be temporarily disconnected to bring the patient to the diagnostic imaging department. Before discontinuing the suction, obtain approval from the nurse in charge. With his/her permission, turn off the suction, clamp off the tube with a hemostat or special clamp, and then disconnect the tube. Wipe the tube with a tissue or gauze sponge and wrap the tip in a washcloth to catch any leaks. Pin the loose end of the tube to the patient's gown to prevent the tube from being pulled out of position by its own weight. Take care not to remove the gown without first remembering to unfasten the tube. It is very unpleasant for the patient to have the tube reinserted.

Closed Chest Drainage

Closed chest drainage is a method used to remove fluid or air that has accumulated in the pleural space. It consists of a tube placed within the pleural cavity and connected to a suction device through a drainage receptacle. Chest tubes are inserted in different locations depending on the type of treatment desired, although "safe zone" placement is considered to be at the fifth intercostal space, slightly anterior to midaxillae. Tubes inserted through the anterior superior chest wall remove air (Figure 20-13); they are placed through the posterior inferior chest wall to drain fluid that collects at the base of the pleural space (Figure 20-14).

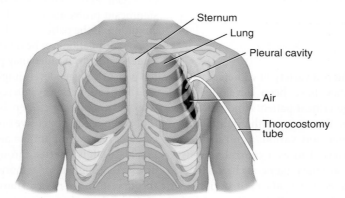

FIG 20-13 A chest tube placed to relieve a pneumothorax.

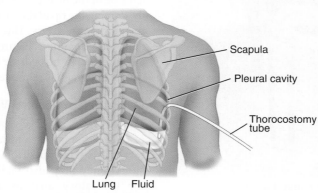

FIG 20-14 A chest tube placed to drain fluid from the pleural space.

A typical drainage system is illustrated in Figure 20-15. Disturbance of the drainage system at either end may result in a rush of air into the pleural space, reversing the intent of the treatment and possibly causing a lung collapse. Use caution, therefore, to avoid disturbing the chest drainage apparatus. The drainage unit must remain below the level of the patient's chest to avoid reverse flow from the unit. Gloves should be worn when taking radiographs of patients with chest tubes to provide protection from potential contact with body fluid from the chest incision. Be aware of the location of chest tubes when positioning patients for chest radiographs, because palpation near the tube insertion area is painful.

> ! Extra caution is required with patients receiving chest suction treatment:
> - Ensure that chest suction and drainage apparatus is not disturbed.
> - Take care that the chest tube is not dislodged when positioning the IR for a chest radiograph.
> - Ensure that the drainage unit remains below the level of the patient's chest.

Specialty Catheters

The radiographer encounters a variety of catheters with specialized functions. They have been developed to help monitor and manage critical patients and patients requiring long-term care. You may see the pulmonary artery Swan–Ganz catheter and various central lines. A central line may be referred to as a **central venous catheter (CVC)**; by a proprietary name such as Hickman, Groshong, Raaf, or Port-A-Cath; or if peripherally inserted, it may be called a **peripherally inserted**

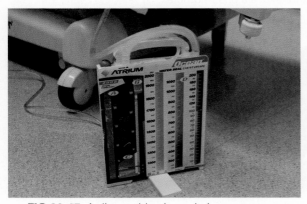

FIG 20-15 A disposable chest drainage system.

central catheter (PICC). In general, all of these catheters are tubes providing access to the circulatory system on a repeated or continuing basis. Because the improper use of these specialized catheters may jeopardize the physical status of patients, only specially trained personnel are permitted to use or care for them.

Pulmonary Artery Flow-Directed Catheters

Pulmonary artery flow-directed catheters such as the Swan–Ganz catheter measure cardiac output, the pressures on the right side of the heart and, indirectly, the left heart and lung pressures. These catheters diagnose right and left ventricular failure and monitor the effects of specific medications, stress, and exercise on heart function. If the pulmonary artery catheter has a fiberoptic infrared sensor, it is also capable of measuring the mixed venous oxygen saturation, which reflects the balance between oxygen supply and demand. This simply means it can reveal the amount of oxygen left in the blood after it has circulated through the body. High or extremely low levels of oxygen on the venous side of circulation could indicate significant problems, depending on the patient's age and condition. If the patient is elderly or very weak, any exercise or stimulation can be detrimental. This may help you understand why a nurse may postpone radiography until the patient's oxygen levels improve.

These catheters are often seen in ICU or CCU patients who have undergone open heart or chest surgery and those who require intensive monitoring. The Swan–Ganz catheter has several lumina and a balloon at its tip (Figure 20-16). It is inserted through the subclavian, internal or external jugular, or femoral vein and advanced until the tip rests in the right atrium. Inflating the balloon with air floats the catheter tip into the right or left pulmonary artery. During the indirect pressure monitoring of the left side of the heart, the balloon is reinflated momentarily, floating the tip of the catheter into a smaller branch of the pulmonary artery. This is called the *pulmonary capillary wedge position* (Figure 20-17). This catheter is usually inserted at the bedside by a physician, and a mobile chest radiograph is requested to verify its placement.

Central Lines or Central Venous Catheters

Central lines or CVCs facilitate the administration of chemotherapy or another long-term drug therapy, total parenteral nutrition, dialysis, or blood transfusions. They may also facilitate the drawing of blood for laboratory analysis and allow central venous pressure monitoring. These catheters share some common characteristics. Almost all are constructed of special materials providing the necessary rigidity for placement and lowering the incidence of blood clot formation. They all possess radiopaque strips or have radiopaque distal ends, allowing radiographic verification of their placement. Depending on their purpose, they may have either single or multiple lumina. Their distal tips all rest in the vena cava near the right atrium.

Central venous catheters can be classified as follows:

- Short- or long-term nontunneled external catheters
- Long-term tunneled external catheters
- Long-term implanted infusion ports

Short- or long-term nontunneled external catheters are frequently inserted at the bedside. They are placed through the skin and directly into a vein in the neck, shoulder, groin, or antecubital fossa. To prevent dislodgment, they are secured at the point of insertion with sutures or a dressing. This helps provide protection from infection. The PICC is inserted into a vein in the patient's arm, at or superior to the antecubital fossa, and advanced until its tip lies in the superior vena cava (Figure 20-18). This catheter is used to administer medication and fluids and to draw blood. The PICC can be used for short or long-term therapy. The CVC is inserted into a vein in the patient's arm, neck, shoulder, or groin and advanced into the vena cava (Figure 20-19). It is used to administer medication and fluids, to draw blood, or to monitor the pressure of the blood as it returns to the right atrium, aiding in the evaluation of right heart function. This CVC is usually used for short-term therapy.

Long-term tunneled external catheters are surgically placed beneath the skin and directed to the desired vein

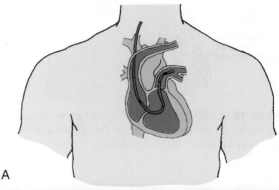

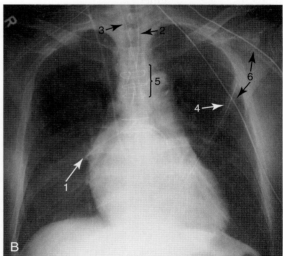

FIG 20-17 **A,** A Swan–Ganz catheter placement. **B,** Anteroposterior (AP) chest radiograph showing (1) the tip of the Swan–Ganz catheter advanced into the right pulmonary artery, (2) an endotracheal tube, (3) a nasogastric tube, (4) a chest tube, (5) sternal wires from open heart surgery, (6) monitor lines (external).

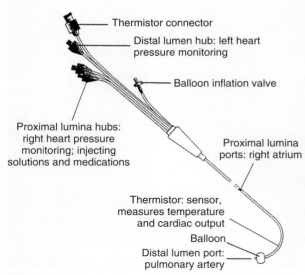

FIG 20-16 An example of a pulmonary artery catheter. This quadruple-lumen catheter measures the cardiac output, heart pressures, and core temperature. It has two lumina for the administration of fluids and medication.

(Figure 20-20). Their access ends are generally located midway between the nipple and the sternum. New tissue formation secures the catheter's Dacron cuff in place, preventing accidental dislodgment while providing a barrier to infection. The Hickman, Groshong, and Raaf catheters are examples of tunneled central venous catheters. All are advanced into the superior vena cava. The Hickman is used for patients requiring long-term parenteral nutrition. The Groshong is a single- or double-lumen catheter used to administer medications and fluids or to draw blood. The Raaf is a large, double-lumen catheter used for dialysis.

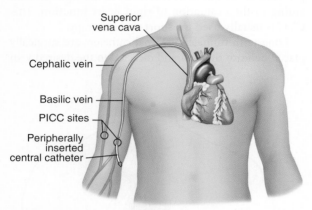

FIG 20-18 A PICC line placed from an antecubital insertion point. (From Lewis SL et al: *Medical-surgical nursing*, ed 9, St. Louis, 2014, Elsevier.)

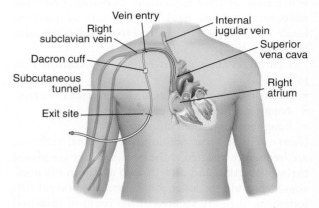

FIG 20-20 The tunneled placement of a catheter for long-term use (e.g., Groshong, Hickman). (From Lewis SL et al: *Medical-surgical nursing*, ed 9, St. Louis, 2014, Elsevier.)

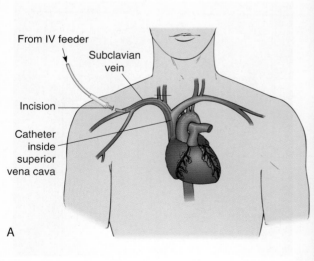

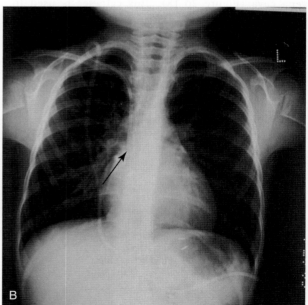

FIG 20-19 **A,** A nontunneled central venous catheter with its tip in the superior vena cava. (From Perry AG, Potter PA, Ostendorf WR: *Clinical nursing skills & techniques*, ed 8, St. Louis, 2014, Elsevier.) **B,** A posteroanterior (PA) chest radiograph showing the proper placement of the CVC.

Long-term implanted infusion ports, also known as venous access ports (Figure 20-21), are used for patients who need intermittent infusion of medication or chemotherapy, blood transfusions, or the sampling of blood from the superior vena cava. The port, encased in plastic or metal (usually titanium), and an attached venous catheter are surgically implanted and sutured under the skin of the upper chest or arm. The other end of the venous catheter is placed in the superior vena cava. The port is externally visible only as a raised portion of skin and can easily be felt under the skin. A specially designed needle called the *Huber needle* is used to access its self-sealing port. An example of a commonly used infusion port is the Port-A-Cath. Other similar products include the InfusaPort, Mediport, and Lifeport catheters.

Mobile C-arm fluoroscopy may be requested to guide specialty catheter tips into place. Chest radiographs are performed to check their position and ensure that no pneumothorax is present. As mentioned previously, watch out for these lines and use caution as you place the IR for radiography. It may be necessary to move any external wires (fiberoptic sensors) out of the way to avoid artifacts on the image.

> Central venous catheters come in many configurations for different purposes, and there are several possible points of access, depending on the catheter. The tip should always be located in the superior vena cava.

Pacemakers

The artificial pacemaker is an electromechanical device that regulates the heart rate by providing low levels of electrical stimulation to the heart muscle to replace the stimulation which is normally provided by nerve impulses. Pacemakers are used primarily to treat conduction defects. If the conduction system of the heart is unable to maintain an effective rate and rhythm, the pacemaker will electrically stimulate the heart to maintain an adequate rate.

The pacemaker system consists of a battery-powered energy source and a wire or catheter delivering electrical stimulation to the heart. Internal pacemakers are surgically implanted inside the patient's chest; external pacemakers are usually temporary, and the bulk of the instrument remains outside the patient's chest in a "pocket" under the skin. When

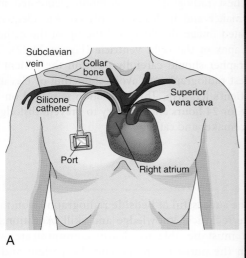

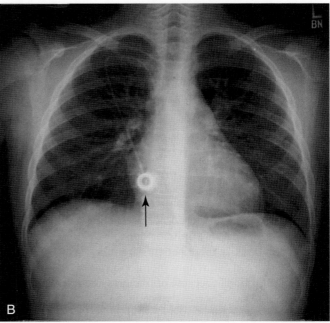

FIG 20-21 A, The placement of a subcutaneous venous access port. **B,** A chest radiograph shows the venous access port *(arrow)*. (A From Perry AG, Potter PA, Ostendorf WR: *Clinical nursing skills and techniques*, ed 8, St. Louis, 2014, Mosby.)

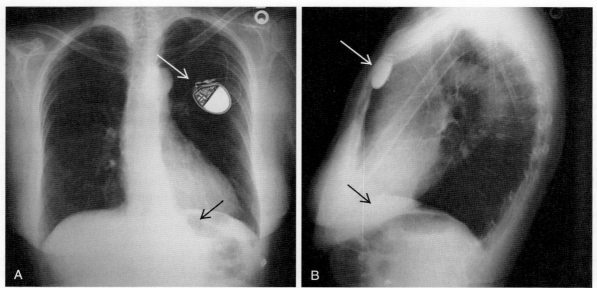

FIG 20-22 Chest radiographs following pacemaker insertion. **A,** A PA projection shows the pacemaker and catheter placement. **B,** Lateral projection. Note the left arm is superimposed on the thorax; elevation of the arm above shoulder level within the first 24 hours risks disturbing the placement of the catheter or pacemaker. *White arrows* indicate catheter placement; *black arrows* indicate the end of the catheter lead.

the pacemaker is inserted under fluoroscopic control in the cardiac catheterization lab or imaging department, a radiographer is part of the team and may assist the cardiologist with patient care procedures and with the technical aspects of fluoroscopic imaging. Pacemakers are also inserted in the operating room and in the ICU or CCU. The C-arm fluoroscope is used when the procedure is performed outside the imaging department.

A chest radiograph is commonly requested after a pacemaker and its leads are placed. An adequately penetrated image should reveal the tip of the catheter in the apex of the right ventricle (Figure 20-22). The radiographer should carefully position the patient for the chest radiograph and avoid abducting or elevating the patient's left arm. This restriction is placed on the patient for 24 hours after surgery to prevent dislodging the pacemaker and catheter.

▌ SUMMARY

- It is more advantageous to do bedside radiography for patients in special care units, orthopedic traction, and isolation because these patients are in a critical condition and need continuous monitoring and care. They may be immobile because of fractures and traction, have infectious diseases that could be transmitted to others, or be immunocompromised and need protective precautions.
- Special care units include intensive care, coronary care, neonatal intensive care, postanesthesia care, and trauma units in the emergency department.

- To be successful at bedside radiography, you must have technical knowledge and skill. Additionally, you must be able to clearly communicate with both the nurse in charge and the patient and be able to assess and adapt to the patient as needed. You must also note the location of the patient's lines, tubes, drainage receptacles, monitoring and support equipment before you set up your x-ray equipment and place the IR. Bedside radiography requires close attention to detail and a high level of performance.

- A tracheotomy is a surgical procedure creating an opening into the trachea to provide a temporary or permanent artificial airway. This opening, through which a tube may be placed, is called a *tracheostomy*. Tracheostomy patients require frequent suctioning and close monitoring and will usually be accompanied by a nurse when brought to the imaging department.
- Patients requiring mechanical assistance with respiration will have either an endotracheal tube or a tracheostomy connected to a ventilator. When doing an x-ray examination, ventilators should never be turned off to eliminate respiratory motion, and care must be used to prevent applying tension to the tubing or disconnecting the endotracheal or tracheostomy tube from the ventilator.
- Nasogastric tubes are passed into the stomach and are used for feeding, the removal of gas and secretions using suction, and for the radiographic examination of the stomach. Dobbhoff, Levin, and Salem–Sump are the names of common nasogastric tubes. Nasoenteric tubes are passed into the stomach, and peristalsis advances them into the small intestine. They are used for decompression, feeding, and the radiographic examination of the small intestine. Cantor, Harris, and Miller–Abbott are the names of some common nasoenteric tubes.
- Closed chest drainage consists of a tube placed in the pleural cavity and connected to a suction device through a drainage receptacle. Tubes are placed in different locations to remove air or fluid. Caution must be exercised during radiography to see that the suction and drainage apparatus is not disturbed at either end,

the chest tube is not dislodged, and the drainage unit always remains below the level of the patient's chest.
- The Swan–Ganz catheter and various central venous catheters are specialty catheters that provide access to the circulatory system on a repetitive basis. The Swan–Ganz catheter is correctly placed when its tip lies in the right or left pulmonary artery. Inflation of the balloon at the tip of the catheter floats the catheter momentarily into a wedged position in a pulmonary artery branch to obtain indirect pressure readings of the left side of the heart. This catheter also measures cardiac output, both pulmonary and right heart pressures, and has other functions as well. Central venous catheters are advanced into the vena cava and facilitate the administration of long-term drug therapy, total parenteral nutrition, dialysis, blood transfusions, the drawing of blood, and central venous pressure monitoring. These catheters may be inserted for short- or long-term use and are tunneled, nontunneled, or designed to attach to implantable infusion ports. Imaging is often requested to check their position or assist in their placement.
- The pacemaker system consists of a battery-powered energy source and a wire or catheter delivering electrical stimulation to the heart to regulate its rate. Pacemakers may be temporary or permanent, and are inserted in surgery, ICU, CCU, cardiac catheterization lab, or the imaging department. Fluoroscopic guidance or a chest x-ray taken following insertion confirms correct placement. You should not elevate or abduct the patient's left arm for 24 hours after surgery to prevent dislodging the pacemaker and catheter.

REVIEW QUESTIONS

1. Which precaution must be followed when obtaining a bedside chest x-ray on a patient who has recently had a pacemaker implanted?
   A. Do not abduct the left arm.
   B. Do not abduct the right arm.
   C. Do not allow the patient to sit upright.
   D. Do not allow the patient to lie flat.
2. Which of the following actions is/are essential before performing a bedside radiographical examination?
   A. Check with the nurse in charge to inquire about the patient's condition.
   B. Confirm the order in the patient's chart.
   C. Greet the patient, check the armband, and prepare the room.
   D. All of the above

3. Nasogastric tubes are placed in patients for the purpose of:
   A. feeding
   B. decompression of gas and fluids
   C. imaging
   D. all of the above
4. An example of a nasogastric tube used to feed the patient is a _____ tube.
   A. Dobbhoff
   B. Miller–Abbott
   C. Harris
   D. Cantor

5. The tip of a PICC or any central venous catheter should be visualized in the:
   A. pulmonary artery
   B. right atrium
   C. right ventricle
   D. vena cava

6. When a Swan–Ganz catheter is in a wedged capillary position, it lies in:
   A. the right or left pulmonary artery
   B. the right ventricle
   C. a branch of the pulmonary artery (lung)
   D. the left atrium

7. Which of the following is NOT a central venous catheter?
   A. Hickman
   B. Groshong
   C. Swan–Ganz
   D. PICC

8. Bedside radiography may be advantageous for patients in:
   A. special care units
   B. isolation
   C. orthopedic traction
   D. all of the above

9. An implanted device that electrically stimulates the heart to control its rate is called a:
   A. pacemaker
   B. Salem–Sump
   C. central venous catheter
   D. mechanical ventilator

10. A surgical opening into the trachea that provides a temporary or permanent artificial airway is called a:
    A. tracheotomy
    B. tracheostomy
    C. pacemaker
    D. ventilator

Answers can be found in the Answer Key on pages 429-431.

CRITICAL THINKING EXERCISES

1. You have arrived in the ICU to obtain a chest radiograph on Mrs. Squire. On assessing her, you notice that she has a tracheostomy and that a chest tube exiting her left thorax is connected to a suction device below the bed. List the steps you would follow in preparation for taking the radiograph to ensure an optimum image while providing proper care to the patient. List the precautions you would take while obtaining her chest radiograph.

2. Observe an experienced radiographer performing bedside radiography and record the special skills required when obtaining radiographs at a bedside compared with those required in the radiology department.

3. A bedside chest radiograph is ordered for a neonate with pediatric respiratory distress syndrome. Describe the steps you would follow to obtain a diagnostic image while minimizing the risk of infection and hypothermia.

4. While placing the IR for a chest radiograph of Mr. Enriques in the ICU, an alarm begins to sound. Mr. Enriques is still in the same semicomatose state as he was when you entered the room and does not appear distressed. You cannot identify any tubes, lines, or cables that have become disconnected. What should you do?

21

Radiography in Surgery

OBJECTIVES

At the conclusion of this chapter, the student will be able to:

- Define the term *sterile corridor* and explain the significance of this concept to the radiographer.
- List the correct attire for a radiographer preparing for imaging in the operating room.
- Describe the steps to prevent contamination from imaging equipment brought into the operating room from an outside area.
- Correctly identify the furnishings and equipment commonly found in an operating room.

- List the typical members of a surgical team and identify which members must scrub and wear sterile attire.
- Describe the general procedures involved in laparoscopic cholecystectomy and surgical cholangiography and the radiographer's role in this procedure.
- List the ways in which imaging localization is used in surgery.
- List three urologic procedures that involve imaging in the surgical suite.

OUTLINE

Surgical Suite
 Surgical Access and Clothing
 Surgical Environment
 Surgical Team
 Surgical Setup
Surgical Procedures Involving Radiography or Fluoroscopy

 Cholecystectomy
 Open Fracture Reduction
 Surgical Localization
 Urologic Procedures

KEY TERMS

laparoscope
lithotripsy

patent, patency
sterile corridor

trocar

The radiographer has a critical role in the operating room. There are many surgical procedures that require imaging before, during, and/or at the completion of surgical procedures. The radiographer must be skilled at setting up and operating the equipment and obtaining the images with accuracy and efficiency. For this reason, an inexperienced radiographer is not sent to the surgical suite alone. An experienced radiographer as a guide is essential to provide proper orientation.

SURGICAL SUITE

Surgical Access and Clothing

To maintain asepsis, all traffic in the surgical suite is limited to personnel and items with a legitimate reason for being there. In addition, special surgical attire must be worn. Just inside the limited access area is a dressing room where personnel can change into surgical attire (Figure 21-1), often called "scrub clothes." Beyond this

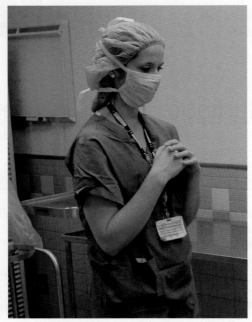

FIG 21-1 Radiographer in scrub clothes for duty in surgery.

point, access is only allowed in clean scrub clothes. Scrub clothes include nonsterile shirt and pants, a mask to cover your nose and mouth, a hat or hood to cover all hair (including a beard if applicable), and shoe covers, which may be optional. Shoe covers will keep your shoes from becoming soiled and may lower the transfer of microorganisms into the operating room. Socks must be worn and shoes with closed heels and toes to protect your feet around moving equipment and from heavy objects that may be accidentally dropped. Gloves are donned to handle anything contaminated with the patient's blood.

Today, many uniforms are very similar to scrub clothes, and it may not be apparent whether someone entering the operating room is in fact wearing clean scrub clothes. For this reason, you may be required to cover your clothes with a disposable gown, even if you are wearing clean scrub clothes. In the past, it was considered good practice to wear a "cover gown" over scrub clothes when leaving the surgical suite temporarily (for example, to consult with the radiologist) or to change into fresh scrub clothes when returning from other hospital areas. Infection control studies reveal that this practice is not necessary for team members, such as radiographers, who do not work in the sterile field. If

you must go outside the surgical suite in scrub clothes, follow the established policy at your institution.

> You are responsible for knowing the proper attire and procedures for your surgical setting and for following them without exception.

Before bringing x-ray equipment into the surgical suite, you must wipe it down with a germicidal solution and place a cover over the portion that will overhang the surgical site. In some hospitals, a mobile x-ray machine is maintained for surgical use only. Some surgical suites also have permanent radiographic installations. While these measures help reduce contamination, the radiographer is still responsible for the cleanliness of the equipment.

Surgical Environment

The average size of a multipurpose operating room (OR) is 400 to 600 square feet (Figure 21-2). Specialty ORs, such as those equipped for trauma or cardiac bypass surgery, may require at least 700 square feet to accommodate advanced minimally invasive technology and larger surgical teams. Because corridors may have higher microbial counts, the doors to the operating room should always remain closed, and the number of times the door is opened should be minimized. Positive air pressure in each of the rooms minimizes air circulation from outside the room. Filtration systems, air exchanges, and circulation provide fresh air, prevent accumulation of anesthesia gases, and reduce airborne contamination in the operating rooms. Ceiling lights provide general illumination, and the overhead operating light provides high-intensity illumination over the operative site. Some rooms have permanent radiographic and fluoroscopic equipment, and PACS monitors suspended from the ceiling or mounted on mobile carts.

There are several varieties of surgical tables, depending on the type of procedure. Examples include spinal, cystourology, and orthopedic designs. Most are height adjustable and tilt for patient positioning. Some contain a tunnel for placing an image receptor beneath the patient. You will find a wide array of monitoring, surgical, and anesthesia equipment arranged around the room. There will also be strategically placed instrument tables, ring stands with basins, buckets, trash containers, and laundry bags (Figure 21-3).

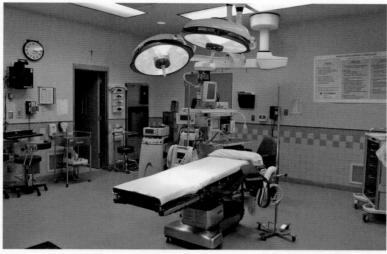

FIG 21-2 A typical operating room. The patient table is in the center. Note the overhead surgical lamps and the anesthesiologist's station beyond the head of the table.

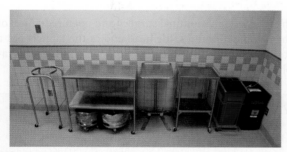

FIG 21-3 Typical operating room equipment, from left to right: a ring stand for basin to hold water, instrument table, Mayo stand, and instrument cart. For waste disposal, two containers are on the right, and two, wheeled "kick buckets" for waste are under the instrument table.

The surgical suite may seem to have a mysterious quality because there is usually a great deal of activity with very little noise. Sudden noises or loud conversations are distracting to the surgical team and may make it difficult for the anesthesiologist to hear heart sounds. Remember that the surgical patient is always at some degree of risk. Prolonged anesthesia increases the risk of surgical complications. This places pressure on the surgical team to work quickly.

Surgical Team

The surgical team is subdivided according to function and consists of both sterile and nonsterile members. The sterile members perform a surgical scrub, don sterile attire, and work within the sterile field. This group may include the following:

- Surgeon
- Assistant to the surgeon (physician)
- Assistant to the physician (PA)
- Scrub person (registered nurse, licensed vocational nurse, or surgical technologist)

The nonsterile members perform their tasks outside the sterile field. This group may include the following:

- Anesthesiologist or anesthetist
- Circulating nurse or surgical technologist
- Various other representatives and/or technologists (biomedical, orthopedic, and radiologic)

The surgical team generally works best in a low-key environment and strives to maintain this type of atmosphere. The tension level may escalate, however, when things are not going well or when errors cause delays. You know how difficult it is to wait patiently when you are tense and anxious. The surgeon and surgical staff may have this state of mind as they wait for you to set up equipment and produce the images. Their work is "on hold," because they cannot proceed without the information your images provide. When the stress levels are high, they may urge you to hurry or have an impatient attitude or tone of voice. At these times, remain focused on your work and do not respond to sharp comments with a similar attitude.

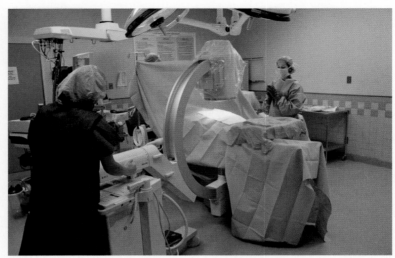

FIG 21-4 Radiographer carefully moves a C-arm mobile fluoroscope into position in operating room. Note wrapping of image intensifier to prevent contamination of sterile field by dust from equipment.

> Your ability to proceed confidently and speak calmly will help insulate you from stress in the operating room, allowing you to complete your work quickly and accurately.

Surgical Setup

When mobile equipment is used, it is usually kept at the ready inside the surgical suite. For some procedures, however, the equipment may be positioned in advance and the tube head covered with sterile drapes during the setup (Figure 21-4). You must be familiar with the institution's policies and the surgeon's preferences.

When working in the OR, be aware of sterile fields and use caution not to contaminate them with your clothing or the equipment. Do not wear dangling jewelry or other loose items around your neck or wrists. Do not fill your shirt pockets with items that could fall out as you work around the surgical table. Also, watch the cables as you manipulate the equipment. If you need to walk near the surgeon or other surgical personnel dressed in sterile attire, pass behind them rather than in front of them to prevent accidental contamination of their gowns or gloves.

The area between the drape over the patient and the instrument table is maintained as a "sterile corridor" and is the province of those wearing sterile gowns and gloves. The radiographer is excluded from this part of the room. For abdominal surgery and open reduction of the lower extremities, the head end of the table is not a sterile field. This is a safe area from which the radiographer may assess the situation.

> Nonscrubbed persons in the operating room, including radiographers, must not pass in front of scrubbed persons or enter the sterile corridor. Be aware of the location of the sterile field so that you do not accidentally contaminate the area.

Image receptors (IRs) are sometimes positioned via a tunnel in the operating table that can be reached from the nonsterile area. Otherwise, they are placed in a sterile cover with the assistance of the scrub nurse or surgeon and positioned by the surgeon. The technique for IR transfer to a sterile cover is the same as that used for protective precautions (see Chapter 9).

SURGICAL PROCEDURES INVOLVING RADIOGRAPHY OR FLUOROSCOPY

Cholecystectomy

One study performed by the radiographer in the surgical suite is the surgical cholangiogram, an adjunct to cholecystectomy. The basis for this radiographic examination is explained in Chapter 19 as part of the discussion on T-tube cholangiography.

The cholecystectomy is a laparoscopic procedure in which three or four small incisions are made in the upper right quadrant between the levels of the xiphoid process and the umbilicus. Trocars (long metal tubes) and a rigid fiberoptic laparoscope (a device for viewing inside the abdominal cavity) are inserted through these incisions. The peritoneal cavity is insufflated with carbon dioxide through one of the trocars to increase its size. The other trocars are used for passing instruments and equipment into the peritoneal cavity to grasp and remove the gallbladder. The scope is connected to a camera that projects the operative site onto a monitor located at the head of the surgical table. This allows the surgeon to observe and manipulate the instruments during the procedure. Following removal of the gallbladder, the C-arm fluoroscope is used to record images of the biliary ducts to verify that they are patent, that is, their passageways are open to the flow of bile (Figure 21-5). A T-tube is not needed for a laparoscopic surgical cholangiogram because contrast can be injected via the laparoscope.

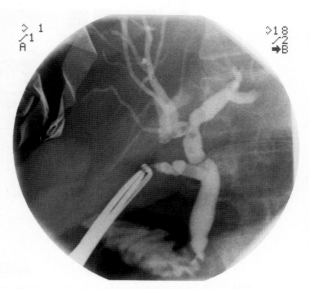

FIG 21-5 Operative cholangiogram. (From Frank ED, Long BW, Smith BJ: *Merrill's atlas of radiographic positions and radiologic procedures*, ed 12, St Louis, 2011, Mosby.)

> A surgical cholangiogram enables the surgeon to identify any remaining gallstones in the biliary ducts and to determine the patency of the ducts before closing the surgical incision.

Open Fracture Reduction

Another common surgical application of radiography is the open reduction of fractures. Plaster or fiberglass casts are used to hold many fractures in position while healing occurs. Some fractures, however, require surgical intervention to align the bone fragments. Internal or external fixation by means of rods, nails, plates, or screws maintains the alignment securely. This method is used to stabilize hip fractures and may also be used for many other types of fracture. Reconstructive orthopedic surgery to correct crippling from developmental defects, previous injuries, or degenerative diseases may also require imaging. A radiographer may be present during these procedures, using the C-arm unit to provide fluoroscopic guidance for aligning bone fragments and placing hardware. A radiographic record is made of the final position of the bones and fixation devices.

Surgical Localization

Localization is the reason for several types of surgical radiography. Radiographs or fluoroscopic visualization may help determine the exact location of foreign bodies, such as bullets, sewing needles, or industrial steel fragments, during their surgical removal.

A spinal needle can be positioned in an intervertebral disk space and radiographed to establish the accuracy of the spinal level before proceeding with the surgical intervention. The C-arm fluoroscope or one of the newer surgical navigation and imaging systems can enable surgeons to visualize the anatomy of the patient's spine during surgery. Some navigation systems permit precise tracking of surgical instruments in relation to the patient's anatomy in three dimensions. These technologies allow surgeons to work more precisely and perform less invasive procedures while reducing radiation exposure to themselves and the staff.

A radiograph can be used to locate a surgical sponge or instrument within the abdominal cavity if the surgical count indicates that an item is missing before the final closure of the incision. C-arm fluoroscopy may guide the surgical positioning of internal pacemakers or catheters. Sonography is used in surgery to precisely

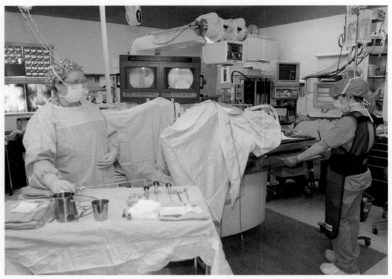

FIG 21-6 Urologic surgical room during procedure. Scrub nurse is standing in the sterile corridor between the patient and the instrument table while radiographer places image receptor in table. (From Frank ED, Long BW, Smith BJ: *Merrill's atlas of radiographic positions and radiologic procedures,* ed 12, St Louis, 2011, Mosby.)

localize tumors in the brain, spine, thyroid, parathyroid, liver, and other organs, enabling the surgeon to obtain an accurate biopsy.

Urologic Procedures

Retrograde urograms (see Chapter 19), ureteral stent placements, stone extractions, and lithotripsy (stone fragmentation by laser, ultrasound, or some other energy) are urologic procedures requiring radiography in the operating room. Newer cystourology rooms (Figure 21-6) are installed with permanent fluoroscopic and radiographic equipment. Preliminary and/or postcontrast images of the kidneys, ureters, and bladder can be obtained.

SUMMARY

- Many surgical procedures require imaging. Before entering the surgical suite, you must don clean scrub clothes, to include nonsterile shirt and pants, a mask, and hat or hood to cover all your hair. Shoe covers are usually optional. If the mobile x-ray equipment is not dedicated for surgical use, you must also wipe the machine with a germicidal solution before bringing it into the surgical suite.

- The size of the operating room ranges from 400 to 750 square feet. Filtration systems, air exchanges, and circulation provide fresh air, prevent airborne contamination, and minimize the accumulation of anesthesia gases. Some rooms have permanent radiographic and fluoroscopic equipment and monitors to view the images. The surgical tables vary in design

according to the type of procedure. Most are height adjustable and tilt; some contain a tunnel for placement of an IR. The rooms contain instrument tables, buckets, ring stands with basins, and monitoring, surgical, and anesthesia equipment.

- The OR team consists of both sterile and nonsterile members. The sterile members perform a surgical scrub, don sterile attire, and work within the sterile field. The nonsterile members work outside the sterile field and include the anesthesiologist or anesthetist, the circulating nurse, the radiographer, and other technologists.

- Depending on the surgical procedure, x-ray equipment may be set up before the procedure or brought in after the procedure begins. You must use care in setting up your equipment to avoid contaminating the sterile field. Radiographers must also avoid entering the sterile corridor, the area between the draped patient and the instrument table.

- A variety of surgical procedures requires radiography. A cholecystectomy may require imaging to ensure the biliary ducts are free of stones. C-arm fluoroscopic guidance is needed for open reduction of fractures, internal fixation of fractures, and reconstructive orthopedic surgery. Localization of foreign bodies, misplaced surgical sponges and instruments, or a spinal needle used to verify the level of an intervertebral disk space are other reasons for surgical radiography. Retrograde urograms, ureteral stent placement, and stone extractions are urologic procedures requiring radiography in the operating room.

REVIEW QUESTIONS

1. Which of the following individuals is not one of the sterile members of the surgical team?
   A. Scrub nurse
   B. Circulating nurse
   C. Surgeon
   D. Assistant to the surgeon
2. Before entering the surgical suite, the radiographer must don the required surgical attire that includes:
   A. nonsterile shirt and nonsterile pants, a mask, and cap or hood.
   B. sterile shirt and pants, a mask, and cap or hood.
   C. nonsterile shirt and shoe covers only.
   D. sterile gown and cap or hood.
3. Which of the following members of the surgical team is most likely to assist you with placing the IR in the table's image receptor opening or slot?
   A. Anesthesiologist
   B. Circulating nurse
   C. Surgeon
   D. Another radiologic technologist
4. A surgical cholangiogram is performed to demonstrate:
   A. the gallbladder.
   B. the common bile duct.
   C. the pancreatic duct.
   D. the ductus arteriosus.

5. When performing a laparoscopic surgical procedure, the peritoneal cavity is insufflated with:
   A. room air.
   B. oxygen.
   C. nitrogen.
   D. carbon dioxide.
6. Imaging may be required in surgery to localize:
   A. a foreign body.
   B. an instrument or sponge that is missing when these items are counted.
   C. the disc space where a spinal procedure will be located.
   D. any of the above.
7. The sterile corridor in the operating room is the area between the patient and:
   A. surgeon.
   B. instrument tray.
   C. anesthesiologist.
   D. x-ray machine or C-arm fluoroscope.
8. A rigid fiberoptic device for viewing inside the abdominal cavity is called a:
   A. gastroscope.
   B. colonoscope.
   C. laparoscope.
   D. bronchoscope.

Answers can be found in the Answer Key on pages 429-431.

CRITICAL THINKING EXERCISES

1. You are sent to the surgical suite and asked to set up the C-arm fluoroscope for a laparoscopic cholecystectomy. The surgeon needs to check for possible residual stones in the biliary ducts. List the precautions you would take in preparing, setting up, and aligning your equipment.

2. You have been sent to the surgical suite alone for the first time, expecting a routine open reduction of the leg, a procedure with which you are familiar. When you arrive, you discover that the approach and procedure are very different from what you expected, and you are not sure how to proceed. What should you do?

22

Special Imaging Modalities

OBJECTIVES

At the conclusion of this chapter, the student will be able to:

- List specific angiographic examinations and name the blood vessels that are demonstrated with each.
- Describe Seldinger technique and state its purpose.
- List five specific procedures classed as interventional radiology and state the purpose of each.
- Identify and state the purpose of each of the principal parts of a computed tomography (CT) scanner.
- List advantages of spiral and multislice spiral/helical scanners in comparison with conventional CT scanners.
- Discuss the use of oral and intravenous (IV) contrast media in CT and list precautions to take to avoid extravasation of IV contrast agents.
- List common diagnostic applications of magnetic resonance imaging (MRI).
- List safety precautions for personnel working in the area of an MRI scanner.

- Explain the use of contrast agents and medications in MRI and the procedures for monitoring sedated patients during MRI examinations.
- Compare and contrast conventional nuclear medicine procedures, positron emission tomography (PET), single photon emission computed tomography (SPECT) scans, and fusion imaging.
- Compare and contrast nuclear medicine procedures with other imaging modalities.
- Describe in simple terms the process of acquiring ultrasound images and list common diagnostic applications for both conventional and Doppler ultrasound.
- Describe the procedure for routine mammography and explain the patient care considerations that are significant with this modality.

OUTLINE

OUTLINE—cont'd

KEY TERMS

amniocentesis
angiocardiogram
angiography
angioplasty
aortogram
arteriogram
atherectomy
atheroma
atherosclerosis
computed tomography (CT)
echocardiography
endovenous laser therapy (EVLT)

fusion imaging
gantry
half-life
magnetic resonance imaging (MRI)
mammography
nuclear medicine
percutaneous
positron emission tomography (PET)
radiofrequency ablation (RFA)
radionuclide

sestamibi
single photon emission computed tomography (SPECT)
stenosis
stent
thrombus (*pl.* thrombi)
transcatheter embolization
transducer
venogram

The imaging techniques in this chapter are not used in every health care institution. They are performed by technologists with advanced training who may also have advanced level certification. These topics provide beginner radiographers with an introduction to the nature and purpose of these imaging modalities. The applicable safety procedures and patient care issues are highlighted. As a student, you should know about these procedures and be able to provide preliminary explanations when patients inquire about them. You should also be prepared to assist with the more routine aspects of patient care if you have scheduled rotations into these specialty areas.

Technological advancements in computers, electronic engineering, and diagnostic pharmaceuticals are producing rapid changes in all of the imaging modalities discussed in this chapter. A scanner that combines positron emission tomography (PET) with computed tomography (CT) combines the speed and flexibility of x-ray CT with data on physiologic functions from nuclear medicine techniques. Gamma cameras with huge overhead gantries are being replaced with hand-held models for some specific applications, such as breast imaging and sentinel node localization. Computer-aided detection (CAD) is enhancing the value of screening mammography, as is the use of CT laser mammography (CTLM). Tiny ultrasound transducers affixed to endoscopes are used to produce sonograms from inside the digestive tract. New contrast media, techniques, and equipment are expanding the diagnostic scope of ultrasound imaging, and new radionuclides are expanding possibilities in PET scanning. Three-dimensional images from various modalities are increasing the speed and accuracy of surgical procedures, while angiographic and endoscopic procedures that were once exclusively diagnostic are now also used for treatment, often eliminating the need for surgery. These advances in imaging provide challenges and avenues of specialization for technologists. We hope that this information will encourage you to conduct additional research and explore these areas further.

CARDIOVASCULAR AND INTERVENTIONAL RADIOGRAPHY

Angiography

Conventional Catheter Angiography

Radiographic procedures that demonstrate vessels are collectively known as angiography. A cerebral angiogram, for example, shows the vessels of the brain (Figure 22-1), while renal angiograms show the arteries and veins of the kidneys. An angiocardiogram is a contrast study visualizing the interior of the heart chambers and the great vessels that enter and exit the heart (Figure 22-2). Selective angiocardiography can be used to demonstrate the coronary arteries. An aortogram, as the name implies, is a procedure that shows the aorta. An arch aortogram shows the thoracic portion and the branches that provide circulation to the head and arms (Figure 22-3); an abdominal aortogram shows the portion between the diaphragm and the iliac bifurcation (Figure 22-4). Arteriograms are studies of specific arteries (Figure 22-5) while venograms are studies of veins (Figure 22-6).

For all of these examinations, water-soluble iodine compounds are used for radiographic contrast, and a rapid series of images is taken using highly specialized equipment. The contrast medium used for angiography is chosen according to the requirements of the specific procedure (Table 19-1). There is some diversity of technical methods among imaging departments, but it is not necessary to explore these variations here, because all angiographic procedures are quite similar from a patient care standpoint. Informed consent is required for these procedures

> Aqueous iodine compounds are injected into the circulatory system for angiographic imaging procedures.

Direct **percutaneous** (through the skin) injection may be used for some angiographic studies, such as those of the extremities, but the preferred injection method for angiocardiography, aortography, and most arteriography is to use a catheter. Angiographic catheters include a radiopaque strip for visibility under the fluoroscope and come in a variety of lengths, gauges, and tip configurations. Catheter insertion is accomplished by the Seldinger technique (Figure 22-7). A large artery, usually the femoral

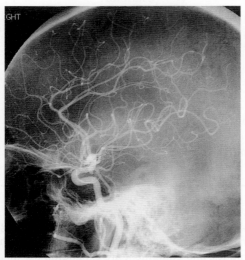

FIG 22-1 A cerebral angiogram. (From Frank ED, Long BW, Smith BJ: *Merrill's atlas of radiographic positions and radiologic procedures,* Volume 3, ed 12, St Louis, 2012, Elsevier.)

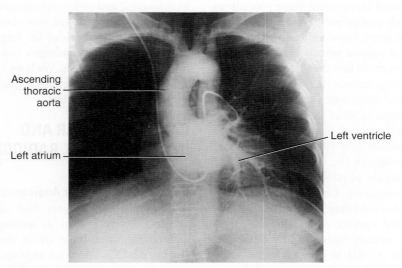

FIG 22-2 An angiocardiogram. (From Ballinger PW: *Merrill's atlas of radiographic positions and radiologic procedures,* ed 9, St Louis, 1999, Mosby.)

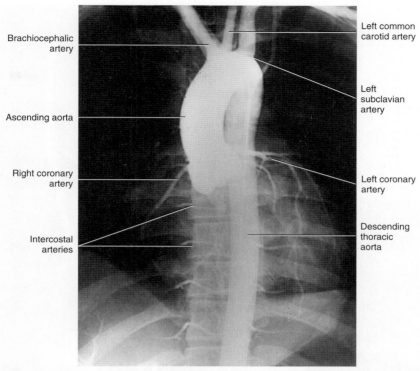

Brachiocephalic artery

Ascending aorta

Right coronary artery

Intercostal arteries

Left common carotid artery

Left subclavian artery

Left coronary artery

Descending thoracic aorta

FIG 22-3 An arch aortogram. (From Frank ED, Long BW, Smith BJ: *Merrill's atlas of radiographic positions and radiologic procedures,* Volume 3, ed 12, St Louis, 2012, Elsevier.)

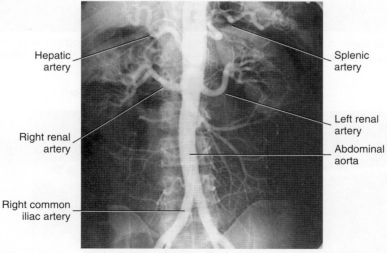

Hepatic artery

Right renal artery

Right common iliac artery

Splenic artery

Left renal artery

Abdominal aorta

FIG 22-4 Abdominal aortogram. (From Long BW, Rollins JH, Smith BJ: *Merrill's atlas of radiographic positioning & procedures,* ed 13, St Louis, 2016, Elsevier.)

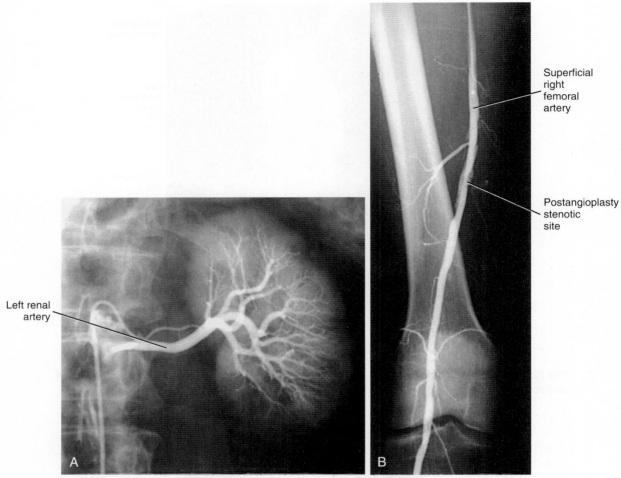

FIG 22-5 Arteriograms. **A,** Selective renal arteriogram **B,** Femoral arteriogram. (From Ballinger PW: *Merrill's atlas of radiographic positions and radiologic procedures,* ed 8, St Louis, 1999, Mosby.)

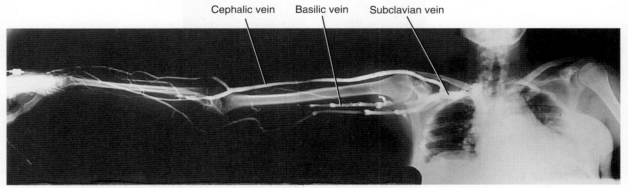

FIG 22-6 Venogram, normal upper extremity. (From Long BW, Rollins JH, Smith BJ: *Merrill's atlas of radiographic positioning & procedures,* ed 13, St Louis, 2016, Elsevier.)

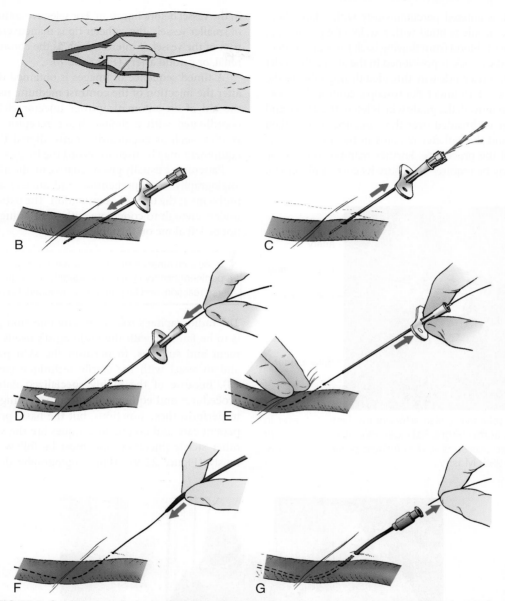

FIG 22-7 Seldinger technique. **A,** An ideal arteriotomy occurs in the femoral artery just below the inguinal ligament. **B,** A beveled compound needle containing an inner cannula pierces through the artery. **C,** The needle's solid inner cannula is removed and the needle is retracted until blood flow indicates placement of the tip within the lumen of the artery. **D,** A flexible guide wire is inserted into the artery through the needle. **E,** The needle is removed; pressure fixes the wire and reduces hemorrhage. **F,** The catheter is slipped over the wire into the artery. **G,** The guide wire is removed, leaving the catheter in the artery. (From Long BW, Rollins JH, Smith BJ: *Merrill's atlas of radiographic positioning & procedures,* ed 13, St Louis, 2016, Elsevier.)

or brachial, is entered percutaneously with a large-bore needle. The needle is fitted with a stylet of equal length, which prevents blood from flowing back through the needle. When the needle is positioned in the artery, the stylet is removed, and a guide wire threaded through the needle and into the artery under fluoroscopic control. The needle is then removed, the guide wire is left in the vessel, and the catheter is threaded over the wire. The wire is then removed, and the catheter remains in the artery for the duration of the procedure. Further manipulation of the catheter may be required to ensure its correct placement

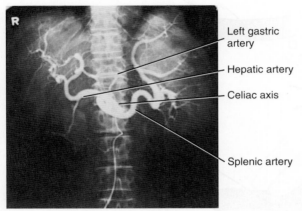

FIG 22-8 Selective celiac arteriogram. Note catheter in abdominal aorta. (From Ballinger PW: *Merrill's atlas of radiographic positions and radiologic procedures*, ed 8, St Louis, 1995, Mosby.)

in the vessel before injection. For selective catheterization of smaller vessels, the catheter tip is maneuvered into the root of the vessel of interest, such as the coronary, celiac, renal, or carotid artery (Figure 22-8).

A timed sequence of images is obtained during and after the injection of the contrast medium, usually with the aid of an automatic power injector electronically coordinated with a digital image receptor. For some studies, such as angiocardiograms, digital fluoroscopy equipment may be used to record the images.

Patients are usually given sedative medications before angiography, so apprehension and anxiety are seldom problems at the time of examination. The patient usually is alert enough to cooperate with positioning, but must not be left alone on the table.

> **!** As with other contrast media injections, you must take a pertinent history in advance, identify any signs of an adverse reaction, and be prepared to respond if one occurs.

The radiographer's role, as in any injection procedure, is to be familiar with the radiologist's needs for equipment and supplies, to perform the skin preparation, and to assist with the sterile technique (see Chapter 18). Because of the highly specialized nature of the procedures and equipment, specific training is needed to perform these functions, but the basic principles of patient care and aseptic techniques are the same as for other sterile injections and must be followed meticulously (Figure 22-9). Many angiography departments

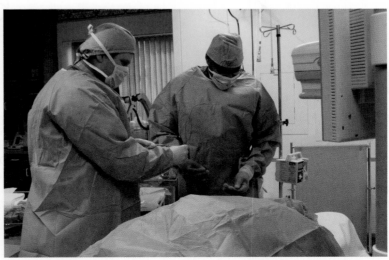

FIG 22-9 Technologist assists radiologist during angiography procedure.

are staffed with nurses or cardiovascular technicians who assist the physician and handle patient care duties. When this is the case, the technologist's duties are mainly technical.

Follow-up care is very important after angiography to avoid the possibility of hemorrhage or hematoma at the puncture site. Until quite recently, the procedure for accomplishing hemostasis following arterial puncture was to apply firm, continuous pressure to the injection site for 5 to 10 minutes, followed by the application of a pressure dressing, which was monitored by the nursing service. The patient was not permitted to walk for up to 24 hours. The pressure dressing may be a thick gauze dressing held in place by tape, or an inflatable ball may be positioned over the artery and held in place by a belt. A pressure dressing is also applied after studies involving the puncture of a large vein. Some new products called *vascular closure devices* (VCDs) make it possible to achieve hemostasis in 5 minutes or less and permit patient activity after only 1 hour. One type consists of a nickel-titanium clip implanted in the artery with a special applicator (Figure 22-10). Another type consists of an application device and sheath that facilitates vessel closure with sutures (Figure 22-11).

> **!** Following arterial puncture, be aware that the extremity where the catheter was inserted must be kept from bending for a certain period of time as specified in the protocol.

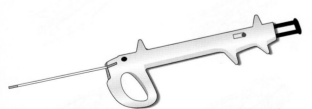

FIG 22-10 Vascular closure device. Star clip with applier, Abbott Labs.

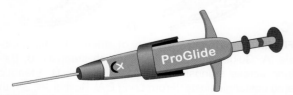

FIG 22-11 Application device and sheath to facilitate vessel closure with sutures, Abbott Labs.

Conventional angiography is not without risk. Potential complications include damage to the artery during manipulation of the guide wire or catheter, reaction to contrast media, hemorrhage or hematoma at the puncture site, and thrombosis (clotting) within the vessel following the procedure. Because of these risks, as well as the differential in cost, angiography has been supplanted to some degree by technological advances in Doppler ultrasound, nuclear medicine, magnetic resonance angiography (MRA), and CT angiography (CTA). Despite these advances, angiography continues to be used because it provides the best anatomic demonstration of structures within the circulatory system and also offers the opportunity for immediate therapeutic interventions to treat any problems identified (see section on interventional radiology later in this chapter).

Digital Subtraction Angiography

Computerized imaging equipment is used in imaging centers to perform digital subtraction angiography (DSA). Angiographic images are recorded in digital format on a computer. The images can then be manipulated to enhance contrast and decrease visibility of the superimposing structures. The resulting images are managed by a picture archiving and communication system (PACS) as with other digital images. In the subtraction process, two radiographic or fluoroscopic runs in the same projection are used: one with contrast and one without. The computer then eliminates structures from the contrast image that are common to both images, leaving only the image of the contrast-enhanced vessels (Figure 22-12).

DSA can be performed using either conventional arterial catheterization or intravenous (IV) contrast injection. IV contrast administration is less invasive than arterial catheterization and is therefore less hazardous. It is relatively painless and can safely be used in patients at high risk for arterial catheterization. IV contrast is used less often, however, because of the relatively poor anatomic detail obtained compared with arterial injections.

Interventional Radiology

While the use of angiography for diagnosis has decreased somewhat with the increasing use of other modalities, the use of angiographic techniques for interventional radiology is expanding. Interventional radiology refers to the nonsurgical treatment or correction of a vascular problem, often at the time it is diagnosed and/or located radiographically. When the nature and precise location of a vascular constriction or bleed have been established using angiography, and a specialized catheter is in place within the vessel, the catheter can be utilized to provide treatment. Most interventional radiology is performed in the angiography suite by the angiography team, usually in conjunction with a diagnostic angiographic procedure.

Percutaneous Transluminal Angioplasty

Percutaneous transluminal angioplasty (PTA) is an interventional technique commonly associated with arteriography. The term angioplasty means "vessel repair." PTA is used extensively as a treatment for atherosclerosis, narrowing or blockage of an artery caused by the buildup of fatty plaque. Arteries may also become constricted because of calcium deposits and/or thrombi (blood clots; singular, thrombus). When arterial stenosis (narrowing) is localized on an arteriogram or with another imaging modality, a variety of nonsurgical techniques can be utilized to open the constricted area and increase blood flow.

Balloon angioplasty is a technique commonly employed to treat atherosclerosis. A balloon-tipped catheter with a double lumen is used. The balloon is inflated with a dilute contrast medium, and the pressure from the expanding balloon extends the artery wall, enlarging the lumen of the artery (Figure 22-13). Patient care is comparable to that described for arteriography in the preceding section. Similar techniques can be used to dilate veins, ureters, bile ducts, and portions of the gastrointestinal tract.

Percutaneous **atherectomy** is a PTA method in which the blocking plaque material is cut away. The term atherectomy refers to the removal of an **atheroma** (plaque deposit). Several types of specialized catheters have been developed for this purpose, but the one most commonly used is fitted with an abrasive burr- or cone-shaped rotational head that functions with a liquid spray to pulverize the atheromatous material. Balloon angioplasty is sometimes used in combination with percutaneous atherectomy to provide a wider and smoother lumen in the vessel.

PTA procedures may also involve placement via catheter of a vascular **stent**. A stent device is a flexible plastic or wire mesh tube that is permanently situated within a vessel or other tubular structure to keep it open (Figure 22-14). Stent placement may be used to treat blocked arteries in the heart, kidneys, legs, or groin.

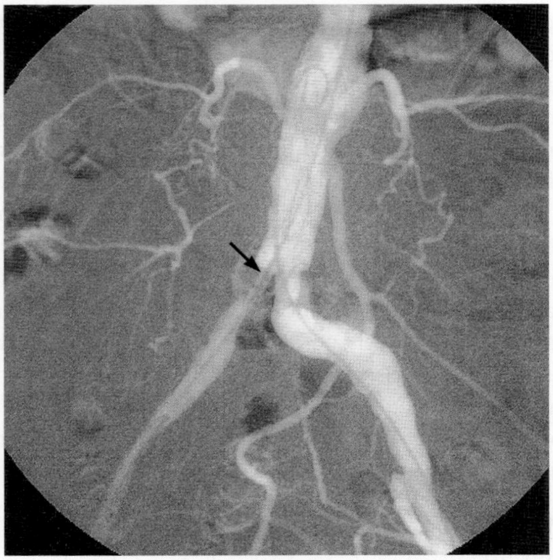

FIG 22-12 Digital subtracted image of high-grade stenosis of right common iliac artery (*arrow*). (From Frank ED, Long BW, Smith BJ: *Merrill's atlas of radiographic positioning and procedures,* Volume 3, ed 12, St. Louis, 2012, Elsevier.)

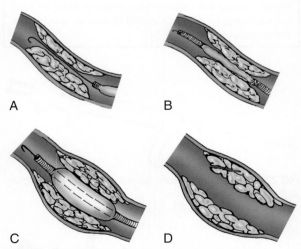

FIG 22-13 Balloon angioplasty of atherosclerotic stenosis. **A,** Guide wire advanced through stenosis. **B,** Balloon across stenosis. **C,** Balloon inflated. **D,** Stenotic area postangioplasty. (From Long BW, Rollins JH, Smith BJ: *Merrill's atlas of radiographic positioning & procedures,* ed 13, St Louis, 2016, Elsevier.)

Special stents called *drug-eluting stents* (DES) have been widely acclaimed as a treatment for coronary artery narrowing. Before the use of DES, artery walls grew at an accelerated rate around the newly implanted stents, forming an excess of normal tissue that caused the artery to narrow again. This process is called intimal hyperplasia. The DES slowly releases a special medication (sirolimus or paclitaxel) over the first month it is in place. This medication prevents the overgrowth of cells in the opened area as it heals. There is controversy over the long-term efficacy of DES compared with bare metal stents. Studies indicate that DES placement is a very safe therapy, but there is not any significant difference in the long-term survival rates or the rates of myocardial infarction between groups receiving the two types of stents.

Transcatheter Embolization

Unlike PTA, the purpose of which is to increase blood flow in a vessel, transcatheter embolization is an interventional technique used to decrease or stop blood flow. There are three principal reasons for performing transcatheter embolization:

1. To stop hemorrhage at an active bleeding site, for example, a bleeding ulcer;
2. To cut off the flow of blood to diseased or malformed areas such as tumors or arteriovenous malformations (AVMs);
3. To reduce blood flow to a specific area to minimize blood loss during surgery.

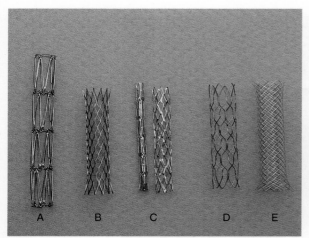

FIG 22-14 Examples of intravascular stents. (From Long BW, Rollins JH, Smith BJ: *Merrill's atlas of radiographic positioning & procedures,* ed 13, St Louis, 2016, Elsevier.)

A variety of liquid, gel, and solid materials can be used to accomplish embolization, and the choice depends on the site and the duration of embolization desired. For example, polyvinyl alcohol (Ivalon), silicone beads, or stainless steel coils can be used to provide permanent vessel occlusion, whereas a special product called *Gelfoam* or a *vasoconstricting drug* such as vasopressin (Pitressin) provides temporary vessel closure. A catheter is placed using the Seldinger technique, and angiography may be used to diagnose hemorrhage, locate the exact site for embolization, and/or confirm the success of the procedure.

Sclerotic Therapy and Radiofrequency Ablation

In the past, venous problems such as occlusion, stenosis, varicosity, and inflammation were treated surgically. The veins were either ligated (tied off) or stripped (removed surgically). Nonsurgical therapies such as chemical injection and interventional radiology now offer minimally invasive treatment options for these types of problems.

Sclerotic therapy involves injections that cause thickening and occlusion of the vein, and it is useful for treating "spider veins" and other small veins of the lower legs. Larger veins, such as the greater saphenous and the accessory saphenous vein systems, can now be treated with two different methods: **radiofrequency ablation (RFA)** and **endovenous laser therapy (EVLT)**. These are minimally invasive technologies, and research indicates that the results are similar for both procedures.

RFA was originally utilized for the treatment of tumors. When using RFA to treat veins, a special device is used consisting of a tiny RF generator associated with a sterile catheter and a collapsible electrode. For EVLT, the procedure is similar except that this method uses energy from an 810 nm diode laser delivered through a fine fiberoptic probe. In both cases, the length of the vein is anesthetized with local injections of lidocaine, and the catheter is positioned in the vein over a guide wire using the Seldinger technique under fluoroscopic control. The treatment is continuously monitored by color Doppler ultrasound to confirm reduction of blood flow in the vein.

Patient care procedures include preparation for injection of lidocaine over the length of the vein to be treated, maintaining hemostasis at the puncture site following the procedure, and providing patient instruction for follow-up care. Care following endovenous treatment of the larger veins may include wearing compression stockings, following a prescribed walking regimen, and avoiding standing for prolonged periods. The patient is usually seen again within 72 hours, after which normal activity is resumed.

COMPUTED TOMOGRAPHY

Computed tomography (CT) is the same modality which was formerly called *computer-assisted tomography* (CAT) scanning. CT produces axial images, slicelike sections in the transverse plane that can be "reconstructed" by the computer to display the anatomic structures in other planes as well. Image characteristics such as brightness and contrast can be manipulated on the computer. The images can be viewed in different formats called *windows* designed to enhance visualization of specific tissues (Figure 22-15). Institutions with PACS digital image management include CT examinations in this system.

Equipment

The CT scanner (Figure 22-16) consists of a movable table with remote control, a circular **gantry** structure

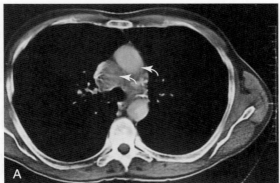
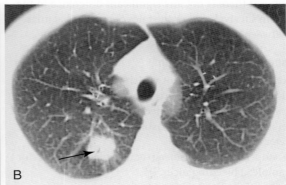

FIG 22-15 Two CT windows demonstrate different structures of the chest from the same image. **A**, Mediastinal structures are demonstrated in the center of the field, but the lungs are not well defined. **B**, "Lung window" demonstrates the blood vessels of the lungs and a lung tumor *(arrow)*. (From Seeram E: *Computed tomography: Physical principles, clinical applications, and quality control*, ed 4, St Louis, 2016, Elsevier.)

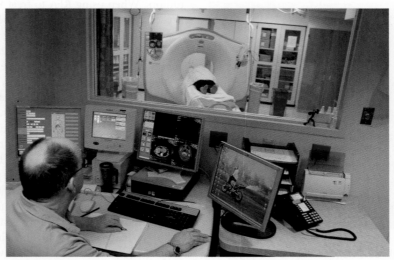

FIG 22-16 Technologist operates CT scanner and monitors patient from control console.

that supports the x-ray tube and detectors, an operator console with a monitor and supporting computer system, and hardware and software to archive and manage data and produce both electronic and hard copies of the images.

During a scan, the x-ray tube (and sometimes also the detectors) rotates around the patient to collect the data. In conventional CT units, the tube makes a complete rotation to gather data for each slice. The table then moves and the tube rotates again to obtain the next slice. A newer generation of scanner, designated as spiral or helical, scans a spiral path around the patient and can collect data on a larger volume of tissue (Figure 22-17). This system permits scanning of a relatively large area during a single breath-hold and reduces scanning time compared with conventional units. The software that supports spiral/helical CT can provide data reconstruction of volume information and render three-dimensional (3-D) images. Scanners designated as *multi-slice spiral/helical scanners* create multiple slices with each rotation of the tube, greatly speeding up the process of image acquisition.

Applications

The versatility of CT is illustrated by its wide range of applications, including studies of the brain, spine, abdomen, pelvis, chest, neck, and paranasal sinuses, plus orthopedic examinations of the extremities and contrast-enhanced vascular studies known as *computed tomography angiography*, or CTA. CT is useful in localizing the lesion and the needle position during needle

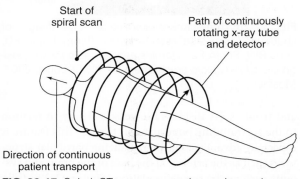

Start of spiral scan

Path of continuously rotating x-ray tube and detector

Direction of continuous patient transport

FIG 22-17 Spiral CT scanners gather volume data as x-ray source and detectors trace a spiral path around the patient. (From Seeram E: *Computed tomography: Physical principles, clinical applications, and quality control,* ed 4, St Louis, 2016, Elsevier.)

aspiration biopsy, a nonsurgical method of obtaining cells for laboratory examination. CT is also a valuable tool for emergency use, especially in the detection of intracerebral or intra-abdominal hemorrhage. Stroke protocols, for example, require a CT scan to rule out brain hemorrhage before initiating thrombolytic therapy. For these reasons, trauma centers usually have at least one CT scanner in the emergency department.

Most CT examinations are noninvasive and are relatively comfortable for the patient. The equipment may cause apprehension, however, and careful explanations are necessary to ensure patient cooperation and a satisfactory study.

Contrast Computed Tomography Examinations

While some CT examinations do not require enhancement with contrast media, the use of contrast agents vastly increases the scope of CT imaging. Studies of the abdomen (Figure 22-18) usually employ oral contrast to help differentiate the GI tract from the surrounding tissues. A special barium compound (such as E-Z-Cat) or an oral aqueous iodine medium (such as Gastrografin mixed with water and flavoring) is ingested by the patient over a specified time period before the study. These are positive contrast agents, in that they are of higher density than the surrounding tissues. In addition, there are negative contrast agents (of lower density) such as Volumen that can also be ingested. The amount of contrast and the time vary depending on whether the examination includes only the upper abdomen or the entire abdomen and pelvis. Outpatients are instructed to fast and arrive early to drink the contrast preparation. Some departments have outpatients take the contrast home with instructions to drink it before reporting for the appointment.

Intravenous injection of an aqueous iodinated contrast medium can also be used to increase the contrast level of the patient's tissues. This is advantageous for studies of the chest, abdomen, and larynx, because it highlights blood vessels and enhances visualization of vascular organs such as the liver and spleen. The contrast also defines the renal collecting system, ureters, and bladder as it is excreted in the urine. IV contrast agents can also be used in CT scans of the head to demonstrate brain lesions (Figure 22-19).

IV contrast is essential in CT angiography. These procedures use spiral/helical scanners to create volumetric 3D images of the arteries and veins of the head

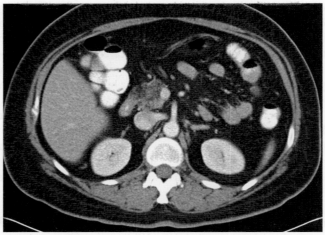

FIG 22-18 Contrast-enhanced axial CT image of the abdomen. (From Long BW, Rollins JH, Smith BJ: *Merrill's atlas of radiographic positioning & procedures,* ed 12, St Louis, 2012, Elsevier.)

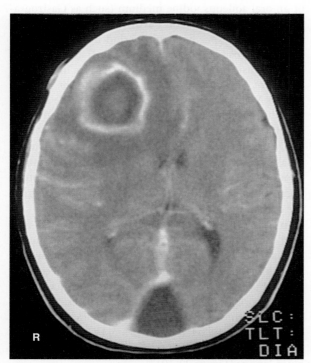

FIG 22-19 CT brain scan with IV contrast agent. (From Frank ED, Long BW, Smith BJ: *Merrill's atlas of radiographic positioning & procedures,* Volume 3, ed 12, St Louis, 2012, Elsevier.)

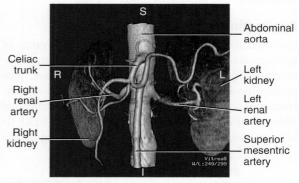

FIG 22-20 Three-dimensional color CTA image of abdominal aorta and renal arteries. (From Frank ED, Long BW, Smith BJ: *Merrill's atlas of radiographic positions and radiologic procedures,* ed 11, St Louis, 2007, Mosby.)

and trunk. CTA displays the vessels clearly in relation to the surrounding bone and soft tissues. This feature is especially advantageous for visualizing particular structures such as the arteries at the base of the brain and systems such as the renal circulation (Figure 22-20). CTA involves less risk than conventional catheter angiography, but provides less image resolution for small vessels.

IV contrast administration often consists of a bolus of the medium injected rapidly at the start of the procedure

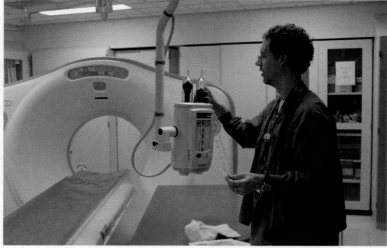

FIG 22-21 Automatic injector controls administration of contrast for CT examinations.

and a continuation of the injection at a much slower rate as the examination proceeds. The initial bolus of contrast medium can be injected with a syringe and followed by a drip infusion. The approach most often used is to connect the IV set to an automatic injector (Figure 22-21) loaded with the contrast medium and programmed to provide the desired flow rates.

The IV line is usually established with an IV catheter and then connected to the syringe, IV tubing, or injector tubing. An intermittent injection port (saline lock) or an established IV line with an injection port may be used. An 18-gauge needle or needleless connector is attached to the injector tubing or syringe and is used to penetrate the port. Once situated, the attachment is secured with tape. If other IV fluids are being administered through the IV line, the tubing must be clamped off to stop the flow during the injection and then released to restore it afterward. The IV line is flushed before and after the contrast injection to avoid mixing the contrast with medication in the tubing or injection port.

The high volume (sometimes as much as 200 mL) of contrast used and the remote location of the technologist during the scan can create significant problems in the event of extravasation of the contrast medium. The use of a powerful automatic injector compounds this hazard. The precautions in Box 22-1 will help minimize this risk.

Review Chapter 14 for additional procedures and precautions related to IV injections. It is customary to

---

BOX 22-1   CT Contrast Injection Precautions

- Select an IV site other than an antecubital vein to avoid the possibility that elbow flexion will compromise the IV line. If an antecubital vein must be used, prevent elbow flexion with an arm board.
- When using an intermittent injection port, flush before connecting the injection tubing to be sure the IV catheter is properly situated in the vein and contains no residual medication.
- Double-check the IV site for possible extravasation at the time the automatic injector is started.
- Instruct the patient to immediately report any sensation of burning, pressure, or other discomfort in the area of the IV site.
- Maintain communication with the patient during and after injection.

---

require informed consent for contrast-enhanced CT examinations.

Computed Tomography Myelography

CT imaging can greatly expand the information obtained with myelography by demonstrating the dural sac and nerve roots in the transverse plane. As soon as the routine myelogram (see Chapter 19) is completed, the patient is brought to the CT scanner for contrast-enhanced images of the spinal canal (Figure 22-22). It is important to minimize delay between the fluoroscopic

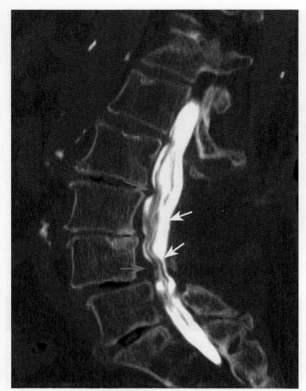

FIG 22-22 CT myelogram of the lumbar spine showing subarachnoid space narrowing *(red arrow)* and cauda equine *(white arrows)*. (From Long BW, Rollins JH, Smith BJ: *Merrill's atlas of radiographic positioning & procedures*, ed 12, St Louis, 2012, Elsevier.)

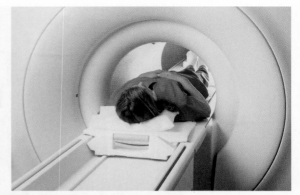

FIG 22-23 Patient inside superconducting 1.5-Tesla magnet for magnetic resonance study. (From Frank ED, Long BW, Smith BJ: *Merrill's atlas of radiographic positions and radiologic procedures*, ed 11, St Louis, 2007, Mosby.)

procedure and the CT examination, because the contrast agent is rapidly absorbed from the spinal fluid into the bloodstream and will not be sufficiently concentrated for good visualization if too much time is lost.

> When routine myelography and CT myelography are combined, it is important to minimize delay between the fluoroscopic procedure and the CT examination.

MAGNETIC RESONANCE IMAGING

Magnetic resonance imaging (MRI) is a noninvasive diagnostic modality that does not use ionizing radiation. A powerful magnetic field and radio frequency (RF) pulses are combined to produce a radio signal in the body that can be detected and processed electronically to provide images on the computer monitor. The computer image is digitized and can be managed

by a PACS. It can also be stored on magnetic tape and photographed with a special camera to produce film copies.

Equipment

MRI equipment includes a patient table, gantry, and console-monitor combination with computer support. The gantry houses the magnet. A conventional gantry is tubular, 5 to 8 feet long, and surrounds most of the patient's body during the scanning process (Figure 22-23). An open configuration in gantry design provides better accommodation for large or claustrophobic patients (Figure 22-24). The open gantry unit has a less powerful magnetic field and does not provide image quality equal to that produced by conventional units without significantly increased scanning time.

RF coils are essential components of the MRI system. They generate radio frequency pulses electronically and are the cause of the loud, hammering sound that is typical of MRI scanners. The coils transmit pulses of RF energy to the patient's body and receive the RF signal emitted by the resonating tissue. The information associated with this signal is digitized, stored in the computer, and used to form the image. Depending on the application, the same or different coils are used for transmitting the RF pulses and receiving the RF signal. The three basic types of coil are body, head, and surface coils. The body coil is a permanent part of the scanner; it completely surrounds the patient's body in conventional, tubular-gantry scanners. The body

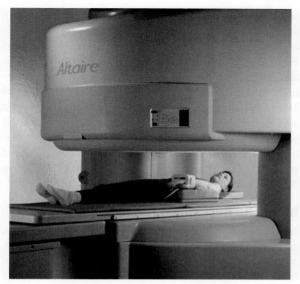

FIG 22-24 Open-gantry MRI unit.

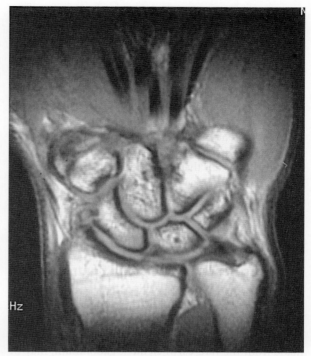

FIG 22-26 Coronal MRI scan of the wrist using a surface coil is an example of an MRI joint study. (From Frank ED, Long BW, Smith BJ: *Merrill's atlas of radiographic positions and radiologic procedures*, ed 10, St Louis, 2003, Mosby.)

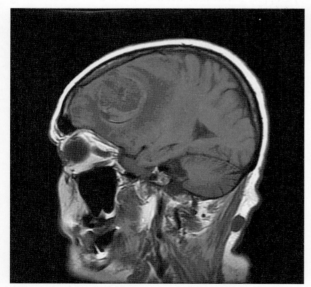

FIG 22-25 Sagittal MRI section through brain showing frontal lobe mass without contrast agent. (From Long BW, Rollins JH, Smith BJ: *Merrill's atlas of radiographic positioning & procedures*, ed 12, St Louis, 2012, Elsevier.)

coil transmits RF pulses for all scans and serves as a receiving coil for RF signals when scanning the trunk of the body. The helmet type of head coil completely surrounds the patient's head and is a receiver coil only; the body coil is used to transmit the RF pulses. Surface coils can be placed directly on or around the anatomic area of interest. They are designed with different shapes corresponding to the requirements of the different body parts. As in the case of the head coil, surface coils are receiver coils only.

Applications

MRI provides excellent imaging of the soft tissues of the nervous system (Figure 22-25) and is useful in the diagnosis of many types of pathology, including brain and spinal cord tumors and diseases such as multiple sclerosis. MRI is used extensively in place of myelography for the diagnosis of herniated intervertebral disks. This modality is also effective in imaging the soft tissue components of joints (Figure 22-26), providing an alternative to arthrography of the knee, shoulder, and temporomandibular joints. Gadolinium contrast for an arthrogram can be introduced into the joint in the radiology department under fluoroscopic control in advance of the MRI study or in conjunction with a routine radiographic arthrogram study.

MRI can also be used to examine the female breasts. Although this application may reveal occult primary tumors, it is not currently practical for breast cancer screening. MRI mammography is used mainly for assessment of primary tumors following mammography and for determining response to treatment.

Typical scan time for a series of slicelike images ranges from 1 to 10 minutes, and several series demonstrating different body planes and using a variety of RF pulse sequences may be included in an examination. It is critically important that the patient remain still during a scan series and for the initial position to be maintained throughout the study. Some pulse sequences allow images to be made in the space of a breath-hold, providing clear visualization of areas such as the lungs and the liver that would otherwise be blurred because of respiratory motion.

Magnetic Resonance Imaging Contrast Media

Although contrast media are not required for many MRI studies, paramagnetic agents such as gadopentetate dimeglumine (Magnevist) and gadoteridol (ProHance), made from the rare-earth element gadolinium, may be injected intravenously. These agents are often called *GBCAs*, a general term referring to gadolinium-based contrast agents. They provide contrast enhancement of certain lesions, particularly brain and spinal cord tumors, and aid in differentiating disk material from scar tissue in postoperative spine examinations.

GBCAs tend to irritate the veins, sometimes causing superficial inflammation of blood vessels and, rarely, blood clots. Allergic reactions to gadolinium contrast agents have been reported, but they are not common, occurring in fewer than one in a thousand cases. Typical allergic responses include rash, sweating, itching, hives, and facial swelling. Severe allergic responses have occurred, but are very rare. See Chapter 16 for emergency response to contrast reactions.

> **!** As when using any contrast medium, a history of allergies and kidney function is taken and emergency supplies must be readily available when GBCAs are in use.

Of greater concern when administering GBCAs is the risk of nephrogenic systemic fibrosis/nephrogenic fibrosing dermopathy (NSF/NFD) in patients who suffer from advanced renal disease. For these patients specifically, the risk is estimated to be about 4%. Symptoms can be noticed within the first 24 hours following the MRI study and include a thickening of the skin that prevents bending and extending joints, resulting in decreased mobility. Fibrosis may spread to other parts of the body, such as the diaphragm, the muscles in the thigh and lower abdomen, and the pulmonary vessels. The clinical course of NSF/NFD is progressive and may be fatal. There is no specific treatment, but several approaches may be used to decrease symptoms. Patients with chronic liver disease and those who have recently received or are about to receive liver transplants are also at risk of developing NSF/NFD if they are experiencing kidney insufficiency.

Magnetic Resonance Angiography

Magnetic resonance angiography (MRA) uses magnetic resonance technology to study the cardiovascular system. MRA is used to detect, diagnose, and aid in the treatment of heart disorders, stroke, and blood vessel diseases. It can be used to confirm the diagnosis of vascular problems detected by Doppler ultrasound methods and is used as a screening tool for patients at risk of aneurysm. Although MRA can provide detailed images of blood vessels without use of contrast media, gadolinium contrast is usually given during a portion of the study to enhance the image detail. MRA encompasses a group of MR methods involving special RF pulse sequences to highlight blood flow and suppress the images of stationary surrounding structures (Figure 22-27).

Magnetic Resonance Spectroscopy and Spectroscopic Imaging

Magnetic Resonance Spectroscopy (MRS) is a specialized MR technique involving the scanning of a volume of tissue to identify and measure the quantities of specific chemicals in the tissue (Figure 22-28). Chemical and physiological information obtained with MRS makes it a particularly useful research tool for the investigation of brain function, but MRS also provides diagnostic information about biochemical and metabolic pathways in the central nervous system. The speed and precision of MRS analyses permit access to unique and transient biochemical events. The most prevalent uses of this technique include differential diagnosis of tumor malignancy, coma, multiple sclerosis, and human immunodeficiency virus (HIV); prognoses in cases of head injury and cerebrovascular accident (CVA); and investigation of neonatal hypoxia and congenital errors in metabolism. MRS also assists in planning surgery for patients with temporal lobe epilepsy and is being used in the investigation of muscle disorders.

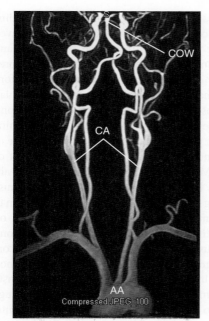

FIG 22-27 Contrast-enhanced MRA shows carotid arteries (CA) from the aortic arch (AA) to the circle of Willis (COW). (From Long BW, Rollins JH, Smith BJ: *Merrill's atlas of radiographic positioning & procedures,* ed 12, St Louis, 2012, Elsevier.)

Magnetic resonance spectroscopic imaging (MRSI) uses phase encoding methods to obtain spectra from multiple regions across the field of view. Instead of the volume information obtained with MRS, MRSI provides an image that maps the location and quantity of specific chemicals. MRSI holds great promise for the future but is still limited by technical problems, causing it to be currently somewhat less reliable than MRS for many applications.

Functional Magnetic Resonance Imaging

Functional Magnetic Resonance Imaging (fMRI) is used to evaluate the function of the brain during a given activity. This form of neuroimaging is based on the concept that normal brain tissues have different vascular flow than injured and diseased tissues. Actions and energy use, such as body part movement, speech, thought and sensation, all trigger different hemodynamic reactions, which are then measured by magnetic strength and computerized into an MRI image (Figure 22-29). This mapping of the brain responses on fMRI images allows a neurosurgeon to determine which parts of the brain are functioning properly, the extent of damaging pathology on body functions, and helps planning for surgery in the event brain surgery is necessary.

Magnetic Resonance Imaging Safety

The unique MRI environment requires special safety precautions. Conditions affecting patient safety involve

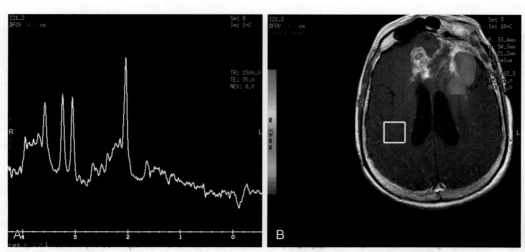

FIG 22-28 Routine spectroscopy in a patient with a primary brain tumor. Voxel shows normal brain spectra in an area unaffected by the brain tumor. **A,** Magnetic resonance spectroscopy (MRS) graph measures certain metabolites. **B,** Indication of specific brain area of MRS measurement. (From Long BW, Rollins JH, Smith BJ: *Merrill's atlas of radiographic positioning & procedures,* ed 13, St Louis, 2016, Elsevier.)

both the powerful magnetic field within the gantry and the thermal effects of RF pulses on certain materials that could overheat and possibly burn the patient. The RF energy used is a form of nonionizing radiation that can heat the tissues of the body. For this reason, the United States Food and Drug Administration (FDA) has established limits on exposure to RF energy that vary according to the anatomy being imaged.

The magnetic field and/or the rapid RF gradients may be hazardous for patients with artificial heart valves, aneurysm clips, neurostimulators, middle ear prostheses, or certain intrauterine devices (IUDs). Special reference directories can be used to determine the safety of specific devices with respect to MRI. Cardiac pacemakers can be a particular hazard, and patients with conventional pacemakers must not enter the scan room, because the magnetic field may cause the device to malfunction. A few fatalities have resulted from overheating of these pacemakers or pericardial wires when patients with implanted devices were scanned. Individuals with conventional pacemakers who come within the influence of the magnetic field should see their cardiologists immediately for evaluation of their pacemaker, because the magnetic field may damage it, causing it to fail without warning, even though the damage may not be immediately apparent. Recently, there have been significant advances with pacemaker engineering and MRI compatibility. MRI is often essential to medically diagnose patients, and as a patient's age

increases, so do the chances of the patient needing a cardiac device. Companies, such as Medtronic, have created MRI-safe pacemakers (e.g. Revo MRI SureScan Pacing System) in order to serve patients better and more safely.

Other conditions that merit assessment before entering the magnetic field include hemolytic anemia, orthopedic pins and screws, metal fragments or shrapnel in the soft tissues, and the presence of tattoos containing ferromagnetic pigments. Most orthopedic hardware is safe in the magnet, although it may cause significant compromise of MRI image quality in the region. Metalworkers who may have slivers of steel in their tissues must have a screening radiographic or CT head examination to detect any fragments that could damage their eyes or brain, because the pull of the magnetic field is so strong that it could cause these fragments to move. Tattoos containing ferromagnetic pigments can cause burns. Although the energies involved in MRI have not been demonstrated to cause complications in pregnancy, the prevailing philosophy is to avoid examination of pregnant patients during the first trimester and for pregnant technologists to avoid entering the magnetic field during a scan.

> **!** The principal means of ensuring patient safety during an MRI is careful patient screening before the procedure. Patients with conventional pacemakers **must not** enter the MRI scan room. Hemolytic anemia, orthopedic pins and screws, and metal fragments or shrapnel in the soft tissues are other conditions that should be identified in MRI patients before they enter the room.

Before the scan begins, the technologist places MRI-safe padding strategically to ensure that the patient's skin does not touch the magnet bore and is well insulated from the potential thermal effects of the RF pulses. Patients are instructed to report any unusual sensation of warmth immediately.

In addition to the magnetic field within the gantry, a significant magnetic field exists throughout the room and may affect anyone who enters. A lesser fringe field extends for some distance into the surrounding area. The magnetic field is present all the time, not just during a scan. All individuals entering the scan room should first be interviewed to determine whether they have surgical implants or metallic foreign bodies that could cause harm.

Loose metal objects must never be carried into the room. A pair of scissors, for instance, may fly from a

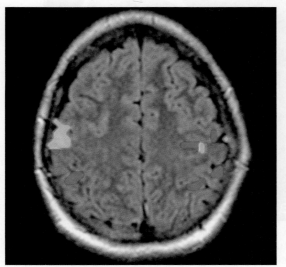

FIG 22-29 A fMRI image depicting brain activity during tongue and lip motion (highlighted areas.)

pocket when entering the magnetic field, endangering bystanders and damaging the gantry (Figure 22-30). Small metal objects such as hairpins or paperclips may be pulled into inaccessible portions of the magnet housing, where they distort the magnetic field and cause degradation of the images. Never enter the scanning room with stretchers, wheelchairs, or crutches that are not made specifically for use with MRI, because the magnetic field is strong enough to pull these items out of control, causing a serious accident. Steel oxygen tanks pose a lethal hazard and must never be taken into the scan room. (Oxygen is available from a wall outlet.)

> **!** Do not enter the MRI room with loose metal objects or with stretchers, crutches, or wheelchairs not made specifically for MRI use.

Individuals should be cautioned not to bring watches, credit cards, magnetized identification badges, hearing aids, or neurostimulators with them when entering the scanning area because the magnet will damage them. No one should

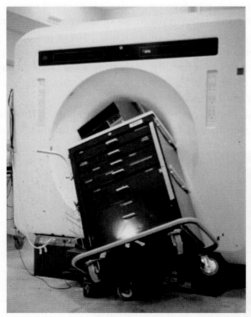

FIG 22-30 A metal emergency cart lodged within the gantry of the MRI machine. Common medical equipment can quickly become projectile objects that lodge in the center of an MRI machine. (From Coté CJ, Lerman J, Todres ID: *A practice of anesthesia for infants and children*, ed 4, Philadelphia, 2009, Saunders Elsevier.)

enter the scan room without the permission of the person responsible for controlling access. Personnel whose work requires them to enter the scan room must receive an orientation including safety instructions specific to this area.

Claustrophobia and Pain Management

The MRI technologist's duties include preparation of the patient for the examination and assistance in dealing with both physical and emotional discomfort. Few people are completely comfortable for any length of time in a tightly enclosed space. Even patients with no history of claustrophobia may feel anxious when entering a conventional tubular MRI gantry. Occasionally this anxiety is so severe that it creates panic, preventing the patient from continuing the examination.

It is important for the patient to know in advance that the table will move into the gantry, that plenty of air is available and that no physical discomfort will occur other than the need to lie still. The machine will make a loud "knocking" noise during the scanning process. Earplugs or earphones with recorded music may be offered. Patients may be reassured to know that they can communicate with the technologist through an intercom and that the technologist is watching them and listening to them at all times during the procedure. Because no radiation danger exists, a friend or family member may be allowed to accompany the patient into the room and stay throughout the procedure if desired. Remember that everyone who enters the scan room must be screened for pacemakers, pregnancy, loose metal objects, and items that could be damaged by the magnet.

A severely claustrophobic patient can be rescheduled at a facility with an open-gantry MRI or be given an antianxiety medication. Medication may also be required for patients whose pain makes it impossible to lie still for the duration of the study. For patients who require medication, an IV catheter with an intermittent injection port is established first. This provides access throughout the procedure in case it is needed for repeat doses, administration of contrast, or emergency drug administration. The radiologist selects and administers the drug(s), and the technologist assists.

Morphine sulfate (MS Contin) or meperidine (Demerol) or fentanyl (Sublimaze) may be administered for analgesia. Ativan (Lorazepam), midazolam (Versed), and diazepam (Valium) are antianxiety drugs used to treat claustrophobia. Fentanyl and midazolam are often preferred over other options for pain and anxiety control because they are relatively short-acting and patients tend to be alert soon after the study. Patients receiving sedation should be instructed not to drive after the procedure and not to ingest alcohol for 24 to 48 hours. Remember that both analgesic and tranquilizing drugs act as respiratory depressants. Patients who have received these medications must be monitored with a pulse oximeter during the procedure, as it is not possible for them to be monitored directly. Make sure that antagonists to reverse the effects of these drugs are available, as well as emergency supplies in the event of adverse reaction. (Review Chapters 13 and 14 for information on sedation and administration of medication and Chapter 16 for responses to emergency situations.)

> **!** Patients who have received analgesic or tranquilizing medications must be monitored with a pulse oximeter during the procedure, as it is not possible for them to be monitored directly.

ULTRASOUND IMAGING

Principles and General Applications

Ultrasound imaging, also called *diagnostic medical sonography*, is a noninvasive procedure that is considered to be very safe for the patient. This imaging modality uses high-frequency sound waves to produce echoes within the body. As the echoes return to the sending point, or **transducer,** their strength and timing are interpreted by a computer to produce a map or graphic image of the echo distribution. The transducer is moved over the surface of the body, and the image is viewed in real time on the computer monitor (Figure 22-31).

The ultrasound wave may be focused, refracted, reflected, or scattered at interfaces between different media, such as liquids, gas, and soft tissues. For this reason, any interface between substances or tissues of varying density produces a different ultrasound echo. Simple fluids tend not to reflect echoes, so they appear dark in the image and are said to be *anechoic*. Soft tissues, depending on their density, appear in various shades of gray. Structures that reflect most of the sound are said to be *hyperechoic* and appear bright on the image. These characteristics of sound behavior within the body make sonography an effective technique to visualize the shape, size, and condition of soft tissues, such as the breast (Figure 22-32), and organs such as the heart, spleen, gallbladder, or pancreas (Figure 22-33). Because sonography permits the differentiation of fluid from adipose tissue, the presence of an abscess, cyst, or tumor or abnormal fluid such as ascites can be demonstrated.

Ultrasound imaging of the scrotum is the primary method used to evaluate disorders of the testicles. This application can determine whether a scrotal mass is cystic or solid, assist in diagnosis of trauma to the scrotum, and diagnose causes of testicular pain or swelling, such as torsion of the spermatic cord. It is useful in determining causes of infertility, evaluating a variocele (enlarged vein or veins in the scrotum), and locating the position of an undescended testicle.

Although conventional radiography is the usual first step in skeletal imaging, ultrasound images of the

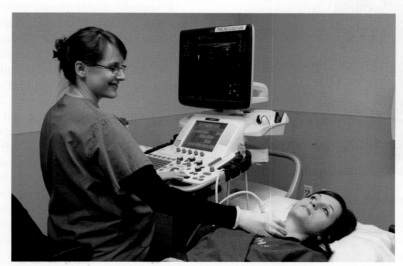

FIG 22-31 Images are viewed in real time during sonography scanning procedure.

musculoskeletal system are useful for visualizing muscles, tendons, ligaments, and joints. These studies are typically used to help diagnose tendon tears, such as those of the rotator cuff in the shoulder or the Achilles tendon in the heel. They can also demonstrate bleeding or other fluid collections within the muscles, bursae, and joints, as well as soft-tissue tumors and the early changes of rheumatoid arthritis.

Obstetrical Ultrasound

Among the more familiar uses of diagnostic sonography are its obstetric applications. Sonography is the

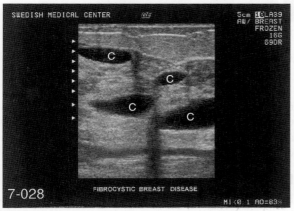

FIG 22-32 Fibrocystic breast disease is demonstrated with several anechoic lesions (fluid-filled cysts) within the breast.

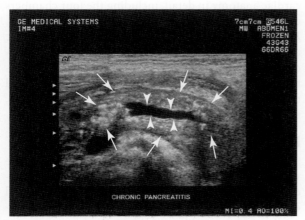

FIG 22-33 Transverse ultrasound scan over the pancreas showing bright echogenic reflections *(arrows)* that represent chronic fibrotic pancreatitis. The dilated pancreatic duct is seen *(arrowheads)*.

principal method used for fetal imaging because of its high level of safety compared with procedures that involve x-rays. A wide range of obstetric information is obtainable using ultrasound methods; the most common studies are done to determine gestational size for age of the fetus, fetal growth and well-being, and to localize needle placement for **amniocentesis** (sampling of amniotic fluid). Obstetrical ultrasound can also be used to establish the presence of a living embryo at an early stage, evaluate the position of the fetus, determine the location of the placenta and the umbilical cord, as well as check the amount of amniotic fluid surrounding the baby.

Conventional sonography displays images in two-dimensional (thin, flat) sections of the body. Technological advances in ultrasound technology include computer integration of data obtained in multiple planes to produce 3-D images that are more lifelike than conventional two-dimensional images (Figure 22-34). A rapid series of 3-D images viewed in sequence provides four-dimensional (4-D) images, which are 3-D images in motion. These methods are used extensively in obstetrical studies to provide prenatal diagnosis of fetal abnormalities, such as heart deformities.

For pelvic and obstetrical studies, the patient is requested to force fluids and not to void for 1 to 2 hours preceding the examination. This preparation provides a full bladder, which is the best "acoustic window" for ultrasound imaging in the pelvic region.

Trauma Applications

Focused assessment with sonography for trauma (FAST) is done in the emergency department as a screening test for blood around the heart (pericardial tamponade) or around the abdominal organs (hemoperitoneum). Four areas are examined for free fluid: the perihepatic space, the perisplenic space, the pericardium, and the pelvis. An extended FAST scan adds bilateral anterior thoracic sonography to the FAST examination for the evaluation of both lungs. These applications of ultrasound technology often reduce the need for CT scans in emergency situations, decreasing the time needed for diagnosis and implementation of life-saving treatments.

Doppler Ultrasound

Doppler ultrasound is a form of sonography that can detect and measure the speed and direction of blood flow. Doppler ultrasound depends on the Doppler effect,

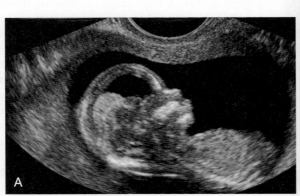 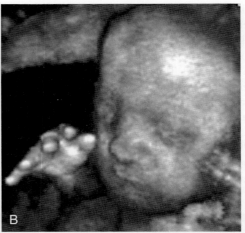

FIG 22-34 Comparison of sonograms of fetus using two-dimensional (**A**) and three-dimensional (**B**) technique. (A From Bontrager KL: *Textbook of radiographic positioning and related anatomy*, ed 7, St Louis, 2009, Mosby; B From Kremkau FW: *Diagnostic ultrasound*, ed 7, St Louis, 2005, Saunders.)

a change in the frequency of a wave resulting from the motion of a reflector, the *red blood cell.*

There are three basic kinds of Doppler ultrasound:

- *Color Doppler*—this technique estimates the average velocity of flow within a vessel by color coding the information. The direction of blood flow is assigned the color red or blue, indicating flow toward or away from the ultrasound transducer.
- *Pulsed Doppler*—this method allows a sampling volume or "gate" to be positioned in a vessel visualized on the gray-scale image and displays a graph of the full range of blood velocities within the gate versus time. The amplitude of the signal is approximately proportional to the number of red blood cells and is indicated, not in color, but simply as a shade of gray.
- *Power Doppler*—this device depicts the amplitude, or power, of Doppler signals rather than the frequency shift. This allows detection of a larger range of Doppler shifts and thus better visualization of small vessels. This method does not record directional and velocity information.

Color Doppler depicts blood flow in a region and is used as a guide for the placement of the pulsed Doppler gate for more detailed analysis at a particular site. Doppler ultrasound has many applications, including the detection and measurement of decreased or obstructed blood flow to the legs. You will recall from earlier in this chapter that color Doppler ultrasound is used to

monitor blood flow for RFA and EVLT. It is also very useful for identifying the location and extent of clots and narrowing in both veins and arteries, including the carotid arteries in the neck (Figure 22-35).

Echocardiography

Echocardiography is the term for ultrasound examinations of the heart. A complete two-dimensional study of the heart is made using color Doppler with pulsed and continuous wave Doppler spectral tracings. With echocardiography it is possible to image the cardiac anatomy in detail, including the four chambers of the heart and the four heart valves (Figure 22-36). Echocardiography is useful in the diagnosis of cardiac pathology, including atherosclerosis, scarring and calcification from previous rheumatic fever, endocarditis, and valvular disease. This technique is also used to diagnose congenital heart conditions in fetuses, neonates, and young children.

Internal Transducers

Specially designed transducers are available for use within the body. For example, a high frequency transducer can be passed from the mouth to the distal esophagus for studies of the heart when routine echocardiograms prove difficult. This method uses the stomach as an acoustic window to achieve excellent imaging of the intracardiac structures.

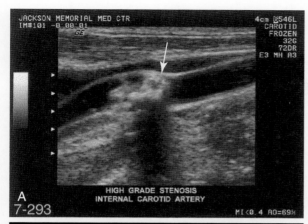

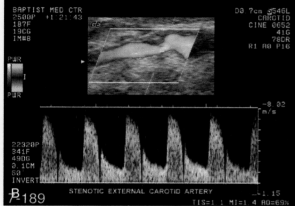

FIG 22-35 A, Longitudinal image of the carotid artery with a high-grade stenosis at the bifurcation *(arrow).* **B,** Color Doppler and spectral waveform demonstrate increased flow velocity in the stenotic external carotid artery. (From Frank ED, Long BW, Smith BJ: *Merrill's atlas of radiographic positions and radiologic procedures,* ed 12, St Louis, 2012, Mosby.)

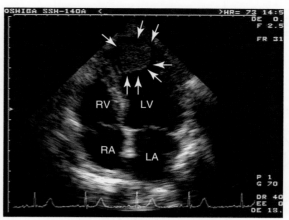

FIG 22-36 Echocardiogram showing the four chambers of the heart and a large thrombus in the left apex *(arrows).* (From Long BW, Rollins JH, Smith BJ: *Merrill's atlas of radiographic positioning & procedures,* ed 13, St Louis, 2016, Elsevier.)

A transrectal transducer is placed in the rectum for optimal imaging of the prostate gland to detect any enlargement or disorders of the prostate or abnormal growth within it. It may also be useful in diagnosing the cause of male infertility.

A transvaginal transducer assists with visualization of the cervix, uterus, and rectouterine recess (Figure 22-37).

Contrast-Enhanced Ultrasound

Contrast-enhanced ultrasound (CEUS) is the application of special ultrasound contrast media to traditional ultrasound imaging. The contrast media are gas-filled microbubbles that are injected intravenously into the systemic circulation. These media are available in several different types that vary with respect to the makeup of the shells of the bubbles and their gas cores. Examples of products include Optison, SonoVue, and Levovist. Microbubbles have a high degree of echogenicity; that is, they have a greater ability to reflect ultrasound waves than soft tissues. This increased echo backscatter greatly enhances image contrast.

Currently under development are targeted microbubbles that have *ligands,* specific proteins that bind them to certain cell types of interest, for example, cancer cells or inflamed cells. These are not yet commercially available.

NUCLEAR MEDICINE

Conventional Nuclear Medicine Techniques

The term **nuclear medicine** refers to the medical use of radioactive isotopes or **radionuclides,** unstable isotopes that give off radiation in their attempt to reach stability. Radionuclides are frequently *tagged* (attached) to pharmaceuticals, forming radiopharmaceuticals that have specific biodistribution patterns that match the organs or systems to be imaged. The technologist administers these radiopharmaceuticals in a variety of ways, depending upon the part of the body to be imaged. For example, some

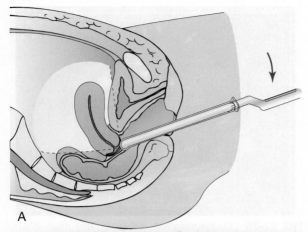

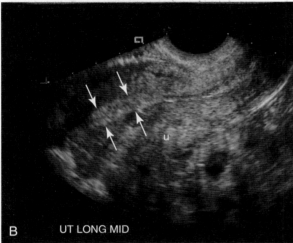

FIG 22-37 A, Transducer placement for transvaginal sagittal scan of the uterus. **B,** Transvaginal midline sagittal image of the uterus. The thickened endometrium is seen as an echogenic line *(arrows)* in the left central part of the uterus (u). (From Frank ED, Long BW, Smith BJ: *Merrill's atlas of radiographic positions and radiologic procedures,* ed 11, St Louis, 2007, Mosby.)

radiopharmaceuticals may be ingested, many are injected, and some are in a gaseous form and are inhaled. Gamma cameras are sensitive to the energies released by radioisotopes and radiopharmaceuticals and can follow their movement through the body. Radiopharmaceuticals are usually short-lived and result in a lower radiation dose than that of radiographic procedures. They are metabolized and excreted primarily in urine or in feces.

Nuclear medicine differs from most other imaging methods in that it provides information about the *function* of organs and tissues. Depending on the isotope used, it is taken up in the target organ within a period ranging from 30 minutes to a few days. It can then be detected and its location recorded by a gamma camera or measured by a scintillation detector. Abnormal tissues are demonstrated on images because the radionuclide is metabolized at a different rate, at a different location, or to a greater or lesser extent than in normal tissue.

Most commonly used radiopharmaceuticals are tagged with Technetium-99 m (^{99m}Tc). It has a **half-life** (the time it takes for its radioactivity to decrease by half) of about 6 hours and can be used with a variety of pharmaceuticals. ^{99m}Tc-tagged pharmaceuticals can be used to image most tissues and systems of the body, including brain, lung, liver, and bone. In bone scanning, for example, ^{99m}Tc is tagged to methylene diphosphonate, a phosphorous compound that is a calcium analog. Thus, it accumulates in active bone tissue with increased uptake in bone that has been damaged by pathologic processes or trauma. These regions of increased accumulation are seen as brighter areas on the monitor screen and darker areas on the permanent images. Bone imaging can reveal many kinds of trauma or pathology, including hairline fractures and metastatic cancer.

> Nuclear medicine differs from most other imaging methods in that it provides information about the *function* of organs and tissues.

Structures that can be demonstrated by nuclear medicine techniques include the thyroid gland, liver, lungs, brain, skeletal system (Figure 22-38), kidneys, heart, and blood vessels. One form of radiopharmaceutical flows in the blood, allowing visualization of blood vessels to detect clots and other abnormalities. Gallium scans are used for diagnosis and follow-up of tumors and are used to evaluate organs suspected of involvement in inflammatory processes. Sentinel node scintigraphy (lymphoscintigraphy) is used to identify lymph drainage pathways and is valuable in staging cancer. Thallium stress studies of the heart are particularly useful in the evaluation of coronary artery disease.

Special injection and disposal procedures required for the safe use of radioactive isotopes are beyond the scope of this text. For further information on this subject, consult a suitable nuclear imaging text.

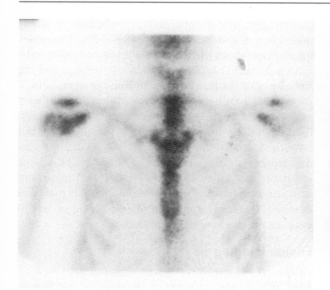

FIG 22-38 Nuclear medicine bone scan shows increased radiopharmaceutical uptake in right shoulder *(image left)*, indicating inflammation due to joint impingement.

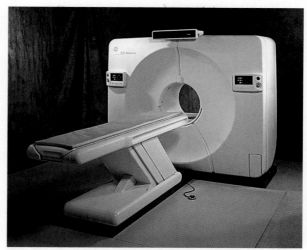

FIG 22-39 Typical whole-body PET scanner. The bed is capable of moving in and out of the gantry to measure the distribution of PET radiopharmaceuticals throughout the body. Data is viewed and analyzed at sophisticated computer workstations. (Courtesy GE Medical Systems, Milwaukee, Wisconsin.)

Positron Emission Tomography

Positron emission tomography (PET) is a highly specialized nuclear medicine technique. Clinical use of PET is expanding, and research continues to increase the useful applications of this modality. It is similar to other nuclear medicine methods in that radioactive substances from within the body are detected and mapped by specialized equipment to obtain information about the function of organs, tissues, or systems. The PET scanner is similar in appearance to a CT scanner (Figure 22-39). A gamma detector array in the PET gantry surrounds the patient and obtains axial images that can be reconstructed by the computer to display the images in other planes. The radioactivity level can be represented on the monitor screen in colors (Figure 22-40).

PET centers are not as accessible as other imaging modalities because they must be located near a particle accelerator to obtain the special radionuclides that are used with PET. The increasing application of PET imaging is fostering the development of new facilities to provide these radionuclides, which are quite different from those used in conventional nuclear medicine. Radioactive atoms such as ^{11}C (carbon), ^{13}N (nitrogen), ^{15}O (oxygen), and ^{18}F (fluorine) are made by bombarding normal chemicals with neutrons to produce radionuclides with very short half-lives. As they decay, they produce pairs of subatomic particles, each pair consisting of a positron and an electron. These particles interact with atoms in the body to produce simultaneous pairs of gamma rays called *annihilation photons*. The radionuclides used in PET are nearly identical to substances that are common in the body and are therefore capable of many chemical interactions and metabolic functions not possible with conventional radionuclides and tagged pharmaceuticals. For example, a commonly used radiopharmaceutical for PET is FDG, a form of glucose, allowing measurement of the metabolism and distribution of sugar. PET is used extensively to study the brain and is also used routinely for measurements of metabolism and blood flow. These measurements may indicate tumors in tissues with abnormally increased metabolism, even when no abnormality can be seen with other imaging modalities. Scanners are designed to acquire data from the top of the head to the base of the trunk, so studies can be performed on the brain, heart, lung, and abdominal structures. PET is a superior method for detecting and staging malignancies such as melanoma (in which case the entire body may be scanned) and tumors of the lung. Other types of tumors and organ transplants can also be studied using PET.

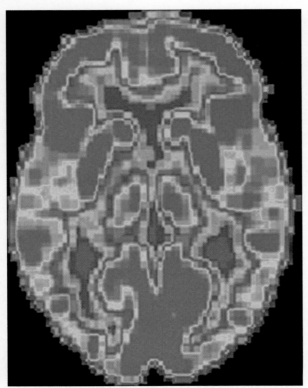

FIG 22-40 PET image of brain. (From Lundy-Elkman L: *Neuroscience: Fundamentals for rehabilitation,* ed 3, St Louis, 2007, Saunders.)

PET is a superior method for detecting and staging malignancies such as melanoma and tumors of the lung.

Single Photon Emission Computed Tomography

Single photon emission computed tomography (SPECT) is a nuclear medicine modality similar to PET, but using different radiopharmaceuticals. The isotopes most commonly used with SPECT are ^{133}Xe (xenon), ^{99m}Tc, and ^{123}I (iodine). These radionuclides result in the emission of single gamma photons instead of pairs and have a longer decay time than those used in PET. The images provide less sensitivity and less detail than PET, but the procedure is less expensive and more accessible because SPECT centers do not have to be located near a particle accelerator.

The principal applications of SPECT imaging are studies of the brain and heart. Brain perfusion studies have proved to be helpful in the diagnosis and classification of dementia and in evaluation of attention deficit disorders. In heart studies, SPECT provides information about the blood flow levels and other indications of cardiac health such as aortic stenosis and the sufficiency of the heart valves. In some centers, SPECT scans are a routine aspect of evaluations for coronary artery disease. In the past, radioactive thallium has been used extensively for perfusion studies of the heart, but now the most common radiopharmaceutical for cardiac studies is Cardiolite, a brand of sestamibi, a large synthetic molecule labeled with ^{99m}Tc. The patient is scanned following exercise, and if abnormality is detected, the scan is repeated after a period of rest to evaluate the extent of the condition.

Fusion Imaging

Advanced nuclear medicine procedures such as PET and SPECT are exceptional modalities for assessing organ function, while CT and MRI scans provide superior anatomic imaging. Until quite recently, it was necessary to do both types of studies separately and correlate the results to obtain both structural and functional information. The development of hybrid imaging systems blends equipment of both types into one unit that scans for both functional and imaging information and automatically correlates the results in a single procedure. These dual processes are called fusion imaging. The basic types are PET-CT, PET-MRI, and SPECT-CT.

These new systems present technical challenges for imaging technologists, and many facilities are finding that cross-training in nuclear medicine and imaging modalities eliminates the need for two technologists to perform a single study. The first fusion imaging system became available commercially in the year 2000, and these modalities are rapidly growing in both popularity and availability.

MAMMOGRAPHY

Mammography is a radiographic procedure that uses special equipment to produce images of high contrast and high resolution for the diagnosis of breast lesions (Figure 22-41). High-quality images are required to ensure that subtle but significant findings are not overlooked, because deficiencies in equipment, technique, or interpretation could result in failure to identify a life-threatening tumor. To assure patients and referring physicians that a facility meets the necessary quality requirements, the American College of Radiology and the FDA cooperate to provide

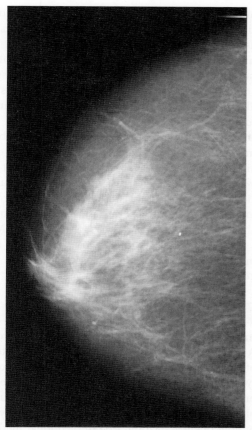

FIG 22-41 Mediolateral projection of normal breast with a low-dose, film-screen mammogram.

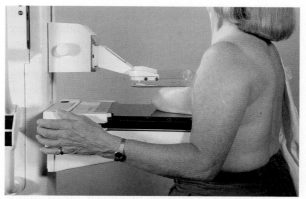

FIG 22-42 Craniocaudal projection of the patient's left breast utilizing compression. (From Long BW, Rollins JH, Smith BJ: *Merrill's atlas of radiographic positioning & procedures,* ed 13, St Louis, 2016, Elsevier.)

certification for mammography departments demonstrating adherence to high standards of excellence. To qualify for this certification, the facility must be staffed by radiographers who have received specialized training and are certified in mammography by the American Registry of Radiologic Technologists.

The American Cancer Society recommends annual mammograms beginning at age 40, although recommendations sometimes vary among organizations and agencies.

In preparing for mammography, patients are instructed not to use underarm deodorant and not to apply powder or lotions on the breasts or axillary areas. These products may contain ingredients that produce metallic artifacts on mammographic images. This is especially true of antiperspirants that contain aluminum salts.

Before the study, the mammographer obtains a pertinent patient history. This usually includes information about previous mammograms, the date of the last menstrual period, number of pregnancies, date of last pregnancy, whether the patient takes any hormones (including birth control tablets), and whether the patient has noticed any breast pain, breast lump(s), or nipple discharge. The precise locations of tenderness or lumps can be indicated on breast diagrams.

> When previous mammograms are available, every effort must be made to obtain them, because comparative evaluation is often significant in radiologic diagnosis.

Some departments include manual breast examinations during the mammography appointment. Mammography also provides an opportunity for patient instruction in breast self-examination (BSE). Although this may be provided for patients in a video format, mammographers must be familiar with the program's content to provide further instruction and answer questions.

Because the breasts must be uncovered for this examination, a comfortable temperature must be maintained in the radiography room. To respect the patient's modesty, drape the upper torso with a gown or sheet except during actual positioning and radiographic exposure (Figure 22-42). Take care to avoid accidental intrusion by others during the examination. A simple door sign reading "Examination in Progress: Do Not Enter" is very helpful.

Mammography units include a compression device that briefly presses the breast tightly against the image receptor during each exposure. Firm compression greatly improves image quality, allowing more accurate interpretation and a reduction in the amount of radiation required for an adequate exposure. Compression of the breast may cause patients discomfort and apprehension, but it does not usually cause pain. Patients with very tender breasts, often from fibrocystic breast disease, may experience pain during compression or during the 24 hours that follow. Aspirin or acetaminophen is recommended for the treatment of postmammography pain and may also be taken in advance of the examination to minimize discomfort. In addition to routine screening examinations and studies for the evaluation of known breast lumps,

> Schedule mammograms on premenopausal women during the first 2 weeks of the menstrual cycle because their breasts are less likely to be tender during this period.

mammographic techniques may also be used to localize needle placement for breast biopsies. A breast biopsy is a minor surgical procedure that requires sterile technique but does not require surgical scrubbing and gowning. The radiographer assists the radiologist as directed. The necessary skills are similar to those needed when assisting with lumbar puncture.

Digital mammography systems offer the ability to manipulate, archive, and read these images electronically with a PACS. Mammography is not the only modality used for breast imaging. When lumps are identified, ultrasound studies are useful for differentiating tumors from cysts and may also provide localization for biopsies. CT laser techniques, MRI, and nuclear medicine studies are also used to supplement mammograms in breast assessment and diagnosis.

▌ SUMMARY

- Radiography that demonstrates blood vessels is called *angiography*. This group of procedures includes arteriograms (images of specific arteries), aortograms (images of the aorta), angiocardiograms (contrast studies of the heart and great vessels), and venograms (radiography of veins). These studies require injection of aqueous iodinated contrast agents and involve multiple images taken in rapid series with specialized equipment.

- The Seldinger technique is the method used to place catheters in specific vessels for angiography. An artery is entered percutaneously with a large needle, and a guide wire is threaded through the needle. The needle is then removed, and a catheter is inserted over the guidewire, which is then removed. The placement of guidewire and catheter tip is guided fluoroscopically.

- Digital subtraction angiography may be accomplished by means of either arterial or IV contrast injection. Digital images of anatomic structures, with and without contrast media, are manipulated to eliminate the image of bones and provide a clearer visualization of the vessels.

- Interventional radiography refers to the repair of vessels by means of specialized catheters in conjunction with angiography. In PTA, a balloon may be used to widen the artery, or an abrasive burr- or cone-shaped

rotational head may serve to pulverize an atheroma. A stent may be inserted to help maintain patency of the vessel. Transcatheter embolization is another type of interventional radiography that is used to prevent hemorrhage, reduce blood flow, or cut off blood supply to a diseased area. Sclerotic therapy and radiofrequency ablation are interventional methods that have largely replaced surgery in the treatment of vein problems such as occlusion, stenosis, varicosity, and inflammation.

- CT is a computerized x-ray technique that produces slicelike axial images. It is used for all parts of the body and often involves the use of contrast agents, either intravenous or oral. CT angiography is the term for volumetric three-dimensional images of the arteries of the head, neck, and torso produced by spiral/helical scanners. CT myelography produces images of the spine, dural sac, and nerve roots following intrathecal injection of a contrast agent.

- MRI is a computerized scanning technique that uses a powerful magnetic field and radiofrequency pulses to produce images of all parts of the body in any body plane. Paramagnetic agents containing gadolinium compounds are used as contrast media for some types of MRI scans. Tranquilizers may be prescribed to prevent claustrophobia in tubular gantry scanners, and narcotic analgesics are sometimes necessary to relieve pain so that patients can lie still for the duration of a scan. The magnetic field surrounding the scanner poses potential hazards, and those working in the area must receive instruction in MRI safety. MRS and MRSI studies provide chemical and physiological information about biochemical and metabolic pathways in the central nervous system. MRA is a technique for studying the cardiovascular system. fMRI studies demonstrate the function of the brain during an activity.

- Diagnostic medical sonography is a noninvasive imaging method that uses high-frequency sound waves to produce computerized images of soft tissues. The method is useful for fetal imaging, abdominal imaging, and breast studies. Doppler ultrasound methods are used to study arteries and veins, and echocardiology is the term for ultrasound examinations of the heart.

- Nuclear medicine is the science of using radioactive isotopes that are often tagged to pharmaceuticals. This imaging provides functional information about various parts of the body. Radionuclides or radiopharmaceuticals can be injected, inhaled, or ingested. The movement of these substances can then be followed through the body using a gamma camera or PET scanner to reveal abnormal patterns of uptake. The bones, thyroid gland, liver, lymph nodes, and other structures can be studied using this modality.

- PET is a specialized, computerized nuclear medicine technique that maps radiopharmaceutical substances within the body to provide information about chemical interactions and metabolic functions of the head, heart, and lungs. It is useful in staging certain types of cancer and for the study of tumors and transplants.

- SPECT is similar to PET imaging but uses different radiopharmaceuticals. SPECT is particularly useful for studying certain types of problems of the heart and the brain.

- Fusion imaging is a recent development in hybrid technology that combines the functional information of SPECT and PET systems with the anatomic imaging of CT or MRI. The resulting hybrid scanners are termed PET-CT, PET-MRI, and SPECT-CT.

- Mammography is radiographic imaging of the breast using specialized x-ray equipment. It is useful for investigating breast lumps and as a screening tool for early detection of breast cancer. Compression of the breast during exposure is essential for image quality. Mammography or sonography may be used to localize needle placement for breast biopsy procedures and to place wires for three-dimensional localization of tumors during surgery.

REVIEW QUESTIONS

1. Which of the following procedures is NOT useful in the diagnosis of atherosclerosis?
   A. Doppler ultrasound
   B. DSA
   C. MRA
   D. CT myelography
2. Which of the following procedures must be done in order to treat a stenosis with angioplasty?
   A. Doppler ultrasound of the carotid artery
   B. Arteriogram
   C. MRI spectroscopy
   D. Amniocentesis
3. Which of the following is NOT a nuclear medicine procedure?
   A. Bone scan
   B. SPECT scan
   C. CT scan
   D. Thallium stress test
4. A contrast agent that contains microscopic bubbles is used to enhance visualization in which of the following modalities?
   A. CT
   B. Sonography
   C. MRI
   D. PET
5. Which of the following modalities is useful for imaging the soft tissue structures of joints?
   A. CT
   B. MRI
   C. Sonography
   D. Mammography
6. An aortogram is a specific type of:
   A. angiogram.
   B. nuclear medicine scan.
   C. ultrasound procedure.
   D. MRI scan.

7. Physical compression of the tissue being imaged is essential in which of the following modalities?
   A. CTA
   B. MRI
   C. Mammography
   D. PET
8. The imaging modality that provides localization for amniocentesis is:
   A. CT myelography.
   B. sonography.
   C. mammography.
   D. scintigraphy.

9. Which of the following modalities does NOT involve the use of ionizing radiation?
   A. Mammography
   B. SPECT
   C. MRI
   D. Angiography
10. Doppler methods for assessing blood flow in arteries and veins are aspects of which of the following imaging modalities?
    A. PET
    B. Sonography
    C. CTA
    D. Venography

Answers can be found in the Answer Key on pages 429-431.

CRITICAL THINKING EXERCISES

1. Marjorie Nolan got lost on her way to the diagnostic sonography department and arrived in the radiography suite by mistake. Marjorie is 5 months pregnant and is very anxious about having an obstetrical ultrasound procedure. What can you say to her to reassure her as you show her the way to her appointment?
2. Your instructor has asked you to observe a balloon angioplasty of a coronary artery when you rotate through the angiography department. You must answer the following questions about the examination:
   A. What is the indication and purpose of this procedure?
   B. Name and describe the technique used to place the catheter.
   C. Name an artery that might be used to insert the catheter.

   D. What should be done after the catheter is removed to prevent hemorrhage?
3. Dr. MacDougal, the radiologist, has not answered his pager, and your supervisor has told you to go to the MRI department and ask him to return to the x-ray department. When you arrive in MRI, the scan room door is closed. Through the window you can see Dr. MacDougal inside visiting with a patient. What should you do?
4. Today your clinical assignment is to assist the technologist in the mammography department. Mrs. Georgia Bates is 73 years old and has just had her first mammogram. She complains that the procedure was very painful and that her breasts still hurt. She wants to know why the technologist hurt her like that. What should you say to Mrs. Bates?

ANSWER KEY

CHAPTER 1

1. C
2. A
3. A
4. B
5. C
6. B
7. B
8. B
9. C
10. A
11. B
12. B

CHAPTER 2

1. B
2. C
3. D
4. A
5. A
6. A
7. C
8. D
9. B
10. A

CHAPTER 3

1. D
2. C
3. A
4. A
5. C
6. D
7. D
8. B
9. C
10. B

CHAPTER 4

1. C
2. C
3. D
4. B
5. B
6. C
7. A
8. C
9. B.
10. A

CHAPTER 5

1. B
2. C
3. B
4. B
5. C
6. A
7. B
8. D
9. A
10. C

CHAPTER 6

1. C
2. D
3. D
4. D
5. A
6. C
7. D
8. D
9. C
10. A

CHAPTER 7

1. D
2. A
3. B
4. A
5. C
6. C
7. B
8. C

9. A
10. D

CHAPTER 8

1. C
2. D
3. B
4. C
5. A
6. D
7. A
8. B
9. B
10. A
11. D

CHAPTER 9

1. B
2. A
3. D
4. C
5. D
6. A
7. B
8. A
9. C
10. C

CHAPTER 10

1. C
2. D
3. D
4. C
5. B
6. C
7. D
8. D
9. A
10. B

CHAPTER 11

1. B
2. A
3. D
4. C

5. C
6. B
7. C
8. D

CHAPTER 12

1. C
2. B
3. C
4. A
5. B
6. B
7. B
8. D
9. B
10. A

CHAPTER 13

1. B
2. D
3. A
4. B
5. A
6. C
7. D
8. D
9. B
10. B

CHAPTER 14

1. C
2. C
3. B
4. B
5. C
6. B
7. D
8. B
9. A
10. C

CHAPTER 15

1. B
2. B

3. A
4. C
5. D
6. A
7. D
8. B
9. A
10. B

CHAPTER 16

1. B
2. C
3. D
4. B
5. D
6. A
7. B
8. C
9. A
10. A

CHAPTER 17

1. D
2. A
3. C
4. C
5. C
6. B
7. A
8. B
9. C
10. C

CHAPTER 18

1. D
2. B
3. C
4. C
5. D
6. B
7. A
8. B
9. B
10. D

CHAPTER 19

1. B
2. C
3. A
4. C
5. B
6. C
7. D
8. A
9. B
10. D

CHAPTER 20

1. A
2. D
3. D
4. A
5. D
6. A
7. C
8. D
9. A
10. B

CHAPTER 21

1. B
2. A
3. C
4. B
5. D
6. D
7. B
8. C

CHAPTER 22

1. D
2. B
3. C
4. B
5. B
6. A
7. C
8. B
9. C
10. B

3M: *3M Particulate Respirators 8511 with Cool Flow Exhalation Valve.* http://www.soscleanroom.com/ 3mparticulaterespirators8511withcoolflowexhala tionvalve-10bx.aspx?gclid=CKWDlejW9KkCFRVgg wodPy-29YA.

Administration on Aging (AoA): *What is Elder Abuse?* 10–8–09 http://www.aoa.gov/aoaroot/aoa_programs/ elder_rights/ea_prevention/whatisea.aspx.

Amersham Health X-Ray Products: *Clinical references, glucophage (metformin) and iodinated contrast media,* http://www.ashp.org/Import/ PRACTICEANDPOLICY/ PracticeResourceCenters/ ContrastMedia/ QuickGuidetoContrastMedia.aspx, November 2002.

ASRT Task Force on Governance Restructuring: *Recommended governance structure,* www.asrt.org, November 2002.

Bonewit-West K: *Clinical procedures for medical assistants,* ed 9, St Louis, 2014, Elsevier.

Bracco imaging pharmaceutical products: *Contrast media,* http://www.braccoimaging.com/, November 2002.

Centers for Disease Control and Prevention: *Flu Activity & Surveillance.* http://www.cdc.gov/flu/weekly/ fluactivitysurv.htm.

Centers for Disease Control and Prevention: Guideline for isolation precautions: preventing transmission of infectious agents in healthcare settings 2007, Part II. November 2006. In *Fundamental elements needed to prevent transmission of infectious agents in healthcare settings,* (serial online) www. cdc.gov/ncidod/dhqp/pdf/ guidelines/Isolation2007.pdf.

Centers for Disease Control and Prevention: *Healthcare-associated Infections (HAI).* http://www.cdc.gov/ ncidod/dhqp/pdf/isolation2007.pdf isolation.

Centers for Disease Control and Prevention: *HIV in the United States: At A Glance,* http://www.cdc.gov/ hiv/resources/factsheets/us.htm, March 14, 2012.

Centers for Disease Control and Prevention: *HIV/AIDS Surveillance Report.* http://www.cdc.gov/hiv/topics/ surveillance/resources/reports/print/.

Centers for Disease Control and Prevention: rev ed, *HIV/ AIDS surveillance report, 2005,* Vol. 17. Atlanta, 2007, U.S. Department of Health and Human Services, pp 1–54 (serial online). http://www.cdc.gov/hiv/surveillance/ resources/reports/2005report. November 2006.

Centers for Disease Control and Prevention: *PEP for HIV exposure in health care workers,* Morbidity and Mortality Weekly Report, Recommendations and Reports September 30, 2005/Vol. 54/No. RR-9.

Centers for Disease Control and Prevention: *Reported tuberculosis in the United States, 2006,* Atlanta, 2007, U.S. Department of Health and Human Services (serial online) www.cdc.gov/tb/surv/surv2006.

Centers for Disease Control and Prevention: Trends in tuberculosis morbidity—United States, 1992-2002, *MMWR Morb Mortal Wkly Rep* 52:217–222, 2003. (serial online) www.cdc.gov/mmwr/preview/ mmwrhtml/mm5211a2.htm. November 2006.

Chobanian AV, et al.: The seventh report of the Joint National Committee on Prevention, Detection, Evaluation, and Treatment of High Blood Pressure, *J Am Med Assoc* 289:2560–2572, 2003.

Death with Dignity Acts, www.deathwithdignity.org/, 2012.

Durand KS: *Critical thinking: developing skills in radiography,* Philadelphia, 1999, FA Davis.

Enrollment snapshot of radiography, radiation therapy and nuclear medicine programs, American Registry of Radiologic Technologists, November 2002 (website). www.asrt.org.

Furlow B: Ergonomics in the health care environment, *Radiol Technol* 74:137–150, 2002.

Jensen SC, Peppers MP: *Pharmacology and drug administration for imaging technologists,* ed 2, St Louis, 2006, Mosby.

Joyce EV, Villanueva ME: *Say it in Spanish,* ed 3, St Louis, 2004, Saunders.

Kimmel N: *Therapeutic Communication in the Nursing Profession,* http://ezinearticles.com/? Therapeutic-Communication-in-the-Nursing- Profession&id=594747, March 2007.

Kremkau FW: *Sonography principles and instruments,* ed 9, St Louis, 2010, Mosby.

Long BW, Rollins JH, Smith BJ: *Merrill's atlas of radiographic positioning & procedures,* ed 13, St Louis, 2016, Mosby.

Occupational Safety and Health Administration: *2153. Occupational exposure to tuberculosis,* (website) www. osha.gov/pls/oshaweb/owadisp.show_document?p_ table=UNIFIED_AGENDA&p_id=4120, November 2002.

Occupational Safety and Health Administration: *Clinical Services, Radiology: Bloodborne Pathogens.* http://www. osha.gov/SLTC/etools/hospital/clinical/radiology/ radiology.html#BloodbornePathogens.

Occupational Safety and Health Administration: *Clinical Services, Radiology: Ergonomics.* http://www.osha. gov/SLTC/etools/hospital/clinical/radiology/ radiology. html#Ergonomics.

Occupational Safety and Health Administration: *Clinical Services, Radiology: Slips, Trips and Falls*. www.osha.gov/SLTC/etools/hospital/clinical/radiology/radiology.html#Slips/Falls.

Occupational Safety and Health Administration: *Clinical Services, Radiology: Tuberculosis*. http://www.osha.gov/SLTC/etools/hospital/clinical/radiology/radiology.html#Tuberculosis.

Occupational Safety and Health Administration: *Revision to OSHA's bloodborne pathogens standard: technical background and summary*, (website) www.osha.gov/needlesticks/needlefact.html, 2001.

Occupational Safety and Health Administration: *Tuberculosis*. http://www.osha.gov/SLTC/tuberculosis/.

Ouellette DR: *Pulmonary Embolism*, eMedicine, Medscape. emedicine.medscape.com/article/300901-overview.

Parelli RJ: *Medicolegal issues for radiographers*, ed 3, Delray Beach, Fla, 1997, GR/St Lucie Press.

Perry AG, Potter PA, Ostendorf WR: *Clinical nursing skills & techniques*, ed 8, St Louis, 2014, Mosby.

Perry AG, Potter PA, Ostendorf WR: *Nursing interventions and clinical skills*, ed 6, St Louis, 2016, Mosby.

Potter PA, Perry AG, Stockert PA, Hall A: *Fundamentals of nursing*, ed 8, St Louis, 2013, Mosby.

Purtilo R: *Ethical dimensions in the health professions*, ed 4, Philadelphia, 2005, Elsevier–Saunders.

Sanchez T: Care targets workplace and patients, *ASRT Scanner* 33:35, 2001.

Seeram E: *Computed tomography*, ed 3, St Louis, 2008, Saunders.

Sprawls P: *Magnetic resonance imaging principles, methods and techniques*, Madison, Wis, November 2002, Medical Physics Publishing.

Spry C: Low-temperature sterilization, *Infection Control Today*, May 2001. (website) www.infectioncontroltoday.com/articles/412/412_151steriliz.html.

Tortorici M: *Administration of imaging pharmaceuticals*, Philadelphia, 1997, Saunders.

Tortorici M, Apfel P: *Advanced radiographic and angiographic procedures*, Philadelphia, 1995, FA Davis.

World Health Organization: *Patient Safety: WHO Guidelines on Hand*. http://whqlibdoc.who.int/publications/2009/9789241597906_eng.pdf.

A | APPENDIX

The Practice Standards for Medical Imaging and Radiation Therapy: Radiography Practice Standards

PREFACE TO PRACTICE STANDARDS

A profession's practice standards serve as a guide for appropriate practice. The practice standards define the practice and establish general criteria to determine compliance. Practice standards are authoritative statements established by the profession for judging the quality of practice, service, and education provided by individuals who practice in medical imaging and radiation therapy.

Practice standards can be used by individual facilities to develop job descriptions and practice parameters. Those outside the imaging, therapeutic, and radiation science community can use the standards as an overview of the role and responsibilities of the individual as defined by the profession.

The individual must be educationally prepared and clinically competent as a prerequisite to professional practice. Federal and state laws, accreditation standards necessary to participate in government programs, and lawful institutional policies and procedures supersede these standards.

Format

The Practice Standards for Medical Imaging and Radiation Therapy are divided into six sections: introduction, scope of practice, clinical performance, quality performance, professional performance, and advisory opinion statements.

Introduction

The introduction provides definitions for the practice and the education and certification for individuals, in addition to an overview of the specific practice.

Scope of Practice

The scope of practice delineates the parameters of the specific practice.

Clinical Performance Standards

The clinical performance standards define the activities of the individual in the care of patients and delivery of diagnostic or therapeutic procedures. The section incorporates patient assessment and management with procedural analysis, performance, and evaluation.

Quality Performance Standards

The quality performance standards define the activities of the individual in the technical areas of performance including equipment and material assessment, safety standards, and total quality management.

Professional Performance Standards

The professional performance standards define the activities of the individual in the areas of education, interpersonal relationships, self-assessment, and ethical behavior.

Advisory Opinion Statements

The advisory opinions are interpretations of the standards intended for clarification and guidance for specific practice issues.

Each performance standards section is subdivided into individual standards. The standards are numbered and followed by a term or set of terms that identify the standards, such as "assessment" or "analysis/determination." The next statement is the expected performance of the individual when performing the procedure or treatment. A rationale statement follows and explains why an individual should adhere to the particular standard of performance.

Criteria

Criteria are used in evaluating an individual's performance. Each set is divided into two parts: the general criteria and the specific criteria. Both criteria should be used when evaluating performance.

General Criteria

General criteria are written in a style that applies to imaging and radiation science individuals. These criteria are the same in all of the practice standards, with the exception of limited x-ray machine operators, and should be used for the appropriate area of practice.

Specific Criteria

Specific criteria meet the needs of the individuals in the various areas of professional performance. Although many areas of performance within imaging and radiation sciences are similar, others are not. The specific criteria are drafted with these differences in mind.

INTRODUCTION TO RADIOGRAPHY PRACTICE STANDARDS

Definition

The practice of radiography is performed by health care professionals responsible for the administration of ionizing radiation for diagnostic, therapeutic, or research purposes. A radiographer performs radiographic procedures at the request of and for interpretation by a licensed independent practitioner.

The complex nature of disease processes involves multiple imaging modalities. Although an interdisciplinary team of clinicians, radiographers, and support staff plays a critical role in the delivery of health services, it is the radiographer who performs the radiographic procedure that creates the images needed for diagnosis.

Radiography integrates scientific knowledge, technical skills, patient interaction, and compassionate care resulting in diagnostic information. Radiographers recognize patient conditions essential for successful completion of the procedure. Radiographers must demonstrate an understanding of human anatomy, physiology, pathology, and medical terminology.

Radiographers must maintain a high degree of accuracy in radiographic positioning and exposure technique. They must possess, use, and maintain knowledge of radiation protection and safety. Radiographers independently perform or assist the licensed independent practitioner in the completion of radiographic procedures. Radiographers prepare, administer, and document activities related to medications in accordance with state and federal regulations or lawful institutional policy.

Radiographers are the primary liaison between patients, licensed independent practitioners, and other members of the support team. Radiographers must remain sensitive to needs of the patient through good communication, patient assessment, patient monitoring, and patient care skills. As members of the health care team, radiographers participate in quality improvement processes and continually assess their professional performance.

Radiographers think critically and use independent, professional, and ethical judgment in all aspects of their work. They engage in continuing education to include their area of practice to enhance patient care, public education, knowledge, and technical competence.

Education and Certification

Radiographers prepare for their role on the interdisciplinary team by successfully completing an accredited educational program in radiologic technology and attaining appropriate primary certification by the American Registry of Radiologic Technologists. Those passing the ARRT examination use the credential R.T.(R). To maintain ARRT certification, radiographers must complete appropriate continuing education and meet other requirements to sustain a level of expertise and awareness of changes and advances in practice.

Overview

An interdisciplinary team of radiologists, radiographers, and other support staff plays a critical role in the delivery of health services as new modalities emerge and the need for imaging procedures increases. A comprehensive procedure list for the radiographer is impractical because clinical activities vary by practice needs and expertise of the radiographer. As radiographers gain more experience, knowledge, and clinical competence, the clinical activities for the radiographer may evolve.

State statute, regulation, or lawful community custom may dictate practice parameters. *Wherever there is a conflict between these standards and state or local statutes or regulations, the state or local statutes or regulations supersede these standards.* A radiographer should, within the boundaries of all applicable legal requirements and restrictions, exercise individual thought, judgment, and discretion in the performance of the procedure.

RADIOGRAPHER SCOPE OF PRACTICE

The scope of practice of the medical imaging and radiation therapy professional includes the following:

- Receiving, relaying, and documenting verbal, written, and electronic orders in the patient's medical record.
- Corroborating patient's clinical history with procedure, and ensuring information is documented and available for use by a licensed independent practitioner.
- Verifying informed consent.
- Assuming responsibility for patient needs during procedures.
- Preparing patients for procedures.
- Applying principles of ALARA to minimize exposure to patient, self, and others.
- Performing venipuncture as prescribed by a licensed independent practitioner.
- Starting and maintaining intravenous access as prescribed by a licensed independent practitioner.
- Identifying, preparing, and/or administering medications as prescribed by a licensed independent practitioner.
- Evaluating images for technical quality, and ensuring proper identification is recorded.
- Identifying and managing emergency situations.
- Providing education.
- Educating and monitoring students and other health care providers.
- Performing ongoing quality assurance activities.

The scope of practice of the radiographer also includes the following:

1. Performing diagnostic radiographic and noninterpretive fluoroscopic procedures as prescribed by a licensed independent practitioner.
2. Determining technical exposure factors.
3. Assisting licensed independent practitioner with fluoroscopic and specialized radiologic procedures.
4. Applying the principles of patient safety during all aspects of radiographic procedures, including assisting and transporting patients.

RADIOGRAPHY CLINICAL PERFORMANCE STANDARDS

Standard One—Assessment

The radiographer collects pertinent data about the patient and the procedure.

Rationale

Information about the patient's health status is essential in providing appropriate imaging and therapeutic services.

General Stipulation

The individual must be educationally prepared and clinically competent as a prerequisite to professional practice. Federal and state laws, accreditation standards necessary to participate in government programs, and lawful institutional policies and procedures supersede these standards.

General Criteria

The radiographer:

1. Gathers relevant information from the patient, medical record, significant others, and health care providers.
2. Reconfirms patient identification and verifies the procedure requested or prescribed.
3. Reviews the patient's medical record to verify the appropriateness of a specific examination or procedure.
4. Verifies the patient's pregnancy status.
5. Assesses factors that may contraindicate the procedure, such as medications, patient history, insufficient patient preparation, or artifacts.
6. Recognizes signs and symptoms of an emergency.

Specific Criteria

The radiographer:

1. Assesses patient risk for allergic reaction to medication prior to administration.
2. Locates and reviews previous examinations for comparison.
3. Identifies and removes artifact-producing objects.

RADIOGRAPHY CLINICAL PERFORMANCE STANDARDS

Standard Two—Analysis/Determination

The radiographer analyzes the information obtained during the assessment phase and develops an action plan for completing the procedure.

Rationale

Determining the most appropriate action plan enhances patient safety and comfort, optimizes diagnostic and therapeutic quality, and improves efficiency.

General Stipulation

The individual must be educationally prepared and clinically competent as a prerequisite to professional practice. Federal and state laws, accreditation standards necessary to participate in government programs and lawful institutional policies and procedures supersede these standards.

General Criteria

The radiographer:
1. Selects the most appropriate and efficient action plan after reviewing all pertinent data and assessing the patient's abilities and condition.
2. Uses professional judgment to adapt imaging and therapeutic procedures to improve diagnostic quality and therapeutic outcome.
3. Consults appropriate medical personnel to determine a modified action plan.
4. Determines the need for and selects supplies, accessory equipment, shielding, and immobilization devices.
5. Determines the course of action for an emergency or problem situation.
6. Determines that all procedural requirements are in place to achieve a quality diagnostic or therapeutic procedure.

Specific Criteria

The radiographer:
1. Reviews lab values prior to administering medication and beginning specialized radiologic procedures.
2. Determines type and dose of contrast agent to be administered, on the basis of the patient's age, weight, and medical/physical status.

3. Verifies that exposure indicator data for digital radiographic systems has not been altered or modified.
4. Analyzes digital images to determine use of appropriate imaging parameters.

RADIOGRAPHY CLINICAL PERFORMANCE STANDARDS

Standard Three—Patient Education

The radiographer provides information about the procedure and related health issues according to protocol.

Rationale

Communication and education are necessary to establish a positive relationship.

General Stipulation

The individual must be educationally prepared and clinically competent as a prerequisite to professional practice. Federal and state laws, accreditation standards necessary to participate in government programs, and lawful institutional policies and procedures supersede these standards.

General Criteria

The radiographer:
1. Verifies that the patient has consented to the procedure and fully understands its risks, benefits, alternatives, and follow-up. The radiographer verifies that written or informed consent has been obtained.
2. Provides accurate explanations and instructions at an appropriate time and at a level the patients and their care providers can understand. Addresses patient questions and concerns regarding the procedure.
3. Refers questions about diagnosis, treatment, or prognosis to a licensed independent practitioner.
4. Provides related patient education.
5. Explains precautions regarding administration of medications.

Specific Criteria

The radiographer:
1. Consults with other departments for patient services.
2. Instructs patients regarding preparation prior to imaging procedures, including providing information about oral or bowel preparation and allergy preparation.

RADIOGRAPHY CLINICAL PERFORMANCE STANDARDS

Standard Four—Performance

The radiographer performs the action plan.

Rationale

Quality patient services are provided through the safe and accurate performance of a deliberate plan of action.

General Stipulation

The individual must be educationally prepared and clinically competent as a prerequisite to professional practice. Federal and state laws, accreditation standards necessary to participate in government programs, and lawful institutional policies and procedures supersede these standards.

General Criteria

The radiographer:
1. Performs procedural timeout.
2. Implements an action plan.
3. Explains each step of the action plan to the patient as it occurs and elicits the cooperation of the patient.
4. Uses an integrated team approach.
5. Modifies the action plan according to changes in the clinical situation.
6. Administers first aid or provides life support.
7. Utilizes accessory equipment.
8. Assesses and monitors the patient's physical, emotional, and mental status.
9. Applies principles of sterile technique.
10. Positions patient for anatomic area of interest, respecting patient ability and comfort.
11. Immobilizes patient for procedure.
12. Monitors the patient for reactions to medications.

Specific Criteria

The radiographer:
1. Employs proper radiation safety practices.
2. Utilizes technical factors according to equipment specifications to meet the ALARA principle.
3. Uses pre-exposure collimation and proper field-of-view selection.
4. Uses appropriate pre-exposure radiopaque markers for anatomic and procedural purposes.
5. Selects the best position for the demonstration of anatomy.
6. Injects medication into peripherally inserted central catheter lines or ports.

RADIOGRAPHY CLINICAL PERFORMANCE STANDARDS

Standard Five—Evaluation

The radiographer determines whether the goals of the action plan have been achieved.

Rationale

Careful examination of the procedure is important to determine that expected outcomes have been met.

General Stipulation

The individual must be educationally prepared and clinically competent as a prerequisite to professional practice. Federal and state laws, accreditation standards necessary to participate in government programs, and lawful institutional policies and procedures supersede these standards.

General Criteria

The radiographer:
1. Evaluates the patient and the procedure to identify variances that may affect the expected outcome.
2. Completes the evaluation process in a timely, accurate, and comprehensive manner.
3. Measures the procedure against established policies, protocols, and benchmarks.
4. Identifies exceptions to the expected outcome.
5. Develops a revised action plan to achieve the intended outcome.
6. Communicates revised action plan to appropriate team members.

Specific Criteria

The radiographer:
1. Evaluates images for positioning to demonstrate the anatomy of interest.
2. Evaluates images for optimal technical exposure factors.
3. Reviews images to determine whether additional images will enhance the diagnostic value of the procedure.

RADIOGRAPHY CLINICAL PERFORMANCE STANDARDS

Standard Six—Implementation

The radiographer implements the revised action plan.

Rationale

It may be necessary to make changes to the action plan to achieve the expected outcome.

General Stipulation

The individual must be educationally prepared and clinically competent as a prerequisite to professional practice. Federal and state laws, accreditation standards necessary to participate in government programs, and lawful institutional policies and procedures supersede these standards.

General Criteria

The radiographer:
1. Bases the revised plan on the patient's condition and the most appropriate means of achieving the expected outcome.
2. Takes action based on patient and procedural variances.
3. Measures and evaluates the results of the revised action plan.
4. Notifies appropriate health care provider when immediate clinical response is necessary based on procedural findings and patient condition.

Specific Criteria

The radiographer:
1. Obtains additional images that will produce the expected outcomes based on patient condition and procedural variances.

RADIOGRAPHY CLINICAL PERFORMANCE STANDARDS

Standard Seven—Outcomes Measurement

The radiographer reviews and evaluates the outcome of the procedure.

Rationale

To evaluate the quality of care, the radiographer compares the actual outcome with the expected outcome.

General Stipulation

The individual must be educationally prepared and clinically competent as a prerequisite to professional practice. Federal and state laws, accreditation standards necessary to participate in government programs, and lawful institutional policies and procedures supersede these standards.

General Criteria

The radiographer:
1. Reviews all diagnostic or therapeutic data for completeness and accuracy.
2. Uses evidenced-based practice to determine whether the actual outcome is within established criteria.
3. Evaluates the process and recognizes opportunities for future changes.
4. Assesses the patient's physical, emotional, and mental status prior to discharge.

Specific Criteria

None added.

RADIOGRAPHY CLINICAL PERFORMANCE STANDARDS

Standard Eight – Documentation

The radiographer documents information about patient care, the procedure, and the final outcome.

Rationale

Clear and precise documentation is essential for continuity of care, accuracy of care, and quality assurance.

General Stipulation

The individual must be educationally prepared and clinically competent as a prerequisite to professional practice. Federal and state laws, accreditation standards necessary to participate in government programs, and lawful institutional policies and procedures supersede these standards.

General Criteria

The radiographer:
1. Documents diagnostic, treatment, and patient data in the medical record in a timely, accurate, and comprehensive manner.
2. Documents exceptions from the established criteria or procedures.
3. Provides pertinent information to authorized individual(s) involved in the patient's care.
4. Records information used for billing and coding procedures.

5. Archives images or data.
6. Verifies patient consent is documented.
7. Documents procedural timeout.

Specific Criteria

The radiographer:
1. Documents fluoroscopic time.
2. Documents radiation exposure.
3. Documents the use of shielding devices and proper radiation safety practices per institutional policy

RADIOGRAPHY QUALITY PERFORMANCE STANDARDS

Standard One—Assessment

The radiographer collects pertinent information regarding equipment, procedures, and the work environment.

Rationale

The planning and provision of safe and effective medical services relies on the collection of pertinent information about equipment, procedures, and the work environment.

General Stipulation

The individual must be educationally prepared and clinically competent as a prerequisite to professional practice. Federal and state laws, accreditation standards necessary to participate in government programs, and lawful institutional policies and procedures supersede these standards.

General Criteria

The radiographer:
1. Determines that services are performed in a safe environment, minimizing potential hazards, in accordance with established guidelines.
2. Confirms that equipment performance, maintenance, and operation comply with manufacturer's specifications.
3. Verifies that protocol and procedure manuals include recommended criteria and are reviewed and revised.

Specific Criteria

The radiographer:
1. Maintains controlled access to restricted area during radiation exposure.
2. Follows federal and state guidelines to minimize radiation exposure levels.

3. Maintains and performs quality control on radiation safety equipment such as aprons, thyroid shields, etc.
4. Develops and maintains standardized exposure technique guidelines for all equipment.
5. Participates in radiation protection, patient safety, risk management, and quality management activities.
6. Reviews digital images for the purpose of monitoring radiation exposure.
7. Wears one or more personal radiation monitoring devices at the level indicated on the personal radiation monitoring device or as indicated by the radiation safety officer or designee.

RADIOGRAPHY QUALITY PERFORMANCE STANDARDS

Standard Two—Analysis/Determination

The radiographer analyzes information collected during the assessment phase to determine the need for changes to equipment, procedures, or the work environment.

Rationale

Determination of acceptable performance is necessary to provide safe and effective services.

General Stipulation

The individual must be educationally prepared and clinically competent as a prerequisite to professional practice. Federal and state laws, accreditation standards necessary to participate in government programs, and lawful institutional policies and procedures supersede these standards.

General Criteria

The radiographer:
1. Assesses services, procedures, and environment to meet or exceed established guidelines and adjusts the action plan.
2. Monitors equipment to meet or exceed established standards and adjusts the action plan.
3. Assesses and maintains the integrity of medical supplies such as a lot/expiration, sterility, etc.

Specific Criteria

None added.

RADIOGRAPHY QUALITY PERFORMANCE STANDARDS

Standard Three—Education

The radiographer informs the patient, public, and other health care providers about procedures, equipment, and facilities.

Rationale

Open communication promotes safe practices.

General Stipulation

The individual must be educationally prepared and clinically competent as a prerequisite to professional practice. Federal and state laws, accreditation standards necessary to participate in government programs, and lawful institutional policies and procedures supersede these standards.

General Criteria

The radiographer:
1. Elicits confidence and cooperation from the patient, the public, and other health care providers by providing timely communication and effective instruction.
2. Presents explanations and instructions at the learner's level of understanding.
3. Educates the patient, public, and other health care providers about procedures along with the biologic effects of radiation, sound wave or magnetic field, and protection.
4. Provides information to patients, health care providers, students, and the public concerning the role and responsibilities of individuals in the profession.

Specific Criteria

None added.

RADIOGRAPHY QUALITY PERFORMANCE STANDARDS

Standard Four—Performance

The radiographer performs quality assurance activities.

Rationale

Quality assurance activities provide valid and reliable information regarding the performance of equipment, materials, and processes.

General Stipulation

The individual must be educationally prepared and clinically competent as a prerequisite to professional practice. Federal and state laws, accreditation standards necessary to participate in government programs, and lawful institutional policies and procedures supersede these standards.

General Criteria

The radiographer:
1. Maintains current information on equipment, materials, and processes.
2. Performs ongoing quality assurance activities.
3. Performs quality control testing of equipment.

Specific Criteria

The radiographer:
1. Consults with medical physicist when performing the quality assurance tests.
2. Monitors image production to determine technical acceptability.
3. Performs routine archiving status checks.

RADIOGRAPHY QUALITY PERFORMANCE STANDARDS

Standard Five—Evaluation

The radiographer evaluates quality assurance results and establishes an appropriate action plan.

Rationale

Equipment, materials, and processes depend on ongoing quality assurance activities that evaluate performance on the basis of established guidelines.

General Stipulation

The individual must be educationally prepared and clinically competent as a prerequisite to professional practice. Federal and state laws, accreditation standards necessary to participate in government programs, and lawful institutional policies and procedures supersede these standards.

General Criteria

The radiographer:
1. Validates quality assurance testing conditions and results.
2. Evaluates quality assurance results.
3. Formulates an action plan.

Specific Criteria

None added.

RADIOGRAPHY QUALITY PERFORMANCE STANDARDS

Standard Six—Implementation

The radiographer implements the quality assurance action plan for equipment, materials, and processes.

Rationale

Implementation of a quality assurance action plan promotes safe and effective services.

General Stipulation

The individual must be educationally prepared and clinically competent as a prerequisite to professional practice. Federal and state laws, accreditation standards necessary to participate in government programs, and lawful institutional policies and procedures supersede these standards.

General Criteria

The radiographer:
1. Obtains assistance to support the quality assurance action plan.
2. Implements the quality assurance action plan.

Specific Criteria

None added.

RADIOGRAPHY QUALITY PERFORMANCE STANDARDS

Standard Seven—Outcomes Measurement

The radiographer assesses the outcome of the quality management action plan for equipment, materials, and processes.

Rationale

Outcomes assessment is an integral part of the ongoing quality management action plan to enhance diagnostic and therapeutic services.

General Stipulation

The individual must be educationally prepared and clinically competent as a prerequisite to professional practice. Federal and state laws, accreditation standards necessary to participate in government programs, and lawful institutional policies and procedures supersede these standards.

General Criteria

The radiographer:
1. Reviews the implementation process for accuracy and validity.
2. Determines that actual outcomes are within established criteria.
3. Develops and implements a modified action plan.

Specific Criteria

None added.

RADIOGRAPHY QUALITY PERFORMANCE STANDARDS

Standard Eight—Documentation

The radiographer documents quality assurance activities and results.

Rationale

Documentation provides evidence of quality assurance activities designed to enhance safety.

General Stipulation

The individual must be educationally prepared and clinically competent as a prerequisite to professional practice. Federal and state laws, accreditation standards necessary to participate in government programs, and lawful institutional policies and procedures supersede these standards.

General Criteria

The radiographer:
1. Maintains documentation of quality assurance activities, procedures, and results in accordance with established guidelines.
2. Documents in a timely, accurate, and comprehensive manner.

Specific Criteria

None added.

RADIOGRAPHY PROFESSIONAL PERFORMANCE STANDARDS

Standard One—Quality

The radiographer strives to provide optimal patient care.

Rationale

Patients expect and deserve optimal care during diagnosis and treatment.

General Stipulation

The individual must be educationally prepared and clinically competent as a prerequisite to professional practice. Federal and state laws, accreditation standards necessary to participate in government programs, and lawful institutional policies and procedures supersede these standards.

General Criteria

The radiographer:
1. Collaborates with others to elevate the quality of care.
2. Participates in ongoing quality assurance programs.
3. Adheres to standards, policies, and established guidelines.
4. Applies professional judgment and discretion while performing diagnostic study or treatment.
5. Anticipates and responds to patient needs.
6. Respects cultural variations.

Specific Criteria

None added.

RADIOGRAPHY PROFESSIONAL PERFORMANCE STANDARDS
Standard Two—Self-Assessment

The radiographer evaluates personal performance.

Rationale

Self-assessment is necessary for personal growth and professional development.

General Stipulation

The individual must be educationally prepared and clinically competent as a prerequisite to professional practice. Federal and state laws, accreditation standards necessary to participate in government programs, and lawful institutional policies and procedures supersede these standards.

General Criteria

The radiographer:
1. Assesses personal work ethics, behaviors, and attitudes.
2. Evaluates performance and recognizes opportunities for educational growth and improvement.
3. Recognizes and applies personal and professional strengths.
4. Participates in professional societies and organizations.

Specific Criteria

None added.

RADIOGRAPHY PROFESSIONAL PERFORMANCE STANDARDS
Standard Three—Education

The radiographer acquires and maintains current knowledge in practice.

Rationale

Advancements in the profession require additional knowledge and skills through education.

General Stipulation

The individual must be educationally prepared and clinically competent as a prerequisite to professional practice. Federal and state laws, accreditation standards necessary to participate in government programs, and lawful institutional policies and procedures supersede these standards.

General Criteria

The radiographer:
1. Completes education related to practice.
2. Maintains credentials and certification related to practice.
3. Participates in continuing education to maintain and enhance competency and performance.
4. Shares knowledge and expertise with others.

Specific Criteria

None added.

RADIOGRAPHY PROFESSIONAL PERFORMANCE STANDARDS
Standard Four—Collaboration and Collegiality

The radiographer promotes a positive and collaborative practice atmosphere with other members of the health care team.

Rationale

To provide quality patient care, all members of the health care team must communicate effectively and work together efficiently.

General Stipulation

The individual must be educationally prepared and clinically competent as a prerequisite to professional practice. Federal and state laws, accreditation standards necessary to participate in government programs, and lawful institutional policies and procedures supersede these standards.

General Criteria

The radiographer:

1. Shares knowledge and expertise with members of the health care team.
2. Develops collaborative partnerships to enhance quality and efficiency.
3. Promotes understanding of the profession.

Specific Criteria

None added.

RADIOGRAPHY PROFESSIONAL PERFORMANCE STANDARDS
Standard Five—Ethics

The radiographer adheres to the profession's accepted ethical standards.

Rationale

Decisions made and actions taken on behalf of the patient are based on a sound ethical foundation.

General Stipulation

The individual must be educationally prepared and clinically competent as a prerequisite to professional practice. Federal and state laws, accreditation standards necessary to participate in government programs, and lawful institutional policies and procedures supersede these standards.

General Criteria

The radiographer:

1. Provides health care services with respect for the patient's dignity, age-specific needs, and culture.
2. Acts as a patient advocate.
3. Takes responsibility for decisions made and actions taken.

4. Delivers patient care and service free from bias or discrimination.
5. Respects the patient's right to privacy and confidentiality.
6. Adheres to the established practice standards of the profession.

Specific Criteria

None added.

RADIOGRAPHY PROFESSIONAL PERFORMANCE STANDARDS
Standard Six—Research and Innovation

The radiographer participates in the acquisition and dissemination of knowledge and the advancement of the profession.

Rationale

Scholarly activities such as research, scientific investigation, presentation, and publication advance the profession.

General Stipulation

The individual must be educationally prepared and clinically competent as a prerequisite to professional practice. Federal and state laws, accreditation standards necessary to participate in government programs, and lawful institutional policies and procedures supersede these standards.

General Criteria

The radiographer:

1. Reads and evaluates research relevant to the profession.
2. Participates in data collection.
3. Investigates innovative methods for application in practice.
4. Shares information through publication, presentation, and collaboration.
5. Adopts new best practices.
6. Pursues lifelong learning.

Specific Criteria

None added.

Informed Consent Form

☐ **MEDICAL CENTER CAMPUS**   Southwest Washington Medical Center   ☐ **MEMORIAL CAMPUS**
VANCOUVER, WA

SPECIAL CONSENT TO OPERATION, POST OPERATIVE CARE, MEDICAL TREATMENT, ANESTHESIA, OR OTHER PROCEDURE

Patient:_____   Patient No._____

Washington State law guarantees that you have both the right and obligation to make decisions concerning your health care. Your physician can provide you with the necessary information and advice, but as a member of the health care team, you must enter into the decision making process. This form has been designed to acknowledge your acceptance of treatment recommended by your physician.

1. I hereby authorize Dr._____ and/or such associates or assistants as may be selected by said physician to treat the following condition(s) which has (have) been explained to me: (Explain the nature of the condition(s) in professional and lay language.)

_____
_____
_____

2. The procedures planned for treatment of my condition(s) have been explained to me by my physician. I understand them to be: (Describe procedures to be performed in professional and lay language.)

_____
_____
_____

At:_____
(NAME OF HOSPITAL OR MEDICAL FACILITY)

3. I recognize that, during the course of the operation, post operative care, medical treatment, anesthesia or other procedure, unforeseen conditions may necessitate additional or different procedures than those above set forth. I therefore authorize my above named physician, and his or her assistants or designees, to perform such surgical or other procedures as are in the exercise of his, her or their professional judgment necessary and desirable. The authority granted under this paragraph shall extend to the treatment of all conditions that require treatment and are not known to my physician at the time the medical or surgical procedure is commenced.

4. I have been informed that there are significant risks such as severe loss of blood, infection and cardiac arrest that can lead to death or permanent or partial disability, which may be attendant to the performance of any procedure. I acknowledge that no warranty or guarantee has been made to me as to result or cure.

IMPORTANT: HAVE PATIENT SIGN FULL OR LIMITED DISCLOSURE BOX AND SIGNATURE LINE AT BOTTOM.

Full Disclosure

I certify that my physician has informed me of the nature and character of the proposed treatment, of the anticipated results of the proposed treatment, of the possible alternative forms of treatment; and the recognized serious possible risks, complications, and the anticipated benefits involved in the proposed treatment and in the alternative forms of treatment, including non-treatment.

_____
PATIENT/OTHER LEGALLY RESPONSIBLE PERSON SIGN
IF APPLICABLE

Limited Disclosure

I certify that my physician has explained to me that I have the right to have clearly described to me the nature and character of the proposed treatment; the anticipated results of the proposed treatment; the alternative forms of treatment; and the recognized serious possible risks, complications, and anticipated benefits involved in the proposed treatment, and in the alternative forms of treatment, including non-treatment.

I do not wish to have these risks and facts explained to me.

_____
PATIENT/OTHER LEGALLY RESPONSIBLE PERSON SIGN
IF APPLICABLE

Any sections below which do not apply to the proposed treatment may be crossed out. All sections crossed out must be initialed by both physician and patient.

5. I consent to the administration of anesthesia by my attending physician, by an anesthesiologist, or other qualified party under the direction of a physician as may be deemed necessary. I understand that all anesthetics involve risks of complications and serious possible damage to vital organs such as the brain, heart, lung, liver and kidney and that in some cases may result in paralysis, cardiac arrest and/or brain death from both known and unknown causes. I understand there is a risk of dental injury during airway management.

6. I consent to the use of transfusion of blood and blood products as deemed necessary, and potential complications associated with this procedure have been explained by my physician.

7. Any tissues or parts surgically removed may be disposed of by the hospital or physician in accordance with accustomed practice.

I certify this form has been fully explained to me, that I have read it or have had it read to me, that the blank spaces have been filled in, and that I understand its contents.

DATE:_____ TIME:_____ A.M. P.M.

_____
PATIENT/OTHER LEGALLY RESPONSIBLE PERSON SIGN

WITNESS:_____

_____
RELATIONSHIP OF LEGALLY RESPONSIBLE PERSON TO PATIENT

Courtesy Southwest Washington Medical Center.

Accepted Abbreviations and Descriptive Terms Used in Charting

Abbreviation	Word or Phrase
Ab	abdomen
ac	before meals
ad lib	freely, as desired
AED	automatic external defibrillator
amt	amount
AP	apical pulse
aq	water
2 i d	two times per day
BP	blood pressure
BRP	bathroom privileges
C or cent	centigrade
$\overline{c}$	with
caps	capsule
CHF	congestive heart failure
cm	centimeter
CPR	cardiopulmonary resuscitation
ECG or EKG	electrocardiogram
ED	emergency department
EEG	electroencephalogram
EENT	eye, ear, nose, and throat
ENT	ear, nose, and throat
ER	emergency room or emergency department
fld	fluid
GB	gallbladder
GI	gastrointestinal
Gm or gm	gram
gtt	drop, drops
GU	genitourinary
gyn	gynecology
(H)	hypodermically
H or hrs	hour, hours
H_2O	water

Abbreviation	Word or Phrase
HA	headache
Hct	hematocrit
Hgb or Hb	hemoglobin
I&O	intake and output
IM	intramuscular
IV	intravenous
Kg or kg	kilogram
KUB	kidneys, ureters, and bladder
L	left
L	liter
lab	laboratory
LBP	low back pain
LLQ	left lower quadrant— abdomen
LP	lumbar puncture
LUQ	left upper quadrant— abdomen
MI	myocardial infarction
mcg	microgram
mg	milligram
mL	milliliter
MVC	motor vehicle crash
noct	at night
NPO	nothing by mouth
NS	normal saline solution
OB or obs	obstetrics
OD	right eye
OJ	orange juice
OPC	outpatient clinic
OR	operating room
OS	left eye
P or $\overline{P}$	after
pc	after meals
pH	hydrogen ion concentration

Abbreviation	Word or Phrase
PO	by mouth
PP	postprandial, after meals
prn	when necessary, as needed
qh	every hour
q 2 h	every 2 hours
4 i d	four times per day
qs	quantity sufficient
qns	quantity not sufficient
RBC	red blood cells or red blood cell count
RLQ	right lower quadrant—abdomen
RUQ	right upper quadrant—abdomen
Rx	therapy

Abbreviation	Word or Phrase
s̄	without
SOB	short of breath
spec	specimen
subcut.	subcutaneous
STAT	at once
3 i d	three times per day
TPR	temperature, pulse, respiration
URI	upper respiratory infection
UTI	urinary tract infection
WBC	white blood cells or white blood cell count
WC	wheelchair
wt	weight
×	times

Do Not Use the Following Dangerous Abbreviations and Dose Designations

Abbreviation or Expression	Intended Meaning	Misinterpretation	Correction
@	At	Mistaken for number 2	Write "at"
>	Greater than	Mistaken for number 7	Write "greater than"
<	Less than	Mistaken for letter L	Write "less than"
μg	Microgram	Mistaken for mg	Write "mcg"
/ (slash mark)	Separates two doses or indicates "per"	Mistaken for the number 1	Do not use slash mark to separate doses. Write out "per"
cc	Cubic centimeters	Misread as "U" (units)	Write "mL" or "milliliters"
D/C	Discharge, discontinue	Two meanings confused	Write out "discharge" or "discontinue"
IU	International Unit	Mistaken for IV or the number 10	Write "International Unit"
MS, MSO_4, $MgSO_4$	Morphine sulfate or magnesium sulfate	Confused for one another	Write "$MgSO_4$," "morphine sulfate," or "magnesium sulfate"
Q.D., QD, q.d., qd	Daily	Misread or mistaken for QOD	Write "daily"
Q.O.D., QOD, q.o.d., qod	Every other day	Misread or mistaken for QD	Write "every other day"
qhs	Nightly at bedtime	Misread as every hour	Write "nightly"
SC	Subcutaneous	Mistaken for SL (sublingual)	Write "subcut" or "subcutaneous"
ss	Sliding scale (insulin) One-half (apothecary)	Mistaken for 55	Spell out "sliding scale" Write "one-half" or "1/2"
sub q	Subcutaneous	"q" is mistaken to mean "every"	Write "subcut" or "subcutaneous"
U or u	Unit or units	May be read as a 0 or a 4	There is no acceptable abbreviation; write "unit"
Zero after decimal point (1.0)	1 mg	Misread as 10 mg if decimal point is not seen	Do not use terminal zeros after whole numbers
No zero before decimal dose (.5 mg)	0.5 mg	Misread as 5 mg if decimal point is not seen	Always use zero before decimal point when dose amount is less than a whole number

Descriptive Terms Typically Used in Charting

Area of Concern	Factor to be Charted	Suggested Terms to Use
Abdomen	Hard, boardlike Appears swollen, rounded Soft, flabby, flat Area or region	Hard, rigid Distended Relaxed, flaccid, flat **Region** 1. Right hypochondriac 2. Epigastric 3. Left hypochondriac 4. Right lumbar 5. Umbilical 6. Left lumbar 7. Right iliac 8. Hypogastric 9. Left iliac region 1. Right upper quadrant 2. Left upper quadrant 3. Right lower quadrant 4. Left lower quadrant

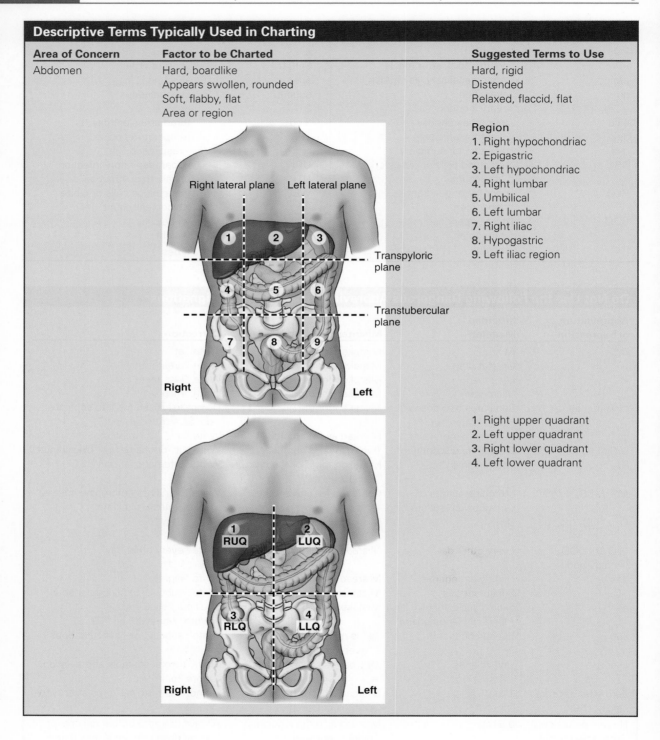

Descriptive Terms Typically Used in Charting—cont'd

Area of Concern	Factor to be Charted	Suggested Terms to Use
Amounts	Large amount	Excessive, profuse, copious
	Moderate amount	Moderate, usual
	Small amount	Scanty, slight
Appearance, general	Thin and undernourished	Emaciated
	Fat, greatly overweight	Obese
	Seems very sick	Acutely ill
Appetite	Loss of appetite	Anorexia
	Would not eat	Refused food (state reason)
Attitude (mental state)	Has "don't care" attitude	Apathetic
	Afraid, worried	Anxious, apprehensive
	Feeling blue, sad	Depressed
		Other characteristic terms: anxiety, defiance, anger, pain, boredom, happiness, dissatisfaction, irritability, worry
Back regions	Upper back	Thoracic region, dorsal region
	Small of the back	Lumbar region
	Lower spine	Sacral region
	Buttocks	Gluteal area
Bleeding	Very little	Oozing
	Abnormal bleeding	Hemorrhage
	Nosebleed	Epistaxis
	Blood in vomitus	Hematemesis
	Blood in urine	Hematuria
	Coughing or spitting up blood	Hemoptysis
	Bleeding stopped	Hemorrhage controlled, hemostasis
Breathing	Breathing	Respiration
	Act of inhaling	Inspiration
	Act of exhaling	Expiration
	Difficulty in breathing	Dyspnea, dyspneic
	Unable to breathe lying down	Orthopnea
	Cessation of breathing for short periods	Apnea
	Rapid breathing	Hyperpnea
	Increasing dyspnea with periods of apnea	Cheyne-Stokes respiration
	Large amount of air inspired or expired	Deep breathing
	Small amount of air inspired or expired	Shallow breathing
	Abnormal variations in rhythm	Irregular respiration
Chill	Blanket applied to keep warm	External heat applied
	Severity (degree of)	Severe, moderate, slight
	Long lasting	Persistent, long duration
	Lasting only briefly	Short duration
	Came on suddenly	Sudden onset
Level of consciousness	Fully conscious, aware of surroundings	Alert, fully conscious
	Only partly conscious	Stuporous
	Unconscious, but can be aroused	Semicomatose
	Unconscious, cannot be aroused	Comatose

Images from Bontrager KL, Lampignano JP: *Textbook of radiographic positioning and related anatomy*, ed 8, St Louis, 2014, Mosby.

Incident Report Form

Redland Valley Hospital INCIDENT REPORT	(Patient ID Imprint)

(Not a part of medical record)

Incident date _____ Time _____

Affected person ☐ Patient ☐ Employee ☐ Visitor ☐ Other _____

Name _____ Gender _____ Address _____

Phone _____

Location of incident: _____

_____

_____

_____

Description of occurrence: _____

_____

Condition of victim:

  Before incident: _____

  After incident: _____

Seen by physician: ☐ Yes ☐ No   Physician name: _____

Date _____ Time _____

Action taken: _____

_____

_____

Name: _____	Witness: _____
Signature: _____	Signature: _____
Title: _____	Witness: _____
	Signature: _____

Facility copy original (White)   Attorney copy (Blue)   Insurance copy (Yellow)

Courtesy Southwest Washington Medical Center.

Abbreviated List of Useful Clinical Phrases in Spanish*

SPANISH

Bold face type indicates accented syllables.

1. Good morning!
   ¡Buenos días!
   Boo-**eh**-nohs   **dee**-ahs!

2. Hello, Mr. Martinez.
   Hola, señor Martinez.
   Oh-lah,   seh-**nyohr**   Mahr-**tee**-nehs.

3. My name is _____.
   Me llamo _____.
   May **yah**-moh _____.

4. I am the x-ray technologist.
   Soy la radiografía tecnólogo.
   Soy lah   rah-dee-oh-**grah**-fee-ah   teck-**noh**-loh-goh.

5. What is your name?
   ¿Cómo se llama?
   Coh-moh   say   **yah**-mah?

6. What is your last name?
   ¿Cuál es su appellido?
   Koo-**ahl** ehs   soo   ah-peh-**yee**-doh?

7. How old are you?
   ¿Quántos años tiene?
   Koo-**ahn**-tohs   **ah**-nyohs   tee-**eh**-neh?

8. What is your birthdate?
   ¿Cuál es la fecha de nacimiento?
   Koo-**ahl** ehs   lah   **feh**-chah   deh   nah-see-mee-**ehn**-toh?

9. Please sit here.
   Sientese aquí por favor.
   See-**en**-teh-seh   ah-**kee**   pore   fah-**bore.**

10. Are you pregnant?
    ¿Está embarazada?
    Ess-**tah**   em-bah-rah-**sah**-dah?

11. When was your last menstrual period?
    ¿Cuándo tuvo su último menstruación?
    Koo-**ahn**-doh   **too**-boh   soo   **ool**-tee-moh   mehns-troo-ah-see-**ohn?**

12. Do you have pain?
    ¿Tiene dolor?
    Tee-**eh**-neh   doh-**lohr?**

13. Where does it hurt?
    ¿Dónde le duele?
    Dohn-deh   leh   doo-**eh**-leh?

14. What symptoms do you have?
    ¿Qué sintomas tiene?
    Keh   seen-**toh**-mahs tee-**eh**-neh?

15. Do you have allergies?
    ¿Tiene alergias?
    Tee-**eh**-neh   ah-**lehr**-ghee-ahs?

16. What allergies do you have?
    ¿Qué alergias tiene?
    Keh   ah-**lehr**-ghee-ahs   tee-**eh**-neh?

17. Do you have medical problems?
    ¿Tiene problemas médicos?
    Tee-**eh**-neh   proh-**bleh**-mahs   **meh**-dee-kohs?

18. Do you have cardiac problems?
    ¿Tiene problemas cardíacos?
    Tee-**eh**-neh   proh-**bleh**-mahs   kahr-**dee**-ah-kohs?

19. Do you have respiratory problems?
    ¿Tiene problemas respiratorios?
    Tee-**eh**-neh   proh-**bleh**-mahs   rehs-peer-eh-**toh**-ree-ohs?

20. Do you have kidney problems?
    ¿Tiene problemas de riñón?
    Tee-**eh**-neh   proh-**bleh**-mahs   de   ree-**nyohn?**

*Modified from Joyce EV, Villanueva ME: *Say It in Spanish,* ed 3, St. Louis, 2004, Saunders.

21. Please come with me.
Favor de venir conmigo.
Fah-**bore** day veh-**neer** kohn-**mee**-goh.
22. Please remove all your clothing and put on the gown.
Favor de quitar toda la ropa y vestirse en la bata.
Fah-**bore** deh kee-**tar** **toh**-dah lah **roh**-pah ee vess-**teer**-she en lah **bah**-tah.
23. Please remove your clothing to the waist and put on the gown.
Favor de quitar la ropa hasta la cintura y vestirse en la bata.
Fah-**bore** deh kee-**tar** lah **roh**-pah ah-stah lah sin-**too**-rah ee vess-**teer**-seh en lah **bah**-tah.
24. I'm going to take x-rays.
Le tomaré radiografías.
Leh toh-mah-**reh** rah-dee-oh-**grah**-fee-ahs.
25. Can you stand?
¿Puede usted estar parado?
Poo-**eh**-deh oo-**sted** ess-**tahr** pah-**rah**-doh?
26. Please face this board.
Haga frente por favor a este tablero.
Ah-gah **fren**-teh pore fah-**bore** ah **ehs**-teh tah-**bleh**-roh.
27. Stand here, please.
Parese aquí por favor.
Pah-**reh**-seh ah-**kee** pore fah-**bore.**
28. Lift your arms.
Levante los brazos.
Leh-**vahn**-teh los **brah**-sohs.
29. Please turn to your right/left.
Dé vuelta por favor a su derecho/a la izquierda.
Deh boo-**ehl**-tah pore fah-**bore** ah soo deh-**reh**-cho/ah lah ees-kee-**air**-dah.
30. Please lie down on the table.
Acuestese en la mesa por favor.
Ah-**quest**-eh-seh en lah **meh**-sah pore fah-**bore.**
31. Please lie on your back/stomach.
Por favor mentira en su trasero/estómago.
Pore fah-**bore** men-tee- rah en soo trah-**seh**-roh/ehs-**toh**-mah-goh.
32. Don't move.
No se mueva.
Noh seh moo-**ay**-vah.
33. When I tell you, hold your breath.
Cuándo le avise, no respire.
Kwan-doh leh ah-**vee**-seh, noh reh-**spee**-reh.

34. Stop breathing.
No respire.
Noh reh-**spee**-reh.
35. You can breathe now.
Ya puede respirar ahora.
Yah poo-**ay**-deh reh-spee-**rahr** ah-**ohr**-ah.
36. Sit back in the chair.
Siéntese detrás en la silla.
See-**en**-teh-seh deh-**trahs** en lah **see**-yah.
37. Move onto the stretcher.
Muévase sobre el ensanchador.
Moo-**eh**-veh-she **soh**-breh ell en-sahn-chah-**dohr.**
38. Remain here.
Quedese aquí.
Keh-**deh**-seh ah-**kee.**
39. I will return shortly.
Regresarse en seguida.
Reh-greh-**sahr**-seh en seh-**ghee**-dah.
40. One time more.
Uno vez mas.
Oo-noh vehs mahs.
41. You need to drink water.
Necesita tomar agua.
Neh-**seh**-see-tah toh-**mahr ah**-goo-ah.
42. You cannot smoke here.
No puede fumar aquí.
Noh poo-**eh**-deh foo-**mahr** ah-**kee.**
43. I am finished. That's all.
Ya termine. Es todo.
Yah tare-**mee**-neh. Ehs **toh**-doh.
44. Now you can get dressed.
Ahora se puede ponar su ropa.
Ah-**ohr**-ah seh poo-**ay**-day poh-**nahr** soo **roh**-pah.
45. The doctor will talk to you.
El doctor hablara con usted.
Ell dock-**tohr** ah-**blah**-rah kohn oo-**sted.**
46. Thank you. Goodbye.
Gracias. Adiós.
Grah-see-ahs. Ah-dee-**ohs.**
47. You are welcome.
De nada.
Deh **nah**-dah.

Radiology Department Infection Control Procedures

ROUTINE DEPARTMENTAL CLEANING

Counters and Surfaces Frequently Contacted by Personnel Who Handle Patients

- Any hospital-grade disinfectant-detergent registered by the U.S. Environmental Protection Agency (EPA) may be used for cleaning counters and surfaces. Additionally, the use of a dilute bleach solution* or commercially prepared germicide-impregnated disposable cloths may be used.
- Wipe down twice daily using disinfectant, dilute bleach,* or germicide cloths. (NOTE: These surfaces are to include counters and work areas in radiography rooms, counters surrounding reception desk, image processing counters, and counters in image-viewing areas.)

Closed Storage Areas Containing Linen and Nonsterile Medical Supplies

- Wipe shelves and doors weekly with disinfectant, dilute bleach,* or germicide cloths.

Storage Areas Containing Sterile Supplies

- Dust daily; remove all items from shelves weekly and wash surfaces using disinfectant.
- Check expiration dates on all sterile supplies at time of weekly cleaning. Resterilize or replace items as needed.

Lead Aprons and Gloves

- Clean weekly using disinfectant, dilute bleach,* or germicide cloths.
- Clean following contact with blood or body fluids, using recommended disinfectant.

*Use a solution of 5.25% sodium hypochlorite (household bleach) diluted 1:10 with water.

Mobile X-Ray Machines

- Clean after each use using disinfectant, dilute bleach,* or germicide cloth. Pay particular attention to the tube handles, collimator dials, on-button, exposure switch, drive handles, grid cap, and cassettes. A DR image receptor and its cord, if applicable, must also be wiped down, even if placed in a protective cover when used.
- Wipe thoroughly with disinfectant, dilute bleach,* or germicide before entering surgery, newborn nursery, or patient room designated for protective precautions.
- Mobile machines should be thoroughly cleaned weekly.

X-Ray Machines, Tables, Vertical Buckys

- Thoroughly wash radiography table top and vertical bucky with a disinfectant, dilute bleach,* or germicide cloth after each patient contact.
- Change pillowcases, using clean linen for each patient.
- Dust daily the overhead tube, spot film devices, image intensifiers, and television monitors.
- Dust weekly the overhead tracks for ceiling-mounted equipment using a vacuum cleaner.
- Wash weekly the control stands, spot film devices, and the entire radiography table with disinfectant.

Wheelchairs and Stretchers

- Thoroughly clean entire surface of wheelchair and stretcher with a disinfectant, dilute bleach,* or germicide cloth weekly.
- Wipe down patient contact areas after each use.
- Wash down wheelchairs or stretchers used for isolation patients with disinfectant immediately after use.
- Wash down wheelchairs or stretchers contaminated with patient secretions or excretions with a disinfectant or dilute bleach* before being reused.

PERSONNEL PRACTICES

Hand Hygiene

Personnel are instructed to wash hands with either a nonantimicrobial soap or antimicrobial soap and water in the following clinical situations:

- When hands are visibly dirty or contaminated with blood or body fluids
- Before eating and after using a restroom
- After blowing or wiping your nose
- If exposure to *Bacillus anthracis* or *Clostridium difficile* is known or suspected, because the physical action of washing and rinsing hands helps to remove spores

An alcohol-based hand rub, or alternatively hand-washing, may be used in these clinical situations:

- On reporting for duty
- Between examinations of patients
- Before donning sterile gloves
- Before inserting indwelling urinary catheters
- After contact with patient's intact skin (eg, taking a pulse, blood pressure, lifting a patient)
- After contact with inanimate objects, including medical equipment, in the immediate vicinity of the patient
- After removing gloves
- On entering and leaving isolation areas or handling articles for isolation areas
- After handling dressings, sputum containers, urinals, catheters, or bedpans (use handwashing if hands are visibly contaminated)
- If moving from a contaminated body site to a clean body site during patient care
- On completing duty

Standard Precautions

All personnel are to observe Standard Precautions (see Chapter 9 and Appendix G) whenever contact with blood or body fluids is possible.

Good Personal Hygiene

Personnel are directed to practice the following:

- Bathe and wash hair regularly.
- Wear clean uniforms or scrubs and duty shoes.
- Pay particular attention to frequently overlooked items of personal cleanliness, such as fingernails, watchbands, intricate jewelry, and shoelaces.
- Change clothing that is soiled in the process of patient care before continuing work.
- Do not report for duty when affected by the following:
  - Contagious skin diseases
  - Acute upper respiratory infections
  - Any other communicable diseases

Infection Control Guidelines*

STANDARD PRECAUTIONS

Use Standard Precautions for the care of all patients. Assume that every person is potentially infected or colonized with an organism that could be transmitted in the health care setting.

A. Hand Hygiene
   1. Perform hand hygiene after touching blood, body fluids, secretions, excretions, mucous membranes, nonintact skin, potentially contaminated intact skin, and contaminated items, whether or not gloves are worn. Perform hand hygiene immediately after gloves are removed, between patient contacts, and when otherwise indicated to avoid transfer of microorganisms to other patients or environments. It may be necessary to wash hands between tasks and procedures on the same patient to prevent cross-contamination of different body sites.
   2. Wash hands when hands are visibly dirty, contaminated with proteinaceous material, visibly soiled with blood or body fluids, or if contact with *Clostridium difficile* or *Bacillus anthracis* spores is likely to have occurred. Use either a plain (nonantimicrobial) soap and water or an antimicrobial soap and water to wash hands.

   3. If hands are not visibly soiled, alcohol hand rubs may be used to perform hand hygiene.
B. Gloves
   1. Wear gloves (clean, nonsterile gloves are adequate) when touching blood, body fluids, secretions, excretions, mucous membranes, nonintact skin, potentially contaminated intact skin, and contaminated items.
   2. Change gloves between tasks and procedures on the same patient after contact with material that may contain a high concentration of microorganisms.
   3. Remove gloves promptly after use, before touching noncontaminated items and environmental surfaces, and before going to another patient, and perform hand hygiene immediately to avoid transfer of microorganisms to other patients or environments.
C. Mask, Eye Protection, or Face Shield
   Wear a mask and eye protection or a face shield to protect mucous membranes of the eyes, nose, and mouth during procedures and patient-care activities that are likely to generate splashes or sprays of blood, body fluids, secretions, or excretions.
D. Gown
   1. Wear a gown (a clean, nonsterile gown is adequate) to protect skin and to prevent soiling of clothing during procedures and patient-care activities that are likely to generate splashes or sprays of blood, body fluids, secretions, or excretions.
   2. Select a gown that is appropriate for the activity and amount of fluid likely to be encountered.
   3. Remove a soiled gown as promptly as possible, and perform hand hygiene to avoid transfer of microorganisms to other patients or environments.

*From Centers for Disease Control and Prevention: Siegel JD, Rhinehart E, Jackson M, Chiarello L, and the Healthcare Infection Control Practice Advisory Committee, 2007 Guidelines for Isolation Precautions: Preventing Transmission of Infectious Agents in Healthcare Settings, June 2007. Available at http://www.cdc.gov/hicpac/2007IP/2007isolationPrecautions.html

E. Patient-Care Equipment
1. Handle used patient-care equipment soiled with blood, body fluids, secretions, or excretions in a manner that prevents skin and mucous membrane exposures, contamination of clothing, and transfer of microorganisms to other patients and environments.
2. Ensure that reusable equipment is not used for the care of another patient until it has been cleaned and reprocessed appropriately.
3. Ensure that single-use items are discarded properly.

F. Environmental Control
Ensure that the hospital has adequate procedures for the routine care, cleaning, and disinfection of environmental surfaces, beds, bedrails, bedside equipment, and other frequently touched surfaces, and ensure that these procedures are being followed.

G. Linen
Handle, transport, and process used linen soiled with blood, body fluids, secretions, or excretions in a manner that prevents skin and mucous membrane exposures and contamination of clothing, and that avoids transfer of microorganisms to other patients and environments.

H. Needles and Other Sharps and Patient Resuscitation Equipment
1. Take care to prevent injuries when using needles, scalpels, and other sharp instruments or devices; when handling sharp instruments after procedures; when cleaning used instruments; and when disposing of used needles.
2. Never recap used needles, or otherwise manipulate them using both hands, or use any other technique that involves directing the point of a needle toward any part of the body; rather, use either a one-handed "scoop" technique or a mechanical device designed for holding the needle sheath.
3. Do not remove used needles from disposable syringes by hand, and do not bend, break, or otherwise manipulate used needles by hand.
4. Place used disposable syringes and needles, scalpel blades, and other sharp items in appropriate puncture-resistant containers, which are located as close as practical to the area in which the items were used, and place reusable syringes and needles in a puncture-resistant container for transport to the reprocessing area. Use mouthpieces, resuscitation bags, or other ventilation devices as an alternative to mouth-to-mouth resuscitation methods in areas where the need for resuscitation is predictable.
5. Refer to Chapters 7, 9, and 14 for OSHA policies regarding safe medical devices and practices to ensure safety of health care workers.

I. Patient Placement
Place a patient who contaminates the environment, or who does not (or cannot be expected to) assist in maintaining appropriate hygiene or environmental control, in a private room. If a private room is not available, consult with infection control professionals regarding patient placement or other alternatives.
NOTE: Three new elements have been added to Standard Precautions with a focus on patient protection. These new elements are described in J, K, and L.

J. Respiratory Hygiene/Cough Etiquette
The following measures to contain respiratory secretions are recommended for health care facility staff, patients, and visitors with signs and symptoms of respiratory infection.
1. Cover the mouth when sneezing or coughing, using tissues to contain respiratory secretions. If a tissue is unavailable, cough or sneeze into your sleeve or elbow rather than your hands.
2. Dispose of used tissues in no-touch receptacles.
3. Perform hand hygiene after soiling of hands with respiratory secretions.
4. Wear a surgical mask if tolerated or maintain spatial separation of more than 3 feet if possible.
5. Post signs in waiting areas for patients and visitors that encourage respiratory hygiene/cough etiquette.
6. Provide tissues and no-touch receptacles for used tissues.
7. Provide conveniently located dispensers of alcohol-based handrub or, where sinks are available, supplies for handwashing.

K. Safe Injection Practices to Prevent Infections in Patients
1. Do not administer medications from a syringe to multiple patients, even if needle or cannula on the syringe is changed.
2. Use intravenous bags, tubing, and connectors for one patient only and dispose appropriately after use.

3. Use single-dose vials for parenteral medications whenever possible and do not administer medications from single-dose vials to multiple patients.
4. If multidose vials must be used, both the needle or cannula and syringe used to access the vial must be sterile.
5. Multiple dose vials should be reused only for the same patient on the same day due to the high incidence of cross-contamination when they are stored for reuse on another occasion.
L. Infection Control Practices for Special Lumbar Puncture Procedures

Wear a surgical mask when placing a catheter or injecting material into the spinal canal or subdural space (ie, during myelograms, lumbar puncture, and spinal or epidural anesthesia) to prevent droplet spread of oral flora during spinal procedures.

TRANSMISSION-BASED PRECAUTIONS

There are three categories of transmission-based precautions: airborne, droplet, and contact precautions. Transmission-based precautions are used in addition to Standard Precautions for patients with documented or suspected infection or colonization with highly transmissible pathogens. Some infections have multiple routes of transmission and may fall under more than one of these precaution categories. Link to the CDC website to obtain additional information.

Airborne Precautions

In addition to Standard Precautions, use Airborne Precautions for patients known or suspected to have serious illnesses transmitted by airborne droplet nuclei.

Diseases Requiring Airborne Precautions

- Measles
- Varicella (including disseminated zoster)
- Tuberculosis
- Severe acute respiratory syndrome

Precautions

- Wear respiratory protection (N95 or higher level respirator) when entering the room of a patient with known or suspected infectious pulmonary tuberculosis.
- Susceptible persons should not enter the room of patients known or suspected to have measles (rubeola) or varicella (chickenpox) if other immune caregivers are available.
- If susceptible persons must enter the room of a patient known or suspected to have measles or varicella, they should wear respiratory protection (N95 respirator).
- Persons immune to measles (rubeola) or varicella need not wear respiratory protection.

Droplet Precautions

In addition to Standard Precautions, use Droplet Precautions, or the equivalent, for patients known or suspected to be infected with microorganisms transmitted by large particle droplets that can be generated by patients during coughing, sneezing, talking, or the performance of procedures.

Diseases Requiring Droplet Precautions

- Invasive *Haemophilus influenzae* type b disease, including meningitis, pneumonia, epiglottitis, and sepsis
- Invasive *Neisseria meningitidis* disease, including meningitis, pneumonia, and sepsis
- Other serious bacterial respiratory infections spread by droplet transmission, including:
  - Diphtheria (pharyngeal)
  - Mycoplasma pneumonia
  - Pertussis
  - Pneumonic plague
  - Streptococcal (group A) pharyngitis, pneumonia, or scarlet fever in infants and young children
- Serious viral infections spread by droplet transmission, including:
  - Adenovirus
  - Influenza
  - Mumps
  - Parvovirus B19
  - Rubella

Precautions

Wear a surgical mask when working within 3 feet of the patient. Some hospitals may implement the wearing of a mask to enter the room.

Contact Precautions

In addition to Standard Precautions, use Contact Precautions, or the equivalent, for specified patients known or suspected to be infected or colonized with epidemiologically important microorganisms that can be transmitted by direct contact with the patient (hand or skin-to-skin contact that occurs when performing patient-care activities that require touching the patient's dry skin) or indirect contact (touching) with environmental surfaces or patient-care items in the patient's environment.

Diseases Requiring Contact Precautions

- Gastrointestinal, respiratory, skin, or wound infections or colonization with multidrug-resistant bacteria judged by the infection control program, based on current state, regional, or national recommendations, to be of special clinical and epidemiologic significance.
- Enteric infections with a low infectious dose or prolonged environmental survival, including: enterocolitis caused by:
  - *C.difficile,* enterohemorrhagic *Escherichia coli* O157:H7, *Shigella* sp., hepatitis A, and rotavirus for diapered or incontinent patients
  - Respiratory syncytial virus, parainfluenza virus, or enteroviral infections in infants and young children
- Skin infections that are highly contagious or that may occur on dry skin, including:
  - Diphtheria (cutaneous)
  - Herpes simplex virus (neonatal or mucocutaneous)
  - Impetigo
  - Major (noncontained) abscesses, cellulitis, or decubiti
  - Pediculosis
  - Scabies
  - Staphylococcal furunculosis in infants and young children

- Varicella zoster (disseminated or in the immunocompromised host)
- Viral hemorrhagic infections (Ebola, Lassa, or Marburg)

Precautions

- Wear clean, nonsterile gloves.
- A clean, nonsterile gown is also worn whenever you anticipate that your clothing will have substantial contact with the patient, environmental surfaces, or items in the patient's room, or if the patient is incontinent or has diarrhea, an ileostomy, a colostomy, or wound drainage not contained by a dressing.
- During the course of providing care for a patient, change gloves after having contact with infective material that may contain high concentrations of microorganisms (eg, fecal material and wound drainage).
- Remove gown and gloves before leaving the patient's room and wash hands immediately with an antimicrobial agent or a waterless antiseptic agent.
- After glove and gown removal, ensure that clothing does not contact potentially contaminated environmental surfaces to avoid transfer of microorganisms to other patients or environments.

NOTE: Remember to follow Standard Precautions in addition to the Transmission-Based Precautions described above. This includes practicing hand hygiene before and after patient contact, disinfecting equipment and supplies before use on other patients, and proper placement of contaminated disposable items and linen.

Urine Collection

PROCEDURE FOR COLLECTING A URINE SPECIMEN

Because improperly collected urine may yield incorrect test results, urine should always be collected using the clean-catch midstream specimen technique. This technique is based on the concept that the tissues adjacent to the urethral meatus must be cleansed with an appropriate cleansing solution before collection to avoid contamination of the specimen. Only the middle portion of the urine stream is collected for analysis. The initial and final portions of the urine stream are discarded.

Supplies

- Urine specimen containers should be clean and dry and are used only once. A variety of collection containers is available. Some have pour spouts to facilitate filling the urinalysis tubes, and others have caps. Cups with caps should be used if the specimen will not be analyzed immediately after collection. This type is most practical for occasional use in the imaging department.
- Gauze sponges moistened with an appropriate cleansing solution are used to cleanse the patient prior to urine collection. A variety of appropriate cleansing solutions is available, and standard 2- × 2-inch gauze

sponges are adequate. Towelettes premoistened with an appropriate cleansing solution are also available and can be used in place of gauze sponges.

Specimen Collection
Female

A female patient spreads the labia and cleanses in an anterior-to-posterior direction with three separate gauze sponges or towelettes moistened with cleansing solution. A separate sponge is used to cleanse each side of the meatus, and a third sponge is wiped directly over the meatus. A dry sponge is then wiped directly over the meatus. Keeping the labia spread, a small amount of urine is passed into the toilet. At least 15 mL of urine is collected into an appropriate specimen container. The remaining urine in the bladder is then passed into the toilet.

Male

A circumcised male cleanses the glans penis using sponges moistened with cleansing solution, wiping from the center outward. An uncircumcised male must first retract the foreskin and keep it retracted during cleansing and collection. A dry sponge is used to wipe directly over the meatus. At least 15 mL of urine is collected into a specimen container from the middle portion of the urine stream.

Two- And Three-Person Lift

These manual lifts can result in some degree of risk and discomfort to the patient. Mechanical lifts are definitely preferred when they are available.

TWO-PERSON LIFT

If the patient's weight permits, two people can perform the lift from the wheelchair to the table (Appendix Fig. I-1). The stronger of the two is the primary lifter, and the second person assists. First, place the wheelchair parallel to the table and lock the wheels. Next, remove the chair arm that is nearest the table, if possible. Instruct the patient to cross both arms over the chest. The primary lifter then stands behind the chair and reaches around the patient, extending his or her arms through the patient's axillae and grasping the patient's forearms from the top. The assistant kneels on one knee near the patient's feet and cradles the patient's

thighs in one arm and the lower legs in the other. On signal, both lift together and place the patient gently on the table.

THREE-PERSON LIFT

The three-person lift is similar to the two-person lift and is safer if the patient's weight is too much for two people to lift easily (Appendix Fig. I-2). In this case, remove both arms of the wheelchair and position the first two lifters as for the two-person lift. The third lifter kneels on one knee at the side of the chair farthest from the table, placing one arm around the patient's waist and the other under the buttocks. Next, all lift together on signal. The role of the third lifter is primarily to assist in raising the patient from the chair. The wheelchair will block any forward motion of the third lifter; therefore the first two lifters must complete the transfer.

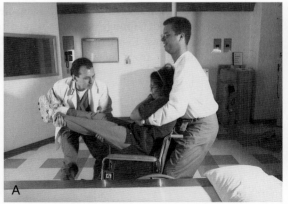
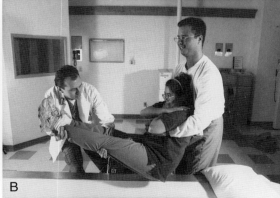

APPENDIX FIG. I-1 Two-person lift. **A,** Primary lifter stands behind the chair and reaches around the patient, extending his arms through the patient's axillae and grasping her arms from the top. The assistant kneels on one knee, cradling the patient's thighs and legs. **B,** On signal, both lift together and place the patient gently on the table.

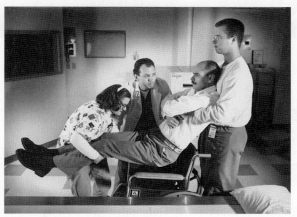

APPENDIX FIG. I-2 Three-person lift. Three-person lift is much like the two-person lift, with the third person helping to raise the patient's hips until they are clear of the chair.

Iodinated Contrast Media Products for Radiography

Trade Name	Generic Name	Iodine (% Weight/ Volume)	Ionic or Nonionic	Osmolality	Approved Uses
Conray	Iothalamate meglumine	28.2	Ionic	High	Multipurpose
Conray-30	Iothalamate meglumine	14.1	Ionic	High	Excretory urography, CT
Conray-43	Iothalamate meglumine	20.2	Ionic	High	Excretory urography, venography, CT, DSA (digital subtraction angiography)
Conray-400	Iothalamate sodium	40	Ionic	High	Angiography
Cysto-Conray II	Iothalamate meglumine	8.1	Ionic	High	Retrograde cystourethrography
Cystografin	Diatrizoate meglumine	14.1	Ionic	High	Retrograde cystourethrography
Cystografin-Dilute	Diatrizoate meglumine	8.5	Ionic	High	Retrograde cystourethrography
Ethiodol	Ethiodized oil	37			Lymphography
Gastrografin	Diatrizoate meglumine and diatrizoate sodium	47.1	Ionic	High	Gastrointestinal studies, CT body scans (oral)
Hexabrix	Sodium meglumine and ioxaglate	32	Ionic	Low	Angiography and multipurpose
Hypaque 76	Diatrizoate meglumine and diatrizoate sodium	34	Ionic	High	Multipurpose
Hypaque Meglumine 60%	Diatrizoate meglumine	30	Ionic	High	Multipurpose
Hypaque Sodium 50%	Diatrizoate sodium	25	Ionic	High	Multipurpose
Hypaque Sodium Oral Powder	Diatrizoate sodium	58	Ionic	High	Gastrointestinal studies

Trade Name	Generic Name	Iodine (% Weight/ Volume)	Ionic or Nonionic	Osmolality	Approved Uses
Hypaque-Cysto 30%	Diatrizoate meglumine	15	Ionic	High	Retrograde cystourethrography
Imagopaque 150	Iopentol	15	Nonionic	Low	Femoral arteriography, ERCP
Imagopaque 200	Iopentol	20	Nonionic	Low	Venography, ERCP
Imagopaque 250	Iopentol	25	Nonionic	Low	Venography, ERCP, hysterosalpingography
Imagopaque 300	Iopentol	30	Nonionic	Low	Angiography, aortography, excretory urography, venography, DSA, CT, arthrography, gastrointestinal studies (oral)
Imagopaque 350	Iopentol	35	Nonionic	Low	Angiocardiography, excretory urography, DSA, CT, arthrography, gastrointestinal studies (oral)
Iomeron 150	Iomeprol	15	Nonionic	Low	Urography infusion, cystourethrography, CT, arterial DSA
Iomeron 200	Iomeprol	20	Nonionic	Low	Venography, CT, arterial DSA, arthrography, hysterosalpingography, ERCP, retrograde urography
Iomeron 250	Iomeprol	25	Nonionic	Low	Excretory urography, venography, CT, IV and arterial DSA
Iomeron 300	Iomeprol	30	Nonionic	Low	Angiocardiography, excretory urography, venography, CT, IV and arterial DSA, arthrography, hysterosalpingography, discography, ERCP
Iomeron 350	Iomeprol	35	Nonionic	Low	Angiocardiography, coronary arteriography, excretory urography, CT, IV and arterial DSA, arthrography, ERCP, hysterosalpingography
Iomeron 400	Iomeprol	40	Nonionic	Low	Angiocardiography, coronary arteriography, excretory urography, CT, IV DSA
Isovue-200	Iopamidol	20	Nonionic	Low	Venography
Isovue-300	Iopamidol	30	Nonionic	Low	Peripheral arteriography
Isovue-370	Iopamidol	37	Nonionic	Low	Selective visceral arteriography
Isovue-M 200	Iopamidol	20	Nonionic	Low	Thoracic myelography
Isovue-M 300	Iopamidol	30	Nonionic	Low	Total column myelography
MD-76	Diatrizoate meglumine and diatrizoate sodium	37	Ionic	High	Excretory urography, angiography, CT

Continued

Trade Name	Generic Name	Iodine (% Weight/ Volume)	Ionic or Nonionic	Osmolality	Approved Uses
MD-Gastroview	Diatrizoate meglumine and diatrizoate sodium	37	Ionic	High	Gastrointestinal studies (oral administration)
Omnipaque 140	Iohexol	14	Nonionic	Low	Arterial DSA
Omnipaque 180	Iohexol	18	Nonionic	Low	Myelography
Omnipaque 240	Iohexol	24	Nonionic	Low	Multipurpose
Omnipaque 300	Iohexol	30	Nonionic	Low	Arteriography, aortography, CT(IV and intrathecal)
Omnipaque 350	Iohexol	35	Nonionic	Low	Aortography, angiocardiography, CT (IV), IV DSA
Optiray 160	Ioversol	16	Nonionic	Low	Arterial DSA
Optiray 240	Ioversol	24	Nonionic	Low	Cerebral arteriography, venography, excretory urography, CT
Optiray 300	Ioversol	30	Nonionic	Low	Arteriography, excretory urography, CT
Optiray 320	Ioversol	32	Nonionic	Low	Angiography
Optiray 350	Ioversol	35	Nonionic	Low	Angiography, excretory urography, IV DSA, CT
Renografin-60	Diatrizoate meglumine and diatrizoate sodium	29.25	Ionic	High	Multipurpose
Reno-30	Diatrizoate meglumine	14.1	Ionic	High	Retrograde urography
Reno-60	Diatrizoate meglumine and diatrizoate sodium	29.25	Ionic	High	Multipurpose
Reno-M-Dip	Diatrizoate meglumine	14.1	Ionic	High	Urography infusion, leg venography
Renovist	Diatrizoate meglumine and diatrizoate sodium	69.3	Ionic	Moderate	Multipurpose
Renovist II	Diatrizoate meglumine and diatrizoate sodium	57.6	Ionic	Moderate	Multipurpose
Renovue-65	Iodamide meglumine	65	Ionic	Moderate	Excretory urography
Renovue-Dip	Iodamide meglumine	24	Ionic	Moderate	Urography infusion

Trade Name	Generic Name	Iodine (% Weight/ Volume)	Ionic or Nonionic	Osmolality	Approved Uses
Sinografin	Diatrizoate meglumine and iodipamide meglumine	47.1	Ionic	High	Hysterosalpingography
Telepaque	Iopanoic acid	66.7	—	—	Cholecystography (oral administration)
Visipaque 270	Iodixanol	27	Nonionic	Very low (isosmolar)	Angiography, cerebral angiography, IV and arterial DSA, excretory urography, venography, CT, arthrography, ERCP, hysterosalpingography
Visipaque 320	Iodixanol	32	Nonionic	Very low (isosmolar)	Angiocardiography, peripheral arteriography, DSA, CT, arthrography, ERCP, hysterosalpingography

CT, computed tomography; *DSA,* digital subtraction angiography; *ERCP,* endoscopic retrograde cholangiopancreatography; *IV,* intravenous.

Catheterization Technique

For routine cystography (both male and female), size 14 or 16 Foley (retention) catheters are recommended. Review Chapter 19 for procedures involving sterile trays, gloving, and aseptic technique.

FEMALE CATHETERIZATION PROCEDURE

Prepare for Catheterization:

- Perform hand hygiene.
- Obtain and assemble equipment: catheter, antiseptic solution, cotton balls, specimen bottle, waste urine receptacle, drapes, forceps, syringe, needle, sterile water, and sterile gloves. (All are commercially available in a sterile, disposable tray.)
- Check patient identification and explain the procedure. Provide privacy.
- Position patient supine with hips and knees flexed and legs separated, exposing perineum. Drape torso and legs.
- Place tray between patient's legs. Open tray, add antiseptic to tray, and don gloves, using sterile technique (see Chapter 19).
- Position sterile drapes by first placing a drape under the buttocks. (Cuff drape around your hands to avoid contaminating gloves.) Place the fenestrated (window) drape over the pubis and genital area, exposing the labia.
- Pour antiseptic over cotton balls. Open sterile lubricant from tray and squeeze some onto the drape.
  - Using nondominant hand, separate the labia to provide a clear view of the urethral orifice (Appendix Fig. K-1). NOTE: This hand is now contaminated and will not be used to handle sterile objects.

Cleanse Genital Area:

- Using your fingers or the small forceps, grasp an antiseptic cotton ball with the dominant hand.

- With a single, firm, downward stroke, cleanse the far side of the labia from pubis to anus; discard cotton ball.
- Repeat the previous step for near side of labia.
- With a third cotton ball, cleanse down the center of the labia, directly over the urethral orifice.

To Insert Catheter:

- Place the distal (wide) end of the catheter in the drainage receptacle.
- With your dominant hand or the large forceps, grasp the catheter approximately 3 inches from its tip.
- Apply lubricant to the tip.
- Still exposing the orifice with the nondominant hand, gently insert the tip of the catheter into the orifice, guiding it posteriorly and superiorly approximately 2 inches (Appendix Fig. K-2). Slight resistance may be encountered at the internal urethral sphincter, which will relax when the patient exhales.
- Release the pressure on the catheter. If urine does not flow, the catheter tip may be lodged against the bladder wall. Rotate the catheter between thumb and forefinger, and insert up to 1 inch farther.

If Specimen is Needed:

- Clamp the catheter after a small amount of urine has drained into the receptacle.
- Transfer the distal end of the catheter into the specimen container.
- Release the forceps, allowing at least 30 mL (1 oz) of urine to flow into the container; reclamp the catheter.
- Transfer the catheter end back to the drainage receptacle; unclamp.
- NOTE: Normally, the bladder is emptied completely in preparation for the cystogram. However, no more than 1000 mL should be removed at one time,

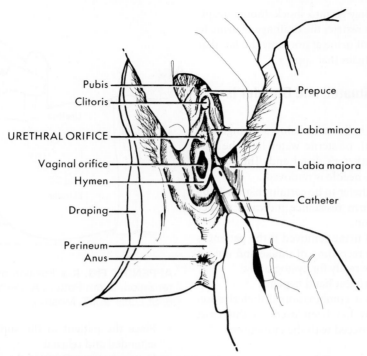

APPENDIX FIG. K-1 Female perineal anatomy, external view.

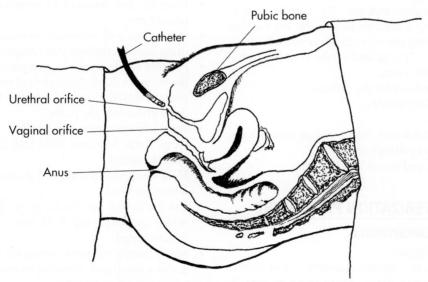

APPENDIX FIG. K-2 Female perineal anatomy, sagittal view.

because the patient may go into shock. (Some hospitals have policies that restrict the drainage of urine to fewer than 1000 mL of urine at one time. Be familiar with institutional policies that apply.)

When Catheter is Situated and Bladder is Empty:

- Inflate the retention balloon by using a syringe and needle to inject 5 mL of sterile water into the balloon valve on the catheter's distal end. The valve is self-sealing when the needle is removed.
- Tug gently on the catheter to be certain that it will be properly retained. Firm resistance indicates proper inflation of the balloon.
- Chart the amount of urine removed if the patient is under orders for the recording of intake and output (I&O). Patient is now ready for cystography.
- Remove gloves, and repeat hand hygiene.
- Discard tray, unless a combination catheterization and cystography tray has been used. In this case, change gloves and proceed with the cystogram.

To Remove Catheter:

- Perform hand hygiene, and don gloves.
- Deflate the retention balloon. This can be accomplished by using a scissors to snip off the balloon valve and allowing the water to drain into a basin or by using a 10-mL syringe and needle to withdraw the water through the valve.
- Place paper towels under the catheter.
- Remove by pulling gently.
- Discard catheter.
- Cleanse the genital area with towel or cotton balls, and attend to the patient's comfort.
- Remove gloves, and repeat hand hygiene.

MALE CATHETERIZATION PROCEDURE

Prepare for Catheterization:

- Perform hand hygiene.
- Obtain equipment: catheter, antiseptic solution, cotton balls, specimen bottle, waste urine receptacle, drapes, forceps, syringe, needle, sterile water, and sterile gloves. (All are commercially available in a sterile, disposable tray.)
- Check patient identification and explain the procedure. Provide privacy.

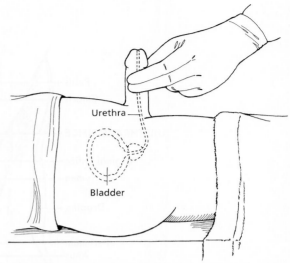

APPENDIX FIG. K-3 Position of penis for male catheterization. (From Potter PA, Perry AG: *Basic nursing*, ed 6, St Louis, 2007, Mosby.)

- Place the patient in the supine position, with legs extended and relaxed.
- Drape the torso down to the pubis, and the legs up to the groin, leaving the penis exposed.
- Place the tray adjacent to patient's hip on the side nearest you.
- Open tray, add antiseptic to tray, and don gloves using sterile technique (see Chapter 19).
- Position sterile drapes by first placing a drape under the buttocks. (Cuff drape around your hands to avoid contaminating gloves.) Place the fenestrated (window) drape over the penis.
- Pour antiseptic over cotton balls.
- Open sterile lubricant from tray, and squeeze some onto the drape.
- Hold the penis in a vertical position with the nondominant hand.
- Use the thumb and forefinger to spread the urinary orifice (Appendix Fig. K-3). NOTE: This hand is now contaminated.
- NOTE: Handle the penis firmly, but not roughly. (Too gentle a touch may stimulate an erection.)

Cleanse Penis:

- Using the dominant hand, pick up an antiseptic cotton ball.
- Cleanse with a circular motion, and work toward the tip; discard cotton ball.

- Use second cotton ball to cleanse firmly but gently over the orifice; discard.

To Insert Catheter:

- Grasp the catheter with the large forceps approximately 4 inches from its tip, and place the distal end in drainage receptacle.
- Lubricate the catheter tip.
- Still holding the penis firmly in the nondominant hand, draw it forward and upward (60 to 90 degrees toward the legs), stretching it slightly. This action will straighten the urethra for easy insertion of the catheter.
- Insert gently and slowly approximately 7 inches. (This will require releasing the catheter and regrasping it approximately 4 inches distal to the original hold.)
- NOTE: Resistance may be felt as the catheter passes the internal urethral sphincter. Use continuous, gentle pressure, and instruct the patient to try to void. Do not force insertion of the catheter. If there seems to be an obstruction or stricture, stop the procedure and call the physician.

If Specimen is Needed:

- Clamp the catheter after a small amount of urine has drained into the receptacle.
- Transfer the distal end of the catheter into the specimen container.
- Release the forceps, allowing at least 30 mL (1 oz) of urine to flow into the container; reclamp the catheter.
- Transfer the catheter end back to the drainage receptacle; unclamp.
- NOTE: Normally the bladder is emptied completely in preparation for the cystogram. However, no more than 1000 mL should be removed at one time, because the patient may go into shock. (Some hospitals have policies that restrict the draining of urine to fewer than 1000 mL of urine at one time. Be familiar with the institutional policies that apply.)

When Catheter is Situated and Bladder is Empty:

- Inflate the retention balloon by using a syringe and needle to inject 5 mL of sterile water into the balloon valve on the catheter's distal end. The valve is self-sealing when the needle is removed.
- Tug gently on the catheter to be certain that it will be properly retained. Firm resistance indicates proper inflation of the balloon.
- Chart the amount of urine removed if the patient is under orders for the recording of I&O. Patient is now ready for cystography.
- Remove gloves. Repeat hand hygiene.
- Discard tray, unless a combination catheterization and cystography tray has been used. In this case, change gloves and proceed with the cystogram.

To Remove Catheter:

- Perform hand hygiene, and don gloves.
- Deflate the retention balloon. This can be accomplished by using a scissors to snip off the balloon valve and allowing the water to drain into a basin, or by using a 10-mL syringe and needle to withdraw the water through the valve.
- Place paper towels under the catheter.
- Remove by pulling gently.
- Discard catheter.
- Cleanse the genital area with towel or cotton balls, and attend to the patient's comfort.
- Remove gloves, and repeat hand hygiene.

GLOSSARY

Abdominal binder a bandage or elasticized wrap that is applied around the lower part of the torso to support the abdomen. It is sometimes applied after abdominal surgery to decrease discomfort and support abdominal muscles.

Abdominal thrust subdiaphragmatic force applied as a treatment for choking. See also *Heimlich maneuver*.

Abduct, abduction to move away from the median plane of the body.

Abrasion a scraping or rubbing away of a surface, such as skin or teeth, by friction.

Abscess a painful, localized collection of pus that can occur as a result of infection.

Acquired immunity infection resistance to a specific organism that occurs after an individual has been infected with the organism, or that is conferred from a vaccine; also called *active immunity* or *acquired resistance*.

Acquired Immune Deficiency Syndrome (AIDS) state 3 HIV infection.

Acute beginning abruptly with marked intensity or sharpness, then subsiding after a relatively short period.

Adduct, adduction to move toward the median axis of the body.

Adult respiratory distress syndrome (ARDS) a respiratory disorder characterized by respiratory insufficiency and hypoxemia.

Advance directive a document that outlines specific wishes about medical care to be followed in the event that an individual loses the ability to make or communicate health care decisions.

Affordable Care Act (ACA) legislation passed in 2010 for the stated purpose of ensuring that all Americans are covered by health insurance; often referred to as "Obamacare."

Ageism a discriminatory attitude toward the elderly that includes a belief that all elderly are ill, disabled, worthless, and unattractive.

Aggravate to worsen.

Aggressiveness undesirable behavior characterized by anger or hostility.

Agonist a drug that produces a specific action and promotes the desired result.

AIDS abbreviation for acquired immune deficiency syndrome.

Airborne contamination mode of transmitting infection by dust containing spores or droplet nuclei, which are particles measuring 5 μm or smaller that contain microorganisms and remain suspended in the air for long periods of time.

ALARA principle a principle that states that all radiation exposure to humans should be limited to levels that are as low as reasonably achievable.

Allergen an agent that causes an allergic response.

Allergic reaction, allergic response an unfavorable physiologic response to an allergen, a substance to which an organism has previously been exposed and to which it has developed antibodies.

Allergy, allergenic a hypersensitive reaction to intrinsically harmless antigens. *Allergenic* describes an individual prone to allergic response.

Alleviate to relieve or to partially remove or correct.

Alzheimer disease a progressive mental deterioration characterized by confusion, memory failure, disorientation, restlessness, agnosia, speech disturbances, inability to carry out purposeful movement, and hallucinosis.

Ambulatory able to walk, hence describing a patient who is not confined to bed or designating a health service for people who are not hospitalized.

Ameba (amoeba) a microscopic, single-cell, parasitic organism.

Amebiasis an infection of the intestine or liver by species of pathogenic amebas acquired by ingesting food or water contaminated with infected feces.

Amniocentesis an obstetric procedure in which a small amount of amniotic fluid is removed for laboratory analysis.

Amplitude with respect to a sine wave, the distance between peak and trough.

Ampule a small, sterile glass or plastic container that usually contains a single dose of a solution.

Analgesic a drug that relieves pain.

Anaphylaxis, anaphylactic, anaphylactoid an exaggerated, life-threatening hypersensitivity reaction to a previously encountered antigen. Penicillin injection and bee stings are the most common causes of anaphylactic shock.

Anastomosis a connection between two vessels or a surgical joining of two ducts, blood vessels, or bowel segments to allow flow from one to the other.

Anemia a decrease in hemoglobin in the blood to a level below 10 g/dL, or a decrease in the number of red blood cells to levels below the normal range of 4.2 million/mm³ to 6.1 million/mm³.

Anesthetic, anesthesia a drug or agent that is capable of producing a complete or partial loss of feeling (anesthesia).

Aneurysm a localized dilation of the wall of a blood vessel.

Angina pectoris a paroxysmal thoracic pain that may radiate down the inner aspect of the left arm and is frequently accompanied by a feeling of suffocation and impending death. It is caused by spasm or occlusion of a coronary artery and is treated by administration of nitroglycerine.

Angiocardiogram a series of radiographs demonstrating vessels of the heart.

Angioedema an acute, painless, dermal, subcutaneous, or submucosal swelling of short duration. It involves the face, neck, lips, larynx, hands, feet, genitalia, or viscera.

Angiogram, angiography a radiograph or examination of a blood vessel into which a contrast medium has been injected.

Angioplasty the reconstruction of blood vessels damaged by disease or injury.

Anode the electrode at which oxidation occurs; also, the electrically positive, target end of an x-ray tube.

Anomaly deviation from what is regarded as normal; a congenital malformation, such as the absence of a limb or the presence of an extra finger.

Anorexia lack or loss of appetite, resulting in the inability to eat.

Anoxia an abnormal condition characterized by a lack of oxygen. It can result from an inadequate supply of oxygen to the respiratory system, an inability of the blood to carry oxygen to the tissues, or an inability of the tissues to absorb the oxygen.

Antagonist a drug that attaches itself to the receptor, preventing the agonist from acting.

Antecubital   in front of the elbow; at the bend of the elbow.

Anthrax   a disease caused by the bacterium *Bacillus anthracis,* affecting primarily farm animals.

Antiallergic   pertaining to a medication used to treat allergies, or one administered in advance to patients who might be expected to have an allergic reaction.

Antibacterial   pertaining to a substance that kills bacteria or inhibits their growth or replication.

Antibiotic   an antimicrobial agent used to treat infections.

Antibody   an immunoglobulin produced by lymphocytes in response to bacteria, viruses, or other antigenic substances. An antibody is specific to an antigen. Antibodies are responsible for acquired immunity and for allergic responses.

Anticholinergic   pertaining to a blockade of acetylcholine receptors that inhibits the transmission of parasympathetic nerve impulses, thus inhibiting secretions.

Anticonvulsant   pertaining to a substance or procedure that prevents or reduces the severity of epileptic or other convulsive seizures.

Antidote   a drug or other substance that opposes the action of a poison.

Antifungal   pertaining to a substance that kills fungi or inhibits their growth or reproduction.

Antigen   a substance, usually a protein, that causes the formation of an antibody that reacts specifically with that antigen.

Antihistamine   any substance capable of reducing the physiologic and pharmacologic effects of histamine. Antihistamines include a wide variety of drugs that block histamine receptors. Used to treat allergies.

Antihypertensive   pertaining to a medication, substance, or procedure that reduces high blood pressure.

Antimicrobial   an agent that kills or inhibits the growth or replication of microorganisms.

Antiseptic   a substance that tends to inhibit the growth and reproduction of microorganisms.

Aortogram, aortography   a radiograph or examination of the aorta made after the injection of a radiopaque contrast medium.

Apathy   lack of interest, enthusiasm, or concern.

Apex, apical   the top, the end, or the tip of a structure, such as the apex of the heart.

Aphasia, aphasic   an abnormal neurologic condition in which language function is defective or absent because of an injury to certain areas of the cerebral cortex.

Aqueous   describing a solution prepared with water.

ARRT (American Registry of Radiologic Technologists)   a national organization of appointees from both ASRT and the American College of Radiology (ACR) that provides certification in radiologic technology.

Arteriogram, arteriography   a radiograph or examination of an artery injected with a radiopaque medium.

Arthritis, arthritic   an inflammatory condition of a joint.

Artifact   something not usually present; a part of a radiographic image that does not represent the intended anatomy.

Arthrography   a method of radiographically visualizing the inside of a joint using a radiolucent or radiopaque contrast medium.

Arthropod   a form of animal life that can cause allergic reactions and serve as a vector for viruses or other disease-causing agents. Arthropods generally are distinguished by a jointed exoskeleton (shell) and paired, jointed legs. This group includes crustaceans, insects, and similar animal forms.

Asepsis   the absence of microorganisms.

Aspirate, aspiration   to withdraw fluid or air from a cavity, or to inhale fluid or a solid object into the lungs.

ASRT (American Society of Radiologic Technologists)   the oldest and largest national professional association for technologists in the radiologic sciences.

Assault   the threat of touching in an injurious way.

Assertiveness   a desirable behavior characterized by a calm, firm expression of feelings or opinions.

Asthma, asthmatic   a respiratory disorder characterized by recurring episodes of paroxysmal dyspnea, wheezing caused by constriction of the bronchi, coughing, and viscous mucoid bronchial secretions.

Asymptomatic   without symptoms.

Asystole   a life-threatening cardiac condition characterized by the absence of electrical and mechanical activity in the heart.

Atelectasis   an abnormal condition characterized by the collapse of a lung or portion of a lung, preventing the respiratory exchange of carbon dioxide and oxygen.

In newborns, it is the term for incomplete lung expansion.

Atherectomy   surgical removal of an atheroma in a major artery.

Atheroma   an abnormal mass of fat or lipids, as in a sebaceous cyst or in deposits in an arterial wall.

Atherosclerosis   a common disorder characterized by yellowish plaques of cholesterol, other lipids, and cellular debris in the inner layers of the walls of arteries.

Atrium   a chamber or cavity, such as the right and left atria of the heart.

Atropine   an alkaloid anticholinergic drug that blocks parasympathetic stimuli by raising the threshold of response of effector cells to acetylcholine.

Attending physician   one who is primarily responsible for managing the care of a hospital patient.

Attenuate, attenuation   the process of reduction, such as the reduction of x-ray beam intensity when it penetrates matter.

Aura   a sensation, as of light or warmth, that may precede an attack of migraine or an epileptic seizure.

Autoclave   an appliance used to sterilize medical instruments or other objects with steam under pressure.

Autoimmune   relating to disease caused by antibodies or lymphocytes produced against substances naturally present in the body.

Automatic exposure control (AEC)   device that terminates the exposure when a specific quantity of radiation has reached the image receptor (IR).

Autonomy   the quality of having the ability or tendency to function independently.

Axilla, axillary   a pyramid-shaped space forming the underside of the shoulder between the upper arm and the side of the chest; also called the *armpit.* An axillary temperature is taken with the thermometer probe in the axilla.

B cell   a lymphocyte with the ability to produce an immune response. Contact with a foreign antigen stimulates B cells to differentiate into plasma cells that release antibodies.

Backscatter   x-rays scattered back in the direction of the incident x-ray beam.

Bacterium (plural, bacteria)   small, unicellular microorganism.

Barbiturate   a derivative of barbituric acid that acts as a sedative or hypnotic by depressing the central nervous system and causing a decrease in the respiratory rate, blood pressure, and temperature.

Barium impaction solidification of barium sulfate suspension in the intestine causing constipation and potential bowel obstruction.

Barium sulfate, "barium" a radiopaque medium used as a diagnostic aid in gastrointestinal radiography.

Base of support the portion of the body in contact with a horizontal surface, such as the floor.

Battered child syndrome the characteristics of physical abuse in a child.

Battery the unlawful use of force against a person.

Benign not recurrent or progressive; not malignant.

Benzodiazepine one of a group of psychotropic agents prescribed to alleviate anxiety or to treat insomnia.

Beta-blocker a popular term for beta-adrenergic blocking agents used to treat hypertension, rapid heart rate, and sometimes migraine headaches.

Bile a bitter, yellow-green secretion of the liver that is stored in the gallbladder and released into the digestive tract to aid in the digestion of fats.

Biliary pertaining to bile or to the gallbladder and bile ducts, which transport bile.

Bilirubin the orange-yellow pigment of bile, formed principally by the breakdown of hemoglobin in red blood cells after termination of their normal life span; also, a measurement of the bilirubin content of blood as a clinical test of biliary function.

Biopsy the removal of a small piece of living tissue from an organ or other part of the body for microscopic examination to confirm or establish a diagnosis, estimate prognosis, or follow the course of a disease.

Bismuth a reddish, crystalline, trivalent metallic element. It is combined with various other elements, such as oxygen, to produce numerous salts used in the manufacture of many pharmaceutical substances.

Body mechanics the principles of proper body alignment, movement, and balance.

Bolus (injection) a quantity of undiluted contrast medium or other fluid injected intravenously over a short period of time.

Bowel obstruction blockage of the intestine. Acute bowel obstruction is very painful and can be life threatening if untreated.

Bradycardia a heart condition in which the ventricles contract at a rate of fewer than 60 beats/min.

Bradypnea an abnormally low respiratory rate.

Bronchodilation an increase in the diameter of the bronchial lumen, allowing increased airflow to and from the lungs.

Bronchoscopy the visual examination of the tracheal and bronchial tree using a flexible fiberoptic instrument called a bronchoscope.

Bronchospasm an abnormal contraction of the smooth muscle of the bronchi, resulting in an acute narrowing and obstruction of the respiratory airway, causing dyspnea.

Buccal pertaining to the inside of the cheek or to the surface of a tooth or the gum beside the cheek. The buccal route of medication administration involves placement of a drug in paste form on the buccal surface of the mouth.

Bucky a moving grid that limits the amount of scatter radiation reaching an image receptor, thereby increasing the image contrast.

BUN (blood urea nitrogen) a clinical laboratory test of kidney function.

Burnout physical or mental collapse caused by stress or overwork.

Cancer a neoplasm characterized by the uncontrolled growth of anaplastic cells that tend to invade surrounding tissue and to metastasize to distant body sites.

Cannula a flexible tube that can be inserted into a vessel, duct, or cavity to deliver medication or drain fluid.

Carcinogenesis the process of initiating and promoting cancer.

Cardiac pertaining to the heart. A cardiac patient is a person who suffers from heart disease.

Cardiac arrest a sudden cessation of cardiac output and effective circulation. It is usually precipitated by ventricular fibrillation or ventricular asystole.

Cardiac tamponade compression of the heart produced by the accumulation of blood in the pericardial sac; also called *cardiac compression.*

Cardiogenic originating in the heart muscle.

Cardiopulmonary resuscitation (CPR) a basic emergency procedure for life support, consisting of artificial respiration and manual external cardiac massage.

Cardioversion the restoration of the heart's normal sinus rhythm through an electric shock delivered by a defibrillator.

Cassette a device used in radiography for holding a sheet of x-ray film and a set of intensifying screens. A cassette also may have a grid to absorb scatter radiation.

Cataractogenesis the process of initiating and promoting cataracts.

Cathartic a laxative preparation.

Catheter a hollow, flexible tube that can be inserted into a vessel or cavity of the body to withdraw or to instill fluids, monitor various types of information, or to visualize a vessel or cavity.

Catheterize, catheterization the introduction of a catheter into a body cavity or organ to inject or remove a fluid.

Cathode negative electrode; the negative side of the x-ray tube, which consists of the focusing cup(s) and the filament(s).

Cathode ray tube (CRT) a vacuum tube that focuses a beam of electrons onto a screen coated with a phosphor, creating a visible image of information on the face of the tube. The CRT provides a means for graphically representing data processed by a computer and is often called a *computer monitor.*

CCU abbreviation for coronary care unit or critical care unit.

Center of gravity the midpoint or center of the weight of a body or object. In the standing adult human, the center of gravity is in the midpelvic cavity.

Centigray (cGy) The most common unit for calculation of radiation doses in the United States (one one-hundredth of a Gray, equal to 1 rad in the British system).

Central nervous system (CNS) one of the two main divisions of the nervous system, consisting of the brain and the spinal cord. The central nervous system processes information to and from the peripheral nervous system and is the main network of coordination and control for the entire body.

Central ray (CR) an imaginary photon in the center of the x-ray beam that is directed toward the center of the object being radiographed.

Central venous catheter (CVC) a central line providing access to the circulatory system on a repeated or continuing basis. Various types are identified by proprietary name, such as Hickman, Groshong, Raaf, or Port-A-Cath.

Cerebrovascular accident (CVA) an abnormal condition of the brain characterized by occlusion of an artery by an embolus or thrombus, or by cerebrovascular hemorrhage, resulting in ischemia of the brain tissues normally perfused by the damaged vessels.

Chart, charting a patient's medical record; to note data in a patient record.

Chemotherapy the treatment of infections and other diseases with chemical agents. In modern usage, chemotherapy entails the use of chemicals to destroy cancer cells on a selective basis, usually resulting in immunosuppression.

Cholangiogram, cholangiography an image or examination of the biliary ducts after injection of a radiopaque contrast medium. It may be performed before or after biliary tract surgery, and may be part of the surgical procedure.

Cholecystectomy the surgical removal of the gallbladder.

Cholecystitis inflammation of the gallbladder.

Cholecystogram, cholecystography a radiograph or examination of the gallbladder, made after the ingestion of a radiopaque substance, a contrast material containing iodine.

Cholera an acute bacterial infection of the small intestine, characterized by severe diarrhea and vomiting, muscular cramps, dehydration, and depletion of electrolytes. The disease is spread by water and food that have been contaminated by feces of infected persons.

Chronic developing slowly and persisting for a long period.

Chronic obstructive pulmonary disease (COPD) a progressive and irreversible condition characterized by diminished inspiratory and expiratory capacity of the lungs. Emphysema and chronic bronchitis are examples of COPD.

Cilia (singular, cilium) small, hairlike processes on the outer surfaces of some cells, aiding metabolism by producing motion, eddies, or current in a fluid.

Circulating nurse an assistant to the scrub nurse and surgeon whose role is to provide necessary supplies, dispose of soiled supplies, and to keep an accurate count of instruments, needles, and sponges.

Claustrophobia, claustrophobic a morbid fear of being in or becoming trapped in enclosed or narrow places.

CNS abbreviation for central nervous system.

Coccidioidomycosis an infectious fungal disease caused by the inhalation of spores of the bacterium *Coccidioides immitis,* which is carried on windborne dust particles.

Coccus (plural, cocci) a bacterium that is round, spherical, or oval, as gonococcus, pneumococcus, staphylococcus, streptococcus.

Code a discreet signal used to summon an emergency response team for a specific purpose signified by the type of code, for example to resuscitate a patient without alarming patients or visitors, as in "Code zero, 3 west" announced over a public address system to summon the team to the west wing of the third floor.

Code team a specially trained and equipped team that is available to provide cardiopulmonary resuscitation or other specific response when summoned by a specific code over the public address system. A cardiopulmonary code team usually includes a physician, one or more registered nurses, respiratory therapist, and electrocardiologist.

Collimator a device for limiting the size and shape of an x-ray beam.

Colostomy surgical creation of an artificial anus (stoma) on the abdominal wall by incising the colon and drawing it out to the surface.

Coma, comatose pertaining to a state of abnormally deep sleep, caused by illness or injury.

Commode a toilet.

Computed radiography (CR) the method of using a photostimulable phosphor plate to record radiographic images and to digitize them for viewing and storage.

Computed tomography (CT) a computerized radiographic technique that produces detailed images of a cross section of an anatomic structure.

Concussion damage to the brain caused by a violent jarring or shaking, such as a blow or an explosion.

Congenital present at birth, as a congenital anomaly or defect.

Congenital megacolon also called *Hirschsprung disease;* the absence at birth of autonomic ganglia in the smooth muscle wall of the colon, which causes poor or absent peristalsis in the involved segment of the colon, accumulation of feces, and dilation of the bowel.

Congestive heart failure (CHF) an abnormal condition that reflects impaired cardiac pumping. It is caused by myocardial infarction, ischemic heart disease, or cardiomyopathy.

Conjunctiva (plural, conjunctivae) the mucous membrane lining the inner surfaces of the eyelids and anterior part of the sclera.

Contaminate, contamination to soil, stain, touch, or otherwise expose to harmful agents, making an object potentially unsafe for use as intended without barrier techniques.

Contraindication the presence of a disease or physical condition that makes it impossible or undesirable to treat a particular client in the usual manner or to prescribe medicines that might otherwise be suitable.

Contrast medium (plural, contrast media), contrast agent a gas or radiopaque substance that is injected into the body, introduced via catheter, or swallowed to facilitate radiographic imaging of internal structures that otherwise are difficult to visualize radiographically.

Contributory negligence an act of negligence in which the behavior of the injured party contributed to the injury.

Controlled substance any drug defined in the five categories of the Federal Controlled Substances Act of 1970. The categories, or schedules, cover opium and its derivatives, hallucinogens, depressants, and stimulants.

Contusion an injury that does not disrupt the integrity of the skin, caused by a blow to the body and characterized by swelling, discoloration, and pain. Also called a *bruise.*

Convulsion the hyperexcitation of neurons in the brain that leads to a sudden, involuntary series of contractions of a group of muscles; also called a *seizure.*

Coronary pertaining to encircling structures, such as the coronary arteries; pertaining to the heart.

Coronary care unit (CCU) a special care unit designed for patients with critical cardiac conditions whose treatment and status require frequent monitoring. It may be subdivided, with patients recovering from cardiac surgery in one area and those receiving medical and nonsurgical treatment in another.

Corporate negligence negligence attributable to a hospital or other corporation as an entity.

Cortical bone the dense outer surface (cortex) of bone that forms a protective layer around the inner cavity and makes up about 80% of skeletal mass.

Corticosteroid any one of the natural or synthetic hormones elaborated by the adrenal cortex (excluding the sex hormones of adrenal origin) that influence or control key processes of the body. A corticosteroid may be prescribed as an antiallergic medication.

Cortisone a glucocorticoid produced in the liver and made synthetically. It may be prescribed as an antiinflammatory drug.

Costal pertaining to one or more ribs; situated near a rib or on a side close to a rib. Costal respirations involve movement of the rib cage.

Coulombs per kilogram (C/kg) the SI unit for measuring radiation intensity.

Credentials documents that attest to qualifications of individuals. Some examples include registration, licenses, permits, and certificates.

Creatinine a substance formed from the metabolism of creatine, commonly found in blood, urine, and muscle tissue. It is measured in blood and urine tests as an indicator of kidney function.

Creutzfeldt–Jakob disease the human variant of mad cow disease (bovine spongiform encephalopathy). A rare, fatal condition of the structure and function of brain tissues caused by an unidentified slow virus or prion.

Crohn disease an autoimmune disease that causes damaging inflammation, most commonly in the colon, but may affect the entire gastrointestinal system.

CRT abbreviation for cathode ray tube, a computer monitor.

CT abbreviation for computed tomography.

CVA abbreviation for cerebrovascular accident. See *stroke*.

Cyanosis, cyanotic bluish discoloration of the skin and mucous membranes caused by an excess of deoxygenated hemoglobin in the blood or a structural defect in the hemoglobin molecule. Typically occurs with *anoxia*.

Cyst, cystic pertaining to a cyst, a fluid-filled sac.

Cystogram contrast imaging of the internal contours of the urinary bladder. The bladder is filled by retrograde injection of a water-soluble iodine medium through a urinary catheter and examined using fluoroscopy or radiographs.

Cytomegalovirus a member of a group of large, species-specific, herpes-type viruses with a wide variety of disease effects. It causes serious illness in persons with human immunodeficiency virus, in newborns, and in people being treated with immunosuppressive drugs and therapy, especially after organ transplantation.

Dacryocystography radiography of the lacrimal drainage system, the passage from the tear duct to the nasopharynx.

Debilitated feeble, weak, or otherwise disabled.

Decompression the removal of pressure caused by gas or fluid in a body cavity, as the stomach or intestinal tract.

Decubitus ulcers lesions that develop over bony prominences when pressure is exerted for any length of time; also called *bedsores*.

Defecate, defecation the elimination of feces from the digestive tract through the rectum.

Defecography an imaging procedure for the evaluation of patients with defecation dysfunction, also known as *evacuation proctography* or *dynamic rectal examination*.

Defendant the party named in a plaintiff's complaint and against whom the plaintiff's allegations are made.

Defibrillate, defibrillation to terminate ventricular fibrillation by delivery of an electrical shock to the patient's chest.

Defibrillator a device that delivers an electrical shock at a preset voltage to the myocardium through the chest wall for the purpose of restoring normal heart rhythm.

Degenerative pertaining to or involving degeneration or change to a lower or dysfunctional form.

Dehiscence the separation of a surgical incision or rupture of a wound closure, typically an abdominal incision.

Dehydrate, dehydration to remove or lose water from a substance. Dehydration of the body is accompanied by a disturbance in the balance of essential electrolytes, particularly sodium, potassium, and chloride.

Dementia disorder of the mental processes caused by brain disease or injury and marked by memory loss, personality change, and impaired reasoning.

Dengue fever an acute arbovirus infection transmitted to humans by the Aedes mosquito and occurring in tropical and subtropical regions.

Dermatitis an inflammatory condition of the skin. Various cutaneous eruptions occur and may be unique to a particular allergen, disease, or infection.

Detent a mechanism that tends to stop a moving part in a specific location. Detents are built into x-ray tube supports to facilitate tube placement at standard locations.

Deterministic describes biologic radiation effects that are predictable; their intensity is dose dependent. These effects occur only after a certain threshold amount of exposure has been received; formerly called *nonstochastic effects*.

Diabetes, diabetic clinical condition characterized by the excessive excretion of urine. The excess may be caused by a deficiency of antidiuretic hormone, as in diabetes insipidus, or it may be the polyuria resulting from the hyperglycemia that occurs in diabetes mellitus.

Diabetic coma a life-threatening condition occurring in persons with diabetes mellitus. It is caused by inadequate treatment, failure to take prescribed insulin, excessive food intake, or, most frequently, infection, surgery, trauma, or other stressors that increase the body's need for insulin.

Diagnosis, diagnostic identification of a disease or condition by a scientific evaluation of physical signs, symptoms, history, laboratory test results, imaging studies, and other procedures.

Dialysis a medical procedure for the removal of certain substances from the blood or lymph by virtue of the difference in their rates of diffusion through an external semipermeable membrane or, in the case of peritoneal dialysis, through the peritoneum. Dialysis is a treatment for chronic kidney failure.

Diaphoresis, diaphoretic the secretion of sweat, especially the profuse secretion associated with an elevated body temperature, physical exertion, exposure to heat, and mental or emotional stress.

Diastole, diastolic pertaining to diastole, the blood pressure at the instant of maximum cardiac relaxation.

Differentiation a process in development in which unspecialized cells or tissues are systemically modified and altered to achieve specific and characteristic physical forms, physiologic functions, and chemical properties.

Digitalis a general term for cardiotonic glycosides used to treat congestive heart failure and atrial fibrillation.

Dilation the process of causing an increase in the diameter of a body opening, blood vessel, or tube.

Diluent a substance, generally a fluid, that makes a solution or mixture less concentrated, less viscous, or more liquid.

Diphtheria an acute contagious disease caused by the bacterium *Corynebacterium diphtheriae*. It is characterized by the production of a false membrane on mucosal surfaces and is usually accompanied by severe prostration.

Direct contact means of disease transmission in which infectious organisms are transferred to a susceptible host by the touch of an infected individual.

Disaster an emergency of huge magnitude that creates an unforeseen, serious, and immediate threat to public health.

Disinfectant liquid chemical applied to objects to eliminate many or all pathogenic microorganisms.

Disinfection the second level of microbial dilution that involves the destruction of pathogens by using chemical materials.

Disposable not designed for reuse; intended to be thrown away after use.

Distal away from or farthest from the point of origin or attachment.

Distortion a variation in the size or shape of the image in comparison to the object it represents.

Diuresis increased or excessive production of urine.

Diuretic a drug or other substance that tends to promote the formation and excretion of urine.

Diverticulitis inflammation of one or more diverticula. The collection of fecal matter in the thin-walled diverticula causes inflammation and abscess formation in the tissues surrounding the colon.

Diverticulosis the presence of pouchlike herniations through the muscular layer of the colon.

Diverticulum (plural, diverticula) a pouchlike herniation through the muscular wall of a tubular organ. A diverticulum may be present in the esophagus, stomach, the small intestine, or most commonly the colon.

DNA abbreviation for deoxyribonucleic acid, the protein substance of genes.

Dominant with respect to genes, describes the gene of a gene pair that is expressed in the individual.

Doppler a sonographic device that allows the evaluation of flowing media, such as blood, by measuring the Doppler shift of the reflected ultrasound beam.

***Dorsalis pedis* pulse** see *pedal pulse.*

Dose equivalent a measurement of the effective dose of radiation as compared to that of 250 keV x-rays; obtained by multiplying the dose in rad or Gray times the weighting factor (WF) of the specific type of radiation involved in the exposure and epressed in units of rem (British system) and Sieverts (SI system).

Dosimeter device for measuring radiation dose; in radiography, a badge worn to measure cumulative occupational exposure.

Dosimeter an instrument to detect and measure accumulated radiation exposure.

Down syndrome a congenital condition characterized by varying degrees of mental retardation and multiple defects; same as trisomy 21.

Draw sheet a single sheet folded in half that is placed under the patient and over the middle third of the bed; may be used to facilitate patient transfer.

Drip infusion the administration of fluids or medications through an intravenous catheter by gravity flow.

Droplet contamination means of disease transmission that occurs across a short distance, usually not more than 3 feet, when an infectious individual coughs, sneezes, speaks, or sings in the vicinity of a susceptible host.

Duodenitis inflammation of the duodenum.

Dysentery an inflammation of the intestine, especially of the colon, that may be caused by chemical irritants, bacteria, protozoa, or parasites and is characterized by diarrhea and abdominal cramping.

Dysphagia difficulty in swallowing, commonly associated with obstructive or motor disorders of the esophagus.

Dyspnea difficult or painful breathing that can be caused by certain heart conditions, lung conditions, asthma, strenuous exercise, or anxiety.

ED limit a level of effective dose of radiation that has been recommended as an upper limit for individuals who are occupationally exposed to radiation.

Edema the abnormal accumulation of fluid in interstitial spaces of tissues. Also called *swelling.*

Efficacy effectiveness.

Elder abuse any knowing, intentional, or negligent act by a caregiver or any other person that causes harm or serious risk of harm to a vulnerable adult.

Electrical ground the connection of an electric circuit to the earth, which becomes a part of the circuit. Grounding "drains off" excess charges, preventing electrical shocks and overheating of the circuit.

Electrocardiogram (ECG) a graphic record produced by an electrocardiograph, a device for recording heart rhythm by measuring electrical conduction through the heart.

Electrode an electrical contact; a connection for conducting an electrical current from the body to physiologic monitoring equipment.

Electrolarynx an electromechanical device that enables a person without a larynx to speak.

Electrolyte an element or compound that, when dissolved in water or another solvent, dissociates into ions, enabling the fluid to conduct an electric current. An appropriate electrolyte balance in blood and body tissues, especially sodium, calcium, and chlorides, is essential to transmission of nerve impulses.

Electromagnetic energy pertaining to magnetism that is induced by an electric current. Also, energy in the form of electromagnetic waves, such as light, x-rays, and radio waves.

Electron stream the flow of negatively charged particles across an x-ray tube, formed when the high positive electrical potential at the target attracts electrons of the space charge, which move rapidly across the tube.

Embolus (plural, emboli) a free-floating clot, air bubble, or other substance in the bloodstream.

Emergency a serious, unexpected event that demands immediate attention.

Emesis the act of vomiting, or a term for vomit.

Empathy the ability to recognize and to some extent share the emotions and state of mind of another and to understand the meaning and significance of that person's behavior.

Emphysema an abnormal condition of the pulmonary system characterized by overinflation and destructive changes of alveolar walls; one type of COPD.

Endemic constantly present within a community; describes diseases and physical or mental disorders.

Endoscope an illuminated optical instrument for the visualization of the interior of a body cavity or organ.

Endospore a form assumed by certain bacteria in which they resist drying and can live for long periods without warmth, moisture, or nutrients.

Endotracheal within or through the trachea.

Endovenous laser therapy (EVLT) a minimally invasive technology that uses energy from an 810-nm diode laser delivered by a fine fiberoptic probe to treat larger veins, such as the greater saphenous and the accessory saphenous vein systems.

Enema the introduction of a liquid into the colon via the rectum for cleansing, diagnostic, or therapeutic purposes.

Enteral within the small intestine, or via the small intestine. The *enteral route* of medication administration refers to the placement of medications within the digestive tract.

Enteric pertaining to the intestine; an enteric coating on an oral medication that prevents it from dissolving before it reaches the small intestine.

Epidemic the appearance of an infectious disease or condition that affects many people at the same time in the same geographic area.

Epilepsy, epileptic a group of neurologic disorders characterized by recurrent episodes of convulsive seizures, sensory disturbances, abnormal behavior, loss of consciousness, or all of these. Common to all types of epilepsy is an uncontrolled electrical discharge from the nerve cells of the cerebral cortex.

Epinephrine an endogenous adrenal hormone and synthetic adrenergic vasoconstrictor. It is an important emergency drug for the treatment of anaphylaxis.

Epistaxis bleeding from the nose (a nosebleed).

Ergonomics the study of the human body in relation to the working environment.

Erythema "radiation burn," redness, or inflammation of the skin or mucous membranes caused by the dilation and congestion of superficial capillaries.

Esophagitis inflammation of the esophagus.

Esophagram radiograph or radiographic examination of the esophagus.

Estrogen one of a group of hormonal steroid compounds that promote the development of female secondary sex characteristics.

Ethical analysis a method of evaluating situations in which the correct action is in question.

Ethics the science or study of moral values or principles, including ideals of autonomy, beneficence, and justice; the term is also applied to the moral values or principles themselves.

Ethics of care theory that recognizes that right actions for one patient in one situation may be wrong for other patients or other circumstances. A caring ethic demands moral judgments that reflect community values such as respect, patience, tact, and kindness.

Ethnic of or relating to a large group of people classed according to common cultural or racial origin.

Euthanasia the deliberate causing of death for humane purposes (e.g., of a person suffering from an incurable disease or condition).

Evisceration the removal of the viscera from the abdominal cavity; disembowelment; also, the removal of the contents from an organ or an organ from its cavity.

Excretion the elimination of drugs from the body after they have been metabolized.

Exocrine gland any of the multicellular glands that open onto the skin surface through ducts in the epithelium, as the sweat glands and the sebaceous glands.

Expiratory pertaining to the exhalation of air from the lungs.

Exposure index (EI) number an exposure indicator number usually displayed on the monitor, also referred to as *S number* or other number, depending on the equipment. This number must be monitored by radiographers to ensure that exposures are of diagnostic quality and are not excessive.

Exposure time (T) a measurement of how long the exposure will continue; measured in seconds, fractions of seconds, or milliseconds.

Extracorporeal pertaining to something that is outside the body.

Extravasation a passage or escape from a blood or lymph vessel into the tissues, usually of blood, serum, or lymph. With respect to intravenous fluids, it is the same as infiltration.

False imprisonment the intentional, unjustified, nonconsensual detention or confinement of a person for any length of time.

Fasting the act of abstaining from food for a specific period, usually for therapeutic or religious purposes, or in preparation for certain diagnostic tests or procedures.

Fee-for-service health care insurance plan in which insurance companies reimburse patients for the costs of their health care within the limits of the policy and the patient is responsible for any costs not covered.

Fellow a graduate student who is paid for services rendered while receiving advanced education; in the health care setting, physicians receiving advanced training in specialized areas may be designated as fellows.

Felony a crime declared by statute to be more serious than a misdemeanor and deserving a more severe punishment.

Fiberoptics a technical process that uses glass or plastic fibers to transmit light through a specially designed tube and reflect a magnified image by which an internal organ or cavity can be viewed.

Fibrillation involuntary recurrent contraction of a single muscle fiber or of an isolated bundle of nerve fibers. Fibrillation of heart muscle is an ineffective quivering motion that replaces normal heart rhythm and may be life threatening.

Fibrocystic breast disease the presence of single or multiple cysts that are palpable in the breasts. The cysts are benign and fairly common, yet must be investigated to distinguish between cysts and potentially malignant growths.

Filament the source of electrons found at the electrically negative cathode end of the x-ray tube. It is made of the element tungsten.

First-pass effect decrease in the therapeutic effect of a drug before it reaches the target tissue as a result of passing first through the liver via the portal circulation.

Fistula, fistulous tract abnormal passage from an internal organ to the body surface or between two internal organs, often the result of infection.

Flail chest a thorax in which multiple rib fractures cause instability in part of the chest wall and paradoxic breathing, with the lung underlying the injured area contracting on inspiration and bulging on expiration.

Flavivirus a genus of a family of Flaviviridae single-stranded positive-sense ribonucleic acid viruses, including species that cause yellow fever, Dengue fever, and St. Louis encephalitis.

Flora microorganisms that live on or within a body; they compete with disease-producing microorganisms and provide a natural immunity against certain infections.

Fluid overload an excessive accumulation of fluid in the body caused by excessive parenteral infusion or deficiencies in cardiovascular or renal fluid volume regulation; same as hypervolemia.

Fluorescence the emission by certain crystals of light of one wavelength when exposed to energy of a different, usually shorter, wavelength.

Fluoroscope a device used to produce a radiographic image on a fluorescent screen or cathode ray tube monitor for visual examination of internal structures in motion in real time.

Flushing, flushed a prolonged reddening of the face such as that caused by a reaction to certain drugs. Also, the process of injecting saline or heparin solution into an intravenous injection port to prevent mixing of medications and to prevent blood clotting in the port.

Focal spot a small area on an x-ray tube target where the electron stream strikes the target and x-rays are produced.

Fog a generalized exposure caused by scatter radiation that compromises the visibility of the anatomic structures on the radiograph.

Fomite nonliving material, such as bed linen, that can transmit microorganisms.

Fontanel the space between the bones of the skull in an infant or fetus, where ossification is incomplete. The main one is between the frontal and parietal bones.

Forceps any of a large variety of surgical instruments, all of which have two handles or sides, each attached to dull blades that move in opposition to each other like scissors.

Fowler position a modification of the supine position in which the patient's upper body is elevated.

Free radical atom with unpaired electron(s) in its outer shell.

Frequency with respect to a sine wave, the number of times per second that a wave crest passes a given point.

Fungus (plural, fungi) a type of organism that requires an external carbon source. The two basic types are molds and yeasts.

Fusion imaging use of computerized hybrid imaging systems that perform dual processes to obtain both anatomic and functional information. The basic types combine PET with CT, PET with MRI, and SPECT with CT.

Gadolinium an element that is a component of certain intensifying screen phosphors and of paramagnetic contrast agents.

Gait belt also called a *transfer belt*; should be used when assisting patients who are weak or unsteady.

Gamma camera a device that uses the emission of light from a crystal struck by gamma rays to produce an image of the distribution of radioactive material in a body organ. The light is detected by an array of light-sensitive electronic tubes and is converted to electric signals for further processing.

Gantry the portion of an MRI, CT, or other scanning unit that surrounds the patient, emits imaging energy, and detects information needed for image formation.

Gas gangrene necrosis tissue death accompanied by gas bubbles in soft tissue after surgery or trauma. It is caused by anaerobic organisms. Gas gangrene causes toxic delirium and is rapidly fatal if untreated.

Gastritis Inflammation of the stomach.

Gastroesophageal reflux disease (GERD) a type of esophagitis that occurs when stomach contents breech the esophageal sphincter, bringing stomach acid into contact with the more delicate mucosa of the esophagus.

Gastrointestinal (GI) pertaining to the organs of the alimentary tract, from mouth to anus.

Gastroscopy the visual inspection of the interior of the stomach by means of a special fiberoptic instrument (a gastroscope) inserted through the mouth and esophagus.

Generic pertaining to a substance, product, or drug that is not protected by trademark.

Genetic effects occur as a result of damage to the reproductive cells of the irradiated person and may be observed as defects in the children or grandchildren of the irradiated individual.

Germicide, germicidal a chemical that kills pathogenic microorganisms.

Gestation, gestational in viviparous animals, the period from the fertilization of the ovum until birth. Gestation varies by species; in humans the average duration is 266 days, or approximately 280 days from the onset of the last menstrual period.

Giardiasis an inflammatory intestinal condition. The source of infection is usually untreated water contaminated with *Giardia lamblia* cysts. Also called *traveler's diarrhea.*

Glucagon a hormone produced by the pancreas that is important in carbohydrate metabolism. An identical commercial preparation is available for the treatment of hypoglycemia and is used in imaging procedures to cause relaxation of the smooth muscle of the gastrointestinal tract.

Glucose a simple sugar found in certain foods, especially fruits, and a major source of energy present in human and animal body fluids.

Grand mal seizure a seizure characterized by loss of consciousness and repeated rigid arching of the back, alternating with periods of relaxation; same as major motor or tonic-clonic seizure.

Granule a particle, grain, or other small, dry mass capable of free movement. Unlike powders, granules are usually free flowing because of small surface forces involved.

Gray (Gy) the SI unit for radiation dose measurement.

Grid a device placed between the patient and the image receptor during a radiographic examination to limit the amount of scatter radiation reaching a radiographic image receptor, thereby increasing the image contrast.

Grid cap a grid mounted in a frame that can be attached to the front of an image receptor (IR) for mobile radiography and other special applications.

Gross negligence negligent acts that involve reckless disregard for life or limb. It denotes a higher degree of negligence than ordinary negligence and results in more serious penalties.

HAI (health care–associated infection) a hospital-acquired infection, also called *nosocomial infection*, defined as those that occur more than 48 hours after being admitted to the hospital.

Half-life the time required for a radioactive substance to lose 50% of its activity through decay.

Hallucinogen a substance that causes excitation of the central nervous system, characterized by hallucination, mood change, anxiety, sensory distortion, delusion, depersonalization; increased pulse, temperature, and blood pressure; and dilation of the pupils.

Hantavirus a genus of viruses in the Bunyaviridae family. Hantavirus is the cause of several different forms of hemorrhagic fever with renal syndrome.

Heimlich maneuver an emergency procedure for dislodging food or other obstruction from the trachea to prevent asphyxiation; also called *abdominal thrust.*

Hematologic blood-related.

Hematoma a collection of extravasated blood trapped in the tissues of the skin or in an organ, resulting from trauma or incomplete hemostasis after surgery.

Hemodynamics the physical aspects of blood circulation, including cardiac function and peripheral vascular physiologic characteristics.

Hemoglobin a complex protein-iron compound in the blood that carries oxygen to the cells from the lungs and carbon dioxide away from the cells to the lungs.

Hemolytic uremia syndrome a rare kidney disorder marked by renal failure, microangiopathic hemolytic anemia, and platelet deficiency. The syndrome, the cause of which is unknown, usually occurs in infancy.

Hemorrhage, hemorrhagic a loss of a large amount of blood in a short period, either externally or internally. Hemorrhage can be arterial, venous, or capillary.

Hemorrhoid a varicosity in the lower rectum or anus caused by congestion in the veins of the hemorrhoidal plexus.

Hemostat a procedure, device, or substance that arrests the flow of blood; common term for small forceps used to clamp blood vessels or tubing.

Hemothorax an accumulation of blood and fluid in the pleural cavity, between the parietal and visceral pleura, that is usually the result of trauma.

Heparin lock a small adapter with a diaphragm that is attached to an intravenous catheter when more than one injection is anticipated; same as intermittent injection port.

Hepatic pertaining to the liver.

Hepatitis any of several different types of inflammatory conditions of the liver, characterized by jaundice, hepatomegaly (liver enlargement), anorexia, abdominal and gastric discomfort, abnormal liver function, clay-colored stools, and tea-colored urine.

Herniation a protrusion of a body organ or portion of an organ through an abnormal opening in a membrane, muscle, or other tissue.

Herpes any of several kinds of diseases caused by herpesvirus and characterized by eruption of blisters on the skin or mucous membranes. Herpes simplex virus 1 (oral herpes: herpes labialis) and herpes simplex virus 2 (genital herpes: herpes genitalis) are forms of the herpes simplex virus (HSV). Herpes zoster is the causative agent of chicken pox and shingles.

Hiatal hernia protrusion of a portion of the stomach upward through the diaphragm. The condition occurs in approximately 40% of the population, and most people display few, if any, symptoms.

HIPAA (Health Insurance Portability and Accountability Act) law enacted under the U.S. Department of Health and Human Services that protects the privacy rights of patients.

Hirschsprung disease see *congenital megacolon.*

Histamine a compound, found in all cells, produced by the breakdown of histidine. It is released in allergic and inflammatory reactions and causes dilation of capillaries, decrease in blood pressure, increase in secretion of gastric juice, and constriction of smooth muscles of the bronchi and uterus.

Histoplasmosis a lung infection caused by inhalation of spores of the fungus *Histoplasma capsulatum.*

HIV abbreviation for human immunodeficiency virus.

Hives blotchy reddening of the skin with itching; same as urticaria.

HMO (health maintenance organization) organization that provides complete and comprehensive health care for the cost of the premium plus a small fee called a *co-payment* for each visit.

Hospice an approach to care for the terminally ill that seeks to provide comfort without treating the underlying disease.

Hospitalist physician specialist, often an internist, who limits practice to treatment of hospital inpatients.

Human immunodeficiency virus (HIV) a retrovirus that causes acquired immunodeficiency syndrome (AIDS). It is transmitted through contact with an infected individual's blood, semen, breast milk, cervical secretions, cerebrospinal fluid, or synovial fluid. HIV infects T helper cells of the immune system and causes infection with a long incubation period before manifesting the symptoms of AIDS.

Hydration a chemical process in which water is taken up by a chemical without disrupting the rest of the molecule; also, the process of supplying water to a person to restore or maintain the body's fluid balance.

Hydrostatic pressure the pressure exerted by a liquid. The hydrostatic pressure of an intravenous infusion is determined by the height of the fluid container with respect to the vein.

Hygroscopic tending to absorb moisture.

Hyperextension the position of maximum extension of a joint.

Hyperglycemia abnormally elevated level of blood glucose that is characteristic of uncontrolled diabetes mellitus.

Hyperosmolar hyperglycemic nonketotic syndrome (HHNK) a severe condition that can occur when patients with neglected type II diabetes mellitis become dehydrated and hyperglycemic. It maybe induced by other serious conditions; it can lead to coma and seizures and is treated with rapid fluid administration.

Hypertension a common, often asymptomatic disorder characterized by elevated blood pressure persistently exceeding 140/90 mm Hg.

Hyperthermia a higher than normal body temperature; same as fever or pyrexia.

Hyperventilation a respiratory rate that is greater than that metabolically necessary for pulmonary gas exchange. It is the result of rapid breathing, an increased tidal volume, or a combination of both, and causes excessive intake of oxygen and elimination of carbon dioxide, with narrowing of the blood vessels that supply the brain; this can cause light-headedness, and, in severe cases, loss of consciousness.

Hypervolemia an abnormal increase in the amount of intravascular fluid, particularly in the volume of circulating blood or its components; same as fluid overload.

Hypodermic pertaining to the area below the skin, such as a hypodermic injection.

Hypoglycemia a less than normal amount of glucose in the blood, usually caused by administration of too much insulin, excessive secretion of insulin by the islet cells of the pancreas, or dietary deficiency.

Hypotension an abnormal condition in which the blood pressure is not adequate for normal perfusion and oxygenation of the tissues. See also shock.

Hypothalamus a portion of the diencephalon of the brain. It activates, controls, and integrates the peripheral autonomic nervous system, endocrine processes, and many somatic functions, such as body temperature, sleep, and appetite.

Hypovolemia an abnormally low circulating blood volume; may be caused by hemorrhage or by severe dehydration.

Hypoxemia, hypoxia insufficient oxygenation of the blood.

Hysterosalpingography a method of producing radiographic images of the uterus and fallopian tubes as part of the diagnosis of abnormalities in the reproductive tract of a nonpregnant woman.

ICP abbreviation for intracranial pressure.

ICU abbreviation for intensive care unit.

Idiosyncratic (reaction) occurs when a patient overreacts or underreacts to a drug or has an unusual reaction.

Ileostomy surgical formation of an opening of the ileum onto the surface of the abdomen, through which fecal matter is expelled.

Image contrast the difference in the optical density of adjacent structures within the image.

Image detail refers to the sharpness of the image.

Image intensifier an electronic device used to produce a fluoroscopic image with a low radiation exposure. A beam of x-rays passing through the patient is converted by a special vacuum tube into a pattern of electrons. The electrons are accelerated and concentrated onto a small fluorescent screen, where they present a bright image that is usually displayed on a television monitor.

Immobilization the use of various devices to keep patients from moving during imaging procedures.

Immunocompromised having an impaired immune system; common in patients with AIDS and those who have received chemotherapy or medication related to organ or bone marrow transplant.

Immunosuppressant an agent that significantly interferes with the ability of the immune system to respond to antigenic stimulation by inhibiting cellular and humoral immunity.

Incision a cut produced surgically by a sharp instrument to create an opening into an organ or space in the body.

Incontinence inability to control urination or defecation.

Incubator a box-like infant crib that may be used because this closed environment provides extra warmth, moisture, and oxygen while reducing exposure to airborne infection.

Incubator a crib for a newborn that provides security and warmth. A closed incubator may be used for premature infants and those at risk to supply moisture and oxygen while reducing exposure to airborne infection.

Inert (of a chemical substance) not taking part in a chemical reaction; (of a medication ingredient) not active pharmacologically; serving only as a bulking, binding, or sweetening agent or other excipient in a medication.

Infectious mononucleosis an acute infection caused by the Epstein-Barr virus. It is characterized by fever, sore throat, swollen lymph glands, atypical lymphocytes, splenomegaly, hepatomegaly, abnormal liver function, and bruising. The disease is usually transmitted by droplet infection, but is not highly or predictably contagious.

Infiltration the process whereby a fluid passes into the tissues, such as when a local anesthetic is administered or an intravenous infusion leaks from a vein.

Inflammation, inflammatory the protective response of body tissues to irritation, infection, or injury; characterized by warmth, redness, swelling, and pain.

Inflammatory bowel disease (IBD) inflammation and ulcerations of the mucosa of the colon.

Influenza highly contagious infection of the respiratory tract caused by a myxovirus and transmitted by airborne droplet contamination.

Informed consent permission obtained from a patient to perform a specific test or procedure. Informed consent is required before performing most invasive procedures and before admitting a patient to a research study. The document used must be written in a language understood by the patient and be dated and signed by the patient and at least one witness.

Infusion the passive introduction of a substance (fluid, drug, or electrolyte) into a vein or between tissues, as by gravitational force; slow or prolonged intravenous delivery of a drug or fluids.

Ingest, ingestion to take substances into the body through the mouth.

Inpatient a patient who has been admitted to a hospital or other health care facility for at least an overnight stay.

Insulin a naturally occurring hormone secreted by the beta cells of the islets of Langerhans in the pancreas in response to increased levels of glucose in the blood; also, a medication administered to patients who lack sufficient natural insulin.

Intensive care unit (ICU) a special care unit designed for patients in critical condition whose treatment and status require frequent monitoring. The ICU can be subdivided into medical, surgical, trauma, neonatal, and pediatric units.

Intercostal space the space between two ribs.

Interferon a natural cellular protein formed when cells are exposed to a virus or another foreign particle of nucleic acid. Also, a medication made from natural interferons that directs the immune system's attack on viruses, bacteria, tumors, and other foreign substances that may invade the body, such as the hepatitis C virus and certain types of cancer.

Intermammillary line a horizontal anatomic line drawn between the nipples.

Intermittent injection port a small adapter with a diaphragm that is attached to an intravenous catheter when more than one injection is anticipated; same as heparin lock or saline lock.

Intern a physician in the first postgraduate year, learning medical practice under supervision before beginning a residency program or practice.

Intraarterial within an artery.

Intradermal within the dermis layer of the skin.

Intramuscular (IM) within muscle tissue.

Intrathecal pertaining to a structure, process, or substance within a sheath, such as within the spinal canal.

Intrauterine device (IUD) a contraceptive device. It consists of a bent strip of radiopaque plastic with a fine monofilament tail and is placed within the uterus.

Intravascular within a blood vessel.

Intravenous (IV) pertaining to the inside of a vein, as in a thrombus, injection, infusion, or catheter.

Intubate, intubation passage of a tube into a body aperture, specifically the insertion of a breathing tube through the mouth or nose into the trachea to ensure a patent airway for the delivery of anesthetic gases or oxygen or both.

Invasive characterized by a tendency to spread, infiltrate, and intrude. Invasive procedures involve penetration of the body wall (e.g., surgery, angiography).

Iodinated refers to substances to which iodine has been added, especially types of contrast media prepared with iodine compounds, which absorb radiation to a greater degree than blood or soft tissues and therefore produce a more clearly visible white or light shadow on the radiographic image.

Ion a charged particle, an atom or group of atoms that has acquired an electrical charge through the gain or loss of one or more electrons.

Ionic pertaining to a compound that separates into charged particles in solution.

Ionize, ionization to separate or change into ions (charged particles).

Irrigate, irrigation to flush with a fluid, usually with a slow steady pressure on a syringe plunger. It may be done to cleanse a wound or to clear tubing.

Irritable bowel syndrome (IBS) chronic irritation and inflammation of the colon causing bouts of diarrhea, cramping, and gas, without physical changes in the bowel tissue.

Isotonic pertaining to a liquid that has the same concentration of solute as human body fluid.

Ischemia a decreased supply of oxygenated blood to a body organ or part.

Ketoacidosis an acidic condition of the blood accompanied by an accumulation of ketones, resulting from extensive breakdown of fats because of faulty carbohydrate metabolism; often seen in cases of uncontrolled diabetes mellitus.

Kilovolt (kV), kilovoltage measure of electrical potential, 1000 volts.

Kilovoltage peak (kVp) potential difference measured at the peak of the electrical cycle; an x-ray control setting that determines the penetrating power of the x-ray beam.

Kyphosis, kyphotic posterior curvature of the spine, characteristic of the thoracic spinal segments. When abnormally exaggerated, kyphosis results in protrusion of the upper back.

Laceration a torn, jagged wound.

Laparoscope a type of fiberoptic instrument consisting of an illuminated tube with an optical system. It is inserted through the abdominal wall for examining the peritoneal cavity, visualizing structures within the peritoneal cavity, and performing minimally invasive abdominal surgery, such as cholecystectomy.

Laryngectomy surgical removal of the larynx to treat cancer of the larynx.

Larynx, laryngeal the organ of voice that is part of the air passage connecting the pharynx with the trachea.

Latent image the unobservable image stored in the silver halide emulsion of film; it is made visible by processing.

Lesion a wound, injury, or pathologic change in body tissue; also any visible, local abnormality of the tissues of the skin, such as a wound, sore, rash, or boil. A lesion can be described as benign, cancerous, gross, occult, primary, or secondary.

Leukemia a broad term given to a group of malignant diseases affecting the bone marrow.

Level of consciousness (LOC) degree of cognitive function involving arousal mechanisms of the reticular formation of the brain.

Libel a false accusation written, printed, typewritten, or presented in a picture or a sign that is made with malicious intent to defame the reputation of a person who is living or the memory of a person who is dead, resulting in public embarrassment, contempt, ridicule, or hatred.

Lidocaine a local anesthetic agent, also given intravenously to treat ventricular tachycardia.

Line of gravity an imaginary line that extends from the center of gravity to the base of support.

Lipoprotein a conjugated protein in which fats or oils form an integral part of the molecule.

Lithotripsy a procedure for crushing and eliminating a calculus in the renal pelvis, ureter, bladder, or gallbladder.

Long-term effects stochastic radiation effects, sometimes referred to as *latent effects*, may not be apparent for as many as 30 years.

Lordosis, lordotic anterior curvature of the spine, characteristic of both the cervical and lumbar spinal segments.

Lumbar puncture (LP) the introduction of a hollow needle and stylet into the subarachnoid space of the lumbar part of the spinal canal; same as a spinal tap.

Lumen (plural, lumina) the interior canal of an organ or catheter.

Lyme disease an acute, recurrent inflammatory infection transmitted by a tick-borne spirochete, *Borrelia burgdorferi*.

Lymphocyte small agranulocytic leukocyte (white blood cell) originating from fetal stem cells and developing in the bone marrow.

Lymphoma neoplasm consisting of lymphoid tissue that originates in the reticuloendothelial and lymphatic systems. It is usually malignant but is benign in rare cases.

Lysozyme an enzyme found in tears and other secretions that acts to destroy some foreign organisms.

Magnetic resonance imaging (MRI) a noninvasive computerized diagnostic modality that uses a magnetic field and pulses of radio waves to produce images on a computer monitor.

Major motor seizure a seizure characterized by loss of consciousness and a repeated rigid arching of the back alternating with periods of relaxation. Same as grand mal or tonic-clonic seizure.

Malaria a severe infectious illness caused by one or more of at least four species of the protozoan genus *Plasmodium*. The disease is transmitted from human to human by a bite from an infected *Anopheles* mosquito. Malarial infection can also be spread by blood transfusion from an infected patient or by the use of an infected hypodermic needle.

Malpractice professional negligence that is the proximate cause of injury or harm to a patient, resulting from a lack of professional knowledge, experience, or skill that can be expected in others in the profession or from a failure to exercise reasonable care or judgment in the application of professional knowledge, experience, or skill.

Mammogram, mammography a radiograph or examination of the soft tissues of the breast to allow identification of various benign and malignant neoplastic processes.

Managed care systems health care contracts that allow private hospitals and physicians to provide private services while also providing care through insurance plans similar to health maintenance organizations.

Manometer a device for measuring the pressure of a fluid, consisting of a tube marked with a scale and containing a relatively incompressible fluid, such as mercury.

Mastectomy surgical removal of one or both breasts, usually to remove a malignant tumor. It can include breast tissue, chest muscle, and axillary lymph nodes.

Medicaid funds provided by the federal government to aid the medically indigent who fall within a designated eligibility group, recognized by the federal and state governments.

Medicare a federal health insurance program in the United States that covers a portion of the medical care costs for those over the age of 65.

Medication pump a pump that automatically delivers measured amounts of drugs through an intravenous catheter.

Meningitis any infection or inflammation of the membranes covering the brain and spinal cord.

Metabolism the aggregate of all chemical processes that take place in living organisms, resulting in growth, generation of energy, elimination of wastes, and other body functions as they relate to the distribution of nutrients in the blood after digestion.

Metabolite a substance produced by metabolic action or necessary for a metabolic process.

Metabolize to change physically and chemically as a result of body processes.

Microbe, microbial a microorganism, pertaining to a living organism too small to be seen by the naked eye.

Microbial dilution the process of reducing the total number of microorganisms, which is accomplished at three levels: cleanliness measures, disinfection, and sterilization.

Microorganism any tiny, usually microscopic, entity capable of carrying on living processes.

Milliampere, milliamperage (mA) a unit of electric current that is one thousandth of an ampere. It is used to measure the rate of current flow in an x-ray tube and to describe the exposure setting of a radiography machine that determines the rate at which x-rays are produced.

Milliampere seconds (mAs) the product obtained by multiplying the electric current in milliamperes by the exposure time in seconds. The mAs is indicative of the total quantity of radiation involved in an exposure and determines the optical density of the radiographic image.

Miscible able to be mixed or blended with another substance.

Misdemeanor a criminal offense that is considered less serious than a felony and carries a lesser penalty, usually a fine or imprisonment for less than 1 year.

Mission statement the role of an organization, hospital, or health care facility stated in a one- or two-paragraph declaration of the institution's basic philosophy and primary goals. This statement provides guidance for the decisions that govern the activities of the organization or facility.

Mitosis, mitotic a type of cell division that occurs in somatic cells and results in the formation of two genetically identical daughter cells containing the diploid number of chromosomes characteristic of the species.

Mold fungus that occurs in long, branched, filament-like structures composed of many cells.

Moral agent the one responsible for implementing an ethical decision.

Motile, motility capable of spontaneous but unconscious or involuntary movement.

MRSA (methicillin-resistant *Staphylococcus aureus*) drug-resistant form of *Staphylococcus aureus* contributes to surgical wound, urinary tract, and bloodstream infections and can cause respiratory infections.

Mucocutaneous pertaining to the mucous membrane and the skin.

Mucosa, mucosal, mucous membrane any one of four major kinds of thin sheets of tissue that cover or line various parts of the body. Mucous membrane lines cavities or canals of the body that open to the outside.

Mutation an unusual change in genetic material occurring spontaneously or by induction.

Myelogram, myelography a radiograph or examination after the injection of a radiopaque medium into the subarachnoid space to demonstrate any distortions of the spinal cord, spinal nerve roots, and subarachnoid space.

Myocardial infarction (MI) a heart attack; necrosis of heart muscle tissue caused by coronary artery thrombosis or occlusion.

Narcotic pertaining to a substance that produces insensibility or stupor.

Nasoenteric (NE) tube tube placed through the nose and into the gastrointestinal tract as far as the small intestine to aspirate gas and fluid that may cause distention. It is often used postoperatively on patients who have undergone abdominal surgery.

Nasogastric (NG) tube a tube placed through the nose, pharynx, esophagus, and into the stomach to allow feeding of a patient directly into the stomach. It can also be connected to a suction device to empty the stomach.

Nebulizer a device for producing a fine spray. Intranasal and respiratory medications are often administered by a nebulizer; also called an *atomizer*.

Necrosis, necrotic the death of living cells or tissues; containing or affected by dead cells or tissues.

Negligence the commission of an act that a prudent person would not have done or the omission of a duty that a prudent person would have fulfilled, resulting in injury or harm to another person.

Neonate, neonatal newborn an infant from birth to 28 days of age; *neonatal* refers to the period immediately after birth.

Neoonatal intensive care unit (NICU) hospital unit for care of premature and low-birth-weight infants and those with health problems that require frequent monitoring.

Nephrogram a radiograph of the kidney; usually refers to an image of the parenchyma of the kidney in the early postinjection phase of an excretory urogram.

Nephrotoxic term to describe certain chemicals and medications that have a poisonous effect on the kidneys.

Neurogenic pertaining to the formation of nervous tissue; originating from the nervous system.

Neurologic pertaining to the nervous system.

Neurology the field of medicine that deals with the nervous system and its disorders.

Neurostimulator an electronic device worn by patients to control pain and muscle spasm.

Nitrile   a substance that is impervious to many hazardous chemicals; gloves of this material are commonly used in the health care setting.

Nonaccidental trauma (NAT)   another term for battered child syndrome or the signs of elder abuse.

Noninvasive   pertaining to a diagnostic or therapeutic technique that does not require the skin to be broken or a cavity or organ of the body to be entered.

Nonionic   pertaining to compounds that do not dissociate into charged particles when in solution.

Nonstochastic   describes biologic radiation effects that are predictable; their intensity is dose dependent. These effects occur only after a certain threshold amount of exposure has been received; also called *deterministic effects*.

Normal saline   a 0.9% weight per volume (w/v) solution of sodium chloride in water that is isotonic with blood. It is available as a sterile solution for intravenous injection.

Nosocomial   pertaining to a hospital.

Nosocomial infection   hospital-acquired disease.

NPO (nil per os, nothing by mouth)   a patient care instruction advising that the patient is prohibited from ingesting food, beverage, or medicine.

Nuclear medicine   the use of radionuclides to produce imaging studies that reveal information about physiology and function.

Nurse practitioner   a registered nurse who has received advanced education in nursing and clinical experience in a specialized area of nursing practice.

Object-image distance (OID)   the distance between the object and the image receptor (IR).

Occlude, occlusion (in anatomy)   a blockage in a canal, vessel, or passage of the body.

Oncology   the branch of medicine concerned with the study, diagnosis, and treatment of malignancy.

Opaque, opacify, opacification   pertaining to a substance or surface that neither transmits nor allows the passage of light; see also *radiopaque*.

Open reduction   a surgical procedure for realigning a fracture or dislocation by exposing the skeletal parts involved.

Ophthalmology   the branch of medicine concerned with the study of the physiology, anatomy, and pathology of the eye and the diagnosis and treatment of disorders of the eye.

Opiate   a narcotic drug that contains opium; a derivative of opium.

Opioid   pertaining to natural and synthetic chemicals that have opium-like effects, regardless of whether they are derived from opium.

Opportunistic infection   an infection caused by normally nonpathogenic organisms in a host whose resistance has been decreased by disorders such as diabetes mellitus, HIV infection, or cancer, or by cancer treatment that causes immunosuppression.

Optical density (OD)   the overall blackness of the image.

Oral   pertaining to the mouth. An oral temperature is measured with the thermometer probe in the mouth, under the tongue; oral medications are swallowed.

Orthopedic   pertaining to the locomotor system of the body, including the skeleton, muscles, and joints.

Orthopedic traction   a mechanical method that uses weights to provide a constant pull on part of the body for therapeutic reasons, such as to maintain alignment of fracture fragments or to relieve pressure caused by spinal injury.

Orthopnea   an abnormal condition in which a person must sit or stand to breathe deeply or comfortably.

Orthostatic hypotension   a transient state of cerebral anoxia and low blood pressure occurring when an individual assumes a standing posture; same as postural hypotension.

OSHA (Occupational Safety and Health Administration)   a federal agency governing safety in the workplace that provides guidelines to ensure a high level of safety for hospital workers.

OSL (optically stimulated luminescence)   type of personal radiation monitoring dosimeter most commonly used in health care situations today.

Osmolality   the concentration of particles in a solution, which determines the osmotic pressure of the solution expressed in osmoles or milliosmoles per kilogram of water. Osmotic pressure influences the passage of water through semipermeable membranes. Normal adult blood osmolality is 285 to 295 mOsm/kg H_2O.

Osmosis   movement of water or other solvent through a semipermeable membrane in the direction of higher solute concentration.

Osseous   consisting of or resembling bone; bony.

OTC (over the counter)   describes a drug available to the consumer without a prescription.

Outpatient   a patient, not hospitalized, who is being treated in an office, clinic, or other ambulatory care facility; a patient seen briefly in a hospital department without being admitted for an overnight stay.

Pacemaker   an electronic device used in most cases to increase the heart rate in severe bradycardia by electrically stimulating the heart muscle.

PACS (picture archiving and communication system)   the software and hardware that supports digital imaging systems and networks.

PACU (postanesthesia care unit)   an area designed and staffed to provide close observation and care of patients following operative procedures requiring an anesthetic agent; also called a *recovery room*.

Palliative   a substance or treatment that soothes or relieves.

Pallor   an unnatural paleness or absence of color in the skin.

Pandemic   a widespread epidemic.

Paralysis   the loss of muscle function, loss of sensation, or both.

Paramagnetic agents   agents with a small but positive magnetic susceptibility, the small addition of which may greatly reduce the MRI relaxation times of a substance and used as a contrast medium in MRI.

Parenteral   pertaining to treatment introduced into the body other than through the digestive system.

Parietal   pertaining to the wall of a cavity (e.g., the parietal pleura lines the interior walls of the thoracic cavity).

Passive immunity   short-term resistance to infection produced by preformed antibodies. Preformed antibodies can be injected in the form of pooled immune globulin from the general population; they are passed to infants in utero or in breast milk.

Patent, patency   a state of being open or exposed; with respect to tubular structures, open to permit liquid to flow.

Pathogen   any microorganism capable of producing disease.

Pedal pulse a count of the heart rate by means of the advancing pressure wave in the *dorsalis pedis* artery on the dorsal aspect (instep) of the foot.

Pediatric pertaining to health care and treatment of children and the study of childhood diseases.

Penicillin any one of a group of antibiotics derived from cultures of species of the fungus *Penicillium* or similar antibiotics produced semisynthetically.

Percutaneous performed through the skin, such as a biopsy performed using a needle.

Perforated ulcer an ulcer (sore) that penetrates the thickness of a wall or membrane.

Pericardium a fibroserous sac that surrounds the heart and the roots of the great vessels.

Peripherally inserted central catheter (PICC) a commonly used type of central venous catheter that is inserted peripherally, usually in the arm.

Peristalsis the coordinated, rhythmic, serial contraction of smooth muscle that forces food through the digestive tract, bile through the bile duct, and urine through the ureters.

Peritonitis inflammation of the membrane lining the abdominal cavity (peritoneum). It is caused by bacteria or irritating substances introduced into the abdominal cavity, by a penetrating wound or perforation of an organ in the gastrointestinal tract or the reproductive tract.

Permeability the degree to which one substance allows another substance to pass through it.

Pertussis an acute, highly contagious respiratory disease characterized by paroxysmal coughing that ends in a loud whooping inspiration; also called *whooping cough*.

Phagocytosis the process by which certain cells engulf and destroy microorganisms and cellular debris.

Pharmacodynamics the study of how a drug acts on a living organism, including the pharmacologic response and the duration and magnitude of response observed.

Pharmacokinetics the study of how drugs enter the body, are absorbed, reach their site of action, are metabolized, and exit the body.

Pharmacology the study of the preparation, properties, uses, and actions of drugs.

Pharyngitis inflammation or infection of the throat.

Phlebitis inflammation of a vein.

Phlebotomist a person with special training in the practice of drawing blood.

Phosphors fluorescent crystals that give off light when exposed to x-rays; see also *fluorescence*.

Photomultiplier tube a device used in many radiation detection and imaging applications that converts low levels of light into electrical pulses.

Photon the smallest quantity of electromagnetic energy. It has no mass and no charge and travels at the speed of light. Photons can occur in the form of light rays, x-rays, gamma rays, and other electromagnetic energies.

Photosensitive reactive to light.

Photostimulable phosphors crystals that store the energy of the remnant x-ray beam and release it as light when stimulated by a laser.

Picture archiving and communication system (PACS) The computer hardware and software technology used to manage digital images in hospitals and health care facilities.

Pixel a minute area of illumination on a display screen, one of many from which an image is composed.

Plaintiff a person who files a civil lawsuit initiating a legal action.

Pleura, pleural a delicate serous membrane covering the lung and lining the thoracic cavity.

Pleural effusion an abnormal accumulation of fluid within the thoracic cavity between the visceral and parietal pleura.

Pleurisy inflammation of the pleura, sometimes resulting in adhesion of pleural membranes and causing dyspnea and pain.

Pneumatic pertaining to air or gas.

Pneumonia an acute inflammation of the lungs, often caused by inhaled pneumococci of the species *Streptococcus pneumoniae*.

Pneumothorax a collection of air or gas in the pleural space causing the lung to collapse.

Polyp abnormal growth of tissue that can be found in any organ that has blood vessels but occurs most commonly in mucous membranes, especially in the colon.

Positron emission tomography (PET) a computerized nuclear medicine scanning modality involving the injection of radionuclides that emit ion pairs.

Postanesthesia care unit (PACU) sometimes referred to as *postanesthesia recovery* (PAR) or the *recovery room*. It is located just outside the surgical suite, allowing for the unimpeded transfer of patients and immediate access to surgeons, anesthesiologists, and operating room nurses.

Postictal describes the immediate period following a seizure.

Postural hypotension a transient cerebral anoxia that occurs when a patient is bedridden for an extended period of time and blood pools in the extremities when the torso is elevated; same as orthostatic hypotension.

Potent, potency active, powerful, or strong.

Practice standards a written statement developed by the ASRT that describes the radiographer's duties and responsibilities.

Precipitate to cause a substance to separate or to settle out of solution; a substance that has separated from or settled out of a solution.

Preferred provider organization (PPO) a health care insurance system that offers care at reduced rates within an established network of providers.

Premedication any sedative, tranquilizer, hypnotic, or anticholinergic medication administered before anesthesia or other procedure.

Primary health care a basic level of health care that includes programs directed at the promotion of health, early diagnosis of disease or disability, and prevention of disease.

Primary x-ray beam the portion of the x-ray beam between the x-ray tube and the patient; it is not attenuated except by air.

Principle-based ethics, principlism a widely accepted standard for selecting and defending solutions to ethical dilemmas in health care communities based upon six moral principles.

Prion the smallest and least understood of all microbes; infectious protein.

Prognosis a prediction of the probable outcome of a disease based on the condition of the person and the usual course of the disease as observed in similar situations.

Prone being in the position of lying face down.

Proprietary medication medicinal substance that is protected from commercial competition because its ingredients or methods of manufacture are kept secret or are protected by trademark or patent.

Prosthesis (plural, prostheses) an artificial replacement for a missing body part, or a device designed and applied to improve function, such as a hearing aid.

Protocol a written plan specifying the procedures to be followed in giving a particular examination, in conducting research, or in providing care for a particular condition.

Protozoan (plural, protozoa) single-cell microorganism of the subkingdom Protozoa.

Proximal nearer to a point of reference or attachment, usually the trunk of the body, than other parts of the body or of the same structure. For example, the elbow is proximal to the wrist.

Psychomotor pertaining to or causing voluntary movements usually associated with neural activity. Psychomotor skill is the ability to move purposefully.

Pulmonary pertaining to the lungs or the respiratory system.

Pulmonary edema the accumulation of extravascular fluid in lung tissues and alveoli, caused most commonly by congestive heart failure.

Pulmonary embolism (PE) a sudden blockage of a lung artery, usually caused by a blood clot that travels to the lung from a vein in the leg.

Pulse oximeter a digital monitor of pulse rate and oxygen saturation of the blood that is connected to the patient by means of a cable and a small probe attached to a finger or earlobe.

Pyloric stenosis a narrowing of the pyloric sphincter at the outlet of the stomach, causing an obstruction that blocks the flow of food into the small intestine.

Pylorospasm an involuntary contraction of the muscle that forms the pyloric sphincter at the outlet of the stomach, as occurs in pyloric stenosis.

Pyrexia the abnormal elevation of body temperature above 37° C (98.6° F); same as fever.

Qualitative pertaining to the quality, value, or nature of something.

Quantitative capable of being measured.

Quantum (plural, quanta) a group or bundle of photons.

Quarantine the process of keeping a person in enforced isolation for a period of time to limit or prevent the spread of disease or infection.

Rad abbreviation for *radiation absorbed dose*, the basic unit of absorbed dose of ionizing radiation in the British system of radiation measurement. One rad is equal to the absorption of 100 ergs of radiation energy per gram of matter.

Radiation field the cross section of the x-ray beam at the point where it is utilized.

Radiofrequency ablation (RFA) a minimally invasive technology that uses a special device that consists of a tiny RF generator associated with a sterile catheter and a collapsible electrode probe to treat larger veins, such as the greater saphenous and the accessory saphenous vein systems.

Radiograph an x-ray image.

Radiographer an allied health professional who performs diagnostic examinations on patients using a variety of modalities, including radiography, computed tomography, magnetic resonance imaging, mammography, and cardiovascular interventional technology.

Radiography the production of images using ionizing radiation.

Radioisotope a radioactive isotope of an element, used for therapeutic and diagnostic purposes.

Radiologic technologist a person who, under the supervision of a physician, operates diagnostic imaging equipment and assists radiologists and other health professionals.

Radiologist a physician who specializes in medical imaging.

Radiology information management system (RIMS) computer system that allows the technologist access to pertinent and limited information about a patient; also allows for ordering and billing of imaging examinations.

Radiolucent pertaining to materials that allow x-rays to penetrate with a minimum of absorption.

Radionuclide an isotope that undergoes radioactive decay; same as radioisotope.

Radiopaque not permitting the passage of x-rays or other radiant energy.

Radiopharmaceutical a radioactive compound produced for use in nuclear imaging.

Rapid Response Team a team that is trained to intervene and assist caregivers before a patient's condition deteriorates to the point that a conventional code is required.

Rapport a sense of harmony and understanding underlying a relationship between two persons, which is an essential bond between a therapist and patient.

Recessive with respect to genes, describes the gene of a gene pair that is not expressed in the individual.

Rectal pertaining to the rectum, the distal portion of the large intestine, approximately 12 cm long, between the sigmoid colon and the anus. A rectal temperature is measured with the thermometer probe inserted into the rectum.

Recumbent lying down or leaning backward.

Regimen a strictly regulated therapeutic program such as a diet or exercise schedule.

Rem (radiation equivalent in man) the radiation dose equivalent unit in the British system of radiation measurement. Its value is obtained by multiplying the absorbed dose in rad by the weighting factor of the specific type of radiation involved.

Remnant radiation the radiation that remains after the x-ray beam passes through an object to produce an image; same as exit radiation.

Renal pertaining to the kidney.

Res ipsa loquitur legal doctrine applied when negligence and loss are so apparent they would be obvious to anyone. Literally, "the thing speaks for itself."

Resident a physician in one of the postgraduate years of clinical training (often specialized) after the first, or internship, year.

Residual pertaining to the part of something that remains after removing the bulk of the substance.

Respiration, respiratory breathing, the process of the molecular exchange of oxygen and carbon dioxide within the body's tissues, from the lungs to cellular oxidation.

Respiratory arrest the cessation of breathing, caused by obstruction of the airway by a foreign object or by tracheal or bronchial edema.

Respite care short-term health services to the dependent older adult to provide relief for the primary caregiver.

Respondeat superior legal doctrine that holds employers responsible for negligent acts of their employees that occur in the course of their work. Literally, "let the master respond."

Restraints wrist and ankle bands and/or a vest with straps tied to the bed or stretcher; are used to prevent patients from injuring themselves or from disengaging therapeutic devices such as intravenous lines or oxygen masks. The application of these physical restraints on an adult patient requires a physician's order.

Resuscitation the process of sustaining the vital functions of a person in respiratory or cardiac failure while reviving him or her, using techniques of artificial respiration and cardiac massage, correcting acid-base imbalance, and treating the cause of failure.

Retention catheter a type of rectal or urinary catheter with an inflatable cuff that holds the catheter securely in place.

Retrograde moving backward; moving or flowing in the opposite direction to that which is considered normal.

Retrovirus any of a family of ribonucleic acid (RNA) viruses containing an enzyme, reverse transcriptase, in the virion.

Rickettsia (plural, rickettsiae) a genus of microorganisms that combine aspects of both bacteria and viruses.

Rights-based ethics system that emphasizes the rights of individuals in a democratic society to be shielded from undue restriction or harm. The rights of some individuals place duties on others.

Rocky Mountain spotted fever (RMSF) a serious tickborne infectious disease occurring throughout the temperate zones of North and South America; caused by *Rickettsia rickettsii*.

Roentgen (R or r) the standard unit of radiation intensity in the British system of radiation measurement. It is a measurement of radiation intensity in air. The roentgen is equal to the quantity of radiation that will produce 2.08×10^9 ion pairs in a cubic centimeter of dry air.

Scatter radiation ionizing radiation that occurs as a result of the interaction between the primary x-ray beam and matter. It is emitted from the matter in all directions during the exposure, tending to fog the image and produce a radiation hazard in the room. The patient is the principal source of scatter radiation that occurs during radiography.

Sclerosis, sclerotic a condition characterized by hardening of tissue resulting from any of several causes, including inflammation, the deposit of mineral salts, and infiltration of connective tissue fibers.

Secondary health care an intermediate level of health care that includes diagnosis and treatment; performed in a hospital having specialized equipment and laboratory facilities.

Sedation an induced state of quiet, calmness, or sleep, as by means of a sedative or hypnotic medication.

Seizure a hyperexcitation of neurons in the brain leading to a sudden, violent, involuntary series of contractions of a group of muscles.

Senile, senility pertaining to or characteristic of old age or the process of aging.

Sepsis, septic microbial infection, contamination.

Sestamibi a radiopharmaceutical used in nuclear imaging to visualize tissues.

Sharps any needles, scalpels, or other articles that could cause wounds or punctures to personnel.

Sharps container a puncture-proof container where used needles with or without attached syringes and other sharps are disposed of.

Shock an abnormal condition of inadequate blood flow to the body's peripheral tissues, with life-threatening cellular dysfunction.

Short-term effects radiation effects observed within 3 months of exposure; deterministic effects.

Shunt to redirect the flow of a body fluid from one cavity or vessel to another, or a device for accomplishing this.

Side effect any reaction to or consequence of a medication or therapy other than the therapeutic effect.

Sievert (Sv) the dose-equivalent unit in the SI system that results when the dose in Gy is multiplied by the WF.

Sigmoidoscope a fiberoptic instrument used to examine the lumen of the sigmoid colon.

Sine wave (sinusoidal form) a visual graphic of changes in the radiation field that occur in the form of a repeating wave.

Single photon emission computed tomography (SPECT) a computerized nuclear medicine scanning modality similar to PET imaging but involving the injection of radionuclides that emit single photons as opposed to ion pairs as in PET.

Sinus rhythm a cardiac rhythm stimulated by the sinus (sinoatrial) node. A rate of 60 to 100 beats/min is normal.

Sinus tachycardia a rapid heartbeat generated by discharge of the sinoatrial pacemaker. The rate may be 100 to 180 beats/min in an adult.

Siphon using atmospheric pressure to withdraw fluid from a cavity through a tube, or the tube used for this purpose.

Slander any words spoken with malice that are untrue and prejudicial to the reputation, professional practice, commercial trade, office, or business of another person.

Slider board a method of patient transfer that uses a strong sheet of smooth plastic large enough to support the patient's body with handholds cut into the edges.

Sliding mat a method of patient transfer that uses a soft, tubular sheet of flexible plastic that features a low friction surface and is used somewhat like a slider board.

Social contract theory the idea that certain persons or groups have relationships that contain inherent expectations, duties, and obligations such as the duty of a professional person to a client or patient.

Solution a mixture of one or more substances dissolved in another substance. The molecules of each of the substances disperse homogenously and do not change chemically.

Somatic effects radiation effects that affect the body of the irradiated individual directly.

Sonography the process of imaging deep structures of the body by measuring and recording the reflection of pulsed or continuous high-frequency sound waves; also called *diagnostic ultrasound*.

Soporific tending to induce drowsiness or sleep.

Source-image distance (SID) the distance between the x-ray tube target and the image receptor, measured along the central ray.

Spasm, spasmodic an involuntary muscle contraction of sudden onset.

Sphygmomanometer an instrument for indirect measurement of blood pressure. It consists of an inflatable cuff that fits around the arm, a bulb for controlling air pressure within the cuff, and a mercury or aneroid manometer.

Spinal tap   a procedure that involves the insertion of a needle into the subarachnoid space to withdraw spinal fluid. It may be performed to inject a contrast medium for myelography; it is the same as a lumbar puncture.

Spontaneous abortion   a termination of pregnancy before the twentieth week of gestation as a result of abnormalities of the conceptus or maternal environment; also called *miscarriage*.

Spontaneous combustion   the occurrence of fire when a chemical reaction in or near a flammable material causes sufficient heat.

Spore   a reproductive unit of some genera of fungi or protozoa; also, a common term for endospore, a form assumed by some bacteria that is resistant to heat, drying, and chemicals.

Standard Precautions   a system recommended by the CDC to protect health care workers from contracting infections from all patients, regardless of diagnosis, by preventing contact with their blood and body fluids.

Standing order   a written document containing rules, policies, procedures, regulations, and orders for the conduct of patient care in various stipulated clinical situations.

STAT   immediately, at once.

Status epilepticus   a medical emergency characterized by continuous seizures occurring without interruptions.

Stenosis   an abnormal condition characterized by the constriction or narrowing of an opening or passageway in a body structure.

Stent   a tubular device for supporting hollow structures during surgical anastomosis or for holding arteries open during or after angioplasty or to maintain the patency of ureters postoperatively.

Sterile, sterilization   free of living microorganisms; the process of destroying all microorganisms.

Sterile conscience   the awareness of sterile technique and the responsibility for notifying those in charge whenever contamination occurs.

Sterile corridor   the area of an operating room between the patient drape and the instrument table. Access to this area is permitted only to those wearing sterile attire.

Sterile field   a specified area, such as within a tray or on a sterile towel, that is considered free of microorganisms.

Sterilization   treatment of items with heat, gas, or chemicals to make them germ-free.

Steroid   any of a large number of hormonal substances with a similar basic chemical structure, produced mainly in the adrenal cortex and gonads, that may be used to treat inflammatory conditions or as antiallergic medication.

Stochastic   describes biologic radiation effects that are random and unpredictable. Their likelihood is dose dependent, but not their severity. There is no threshold amount of exposure necessary to produce these effects.

Stoma   a pore, orifice, or opening on a surface; the external opening of a colostomy or ileostomy.

Stricture   narrowing of the lumen of a tubular structure, such as a blood vessel or a portion of the gastrointestinal tract.

Stridor   an abnormal, high-pitched sound caused by an obstruction in the trachea or larynx, usually heard during inspiration.

Stroke   an abnormal condition of the brain characterized by a rupture or obstruction of an artery of the brain; same as cerebrovascular accident (CVA).

Stupor, stuporous   a state of unresponsiveness in which a person seems unaware of the surroundings.

Subcellular   pertaining to a lower level of organization, structure, and function than that of a cell.

Subcutaneous (SC)   beneath the skin.

Subdiaphragmatic   beneath the diaphragm.

Subliminal   taking place below the threshold of sensory perception or outside the range of conscious awareness.

Sublingual   pertaining to the area beneath the tongue.

Supine   the position in which the patient is lying on his or her back.

Suppository   an easily melted medicated mass for insertion into the rectum, urethra, or vagina.

Surgical asepsis   the process of creating and maintaining an area that is completely free of pathogens.

Surgical hand rub   a specific method of reducing the number of organisms on the hands and forearms and decreasing the rate of microbial growth in the following hours using a nonantimicrobial soap, drying the skin, and applying a surgical alcohol-based skin rub.

Surgical hand scrub   a specific method of reducing the number of organisms on the hands and forearms and decreasing the rate of microbial growth in the following hours using a brush and antimicrobial soap.

Surgical resection   partial removal of a structure or organ by surgery.

Suspension   a liquid in which small particles of a solid are dispersed, but not dissolved, and in which the dispersal is maintained by stirring or shaking the mixture. If left standing, the solid particles settle at the bottom of the container.

Syncope   a brief lapse in consciousness caused by transient cerebral hypoxia; same as fainting.

Synergistic effect   the acting or working together of two or more components, as when medications produce a combined effect.

Syphilis   a sexually transmitted disease caused by the spirochete *Treponema pallidum,* characterized by distinct stages of effects over a period of years.

Systemic effect   one which involves the whole body rather than a localized area or regional part of the body.

Systolic   pertaining to systole, or the blood pressure measured at the peak of ventricular contraction.

Tachycardia   abnormally rapid pulse; a condition in which the heart beats at a rate greater than 100 beats/min.

Tachypnea   an abnormally rapid respiratory rate (more than 20 breaths/min), as seen with hyperpyrexia.

Target   tungsten disk located at the electrically positive anode end of the x-ray tube, the end opposite the filament. The smooth, hard surface of the target is the site to which the electrons travel and is where the x-rays are generated.

Temporal   pertaining to the sides of the skull, anterior to the ears. The temporal arteries lie beneath the sides of the scalp in the temporal region. A temporal artery thermometer measures temperature from the temporal artery by scanning the forehead and temporal region with an infrared sensor.

Tepid   moderately warm to the touch; lukewarm.

Tertiary health care   a specialized, highly technical level of health care that includes diagnosis and treatment of disease and disability in sophisticated, large research and teaching hospitals.

Tetanus an acute, potentially fatal infection of the central nervous system caused by an exotoxin (tetanospasmin) elaborated by an anaerobic bacillus (*Clostridium tetani*).

Therapeutic communication a process in which the health care professional consciously influences a client or helps the client to a better understanding through verbal or nonverbal communication.

Therapeutic effect the desired benefit of a medication, treatment, or procedure.

Therapy, therapeutic the treatment of any disease or pathologic condition.

Thoracentesis surgical removal of fluid from the pleural space.

Thoracotomy a procedure involving a surgical opening into the thoracic cavity.

Thready descriptive of an abnormal pulse that is weak, somewhat difficult to palpate, and often fairly rapid; the artery does not feel full, and the rate may be difficult to count.

Thrombosis an abnormal vascular condition in which a clot (thrombus) develops within a blood vessel of the body.

Thrombus (plural, thrombi) an aggregation of platelets, fibrin, clotting factors, and the cellular elements of the blood attached to the interior wall of a vein or artery.

Topical mode of medication administration in which the medication is applied to the surface of a part of the body.

Tort a civil wrong, such as negligence, false imprisonment, assault, and battery.

Tourniquet a device, usually a wide, constricting band of elastic material, wrapped around a limb to restrict blood flow. It is applied to a limb to control hemorrhage or to enhance accessibility of veins for venipuncture.

Toxicity, toxic poisonous effect resulting from an excess amount of medication in the blood. These effects can be caused by excessive use of medications, overdose, impaired excretion, or an idiosyncratic reaction to the medication.

Toxin, toxic a poison; having a poisonous effect.

Tracheostomy an opening through the neck into the trachea through which an indwelling tube may be inserted to ventilate the patient's lungs.

Tracheotomy the procedure of making an incision into the trachea through the neck below the larynx, performed to gain access to the airway below a blockage caused by a foreign body, tumor, or edema.

Traction the process of putting a limb, bone, or group of muscles under tension by means of weights and pulleys to align or immobilize the part or to relieve pressure on it.

Tranquilizer a drug prescribed to calm anxious or agitated people, ideally without decreasing their consciousnes; a common term for benzodiazepines.

Transcatheter embolization an interventional technique used to decrease or stop blood flow.

Transdermal through the skin; medication administration method using adhesive patches.

Transducer a handheld device, used in diagnostic sonography, that sends and receives a sound wave signal. It changes electrical impulses into sound waves, receives the reflected sound wave, and converts it back into electrical energy.

Transient ischemic attack (TIA) an episode of cerebrovascular insufficiency, usually associated with partial occlusion of an artery by an atherosclerotic plaque or an embolism.

Trauma physical injury caused by violent or disruptive action or by the introduction into the body of a toxic substance.

Tremor rhythmic, purposeless movements resulting from the involuntary alternating contraction and relaxation of opposing groups of skeletal muscles.

Trendelenburg position a supine position in which the patient's head is lower than the feet.

Triage in the case of disaster or multiple victims needing attention, the process of identifying the victims, performing initial examinations, and assigning priorities for further care.

Trichomoniasis a vaginal infection caused by the protozoan *Trichomonas vaginalis*.

Trisomy 21 see *Down syndrome*.

Trocar a sharp, pointed rod that fits inside a tube. It is used to pierce the skin and the wall of a cavity or canal in the body to aspirate fluids, to instill a medication or solution, or to guide the placement of a soft catheter or fiberoptic device.

Tubercle a nodule or a small eminence, such as that on a bone or the nodules caused by tuberculosis.

Tuberculin referring to or related to a tubercle or to tuberculosis.

Tuberculosis (TB) a chronic granulomatous infection caused by the acid-fast bacillus *Mycobacterium tuberculosis*. It is generally transmitted by the inhalation or ingestion of infected droplet nuclei and usually affects the lungs, although infection of multiple organ systems occurs.

Tungsten chemical symbol W; a metallic element. It has the highest melting point of all metals and is used as a target material in x-ray tubes and as filament material in both x-ray tubes and incandescent light bulbs.

Tympanic membrane a thin, semitransparent membrane in the middle ear that transmits sound vibrations to the internal ear by means of the auditory ossicles; same as ear drum. A tympanic thermometer measures temperature by means of a probe inserted into the ear.

Typhoid fever a bacterial infection usually caused by *Salmonella typhi*, transmitted by contaminated milk, water, or food.

Typhus fever any of a group of acute infectious diseases caused by various species of *Rickettsia* and usually transmitted from infected rodents to humans by the bites of lice, fleas, mites, or ticks.

Ulcer lesion or sore affecting the skin or the mucous lining of the gastrointestinal tract.

Ulcerative colitis a chronic, episodic, inflammatory disease of the large intestine and rectum.

Urogram, urography a radiograph or examination of the urinary tract, obtained using an iodinated contrast agent. For excretory urography, the contrast medium is injected intravenously; for retrograde urography, it is instilled by direct retrograde flow through ureteral catheters.

Urticaria a pruritic skin eruption, usually the result of an allergic reaction, characterized by transient wheals of varying shapes and sizes with well-defined erythematous margins and pale centers; same as hives.

Vaccine, vaccination a suspension of attenuated or killed microorganisms administered intradermally, intramuscularly, orally, or subcutaneously to induce active immunity to infectious disease.

Valid choice a selection of options, all of which are acceptable. Offering valid choices to patients increases their sense of autonomy.

Valsalva maneuver any forced expiratory effort against a closed airway, such as when an individual holds the breath and tightens the muscles in a concerted, strenuous effort to move a heavy object.

Value a personal belief about the worth of a given idea or behavior.

Varicose, varicosity abnormally swollen, knotted, or crooked, as a varicose vein; the condition of being varicose.

Varices (singular, varix) enlarged veins

Vascular pertaining to a blood vessel.

Vasoconstriction a narrowing of the lumen of any blood vessel, especially the arterioles and the veins in the blood reservoirs of the skin and the abdominal viscera.

Vasodilation an increase in the diameter of the blood vessels.

Vasovagal reflex a stimulation of the vagus nerve by reflex in which irritation of the larynx, trachea, or rectum results in slowing of the pulse rate.

Vector (of infection) an animal in whose body a pathogen multiplies or develops before becoming infective to a new host.

Vehicle (of infection) any substance, such as food or water, that can serve as a mode of transmission for infectious agents.

Venipuncture the transcutaneous puncture of a vein by a sharp, rigid needle with a stylet, by a cannula carrying a flexible plastic catheter, or by a steel needle attached to a syringe or catheter. Venipuncture provides access to a vein for medication or fluid administration or to draw blood for testing.

Venogram, venography a radiograph or examination of the veins; same as phlebogram.

Ventilation the process by which gases are moved into and out of the lungs.

Ventilator any of several devices used in respiratory therapy to provide assisted respiration and intensive positive-pressure breathing.

Ventricle small cavity, such as the right and the left ventricles of the heart or one of the cavities filled with cerebrospinal fluid in the brain.

Vertigo a sensation of instability, loss of equilibrium, or rotation, caused by a disturbance in the semicircular canal of the inner ear or the vestibular nuclei of the brainstem.

Vesicant tending to cause blistering; an agent that causes blistering.

Vial a glass container with a metal-enclosed rubber seal.

Virion a rudimentary virus particle with a central nucleoid surrounded by a protein sheath or capsid.

Virtue-based ethics theory that places value on virtues and admirable character traits such as caring, faithfulness, trustworthiness, compassion, and courage.

Virulence factors characteristics of certain microorganisms that cause them to be pathogenic and distinguish them from normal flora. These factors enable bacteria to destroy or damage host cells and resist destruction by the host's cellular defenses.

Virus, viral a minute parasitic microorganism much smaller than a bacterium that, having no independent metabolic activity, can replicate only within a cell of a living plant or animal host.

Viscosity, viscous the ability or inability of a fluid solution to flow easily.

Viscus (plural, viscera), visceral an internal organ; pertaining to an organ.

Void to empty, or evacuate, such as urine from the bladder.

Volt, voltage the unit of electrical potential. In an electric circuit, a volt is the force required to send 1 ampere of current through 1 ohm of resistance, or the difference in potential between two points on a conductor carrying a charge of 1 ampere when there is a dissipation of 1 watt between them.

VRE (vancomycin-resistant enterococci) drug-resistant bacteria that contribute to surgical wound, urinary tract, and bloodstream infections.

Wavelength with respect to a sine wave, the distance between a given point on one wave cycle and the corresponding point on the next successive wave cycle.

Weighting factor (WF) an approximate measure of the relative biologic effectiveness of a particular radiation compared with a reference radiation. The reference is 250 keV x-rays. The weighting factor is multiplied by the dose to determine the dose equivalent. Formerly termed *quality factor* (QF).

Yeast any unicellular, usually oval, nucleated fungus that reproduces by budding.

INDEX

Note: Pages followed by "*b*," "*t*", and "*f*" refer to boxes, tables, and figures respectively.